Anatomical Chart Company

ATLAS OF
PATHOPHYSIOLOGY

FOURTH EDITION

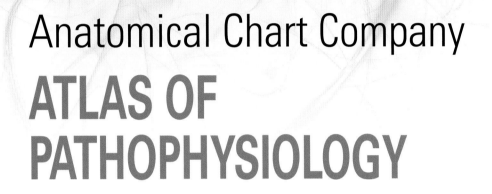

Anatomical Chart Company

ATLAS OF
PATHOPHYSIOLOGY

FOURTH EDITION

Julie G. Stewart, DNP, MPH, MSN, FNP-BC, FAANP

Associate Professor
Sacred Heart University
Fairfield, Connecticut

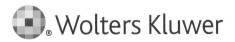 Wolters Kluwer

Philadelphia • Baltimore • New York • London
Buenos Aires • Hong Kong • Sydney • Tokyo

Acquisitions Editor: Nicole Dernoski
Editorial Coordinator: Annette Ferran
Marketing Manager: Linda Wetmore
Production Project Manager: Kim Cox
Design Coordinator: Holly McLaughlin
Manufacturing Coordinator: Kathy Brown
Prepress Vendor: SPi Global

Fourth edition

Library of Congress Cataloging-in-Publication Data
Names: Stewart, Julie G., editor. | Anatomical Chart Co., issuing body.
Title: Anatomical chart company atlas of pathophysiology / [edited by] Julie Stewart.
Other titles: Atlas of pathophysiology.
Description: Fourth edition. | Philadelphia : Wolters Kluwer, [2018] | Preceded by Atlas of pathophysiology. 3rd ed. c2010. | Includes bibliographical references and index.
Identifiers: LCCN 2017038771 | ISBN 9781496370921
Subjects: | MESH: Pathology | Physiology | Atlases
Classification: LCC RB113 | NLM QZ 17 | DDC 616.07022/2—dc23 LC record available at https://lccn.loc. gov/2017038771

LWW.com

CONTRIBUTORS AND CONSULTANTS

Jean Boucher, PhD, RN, ANP-BC, AOCNP
Associate Professor
Graduate School of Nursing
University of Massachusetts Medical School
Worcester, Massachusetts

Nancy Dennert, APRN, MS, MSN, FNP-BC, CDE, BC-ADM
Nurse Practitioner
Endocrine Associates
Trumbull, Connecticut

Heather Ferillo, APRN, MSN, FNP-BC
Clinical Assistant Professor
College of Nursing
Sacred Heart University
Fairfield, Connecticut

Karen Gregory, DNP, APRN, CNS, RRT, AE-C, FAARC
Oklahoma Allergy & Asthma Clinic
Oklahoma City, Oklahoma
Assistant Professor
School of Nursing and Health Studies
Georgetown University
Washington, D.C.

Julie A. Koch, DNP, RN, FNP-BC, FAANP
Assistant Dean of Graduate Nursing
College of Nursing and Health Professions
Valparaiso University
Valparaiso, Indiana

Harry Pomerantz, MSPH, PA-C
Clinical Simulation and Skills Faculty
College of Health Professions
Sacred Heart University
Fairfield, Connecticut

Jagnal Reynold, MBA, PA-C
Director of Clinical Education, Clinical Assistant Professor
College of Health Professions
Sacred Heart University
Fairfield, Connecticut

Sylvie Rosenbloom, DNP, APRN, FNP-BC, CDE
Clinician
Stamford Health Medical Group, Walk-in Center
Stamford, Connecticut

Penny Sessler-Branden, PhD, CNM, RN, CNE
Assistant Clinical Professor
College of Nursing
Sacred Heart University
Fairfield, Connecticut

Mary Lou Siefert, DNSc, RN, AOCN
Assistant Professor
College of Nursing
Sacred Heart University
Fairfield, Connecticut

Frank Tudini, PT, DSc, COMT, OCS, FAAOMPT
Clinical Assistant Professor
College of Health Professions, Physical Therapy
Sacred Heart University
Fairfield, Connecticut

Sherylyn M. Watson, PhD, MSN, RN, CNE
Associate Dean
College of Nursing
Sacred Heart University
Fairfield, Connecticut

FOREWORD

Students seeking to investigate and master the many facets of the human organism need to be well versed in numerous fields before they can begin to understand the intricate physiologic workings of the body. Students must also study how the cells can malfunction and how disease can occur before actually becoming a participant in the healing arts. *Atlas of Pathophysiology*, Fourth Edition, offers a broad overview of pathophysiology while providing sufficient detail to help the learner understand the principles involved. The atlas format adds the power of visual representation to further enhance learning.

Because every discipline involves a unique language, the opening chapters provide a concise review of the vocabulary of pathophysiology. Part I, "Central Concepts," lists and explains the key terms used in the basic disciplines of cancer, infection, genetics, and fluid and electrolyte disorders. Provided in a tabular format, these lists elegantly summarize concepts that students and instructors can reference while building a fundamental knowledge base. The chapter on infectious diseases condenses information on the pathophysiology of over 30 infections, ranging from bacterial to viral to protozoal. The chapters on cancer and genetics explore the rapidly evolving understanding of these disorders. The final chapter on concepts clearly explains fluid, electrolyte, and acid-base disorders.

In Part II, vibrant, full-color illustrations make this volume stand out. The illustrations review essential anatomical structures, vividly depict the changes caused by disease, illuminate pertinent pathology, and clarify and simplify difficult to understand terms. Obviously, visual learners will appreciate and remember the elegant drawings.

The team of authors has drawn on their depth of experience in patient care and teaching medical professionals to compile an impressive array of topics. The 12 chapters encompass all the major organ systems of the body, covering an array of conditions that specifically address issues related to neonates, surgical patients, orthopedics, and the broad field of internal medicine. The book covers nearly 200 conditions, each presented with concisely written text and accompanied by a clinically accurate, vivid illustrations.

Atlas of Pathophysiology, Fourth Edition, fills the need for a factual text for students and a valuable reference for practitioners already providing patient care. Illustrations can be easily shared with patients as an aid to understanding disorders. The contributors and consultants are to be commended for their expertise and the success of their work.

Julie G. Stewart, DNP, MPH, MSN, FNP-BC, FAANP

CONTENTS

Appendix

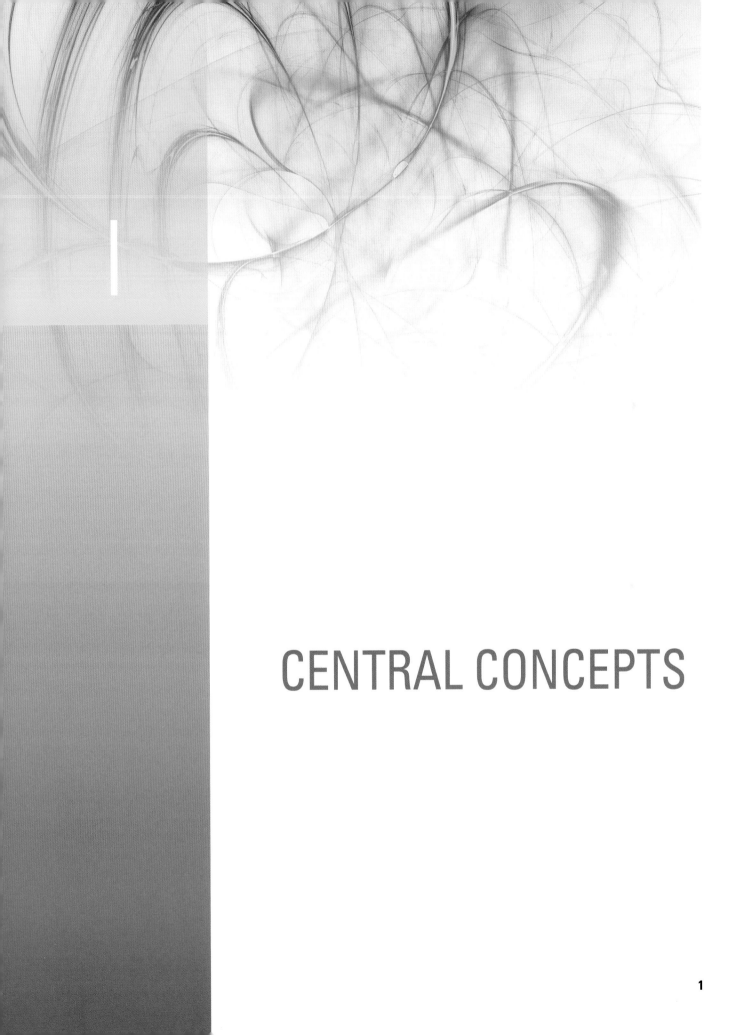

CENTRAL CONCEPTS

CELLS, HOMEOSTASIS, AND DISEASE

The cell is the smallest living component of a living organism. Organisms can be made up of a single cell, such as bacteria, or billions of cells, such as human beings. In large organisms, highly specialized cells that perform a common function are organized into tissue. Tissues, in turn, form organs, which are integrated into body systems.

CELL COMPONENTS

Cells are complex organizations of specialized components, each component having its own specific function. The largest components of a normal cell are the cytoplasm, the nucleus, and the cell membrane. (See *Cell components.*)

Cytoplasm

The cytoplasm consists primarily of a fluid in which the tiny structures that perform the necessary functions to maintain the life of the cell are suspended. These tiny structures, called *organelles*, are the cell's metabolic machinery. Each performs a specific function to maintain the life of the cell. Organelles include:

- *mitochondria* — spherical or rod-shaped structures that are the sites of cellular respiration — the metabolic use of oxygen to produce energy, carbon dioxide, and water. (They produce most of the body's adenosine triphosphate, which contains high-energy phosphate chemical bonds that fuel many cellular activities.)
- *ribosomes* — the sites of protein synthesis
- *endoplasmic reticulum* — an extensive network of two varieties of membrane-enclosed tubules: rough endoplasmic reticulum, which is covered with ribosomes; and smooth endoplasmic reticulum, which contains enzymes that synthesize lipids
- *Golgi apparatus* — synthesizes carbohydrate molecules that combine with protein produced by the rough endoplasmic reticulum and lipids produced by the smooth endoplasmic reticulum to form such products as lipoproteins, glycoproteins, and enzymes
- *lysosomes* — digest nutrients as well as foreign, obsolete, or damaged material in cells. (A membrane surrounding each lysosome separates its digestive enzymes from the rest of the cytoplasm. The enzymes digest nutrient matter brought into the cell by means of endocytosis, in which a portion of the cell membrane surrounds and engulfs matter to form a membrane-bound intracellular vesicle. The membrane of the lysosome fuses with the membrane of the vesicle surrounding the endocytosed material. The lysosomal enzymes then digest the engulfed material. Lysosomes digest the foreign matter ingested by white blood cells [WBCs] by a similar process, *phagocytosis.*)

- *peroxisomes* — contain oxidases, enzymes that chemically reduce oxygen to hydrogen peroxide and hydrogen peroxide to water
- *cytoskeletal elements* — a network of protein structures that maintain the cell's shape and enable cell division and migration
- *centrosomes* — contain centrioles, short cylinders adjacent to the nucleus that take part in cell division
- *microfilaments and microtubules* — enable movement of intracellular vesicles (allowing axons to transport neurotransmitters) and formation of the mitotic spindle, the framework for cell division.

Nucleus

The cell's control center is the nucleus, which plays a role in cell growth, metabolism, and reproduction. Within the nucleus, one or more nucleoli (dark-staining intranuclear structures) synthesize ribonucleic acid (RNA), a complex polynucleotide that controls protein synthesis. The nucleus also stores deoxyribonucleic acid (DNA), the double helix that carries genetic material and is responsible for cellular reproduction or division.

Cell Membrane

The semipermeable cell membrane forms the cell's external boundary, separating it from other cells and from the external environment. The cell membrane consists of a double layer of phospholipids with protein molecules embedded in it. These protein molecules act as receptors, ion channels, or carriers for specific substances.

CELL DIVISION

Each cell must replicate itself for life to continue. Cells replicate by division in one of two ways: mitosis (produces two daughter cells with the same DNA and chromosome content as the mother cell) or meiosis (produces four gametocytes, each containing half the number of chromosomes of the original cell). Most cells divide by mitosis; meiosis occurs only in reproductive cells. Some cells, such as nerve and muscle cells, typically lose their ability to reproduce after birth.

CELL FUNCTIONS

In the human body, most cells are specialized to perform one function. Respiration and reproduction occur in all cells. The specialized functions include:

- *movement* — the result of coordinated action of nerve and muscle cells to change the position of a specific body part, contents within an organ, or the entire organism

- *conduction* — the transmission of a stimulus, such as a nerve impulse, heat, or sound wave, from one body part to another
- *absorption* — movement of substances through a cell membrane (for example, nutrients are absorbed and transported ultimately to be used as energy sources or as building blocks to form or repair structural and functional cellular components)
- *secretion* — release of substances that act in another part of the body
- *excretion* — release of waste products generated by normal metabolic processes.

CELL TYPES

Each of the following four types of tissue consists of several specialized cell types, which perform specific functions.

- *Epithelial cells* line most of the internal and external surfaces of the body. Their functions include support, protection, absorption, excretion, and secretion.
- *Connective tissue cells* are present in skin, bones and joints, artery walls, fascia, and body fat. Their major functions are protection, metabolism, support, temperature maintenance, and elasticity.
- *Nerve cells* constitute the nervous system and are classified as neurons or neuroglial cells. Neurons perform these functions:
  - generating electrical impulses
  - conducting electrical impulses
  - influencing other neurons, muscle cells, and cells of glands by transmitting impulses.
  Neuroglial cells support, nourish, and protect the neurons. The four types include:
  - *oligodendroglia* — produce myelin within the central nervous system (CNS)
  - *astrocytes* — provide essential nutrients to neurons and assist neurons in maintaining the proper bioelectrical potentials for impulse conduction and synaptic transmission
  - *ependymal cells* — involved in the production of cerebrospinal fluid
  - *microglia* — ingest and digest tissue debris when nervous tissue is damaged.
- *Muscle cells* contract to produce movement or tension. The three types include:
  - *skeletal (striated) muscle cells* — extend along the entire length of skeletal muscles. These cells cause voluntary movement by contracting or relaxing together in a specific muscle. Contraction shortens the muscle; relaxation permits the muscle to return to its resting length.
  - *smooth (nonstriated) muscle cells* — present in the walls of hollow internal organs, blood vessels, and bronchioles. By involuntarily contracting and relaxing, these cells change the luminal diameter of the hollow structure and thereby move substances through the organ.
  - *striated cardiac muscle cells* — branch out across the smooth muscle of the chambers of the heart and contract involuntarily. They produce and transmit cardiac action potentials, which cause cardiac muscle cells to contract.

AGE ALERT
In older adults, skeletal muscle cells become smaller and many are replaced by fibrous connective tissue. The result is loss of muscle strength and mass.

PATHOPHYSIOLOGIC CONCEPTS

The cell faces a number of challenges through its life. Stressors, changes in the body's health, disease, and other extrinsic and intrinsic factors can alter the cell's normal functioning.

Adaptation

Cells generally continue functioning despite changing conditions or stressors. However, severe or prolonged stress or changes may injure or destroy cells. When cell integrity is threatened, the cell reacts by drawing on its reserves to keep functioning, by adaptive changes, or by cellular dysfunction. If cellular reserve is insufficient, the cell dies. If enough cellular reserve is available and the body doesn't detect abnormalities, the cell adapts by atrophy, hypertrophy, hyperplasia, metaplasia, or dysplasia. (See *Adaptive cell changes*, page 5.)

Atrophy

Atrophy is a reversible reduction in the size of a cell or organ due to disuse, insufficient blood flow, malnutrition, denervation, or reduced endocrine stimulation. An example is loss of muscle mass after prolonged bed rest.

Hypertrophy

Hypertrophy is an increase in the size of a cell or organ due to an increase in workload. It may result from normal physiologic conditions or abnormal pathologic conditions. Types include:

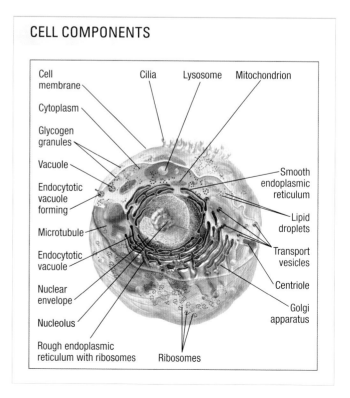

CELL COMPONENTS

- *physiologic hypertrophy* — reflects an increase in workload that isn't caused by disease (for example, the increase in muscle size caused by hard physical labor or weight training)
- *pathologic hypertrophy* — an adaptive or compensatory response to disease; for example, an adaptive response is thickening of heart muscle as it pumps against increasing resistance in patients with hypertension. An example of a compensatory response is when one kidney enlarges if the other isn't functioning or present.

Hyperplasia

Hyperplasia is an increase in the number of cells caused by increased workload, hormonal stimulation, or decreased tissue. Hypertrophy and hyperplasia may occur together and are commonly triggered by the same mechanism. Hyperplasia may be *physiologic, compensatory,* or *pathologic.*

- *Physiologic hyperplasia* is an adaptive response to normal changes — for example, monthly increase in the number of uterine cells in response to estrogen stimulation after ovulation.
- *Compensatory hyperplasia* occurs in some organs to replace tissue that has been removed or destroyed — for example, regeneration of liver cells when part of the liver is surgically removed.
- *Pathologic hyperplasia* is a response to either excessive hormonal stimulation or abnormal production of hormonal growth factors — for example, acromegaly, in which excessive growth hormone production causes bones to enlarge.

Metaplasia

Metaplasia is the replacement of one mature cell type with another differentiated cell type that can better endure the change or stressor. It's usually a response to chronic inflammation or irritation.

- *Physiologic metaplasia* is a normal response to changing conditions and is generally transient. For example, in the body's normal response to inflammation, monocytes migrate to inflamed tissues and transform into macrophages.
- *Pathologic metaplasia* is a response to an extrinsic toxin or stressor and is generally irreversible. For example, after years of exposure to cigarette smoke, stratified squamous epithelial cells replace the normal ciliated columnar epithelial cells of the bronchi. Although the new cells can better withstand smoke, they don't secrete mucus or have cilia to protect the airway. If exposure to cigarette smoke continues, the squamous cells can become cancerous.

Dysplasia

In dysplasia, deranged cell growth of specific tissue results in abnormal size, shape, and appearance. Although dysplastic cell changes are adaptive and potentially reversible, they can precede cancerous changes. Common examples include dysplasia of epithelial cells of the cervix or the respiratory tract.

Cell Injury

Injury to any cellular component can lead to disease as the cells lose their ability to adapt. Cell injury may result from any of several intrinsic or extrinsic causes:

- *toxins* — may be endogenous or exogenous (common endogenous toxins include products of genetically determined metabolic errors and hypersensitivity reactions; exogenous toxins include alcohol, lead, carbon monoxide, and drugs that alter cellular function)
- *infection* — may be caused by viruses, fungi, protozoa, or bacteria

ADAPTIVE CELL CHANGES

Normal cells — Nucleus — Basement membrane

Atrophy

Hypertrophy

Hyperplasia

Metaplasia

Dysplasia

- *physical injury* — disruption of a cell's structure or the relationships among the organelles (for example, two types of physical injury are thermal and mechanical)
- *deficit injury* — loss of normal cellular metabolism caused by inadequate water, oxygen, or nutrients.

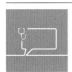

CLINICAL TIP

Oxygen deficiency is the most common cause of irreversible cell injury and cell death.

Injury becomes irreversible when the cell membrane or the organelles can no longer function.

Cell Degeneration

Degeneration is a type of sublethal cell damage that generally occurs in the cytoplasm and doesn't affect the nucleus. Degeneration usually affects organs with metabolically active cells, such as the liver, heart, and kidneys. When changes in cells are identified, prompt health care can slow degeneration and prevent cell death. Unfortunately, many cell changes are unidentifiable, even with the use of a microscope, and early detection of disease is then impossible. Examples of reversible degenerative changes are cervical dysplasia and fatty changes in the liver. Examples of irreversible degenerative diseases include Huntington's chorea and amyotrophic lateral sclerosis.

Cell Aging

During the normal process of aging, cells lose both structure and function. Atrophy may reflect loss of cell structure, hypertrophy or hyperplasia, or lost function. Signs of aging occur in all body systems. Aging can proceed at different rates depending on the number and extent of injuries and the amount of wear and tear on the cell.

Cell Death

Cell death may be caused by internal (intrinsic) factors that limit the cell's life span or external (extrinsic) factors that contribute to cell damage and aging. When stress is severe or prolonged, the cell can no longer adapt and it dies. Cell death may manifest in different ways, depending on the tissues or organs involved. It can involve apoptosis or necrosis.

- *Apoptosis* — genetically programmed cell death — accounts for the constant cell turnover in the skin's outer keratin layer and the lens of the eye. It's characterized by a series of events including chromatin condensation, membrane blebbing, cell shrinkage, and DNA degradation. It's controlled by autodigestion.

There are five types of necrosis:

- *Liquefactive necrosis* occurs when a lytic (dissolving) enzyme liquefies necrotic cells. This type of necrosis is common in the brain, which has a rich supply of lytic enzymes.
- *Caseous necrosis* occurs when necrotic cells disintegrate but the cellular pieces remain undigested for months or years. Its name derives from the resulting tissue's crumbly, cheeselike (caseous) appearance. It commonly occurs in pulmonary tuberculosis.

- *Fat necrosis* occurs when lipase enzymes break down intracellular triglycerides into free fatty acids. These free fatty acids combine with sodium, magnesium, or calcium ions to form soaps. The tissue becomes opaque and chalky white.
- *Coagulative necrosis* commonly follows interruption of blood supply to any organ — generally the kidneys, heart, or adrenal glands — except the brain. It inhibits activity of lysosomal lytic enzymes in the cells, so that the necrotic cells maintain their shape, at least temporarily.
- *Gangrenous necrosis*, a form of coagulative necrosis, typically results from a lack of blood flow and is complicated by an overgrowth and invasion of bacteria. It commonly occurs in the lower limbs as a result of arteriosclerosis or in the GI tract. Gangrene can occur in one of three forms:
  - dry gangrene — occurs when bacterial invasion is minimal. It's marked by dry, wrinkled, dark brown or blackened tissue on an extremity.
  - moist (or wet) gangrene — is accompanied by liquefactive necrosis, which is extensive lytic activity from bacteria and WBCs that produces a liquid center in affected area. It can occur in the internal organs as well as the extremities.
  - gas gangrene — develops when anaerobic bacteria of the genus *Clostridium* infect tissue. It's more likely to follow severe trauma and may be fatal. The bacteria release toxins that kill nearby cells, and the gas gangrene rapidly spreads. Release of gas bubbles from affected muscle cells indicates that gas gangrene is present.

Necrotic cells release intracellular enzymes, which start to dissolve cellular components, and trigger an acute inflammatory reaction in which WBCs migrate to the necrotic area and begin to digest the dead cells.

HOMEOSTASIS: MAINTAINING BALANCE

Every cell in the body participates in maintaining a dynamic, steady state of internal balance, called *homeostasis.*

Pathophysiology results from changes or disruption in normal cellular function. Three structures in the brain are primarily responsible for maintaining homeostasis of the entire body:

- *medulla oblongata* — the part of the brain stem associated with vital functions, such as respiration and circulation
- *pituitary gland* — regulates the function of other glands and, thereby, the body's growth, maturation, and reproduction
- *reticular formation* — a network of nerve cells and fibers in the brain stem and spinal cord that helps control vital reflexes, such as cardiovascular function and respiration.

Each structure that maintains homeostasis through self-regulating feedback mechanisms has three components:

- *sensors* — cells that detect disruptions in homeostasis reflected by nerve impulses or changes in hormone levels
- *CNS control center* — receives signals from the sensor and regulates the body's response to those disruptions by initiating the effector mechanism
- *effector* — acts to restore homeostasis.

Feedback mechanisms exist in two varieties:

- *positive* — moves the system away from homeostasis by enhancing a change in the system
- *negative* — works to restore homeostasis by correcting a deficit in the system and producing adaptive responses.

DISEASE

Although *disease* and *illness* are often used interchangeably, they aren't synonyms. *Disease* occurs when homeostasis isn't maintained. *Illness* occurs when a person isn't in a state of perceived "normal" health. A person may have a disease but not be ill all the time because his body has adapted to the disease.

The cause of disease may be intrinsic or extrinsic. Genetic factors, age, gender, infectious agents, or behaviors (such as inactivity, smoking, or abusing illegal drugs) can all cause disease. Diseases that have no known cause are called *idiopathic*.

The way a disease develops is called its *pathogenesis*. A disease is usually detected when it causes a change in metabolism or cell division that causes signs and symptoms. How the cells respond to disease depends on the causative agent and the affected cells, tissues, and organs. Without intervention, resolution of the disease depends on many factors functioning over a period of time, such as extent of disease and the presence of other diseases. Manifestations of disease may include hypofunction, hyperfunction, or increased mechanical function.

Typically, diseases progress through these stages:

- *exposure or injury* — target tissue exposed to a causative agent or injury
- *latency or incubation period* — no signs or symptoms evident
- *prodromal period* — signs and symptoms generally mild and nonspecific
- *acute phase* — disease reaches full intensity, possibly with complications; called the *subclinical acute phase* if the patient can still function as though the disease weren't present
- *remission* — a second latency phase that occurs in some diseases and is commonly followed by another acute phase
- *convalescence* — patient progresses toward recovery
- *recovery* — return of health or normal functioning; no signs or symptoms of disease remain.

CANCER

Cancer refers to a group of more than 100 different diseases characterized by cellular genetic changes such as DNA mutations and damage that cause abnormal cell growth and development. Malignant cells have two defining characteristics: first, the cells no longer divide and differentiate normally; they can invade surrounding tissues. Secondly, the malignant cells are capable of travel to and growth in distant sites within the body. In the United States, greater than 1.6 million new cases of cancer are expected in 2016; it is the number one cause of death in people younger than age 85, and accounts for more than half a million deaths each year (NIH/NCI, https://www.cancer.gov/about-cancer/understanding/statistics).

CAUSES

Cancer risk factors may include those that can be controlled, such as exposure to substances and certain behaviors, and factors that cannot be controlled, such as age and family history.

Current evidence suggests that cancer develops from either inherited genetic changes or acquired genetic changes resulting from, for example, the exposure to carcinogens (cancer causing agents), such as asbestos, mineral oils, tobacco smoke, and radiation from the sun. Furthermore, additional genetic changes may continue to develop in cells as a result of the cancer itself.

Numerous genetic changes and genes have been identified that may cause cancer or increase one's risk of developing cancer. According to the NCI (https://www.cancer.gov/about-cancer/understanding/what-is-cancer#related-diseases), genetic changes, inherited or acquired, may occur in three major types of genes — proto-oncogenes, tumor suppressor genes, and DNA repair genes. If unchanged, these genes would normally help to halt or prevent the development of cancer.

Proto-oncogenes may develop changes that can cause them to become oncogenes that in turn promote abnormal growth and development in cells that would normally be halted. Tumor suppressor genes may be altered so that cells continue to divide and multiply in an uncontrolled manner that should normally be halted by unaltered tumor suppressor genes. And finally, mutations or changes in DNA repair genes may inhibit DNA repair, and thus, the DNA damage continues and additional mutations develop in other genes allowing or promoting cancer cell growth and development.

Oncogenes provide growth-promoting signals, thereby causing one or more characteristics of cancer cells when overexpressed or mutated.

Proto-oncogenes are genes that can be converted to oncogenes by transforming cells or contributing to tumor formation. *Tumor suppressor genes* are growth-suppressing genes that inhibit tumor development.

Both types of these cancer-related genes can be inherited or acquired. Common causes of acquired genetic damage are viruses, radiation, environmental and dietary carcinogens, and hormones. Other factors that interact to increase a person's likelihood of developing cancer are age, genetics, nutritional status, hormonal balance, and response to stress.

RISK FACTORS

Many cancers are associated with exposure to specific environmental (air pollution, tobacco and alcohol, occupation, and radiation) and lifestyle factors (sexual practices and diet) that may increase one's risk to developing cancer. Accumulating data suggest that some of these factors initiate carcinogenesis, others act as promoters, and some both initiate and promote the disease process. In addition, age and inherited genetics can also determine one's risk of cancer.

Carcinogens

The following section contains a discussion and description of some more common cancer causing substances (carcinogens).

Air Pollution

Environmental factors such as air pollution have been linked to the development of cancer, particularly lung cancer. Many chemicals and other materials used in manufacturing and everyday life contribute to air pollution and are therefore carcinogens, such as arsenic, benzene, hydrocarbons, polyvinyl chlorides, and other industrial emissions as well as motor vehicle exhaust. Other indoor air pollution carcinogens include radon gas, and smoke from tobacco products and burning of cooking fuel. Between 2005 and 2009, there were over 7,000 lung cancer deaths each year due to secondhand smoke exposure (U.S. Department of Health and Human Services, 2014).

Tobacco and Alcohol

Tobacco and many of the chemicals present in tobacco smoke are carcinogenic and responsible for DNA damage in cells associated with cancer. Smoking is responsible for 80% of all lung cancer deaths. The use of tobacco, smoked or smokeless, causes cancer. The risk of lung cancer from cigarette smoking correlates directly with the duration of smoking and the number of cigarettes smoked per day. Research also shows that a person who stops smoking decreases his/her risk of lung cancer.

Although the risk of lung cancer is not strongly associated with pipe and cigar smoking as it is with cigarette smoking, there is evidence that pipe and cigar smoking is associated with oral and other cancers. Smokeless tobacco contains many carcinogens and nicotine and can cause oral and pancreatic cancers (U.S. Department of Health and Human Services, 2014). Inhalation of secondhand smoke, or passive smoking, by nonsmokers also increases the risk of lung and other cancers. The risk of developing an alcohol-related cancer increases with the amount of alcohol consumed regularly over time. Heavy alcohol consumption is an independent risk factor and primary cause of hepatocellular carcinoma. Head and neck, esophageal, breast, and colorectal cancers are also associated with alcohol consumption. Alcohol may increase the risk of cancer through several different mechanisms including those mechanisms that can damage DNA and proteins, and it can impair the absorption and breakdown of nutrients associated with cancer risk. The fermentation and production process for alcoholic beverages may also introduce known carcinogens as a contaminant into the alcoholic beverages. Heavy use of alcohol and cigarette smoking multiplicatively increases the incidence of cancers of the mouth, larynx, pharynx, and esophagus.

Occupation

Certain occupations that expose workers to specific substances increase the risk of cancer. For example, persons exposed to asbestos are at risk for a specific type of lung cancer, called *mesothelioma*. Asbestos also may act as a promoter for other carcinogens. Workers involved in the production of dyes, rubber, paint, and beta-naphthylamine are at increased risk for bladder cancer.

Radiation

Exposure to radiation is a known risk for cancer. Ionizing radiation from X-rays and gamma rays can cause cancer by damaging and changing the cell's DNA. Ultraviolet (UV) radiation, a lower energy radiation than X-rays or gamma rays, mainly causes skin cancer by damaging the DNA in skin cells. Radiation comes from natural sources, such as radon gas and the sun, or can come from man-made sources, such as those for tanning beds, nuclear energy, and imaging studies. The risk of cancer increases with the amount of radiation exposure.

UV sunlight is a direct cause of basal and squamous cell cancers of the skin. The amount and type of exposure to UV radiation correlates with the type of skin cancer that develops. For example, cumulative exposure to UV sunlight is associated with basal and squamous cell skin cancer, and severe episodes of burning and blistering at a young age are associated with melanoma. Ionizing radiation (such as X-rays and gamma rays) is associated with acute leukemia; thyroid, breast, lung, stomach, colon, and urinary tract cancers; as well as multiple myeloma. Low doses of radiation can cause DNA mutations and chromosomal abnormalities, and large doses can inhibit cell division. Ionizing radiation can also enhance the effects of genetic abnormalities. Other compounding variables include the part and percentage of the body exposed, the person's age, hormonal balance, use of prescription drugs, and preexisting or concurrent conditions.

Human Papillomaviruses

Human papillomaviruses (HPVs) are a group of more than 200 related viruses. More than 40 types of HPVs can be transmitted with direct sexual contact from skin and mucous membranes of the infected person to the sexual partner through vaginal, oral, and anal sexual practices. High-risk HPVs are responsible for causing several types of cancer with two types, 16 and 18, responsible for the majority of the HPV-related cancers. HPV is the most common cause of abnormal Papanicolaou (Pap) tests, and cervical dysplasia is a direct precursor to squamous cell carcinoma of the cervix, both of which have been linked to HPV. HPV types 16 and 18 cause 70% of all cervical cancers. More than half of all oral cancers are linked to HPV type 16, and most anal cancers are caused by HPV type 16. Three vaccines have been approved by the Food and Drug Administration (FDA) to prevent HPV infection before sexual activity. The vaccines do not treat HPV infections or related diseases once established.

Dietary Factors

According to the National Cancer Institute (NCI), many studies have been conducted to evaluate the relationship of dietary nutrients or other food-related factors with cancer in humans. Studies to date have not yet been able to show a cause and effect relationship with dietary components that may either cause or prevent cancer. Large epidemiological studies have shown only a correlation or association of dietary components and cancer risk, but not a causal relationship. It is possible or likely that many other factors other than the dietary-related ones in these studies may be responsible for the differences found in the associations of dietary factors and cancer risk.

Age

Age is a major determinant in the development of cancer. The longer men and women live, the more likely they are to develop the disease. For example, because of the long natural history of common cancers, prostate cancer may take up to 60 years to become invasive, while colon cancer may take as long as 40 years to develop into an invasive stage. Possible explanations for the increased incidence of cancer with advancing age include:

- *altered hormonal levels*, which may stimulate cancer
- *ineffective immunosurveillance*, which fails to recognize and destroy abnormal cells
- *prolonged exposure to carcinogenic agents*, which is more likely to produce neoplastic transformation
- *inherent physiologic changes and functional impairments*, which decrease the body's ability to tolerate and survive stress.

Genetics

Genes, through the proteins they encode, are the chemical messages of heredity. Located at specific locations on the 46 chromosomes within the cell's nucleus, genes transmit specific hereditary traits.

Most cancers develop from a complex interplay among multiple genes and between genes and internal or external environmental factors. Phenomenal progress has been made in the fields of cancer genetics and cytogenetics that has established specific chromosomal changes as diagnostic and prognostic factors in acute and chronic leukemias, as diagnostic factors in various solid tumors, and as indicators for the localization and characterization of genes responsible for tumor development.

Moreover, in the past 25 years, research has identified and characterized many of the genetic alterations that lead to tumor transformation at the chromosomal and molecular cell level. The Human Genome Project, started in 1988 to identify the entire sequence of human DNA, has helped to increase knowledge about genetics and cancer carcinogenesis. The Philadelphia (Ph) chromosome was the first identified chromosomal anomaly caused by translocation implicated in a human disease (chronic myelocytic leukemia [CML]). However, it's important to note that not all mutated genes always lead to disease.

As previously discussed, two sets of genes, oncogenes and tumor suppressor genes, participate in the transformation of a normal cell into a malignant cell; however, because multiple, successive changes and distinct cellular genes are required to complete the entire process, the human cell rarely sustains the necessary number of changes needed for tumor transformation. Gene mutations are either *inherited* from a parent (hereditary or germline mutation) or *acquired* (somatic mutation). Inherited gene mutations may account for approximately 5% to 10% of all cancers. Additionally researchers have identified mutations in genes that are associated with greater than 50 malignant syndromes. A cancer syndrome is not a definitive cancer, but rather a disorder that may put an individual at a higher risk for developing a specific cancer (https://www.cancer.gov/about-cancer/causes-prevention/genetics). Acquired mutations are changes in DNA that develop throughout a person's lifetime. Carcinogenic agents, such as radiation or toxins, commonly are able to damage cellular genes, which are present in the cancer cell genome, thereby triggering cancer development.

Hereditary Genes

The list of genetic mutations listed below represents the more commonly inherited cancer syndromes:

- *the adenomatous polyposis coli (APC) suppressor gene*, which is altered by somatic mutations in colonic epithelial cells, permitting the outgrowth of early colonic polyps
- *familial adenomatous polyposis (FAP) or APC*, which acts as an autosomal dominant inherited condition in which hundreds of potentially cancerous polyps develop in the colon and rectum
- *familial cutaneous malignant melanoma gene*, on the distal short arm of chromosome 1
- *expression of the N-myc oncogene* in neuroblastoma, with amplification of this oncogene associated with rapid disease progression in children
- *germline mutation of the P53 gene*, which is mapped to the short arm of chromosome 17 and is associated with Li-Fraumeni syndrome, an extremely rare familial cancer syndrome that increases susceptibility to breast cancer, soft tissue sarcomas, brain tumors, bone cancer, leukemia, and adrenocortical carcinoma
- *human epidermal growth factor receptor-2 (HER-2)/neu proto-oncogene*, which is involved in regulation of normal cell growth. Gene amplification or HER-2/neu overexpression, which occurs in 25% to 30% of human breast cancers and to varying degrees in other tumor types, produces activated HER-2/neu receptors and stimulates cell growth. Tumors positive for the HER-2/neu gene are associated with poor clinical outcomes, shortened disease-free survival, more rapid cancer progression, and poor response to historically standard clinical interventions.
- *retinoblastoma* — The RB1 Gene. Retinoblastoma may be hereditary or nonhereditary and usually occurs in children less than 5 years old.
- *hereditary breast cancer and ovarian cancer syndrome* — The BRCA1 and BRCA2 genes. Mutations in these genes are associated with an increased risk of breast, ovarian, and other cancers.

PATHOPHYSIOLOGIC CONCEPTS

There are three common characteristics of cancer cells: abnormal proliferation (usually rapid), uncontrolled growth with the loss of programmed death (apoptosis), and the ability to metastasize. Metastasis is the ability of the malignant cell to independently spread from a primary site, the site of origin, to other tissues where it establishes secondary foci (metastases). (See *Histologic characteristics of cancer cells*.) Metastasis occurs through transportation of malignant cells in the circulation of the blood or lymphatic fluid. Cancer cells can also spread locally, by invasion of the tissue adjacent to the original tumor. Cancer cells differ from normal cells in terms of cell size, shape, differentiation, function, and ability to travel to distant tissues and organ systems.

Cell Growth

Typically, each of the billions of cells in the human body has an internal clock that tells the cell when it's time to reproduce and die. Mitotic reproduction occurs in a sequence called the *cell cycle*. Normal cell division occurs in direct proportion to cells lost or damaged, thus providing a mechanism for controlling growth and differentiation. These controls are absent in cancer cells, and cell production exceeds cell loss. The loss of control over normal growth is termed *autonomy*. This independence is further evidenced by the ability of cancer cells to break away and travel to other sites in the body (metastasis).

HISTOLOGIC CHARACTERISTICS OF CANCER CELLS

Cancer is a destructive (malignant) growth of cells, which invades nearby tissues and may metastasize to other areas of the body. Dividing rapidly, cancer cells tend to be extremely aggressive and do not possess the normal cellular characteristics of apoptosis and controlled growth.

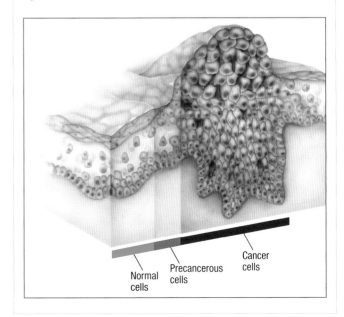

Normal cells   Precancerous cells   Cancer cells

Normal cells reproduce at a rate controlled through the activity of specific control or regulator genes. These genes produce proteins that act as "on" and "off" switches. There is no generalized control gene; different cells respond to specific control genes. In cancer cells, the control genes fail to function normally. The actual control may be lost, or the gene may become damaged. An imbalance of growth factors may occur, or the cells may fail to respond to the suppressive action of the growth factors. Any of these mechanisms may lead to uncontrolled cellular reproduction.

Hormones, growth factors, and chemicals released by cells in close proximity to the malignant cells or by immune or inflammatory cells can influence control gene activity. Substances released by cells can bind to specific receptors on cell membrane and send out signals causing the control genes to stimulate or suppress cell reproduction.

Substances released by nearby injured or infected cells or by cells of the immune system also affect cellular reproduction. For example, interleukin, released by immune cells, stimulates cell proliferation and differentiation, and interferon, released from virus-infected and immune cells, may affect the cell's rate of reproduction.

Additionally, cells that are close to one another appear to communicate with one another through gap junctions (channels through which ions and other small molecules pass). This communication provides information to the cell about the neighboring cell types and the amount of space available. The nearby cells send out physical and chemical signals that control the rate of reproduction. Cancer cells fail to recognize the signals about available tissue space. Instead of forming only a single layer, cancer cells continue to accumulate in a disorderly array.

Cell Differentiation

Normally, during development, cells become specialized — that is, they develop highly individualized characteristics that reflect their specific structure and functions. As the cells become more specialized, their reproduction and development slow down. Eventually, highly differentiated cells become unable to reproduce, and some — skin cells, for example — are programmed to die and be replaced.

Cancer cells lose the ability to differentiate; that is, they enter a state, called *anaplasia*, in which they no longer appear or function like the original cell. Anaplasia occurs in varying degrees. The less the cells resemble the cell of origin, the more anaplastic they are said to be. As anaplastic cells continue to reproduce, they lose the typical characteristics of the original cell. Some anaplastic cells begin functioning as another type of cell, possibly beginning to produce hormones. Anaplastic cells of the same type in the same site exhibit many different shapes and sizes. Mitosis is abnormal, and chromosome defects are common.

Intracellular Changes

The abnormal and uncontrolled proliferation of cancer cells is also associated with numerous changes within the cancer cell itself. These changes affect cell components as follows:

- *Cell membrane* — affects the organization, structure, adhesion, and migration of the cells. Impaired intercellular communication, enhanced response to growth factors, and diminished recognition of other cells causes uncontrolled growth and greatly increases metabolic demand for nutrients.

- *Cytoskeleton* — disrupts protein filament networks, including actin and microtubules. Normally, actin filaments exert a pull on the extracellular organic molecules that bind cells together. Microtubules control cell shape, movement, and division.
- *Cytoplasm* — becomes fewer in number and abnormally shaped. Less cellular work occurs because of a decrease in endoplasmic reticulum and mitochondria.
- *Nucleus* — becomes pleomorphic (enlarged and misshapen) and highly pigmented. Nucleoli are larger and more numerous than normal. The nuclear membrane is often irregular and commonly has projections, pouches, or blebs and fewer pores. Chromatin may clump along the outer areas of the nucleus. Chromosomal breaks, deletions, translocations, and abnormal karyotypes are common and seem to stem from the increased mitotic rate in cancer cells.

Tumor Development and Growth

Typically, a long time passes between an initiating event and the onset of a disease. During this period of time, cancer cells continue to develop, grow, and replicate, each time undergoing successive changes and further mutations.

For a tumor to grow, an initiating event or events must cause a mutation that will transform the normal cell into a cancer cell. After the initial event, the cancer cells continue to grow only if available nutrients, oxygen, and blood supply are adequate and the immune system fails to recognize or respond to the cancer cells.

Two important characteristics affecting tumor growth are (1) the location of the tumor and (2) the available blood supply. The location usually determines the originating cell type, which in turn determines the cell cycle time. For example, epithelial cells have a shorter cell cycle than do connective tissue cells. Thus, tumors of epithelial cells grow more rapidly than do tumors of connective tissue cells.

Tumors need an available blood supply to provide nutrients and oxygen for continued growth and to remove wastes, but a tumor larger than 1 to 2 mm in size has typically outgrown its available blood supply. Some tumors secrete tumor angiogenesis factors, which stimulate the formation of new blood vessels, to meet the blood supply demand.

The degree of anaplasia also affects tumor growth. Remember that the more anaplastic the cells of the tumor, the less differentiated the cells and the more rapidly they divide.

Many cancer cells also produce their own growth factors. Numerous growth factor receptors are present on the cell membranes of rapidly growing cancer cells. The increase in receptors, in conjunction with the changes in the cell membranes, further enhances cancer cell proliferation.

Important characteristics of the host that affect tumor growth include age, sex, overall health status, and immune system function.

AGE ALERT
A person's age is an important factor affecting tumor growth. Relatively few cancers are found in children, and the incidence of cancer correlates directly to increasing age. This suggests that numerous or cumulative events are necessary for the initial mutation to continue, eventually forming a tumor.

Certain cancers are more prevalent in females and others, in males. For example, sex hormones influence tumor growth in breast, endometrial, cervical, and prostate cancers. Researchers believe that sex hormones sensitize the cell to the initial precipitating factor, thus promoting carcinogenesis.

Overall health status is also an important characteristic affecting tumor growth. As tumors obtain nutrients for growth from the host, they can alter normal body processes and cause cachexia. Conversely, if the person is nutritionally depleted, tumor growth may slow down. Chronic tissue trauma has also been linked with tumor growth because healing involves increased cell division. The more rapidly cells divide, the greater the likelihood of mutations.

Metastasis

Between the initiating event and the emergence of a detectable tumor, some or all of the mutated cancer cells may die. The surviving mutated cells, if any, can continue to reproduce creating a tumor. New blood vessels form to support the tumor's continued growth and proliferation. As the cells further mutate and divide more rapidly, they can become more undifferentiated, and the number of cancerous cells soon begins to exceed the number of normal cells. Eventually, the tumor mass invades and can extend beyond the surrounding tissues. When the local tissue is in close proximity to blood or lymph circulation, the tumor can gain access to that circulation. When access is gained, tumor cells that detach may travel to distant sites in the body, where they can survive and form a metastatic tumor in the distant site. This process is called *metastasis*.

Dysplasia

Not all cells that proliferate rapidly go on to become cancerous. Throughout a person's life span, various body tissues experience periods of benign rapid growth such as during wound healing. In some cases, changes in the size, shape, and organization of cells leads to a condition called *dysplasia*. Exposure to a variety of agents including chemicals, viruses, radiation, or chronic inflammation causes dysplastic changes that may be reversed by removing the initiating stimulus or treating its effects. However, if the stimulus isn't removed, precancerous or dysplastic lesions can progress and give rise to cancer.

HOW CANCER METASTASIZES

Cancer cells may invade nearby tissues or metastasize (spread) to other organs. They may move to other tissues by any or all of the three routes described below.

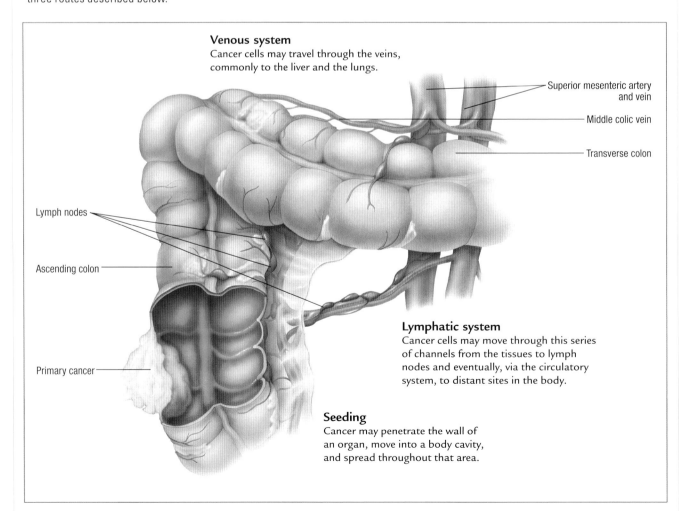

Venous system
Cancer cells may travel through the veins, commonly to the liver and the lungs.

Superior mesenteric artery and vein

Middle colic vein

Transverse colon

Lymph nodes

Ascending colon

Primary cancer

Lymphatic system
Cancer cells may move through this series of channels from the tissues to lymph nodes and eventually, via the circulatory system, to distant sites in the body.

Seeding
Cancer may penetrate the wall of an organ, move into a body cavity, and spread throughout that area.

Localized Tumor

Initially, a tumor remains localized. Recall that cancer cells communicate poorly with nearby cells. As a result, the cells continue to grow and enlarge, forming a mass or clumps of cells. The mass exerts pressure on the neighboring cells, blocking their blood supply, and subsequently causing their death. Tumors can continue to grow locally and may cause pain or other symptoms due to pressure on surrounding structures such as nerves and other organs.

Invasive Tumor

Invasion is growth of the tumor into surrounding tissues and can be the first step in metastasis. Five mechanisms are linked to invasion:

- *cellular multiplication* — By their very nature, cancer cells multiply rapidly.
- *mechanical pressure* — As cancer cells grow, they exert pressure on surrounding cells and tissues, which eventually die because their blood supply has been cut off or blocked. Loss of mechanical resistance opens the way for cancer cells to spread along the lines of least resistance and occupy the space once filled by the dead cells.
- *lysis of nearby cells* — Vesicles on the cancer cell surface contain a rich supply of receptors for laminin, a complex glycoprotein that's a major component of the basement membrane. These receptors permit the cancer cells to attach to the basement membrane, forming a bridgelike connection. Some cancer cells produce and excrete powerful proteolytic enzymes; other cancer cells induce normal host cells to produce them. These enzymes, such as collagenases and proteases, destroy the normal cells and break through their basement membrane, enabling the cancer cells to enter.
- *reduced cell adhesion* — Cancer cells' adhesion decreases, likely the result of deregulation of cell adhesion receptors.
- *increased motility* — Cancer cells secrete chemotactic factors that stimulate motility. Thus, they can move into adjacent tissues and into the circulation, and then to a secondary site. Finally, cancer cells develop fingerlike projections called *pseudopodia* that facilitate cell movement.

Metastatic Tumor

Metastatic tumors are those in which the cancer cells have traveled from the original or primary site to a secondary or more distant site. Most commonly, metastasis occurs through the blood vessels and lymphatic system.

Invasive tumor cells can break down the basement membrane and walls of blood vessels, and the tumor sheds malignant cells into the circulation. Most of the tumor cells die, but a few escape the host defenses and the turbulent environment of the bloodstream. From here, the surviving tumor cells travel through the bloodstream or lymphatic system and commonly lodge in the first capillary bed encountered. When lodged, the tumor cells develop a protective coat of fibrin, platelets, and clotting factors to evade detection by the immune system. Then they become attached to the epithelium, ultimately invading the vessel wall, interstitium, and the parenchyma of the target organ. To survive, the new tumor develops its own vascular network and, when established, may ultimately spread again.

CANCER'S SEVEN WARNING SIGNS

The American Cancer Society has developed a simple way to remember the seven warning signs of cancer. Each letter in the word *CAUTION* represents a possible warning sign that should prompt an individual to see his or her health care provider.

Change in bowel or bladder habits

A sore that doesn't heal

Unusual bleeding or discharge

Thickening or lump in the breast or elsewhere

Indigestion or difficulty swallowing

Obvious change in a wart or mole

Nagging cough or hoarseness

The lymphatic system is the most common route for distant metastasis. Tumor cells enter the lymphatic vessels through damaged basement membranes and are transported to regional lymph nodes. In this case, the tumor becomes trapped in the first lymph node it encounters. The consequent enlargement, possibly the first evidence of a malignancy or metastasis, may be due to the increased tumor growth within the node or a localized immune reaction to the tumor cells. The lymph node may filter out or contain some of the tumor cells, limiting their further spread. The cells that escape can enter the blood from the lymphatic circulation through plentiful connections between the venous and lymphatic systems.

Typically, the first capillary bed, whether lymphatic or vascular, encountered by the circulating tumor cells determines the location of the metastasis. For example, because the lungs receive all of the systemic venous return, they're a frequent site for metastasis.

SIGNS AND SYMPTOMS

In most patients, the earlier the cancer is found, the more effective the treatment is likely to be and the better the prognosis. Some cancers may be diagnosed by a routine physical examination, even before the person develops any signs or symptoms. Others may display some early warning signals. (See *Cancer's seven warning signs.*)

Unfortunately, a person may not notice or heed cancer warning signs. These patients may present with some of the more common signs and symptoms of advancing disease, such as fatigue, cachexia, pain, anemia, thrombocytopenia and leukopenia, and infection. Unfortunately, the seven warning signs are nonspecific and can be attributed to many other disorders.

DIAGNOSTIC TESTS

A thorough history and physical examination should precede sophisticated diagnostic tests. The choice of diagnostic tests is determined by the patient's presenting signs and symptoms and the suspected body system involved. Diagnostic tests serve several purposes, including:

- establishing tumor presence and extent of disease
- determining possible sites of metastasis
- evaluating affected and unaffected body systems
- identifying the stage and grade of tumor.

Useful tests for early detection and staging of tumors include screening tests, X-rays, radioactive isotope scanning (nuclear medicine imaging), computed tomography (CT) scanning, position emission tomography (PET) scanning, endoscopy, ultrasonography, and magnetic resonance imaging (MRI). The single most important diagnostic tool is the biopsy for direct histologic study of the tumor tissue.

- *Screening tests* are perhaps the most important diagnostic tools in the prevention and early detection of cancer. They may provide valuable information about the possibility of cancer even before the patient develops signs and symptoms. Examples of screening tests are colonoscopies mammograms, Pap tests, and fecal occult blood tests.
- *X-rays* are most commonly ordered to identify and evaluate changes in tissue densities. The type and location of the X-ray are determined by the patient's signs and symptoms and the suspected location of the tumor or metastases.
- *Radioactive isotope scanning* involves the use of a specialized camera, which detects radioactive isotopes that are injected into the bloodstream or ingested. The radiologist evaluates their distribution (uptake) throughout tissues, organs, and organ systems. This type of scanning provides a view of organs and regions within an organ that can't be seen with a simple X-ray.
- *CT scanning* evaluates successive layers of tissue by using a narrow-beam X-ray to provide a cross-sectional view of the structure. It can also reveal different characteristics of tissues within a solid organ.
- *PET scans* use radioisotope technology to create a picture of the body in action. Computers construct images from the emission of positive electrons (positrons) by radioactive substances administered to the patient. Unlike other diagnostic methods that simply create images of how the body looks, PET scans provide real-time imaging of the body while it functions. To study cancer spread, PET scans involve injecting the cancer patient with a small amount of radioactive glucose. Cancerous cells metabolize sugar more quickly than do healthy cells, and this process can be viewed on the scanned image. The three-dimensional PET scan pictures show malignancies as having a greater concentration of sugar.
- *Endoscopy* provides a direct view of a body cavity or passageway to detect abnormalities. During endoscopy, the health care provider can excise small tumors, aspirate fluid, or obtain tissue samples for histologic examination.
- *Ultrasonography* uses high-frequency sound waves to detect changes in the density of tissues that are difficult or impossible to observe by radiology or endoscopy. Ultrasound helps to differentiate cysts from solid tumors.
- *MRI* uses magnetic fields and radio frequencies to show a cross-sectional view of the body organs and structures.
- *Biopsy*, removing a portion of suspicious tissue, is the only definitive method to diagnose cancer. Biopsy tissue samples can be taken by curettage, fluid aspiration, fine-needle aspiration, dermal punch, endoscopy, and surgical excision.

The specimen then undergoes laboratory analysis for cell type and characteristics to provide information about the type, grade and stage of the cancer.

Some cancer cells release substances that normally aren't present in the body or are present only in small quantities. These substances, called *tumor markers* or *biologic markers*, are produced either by the cancer cell's genetic material during development and growth or by other cells in response to the presence of cancer. Markers may be found on the cell membrane of the tumor or in body fluids such as blood, cerebrospinal fluid, or urine. Tumor cell markers include hormones, enzymes, genes, antigens, and antibodies. Markers may be helpful in determining the presence of a tumor or the response of a tumor to treatment. Unfortunately, several disadvantages of tumor markers may preclude their use alone as a diagnostic tool for cancer. For example:

- Most tumor cell markers aren't specific enough to identify one certain type of cancer.
- By the time a tumor cell marker level is elevated, the disease may be too far advanced to treat.
- Some nonmalignant diseases, such as pelvic inflammatory disease, pancreatitis, and ulcerative colitis, are also associated with tumor cell markers.
- The absence of a tumor cell marker, perhaps the worst drawback of relying solely on markers, doesn't mean that a person is free from cancer.

TUMOR CLASSIFICATION

Tumors are initially classified as benign or malignant depending on their specific features. Typically, benign tumors are well differentiated; that is, their cells closely resemble those of the tissue of origin. Commonly encapsulated with well-defined borders, benign tumors grow slowly, often displacing but not infiltrating surrounding tissues and, therefore, causing only slight damage. Benign tumors do NOT metastasize.

Conversely, most malignant tumors are undifferentiated to varying degrees, having cells that may closely resemble to those that may differ considerably from those of the tissue of origin. They are seldom encapsulated. Cancer cells rapidly expand in all directions, causing extensive local damage as they infiltrate surrounding tissues. Malignant tumors have the ability to metastasize through the circulatory and/or lymph systems to secondary sites.

Malignant tumors are further classified by tissue type, degree of differentiation (grading), and extent of the disease (staging). High-grade tumors are poorly differentiated and are more aggressive than are low-grade tumors. Early-stage cancers carry a more favorable prognosis than do later-stage cancers that have spread to nearby or distant sites.

TREATMENT

The number of cancer treatments is constantly increasing. They may be used alone or in combination (multimodal therapy), depending on the type, stage, localization, and responsiveness of the tumor and on limitations imposed by the patient's clinical status. Cancer treatment has four goals:

- *cure* — eradicating the cancer and promoting long-term patient survival
- *control* — arresting tumor growth
- *palliation* — alleviating to improve the quality of life throughout the course of the disease
- *Prophylaxis* — providing treatment when no tumor is detectable, although the patient is known to be at high risk of tumor development or recurrence.

Cancer treatment is further categorized by type according to when it's used:

- *Primary* — to eradicate the disease
- *Neo-adjuvant* — treatment given as a first step to shrink a tumor before the primary treatment
- *Adjuvant* — in addition to primary, to eliminate microscopic disease and promote a cure or improve the patient's response
- *Salvage* — Treatment that is given after the cancer has not responded to other treatments (https://www.cancer.gov/publications/dictionaries/cancer-terms).

Any treatment regimen can cause complications. Indeed, many complications of cancer are related to the adverse effects of treatment.

Surgery, once the mainstay of cancer treatment, is now typically combined with other therapies. It may be performed to diagnose the disease, initiate primary treatment, or achieve palliation and is occasionally done for prophylaxis.

Radiation therapy uses high-energy radiation to treat cancer. Used alone or in conjunction with other therapies, it aims to destroy dividing cancer cells while damaging normal cells as little as possible. Two types of radiation are used to treat cancer: *ionizing radiation* and *particle beam radiation.* Radiation therapy has both local and systemic adverse effects, because it affects both normal and malignant cells.

Chemotherapy includes a wide range of antineoplastic drugs, which may induce regression of a tumor and its metastasis. It is used as a primary treatment and is also useful in controlling residual disease and as an adjunct to surgery or radiation therapy. It can induce long remissions and sometimes effect a cure. As a palliative treatment, chemotherapy aims to improve the patient's quality of life by temporarily relieving suffering, and pain and other symptoms (https://www.cancer.gov/publications/dictionaries/cancer-terms?expand=I).

Every dose of a chemotherapeutic agent destroys only a percentage of tumor cells. Therefore, regression of the tumor requires repeated doses of drugs. The goal is to eradicate enough of the tumor so that the immune system can destroy the remaining malignant cells. Unfortunately, chemotherapy also causes numerous adverse effects.

The most commonly used types of chemotherapeutic agents are:

- alkylating agents and nitroureas
- antimetabolites
- antitumor antibiotics
- plant (Vinca) alkaloids
- hormones and hormone antagonists.

Hormonal therapy is based on studies showing that certain hormones can inhibit the growth of certain cancers.

Targeted therapy uses drugs or other agents to "target" or attack specific types of cancer cells producing less collateral harm or damage to normal cells. Targeted therapies can block the action of enzymes, proteins, and other molecules that promote the growth of cancer cells. Most targeted therapies are either small molecule drugs or monoclonal antibodies. An example of a targeted therapy agent is erlotinib, an epidermal growth factor (EGFR) tyrosine kinase inhibitor. Erlotinib is used to treat certain types of non–small cell lung cancer by blocking a protein, EGFR, which may prevent the cancer from growing.

Immunotherapy is a type of biological therapy and may also be a targeted therapy. It is treatment with agents *that may stimulate or repress the immune system response.* Biologic agents are commonly used in combination with chemotherapy or radiation therapy. Types of immunotherapy include cytokines, vaccines, bacillus Calmette-Guerin (BCG), and some monoclonal antibodies. The U.S. Food and Drug Administration has approved several promising drugs for treatment of cancer. For example, rituximab — a monoclonal antibody — is effective to treat relapsed or refractory B-cell non-Hodgkin's lymphoma.

Suggested Reference

U.S. Department of Health and Human Services. (2014). *The Health Consequences of Smoking—50 Years of Progress: A Report of the Surgeon General.* Atlanta, GA: U.S. Department of Health and Human Services, Centers for Disease Control and Prevention, National Center for Chronic Disease Prevention and Health Promotion, Office on Smoking and Health. Accessed August 20, 2015.

INFECTION

Infection is the invasion and multiplication of microorganisms in or on body tissue that cause signs, symptoms, and an immune response. Such reproduction injures the host by causing cell damage from toxins produced by the microorganisms or from intracellular multiplication or by competing with host metabolism. Infectious diseases range from relatively mild illnesses to debilitating and lethal conditions: from the common cold through chronic hepatitis to acquired immunodeficiency syndrome. The severity of the infection varies with the pathogenicity and number of the invading microorganisms and the strength of host defenses.

For infection to be transmitted, these factors must be present: causative agent, infectious reservoir with a portal of exit, mode of transmission, a portal of entry into the host, and a susceptible host.

CAUSES

Microorganisms that are responsible for infectious diseases include viruses, bacteria, fungi, mycoplasmas, rickettsia, chlamydia, spirochetes, and parasites.

Viruses

Viruses are subcellular organisms made up only of a ribonucleic acid (RNA) nucleus or a deoxyribonucleic acid (DNA) nucleus covered with proteins. They're the smallest known organisms, so tiny that only an electron microscope can make them visible. Independent of the host cells, viruses can't replicate. Rather, they invade a host cell and stimulate it to participate in forming additional virus particles. Some viruses destroy surrounding tissue and release toxins. Viruses lack the genes necessary for energy production. They depend on the ribosomes and nutrients of infected host cells for protein production. The estimated 400 viruses that infect humans are classified according to their size, shape, and means of transmission, such as respiratory, fecal, oral, and sexual.

Retroviruses are a unique type of virus that carries their genetic code in RNA rather than the more common carrier DNA. These RNA viruses contain the enzyme reverse transcriptase, which transcribes viral RNA into DNA. The host cell then incorporates the alien DNA into its own genetic material. The most notorious retrovirus known today is human immunodeficiency virus.

Bacteria

Bacteria are simple one-celled microorganisms with a cell wall that protects them from many of the defense mechanisms of the human body. Although they lack a nucleus, bacteria possess all the other mechanisms they need to survive and rapidly reproduce.

Bacteria can be classified according to shape — spherical cocci, rod-shaped bacilli, and spiral-shaped spirilla. They can also be classified according to their need for oxygen (aerobic or anaerobic), their mobility (motile or nonmotile), and their tendency to form protective capsules (encapsulated or nonencapsulated) or spores (sporulating or nonsporulating).

Bacteria damage body tissues by interfering with essential cell function or by releasing exotoxins or endotoxins, which cause cell damage.

Fungi

Fungi have rigid walls and nuclei that are enveloped by nuclear membranes. They occur as yeast (single-cell, oval-shaped organisms) or molds (organisms with hyphae, or branching filaments). Depending on the environment, some fungi may occur in both forms. Found almost everywhere on earth, fungi live on organic matter, in water and soil, on animals and plants, and on a wide variety of unlikely materials. They can live both inside and outside their host.

Mycoplasmas

Mycoplasmas are bacterialike organisms, the smallest of the cellular microbes that can live outside a host cell, although some may be parasitic. Lacking cell walls, they can assume many different shapes ranging from coccoid to filamentous. The lack of a cell wall makes them resistant to penicillin and other antibiotics that work by inhibiting cell wall synthesis.

Rickettsia

Rickettsia are small, gram-negative, aerobic bacterialike organisms that can cause life-threatening illness. They may be coccoid, rod-shaped, or irregularly shaped. Rickettsia require a host cell for replication. They have no cell wall, and their cell membranes are leaky; thus, they must live inside another, better protected cell. Rickettsia are transmitted by the bites of arthropod carriers, such as lice, fleas, and ticks, and through exposure to their waste products. Rickettsial infections that occur in the United States include Rocky Mountain spotted fever, typhus, and Q fever.

Spirochetes

Spirochetes are an atypical type of bacteria that have a helical shape, and the length is many times its width. They have filaments wrapped around the cell wall that propel the spirochete in a corkscrew motion. Spirochetes occur with Lyme disease and syphilis.

Parasites

Parasites are unicellular or multicellular organisms that live on or within another organism and obtain nourishment from the host. They take only the nutrients they need and usually don't kill their hosts. Examples of parasites that can produce an infection if they cause cellular damage to the host include helminths (such as pinworms, roundworms, and tapeworms) and arthropods (such as mites, fleas, and ticks). Helminths can infect the human gut; arthropods commonly cause skin and systemic disease.

RISK FACTORS

A healthy person can usually ward off infections with the body's own built-in defense mechanisms, which include:

- intact skin
- normal flora that inhabit the skin and various organs
- lysozymes secreted by eyes, nasal passages, glands, stomach, and genitourinary organs
- defensive structures such as the cilia that sweep foreign matter from the airways
- a healthy immune system.

However, if an imbalance develops, the potential for infection increases. Risk factors for the development of infection include weakened defense mechanisms, environmental and developmental factors, and pathogen characteristics.

Weakened Defense Mechanisms

The body has many defense mechanisms for resisting entry and multiplication of both exogenous and endogenous microbes. However, a weakened immune system makes it easier for these pathogens to invade the body and launch an infectious disease. This weakened state is referred to as immunodeficiency or immunocompromise.

Impaired function of white blood cells (WBCs), as well as low levels of T cells and B cells, characterizes immunodeficiencies. An immunodeficiency may be congenital or acquired. Acquired immunodeficiency may result from infection, malnutrition, chronic stress, or pregnancy. Diabetes, renal failure, and cirrhosis can suppress the immune response, as can such drugs as corticosteroids and chemotherapy.

Regardless of cause, the result of immunodeficiency is the same. The body's ability to recognize and fight pathogens is impaired. People who are immunodeficient are more susceptible to all infections, are more acutely ill when they become infected, and require a much longer time period to heal.

Environmental Factors

Other conditions that may weaken a person's immune defenses include poor hygiene, malnutrition, inadequate physical barriers, emotional and physical stressors, chronic diseases, medical and surgical treatments, and inadequate immunization.

Good hygiene promotes normal host defenses; poor hygiene increases the risk of infection. Unclean skin harbors microbes, offering an environment for them to colonize, and is more open to invasion. Frequent body washing removes surface microbes and maintains an intact barrier to infection, but it may damage the skin. To maintain skin integrity, lubricants and emollients may be used to prevent cracks and breaks.

The body requires a balanced diet to provide the nutrients, vitamins, and minerals needed for an effective immune system. Protein malnutrition inhibits the production of antibodies, without which the body is unable to mount an effective attack against microbe invasion. Malnutrition has been shown to have a direct relationship to the incidence of nosocomial infections.

Dust can facilitate transportation of pathogens. For example, dustborne spores of the fungus *Aspergillus* transmit the infection. If the inhaled spores become established in the lungs, they're notoriously difficult to expel. Fortunately, most persons with intact immune systems can resist infection with *Aspergillus*, which is usually dangerous only in the presence of severe immunosuppression.

Developmental Factors

Extremely young and old people are at higher risk for infection. The immune system doesn't fully develop until about age 6 months. An infant exposed to an infectious agent usually develops an infection. The most common type of infection in toddlers affects the respiratory tract. When young children put toys and other objects in their mouths, they increase their exposure to a variety of pathogens.

Exposure to communicable diseases continues throughout childhood, as children progress from daycare facilities to schools. Skin diseases, such as impetigo, and lice infestation commonly pass from one child to the next at this age. Accidents are common in childhood as well, and broken or abraded skin opens the way for bacterial invasion. Lack of immunization also contributes to incidence of childhood diseases.

Advancing age, on the other hand, is associated with a declining immune system, partly as a result of decreasing thymus function. Chronic diseases, such as diabetes and atherosclerosis, can weaken defenses by impairing blood flow and nutrient delivery to body systems.

Pathogen Characteristics

A microbe must be present in sufficient quantities to cause a disease in a healthy human. The number needed to cause a disease varies from one microbe to the next and from host to host and may be affected by the mode of transmission. The severity of an infection depends on several factors, including the microbe's pathogenicity, that is, the likelihood that it will cause pathogenic changes or disease. Factors that affect pathogenicity include:

- *specificity* — the range of hosts to which a microbe is attracted (Some microbes may be attracted to a wide range of both humans and animals, while others select only human or only animal hosts.)
- *invasiveness* (sometimes called *infectivity*) — ability of a microbe to invade and multiply in the host tissues (Some microbes can enter through intact skin; others can enter only if the skin or mucous membrane is broken. Some microbes produce enzymes that enhance their invasiveness.)
- *quantity* — the number of microbes that succeed in invading and reproducing in the body
- *virulence* — severity of the disease a pathogen can produce (Virulence can vary depending on the host defenses; any infection can be life threatening in an immunodeficient patient. Infection with a pathogen known to be particularly virulent requires early diagnosis and treatment.)
- *toxigenicity* (related to virulence) — potential to damage host tissues by producing and releasing toxins
- *adhesiveness* — ability to attach to host tissue (Some pathogens secrete a sticky substance that helps them adhere to tissue while protecting them from the host's defense mechanisms.)

- *antigenicity* — degree to which a pathogen can induce a specific immune response (Microbes that invade and localize in tissue initially stimulate a cellular response; those that disseminate quickly throughout the host's body generate an antibody response.)
- *viability* — ability to survive outside its host. Most microbes can't live and multiply outside a reservoir.

STAGES OF INFECTION

Development of infection usually proceeds through four stages. (See *Stages of infection.*)

PATHOPHYSIOLOGIC CONCEPTS

Clinical expressions of infectious disease vary depending on the pathogen involved and the body system affected. Most of the signs and symptoms result from host responses, which may be similar or extremely different from host to host. During the prodromal stage, a person will complain of some common, nonspecific signs and symptoms, such as fever, muscle aches, headache, and lethargy. In the acute stage, signs and symptoms that are more specific provide evidence of the microbe's target. However, some diseases produce no symptoms and are discovered only by laboratory tests.

The inflammatory response is a major reactive defense mechanism in the battle against infective agents. Inflammation may be the result of tissue injury, infection, or allergic reaction. Acute inflammation has two stages: vascular and cellular. In the vascular stage, arterioles at or near the site of the injury briefly constrict and then dilate, causing an increase in fluid pressure in the capillaries. The consequent movement of plasma into the interstitial space causes edema. At the same time, inflammatory cells release histamine and bradykinin, which further increase capillary permeability. Red blood cells and fluid flow into the interstitial space, contributing to edema. The extra fluid arriving in the inflamed area dilutes microbial toxins.

During the cellular stage of inflammation, WBCs and platelets move toward the damaged cells, and phagocytosis of the dead cells and microorganisms begins. Platelets control any excess bleeding in the area, and mast cells arriving at the site release heparin to maintain blood flow to the area.

SIGNS AND SYMPTOMS

Acute inflammation is the body's immediate response to cell injury or cell death. The cardinal signs of inflammation include:

- *redness (rubor)* — dilation of arterioles and increased circulation to the site; a localized blush caused by filling of previously empty or partially distended capillaries
- *heat (calor)* — local vasodilation, fluid leakage into the interstitial spaces, and increased blood flow to the area
- *pain (dolor)* — pain receptors stimulated by swollen tissue, local pH changes, and chemicals excreted during the inflammatory process
- *edema (tumor)* — local vasodilatation, leakage of fluid into interstitial spaces, and blockage of lymphatic drainage
- *loss of function (functio laesa) of a body part* — primarily a result of edema and pain.

CLINICAL TIP
Localized infections produce a rapid inflammatory response with obvious signs and symptoms. Disseminated infections have a slow inflammatory response and take longer to identify and treat, thereby increasing morbidity and mortality.

Fever

Fever follows the introduction of an infectious agent. An elevated temperature helps fight an infection because many microorganisms are unable to survive in a hot environment. When the body temperature rises too high, body cells can be damaged, particularly those of the nervous system.

Diaphoresis (sweating) is the body's method of cooling itself and returning the temperature to normal for that individual. Artificial methods to reduce a slight fever can actually impede the body's defenses against infection.

Stages of Infection	
Stage I	
Incubation	• Duration can range from instantaneous to several years.
	• Pathogen is replicating, and the infected person becomes contagious, thus capable of transmitting the disease.
Stage II	
Prodromal stage	• Host makes vague complaints of feeling unwell.
	• Host is still contagious.
Stage III	
Acute illness	• Microbes actively destroy host cells and affect specific host systems.
	• Patient recognizes which area of the body is affected.
	• Complaints are more specific.
Stage IV	
Convalescence	• Begins when the body's defense mechanisms have contained the microbes.
	• Damaged tissue is healing.

Leukocytosis

The body responds to the introduction of pathogens by increasing the number and types of circulating WBCs. This process is called *leukocytosis.* In the acute or early stage, the neutrophil count increases. Bone marrow begins to release immature leukocytes, because existing neutrophils can't meet the body's demand for defensive cells. The immature neutrophils (called *bands* in the differential WBC count) can't serve any defensive purpose.

As the acute phase comes under control and the damage is isolated, the cellular stage of the inflammatory process takes place. Neutrophils, monocytes, and macrophages begin the process of phagocytosis of dead tissue and bacteria. Neutrophils and monocytes are attracted to the site of infection by chemotaxis, and they identify the foreign antigen and attach to it. Then they engulf, kill, and degrade the microorganism that carries the antigen on its surface. Macrophages, a mature type of monocyte, arrive at the site later and remain in the area of inflammation longer than the other cells. Besides phagocytosis, macrophages play several other key roles at the site, such as preparing the area for healing and processing antigens for a cellular immune response. An elevated monocyte count is common during resolution of any injury and in chronic infections.

Chronic Inflammation

An inflammatory reaction lasting longer than 2 weeks is referred to as chronic inflammation. It may follow an acute process. A poorly healed wound or an unresolved infection can lead to chronic inflammation. The body may encapsulate a pathogen that it can't destroy in order to isolate it. An example of such a pathogen is mycobacteria, one of the species that cause tuberculosis; encapsulated mycobacteria appear in X-rays as identifiable spots in the lungs. With chronic inflammation, permanent scarring and loss of tissue function can occur.

DIAGNOSTIC TESTS

Accurate assessment helps identify infectious diseases, appropriate treatment, and avoidable complications. It begins with obtaining the patient's complete medical history, performing a thorough physical examination, and performing or ordering appropriate diagnostic tests. Tests that can help identify and gauge the extent of infection include laboratory studies, radiographic tests, and scans.

Most commonly, the first test is a WBC count and a differential. An elevation in the overall number of WBCs is a positive result. The differential count is the relative number of each of five types of WBCs — neutrophils, eosinophils, basophils, lymphocytes, and monocytes. This test recognizes only that an immune response has been stimulated. Bacterial infection usually causes an elevation in the counts; viruses may cause no change or a decrease in normal WBC level.

Erythrocyte sedimentation rate may be done as a general test to reveal that an inflammatory process is occurring within the body.

To determine the causative agent, a stained smear from a specific body site is obtained. Stains that may be used to visualize the microorganism include:

- *Gram stain* — identifies gram-negative or gram-positive bacteria
- *acid-fast stain* — identifies mycobacteria and nocardia
- *silver stain* — identifies fungi, legionella, and pneumocystis.

Although stains provide rapid and valuable diagnostic information, they only tentatively identify a pathogen. Confirmation requires culturing. Growth sufficient to identify the microbe may occur in as quickly as 8 hours or as long as several weeks, depending on how rapidly the microbe replicates. Types of cultures that may be ordered are blood, urine, sputum, throat, nasal, wound, skin, stool, and cerebrospinal fluid, but any body substance can be cultured.

A specimen obtained for culture must not be contaminated with any other substance. For example, a urine specimen must not contain debris from the perineum or vaginal area. If obtaining a clean urine specimen isn't possible, the patient must be catheterized to make sure that only the urine is being examined. Contaminated specimens may mislead and prolong treatment.

Additional tests that may be requested include magnetic resonance imaging to locate infection sites, chest X-rays to search the lungs for respiratory changes, and gallium scans to detect abscesses.

TREATMENT

Treatment for infections can vary widely. Vaccines may be administered to induce a primary immune response under conditions that won't cause disease. If infection occurs, treatment is tailored to the specific causative organism. Drug therapy should be used only when it's appropriate. Supportive therapy can play an important role in fighting infections.

- *Antibiotics* work in a variety of ways, depending on the class of antibiotic. Their action is either bactericidal or bacteriostatic. Antibiotics may inhibit cell wall synthesis, protein synthesis, bacterial metabolism, or nucleic acid synthesis or activity, or they may increase cell membrane permeability.
- *Antifungal drugs* destroy the invading microbe by increasing cell membrane permeability. The antifungal binds sterols in the cell membrane, resulting in leakage of intracellular contents, such as potassium, sodium, and nutrients.
- *Antiviral drugs* stop viral replication by interfering with DNA synthesis.

The overuse of antimicrobials has created widespread resistance to some specific drugs. Some pathogens that were once well controlled by medications are again surfacing with increased virulence. One such pathogen is that which is known to cause tuberculosis.

Some diseases, including most viral infections, don't respond to available drugs. Supportive care is the only recourse while the host defenses repel the invader. To help the body fight an infection, the patient should:

- use universal precautions to avoid spreading the infection
- drink plenty of fluids
- get plenty of rest
- avoid people who may have other illnesses
- take only over-the-counter medications appropriate for his symptoms, with full knowledge about dosage, actions, and possible adverse effects or reactions
- follow the health care provider's orders for taking prescription drugs, and be sure to complete the medication as ordered and not share the prescription with others.

DISORDERS

See *Common infectious disorders*, pages xx–xx, which describes a variety of infectious disorders.

Examples of Infectious Disorders

DISORDER	CHARACTERISTICS
Bacterial infections	
Anthrax	Bacterial infection characterized as cutaneous, inhalational, or intestinal • Diagnosis confirmed by isolation of *Bacillus anthracis* from cultures of blood, skin, lesions, or sputum. • Signs and symptoms directly related to the location of infection. Cutaneous anthrax is characterized by a small, elevated, itchy lesion, which develops into a vesicle and then a painless ulcer, along with enlarged lymph glands. Inhalational anthrax is characterized by flulike symptoms initially, followed by severe respiratory difficulty and shock. With intestinal anthrax, fever, nausea, vomiting, and decreased appetite occur, which progress to abdominal pain, hematemesis, and severe diarrhea.
Chlamydia	Typically, a sexually transmitted infection, which is caused by *Chlamydia trachomatis* • Disease pattern depends on the individual infected and the site of infection: usually the eye or genital tract. • If untreated, it can cause blindness in the eye, or if in the genital tract, it can cause pelvic inflammatory disease (PID) in women, which may lead to sterility in a portion of those with PID.
Conjunctivitis	Bacterial or viral infection of the conjunctiva of the eye • Culture from the conjunctiva identifies the causative organism. • Associated with hyperemia of the eye, discharge, tearing, pain, and photophobia.
Gonorrhea	Sexually transmitted infection caused by *Neisseria gonorrhoeae*, a gram-negative, oxidase-positive diplococcus • After exposure, epithelial cells at an infection site become infected, and the disease begins to spread locally. • Disease pattern depends on the individual infected and the site of infection. • As with chlamydia, untreated gonorrhea in women can ascend from the lower genital tract to upper and lead to pelvic inflammatory disease.
Listeriosis	Infection caused by weakly hemolytic, gram-positive bacillus *Listeria monocytogenes* • Primary method of person-to-person transmission is neonatal infection in utero or during passage through an infected birth canal. • Disease may cause abortion, premature delivery, stillbirth, or organ abscesses in fetuses. • Neonates may have tense fontanels due to meningitis, be irritable or lethargic, have seizures, or be comatose.
Lyme disease	Infection caused by spirochete *Borrelia burgdorferi* • Transmitted by ixodid tick, which injects spirochete-laden saliva into the bloodstream. • Stage 1: Tick bite causes a ringlike rash, called *erythema chronicum migrans in 70%–80% of patients*. • Stage 2: Several days to weeks after the initial rash, spirochetes disseminate to other skin sites or organs through the bloodstream or lymphatic system. Patients may develop annular or malar rashes and may have malaise, headache, achiness, and generalized lymphadenopathy. Approximately 15% of patients who are not treated develop neurological issues and a smaller percentage may develop cardiac issues, particularly a heart block. • Stage 3: Spirochetes may survive for years in joints, or they may die after triggering an inflammatory response in the host. Inflammation of one or two joints (often the knee) often occurs in persistent infection; arthritic symptoms tend to resolve over time.
Meningitis	Meningeal inflammation caused by bacteria, viruses, protozoa, or fungi. The most common types are bacterial and viral. • Disease occurs when infecting organisms enter the subarachnoid space and cause an inflammatory response. The organisms gain access to the cerebrospinal fluid, where they cause irritation of the tissues bathed by the fluid. • Characteristic signs include fever, chills, headache, nuchal rigidity, vomiting, photophobia, lethargy, coma, positive Brudzinski's and Kernig's signs, increased deep tendon reflexes, widened pulse pressure, bradycardia, and rash.
Acute otitis media	Inflammation of the middle ear caused by a bacterial infection, most often *S. pneumoniae* or *H. influenzae* • Disease is commonly accompanied by a viral upper respiratory infection. • Viral symptoms occur, generally followed by ear pain.
Peritonitis	Acute or chronic inflammation of the peritoneum caused by microorganism invasion. Secondary peritonitis is the most common cause as a complication of continuous ambulatory peritoneal dialysis (CAPD). • Onset commonly sudden, with severe and diffuse abdominal pain. • Pain intensifies and localizes in the region of infection.

DISORDER	CHARACTERISTICS
Pertussis (whooping cough)	Highly contagious respiratory infection usually caused by the nonmotile, gram-negative coccobacillus *Bordetella pertussis* and, occasionally, by the related similar bacteria *B. parapertussis* or *B. bronchiseptica* • Transmitted by direct inhalation of contaminated droplets from a patient in an acute stage. It may also spread indirectly though soiled linen and other articles contaminated by respiratory secretions. • After approximately 7 to 10 days, *B. pertussis* enters the tracheobronchial mucosa, where it produces progressively tenacious mucus. • Known for its associated spasmodic cough, characteristically ending in a loud, crowing inspiratory whoop. Complications include apnea, hypoxia, seizures, pneumonia, encephalopathy, and death.
Pneumonia	Infection of the lung parenchyma that is bacterial, fungal, viral, or protozoal in origin • The lower respiratory tract can be exposed to pathogens by inhalation, aspiration, vascular dissemination, or direct contact with contaminated equipment. When inside, the pathogen begins to colonize and infection develops. • Bacterial infection initially triggers alveolar inflammation and edema, which produces an area of low ventilation with normal perfusion. Capillaries become engorged with blood, causing stasis. As alveolocapillary membranes break down, the alveoli fill with blood and exudates, causing atelectasis, or lung collapse.
Salmonellosis	Disease caused by a serotype of the genus *Salmonella*, a member of the *Enterobacteriaceae* family • Most common species of *Salmonella* include *S. typhi*, which causes typhoid fever; *S. enteritidis*, which causes enterocolitis; and *S. choleraesuis*, which causes bacteremia. • Nontyphoidal salmonellosis usually follows ingestion of contaminated dry milk, chocolate bars, pharmaceuticals of animal origin, or contaminated or inadequately processed foods, especially eggs and poultry. • Characteristic symptoms include fever, abdominal pain or cramps, and severe diarrhea with enterocolitis.
Shigellosis	Acute intestinal infection caused by the bacteria *Shigella*, a member of the *Enterobacteriaceae* family. It's a short, nonmotile, gram-negative rod. • Transmission occurs primarily through the fecal-oral route. • After an incubation period of 1 to 4 days, *Shigella* organisms invade the intestinal mucosa and cause inflammation. Symptoms can range from watery stools to fever, cramps, and stools with pus, mucus, or blood.
Tetanus	Acute exotoxin-mediated infection caused by the anaerobic, spore-forming, gram-positive bacillus *Clostridium tetani* • Transmission occurs through a puncture wound that is contaminated by soil, dust, or animal excreta containing *C. tetani* or by way of burns and minor wounds. • After *C. tetani* enters the body, it causes local infection and tissue necrosis. It also produces toxins that then enter the bloodstream and lymphatics and eventually spread to central nervous system (CNS) tissue. • Disease is characterized by marked muscle hypertonicity, hyperactive deep tendon reflexes, and painful, involuntary muscle contractions. Severe muscle spasms can last up to 7 days.
Toxic shock syndrome (TSS)	Acute bacterial infection caused by toxin-producing, penicillin-resistant strains of *Staphylococcus aureus*, such as TSS toxin-1 or staphylococcal enterotoxins or exotoxins B and C. It can also be caused by *Streptococcus pyogenes*. • Menstrual TSS is associated with tampon use. • Nonmenstrual TSS is associated with infections, such as abscesses, osteomyelitis, pneumonia, endocarditis, bacteremia, and postsurgical infections. • Signs and symptoms include fever, hypotension, renal failure, and multisystem involvement.
Tuberculosis	Infectious disease transmitted by inhaling *Mycobacterium tuberculosis*, an acid-fast bacillus, from an infected person • Bacilli are deposited in the lungs, the immune system responds by sending leukocytes, and inflammation results. After a few days, leukocytes are replaced by macrophages. Bacilli are then ingested by the macrophages and carried off by the lymphatics to the lymph nodes. Macrophages that infest the bacilli fuse to form epithelioid cell tubercles, tiny nodules surrounded by lymphocytes. • Caseous necrosis develops in the lesion, and scar tissue encapsulates the tubercle. The organism may be killed in the process. • If the tubercles and inflamed nodes rupture, the infection contaminates the surrounding tissue and may spread through the blood and lymphatic circulation to distant sites.

(*Continued*)

DISORDER	CHARACTERISTICS
Urinary tract infection	Infection most commonly caused by enteric gram-negative bacilli • Results from microorganisms entering the urethra and then ascending into the bladder • Commonly causes urgency, frequency, and dysuria

Viral infections

DISORDER	CHARACTERISTICS
Avian influenza	An influenza A virus that typically infects birds • Reported symptoms in humans include fever, cough, sore throat, and muscle aches. • Virus could progress to eye infections, pneumonia, and acute respiratory distress.
Cytomegalovirus infection	A DNA virus that's a member of the herpes virus group • Transmission can occur horizontally (person-to-person contact with secretions), vertically (mother to neonate), or through blood transfusions. • The virus spreads through the body in lymphocytes or mononuclear cells to the lungs, liver, GI tract, eyes, and CNS, where it commonly produces inflammatory reactions.
Herpes simplex virus (HSV)	HSV is an enveloped, double-stranded DNA virus that causes both herpes simplex type 1 and type 2. • Transmission is via mucosal surfaces and infectious secretions: such as oral or cervical secretions. • During exposure, the virus fuses to the host cell membrane and releases proteins, turning off the host cell's protein production or synthesis. The virus then replicates and synthesizes structural proteins. The virus pushes its nucleocapsid (protein coat and nucleic acid) into the cytoplasm of the host cell and releases the viral DNA. Complete virus particles capable of surviving and infecting a living cell are transported to the cell's surface. • Characteristic painful, vesicular lesions are usually observed at the site of initial infection. • Viral shredding can occur at any time, particularly with HSV2 so that asymptomatic transmission of HSV2 can occur with sexual contact.
Herpes zoster	Caused by a reactivation of varicella zoster virus that has been lying dormant in the cerebral ganglia or the ganglia of posterior nerve roots • Small, painful, red, nodular skin lesions develop on areas along nerve paths. • Lesions change to vesicles filled with pus or fluid. • Direct contact with the fluid from a vesicle to a person who has never had varicella (chicken pox) may cause varicella (chicken pox) in that person.
Human immunodeficiency virus (HIV) infection	An RNA retrovirus that causes acquired immunodeficiency syndrome (AIDS) • Virus passes from one person to another through blood-to-blood and sexual contact. In addition, an infected pregnant woman can pass HIV to her baby during pregnancy or delivery as well as through breast-feeding. • Most people with HIV infection develop AIDS; however, current combination drug therapy in conjunction with treatment and prophylaxis of common opportunistic infections can delay the natural progression and prolong survival.
Infectious mononucleosis	Viral illness caused by the Epstein-Barr virus, a B-lymphotropic herpes virus • Most cases spread by the oropharyngeal route, but transmission by blood transfusion or during cardiac surgery is also possible. • The virus invades the B cells of the oropharyngeal lymphoid tissues and then replicates. • Dying B cells release the virus into the blood, causing fever and other symptoms. During this period, antiviral antibodies appear and the virus disappears from the blood, lodging mainly in the parotid gland.
Mumps	Acute viral disease caused by an RNA virus classified as *Rubulavirus* in the *Paramyxoviridae* family • Virus is transmitted by droplets or by direct contact. • Characterized by enlargement and tenderness of parotid gland and swelling of other salivary glands. • With introduction of vaccinations, this is uncommon in countries promoting preventative healthcare and vaccinations.

DISORDER	CHARACTERISTICS
Rabies	Rapidly progressive fatal infection of the CNS caused by an RNA virus in the *Rhabdoviridae* family • Transmitted by the bite of an infected animal through the skin or mucous membranes or, occasionally, in airborne droplets or infected tissue. • The rabies virus begins replicating in the striated muscle cells at the bite site. • The virus spreads along the nerve pathways to the spinal cord and brain, where it replicates again. • The virus moves through the nerves into other tissues, including into the salivary glands.
Respiratory syncytial virus	Infection of the respiratory tract caused by an enveloped RNA paramyxovirus • The organism is transmitted from person to person by respiratory secretions or by touching contaminated surfaces. • Bronchiolitis or pneumonia ensues and, in severe cases, may damage the bronchiolar epithelium. • Interalveolar thickening and filling of alveolar spaces with fluid may occur. • The virus is more common in winter and early spring.
Rubella	An enveloped positive-stranded RNA virus classified as a rubivirus in the *Togaviridae* family • Transmitted through contact with the blood, urine, stool, or nasopharyngeal secretions of an infected person. It can also be transmitted transplacentally. • The virus replicates first in the respiratory tract and then spreads through the bloodstream. • Characteristic maculopapular rash usually begins on the face and then spreads rapidly. • With preventative vaccinations, this disease is uncommon.
Rubeola	Acute, highly contagious paramyxovirus infection that's spread by direct contact or by contaminated airborne respiratory droplets • Portal of entry is the upper respiratory tract. • Characterized by Koplik's spots, a pruritic macular rash that becomes papular and erythematous. • Preventative vaccinations are available.
Smallpox	Acute contagious virus caused by the variola virus, a member of the *Orthopoxvirus* family • Transmitted from person to person by infected aerosols and air droplets. • The incubation period, which is usually 12 to 14 days, is followed by the sudden onset of influenzalike symptoms including fever, malaise, headache, and severe back pain. • Two to three days later, the patient may feel better, however, the characteristic rash appears, first on the face, hands, and forearms and then after a few days progressing to the trunk. Lesions also develop in the mucous membranes of the nose and mouth, then ulcerate and release large amounts of virus into the mouth and throat. • The world was declared free of smallpox in 1980.
Varicella (chickenpox)	Common, highly contagious exanthem caused by the varicella-zoster virus, a member of the herpes virus family • Transmitted by respiratory droplets or contact with vesicles. In utero infection is also possible. • Characterized by a pruritic rash of small, erythematous macules that progress to papules and then to clear vesicles on an erythematous base. • Vaccinations are available for varicella.
Viral pneumonia	Lung infection caused by any one of a variety of viruses, transmitted through contact with an infected individual • The virus first attacks bronchiolar epithelial cells, causing interstitial inflammation and desquamation. • Virus invades bronchial mucous glands and goblet cells and then spreads to the alveoli, which fill with blood and fluid. In advanced infection, a hyaline membrane may form.
Fungal infections	
Histoplasmosis	Fungal infection caused by *Histoplasma capsulatum*, a dimorphic fungus • Transmitted through inhalation of *H. capsulatum* spores or invasion of spores after minor skin trauma. • Initially, infected person may be asymptomatic or have symptoms of mild respiratory illness, progressing into more severe illness affecting several organ systems.

(Continued)

DISORDER	CHARACTERISTICS
Protozoal infections	
Toxoplasmosis	Infection caused by the intracellular parasite *Toxoplasma gondii*, which affects both birds and mammals
	• Transmitted to humans by ingestion of tissue cysts in raw or undercooked meat or by fecal oral contamination from infected cats. Direct transmission can also occur during blood transfusions, organ transplants, or bone marrow transplants.
	• When tissue cysts are ingested, parasites are released, which quickly invade and multiply within the GI tract. The parasitic cells rupture the invaded host cell and then disseminate to the CNS, lymphatic tissue, skeletal muscle, myocardium, retina, and placenta.
	• As the parasites replicate and invade adjoining cells, cell death and focal necrosis occur, surrounded by an acute inflammatory response, which are the hallmarks of this infection.
	• After the cysts reach maturity, the inflammatory process is undetectable and the cysts remain latent within the brain until they rupture.
	• In the normal host, the immune response checks the infection, but this isn't so with immunocompromised or fetal hosts. In these patients, focal destruction results in necrotizing encephalitis, pneumonia, myocarditis, and organ failure.
Trichinosis	Infection caused by the parasite *Trichinella spiralis* and transmitted through ingestion of uncooked or undercooked meat that contains encysted larvae
	• After gastric juices free the larva from the cyst capsule, it reaches sexual maturity in a few days. The female roundworm burrows into the intestinal mucosa and reproduces.
	• Larvae then travel through the lymphatic system and the bloodstream. They become embedded as cysts in striated muscle, especially in the diaphragm, chest, arms, and legs.

GENETICS

Genetics is the study of genes, genetic variation, and heredity in organisms including for human beings. Each individual contains genes that provide instructions regarding physical, biochemical, and functional inherited traits. The Human Genome Project estimates each individual has 20,000 to 25,000 genes, which instruct protein makeup in the human body. Genes are made up of deoxyribonucleic acid (DNA), which transmits sequencing instructions that encode for protein structures. Most of an individual's genetic makeup includes similar genes while a small portion of genes, less than 1%, are somewhat different. These differences are determined by alleles, which provide small differences in DNA sequences that determine characteristics as normally inherited while mutations or abnormalities can occur within the individual as genetic-related disorders or conditions.

GENETIC COMPONENTS

Genes are the instructions for building proteins for the human body. Genetic information carried in genes includes hereditary material as codes formed together in DNA as four bases, adenine (A), thymine (T), cytosine (C), and guanine (G) represented as base pairs in a double helix. Each pair is bound together as A with T and C and G to form a base pair as ladder rungs in the DNA molecule, along with a sugar and phosphate molecule that shape the backbone called a nucleotide. A nucleotide pair is represented as two strands to form a double helix in the DNA. A portion of the nucleotides within a gene instructs the coding of the protein while the gene itself provides other sequencing instructions about the protein makeup itself. DNA is located within the cell nucleus (nuclear DNA) including a small amount in the mitochondria (mitochondrial DNA).

The base pairs of the DNA instruct the function of each individual with over 3 billion bases found in the human body, of which 99% are similar. DNA is responsible for replication and duplication of these base codes to make copies of translated instructions that form an exact copy for the new cells. The human-coding gene can range between 500 letters and over 2.3 million while the average gene is 3,000 letters long. The human genome contains approximately 21,000 protein coding genes, which make up less than 2% of the nucleotides that also code for RNA molecules. The average individual has one to three base pair differences (include over 1.4 million differences) based on shape, function, and sequencing protein differences that make each person unique.

Chromosomes are threadlike structures contained within the nucleus of the DNA molecule. Histones are proteins made up of tightly coiled DNA that support the structure of the chromosome. The chromosome can be described by its constriction point known as the centromere. Each arm of the chromosome is called a chromatid, with the short arm called the "p arm" and long arm

called the "q arm." Telomeres are sections of DNA found at the end of each chromosome that provide distinct structures containing the same sequence of bases repeated over and over again, which play a role in organization, protection, and replication of the chromosome. Chromosomes are only visible under the microscope during cell division where visualization of the location of the centromere describes the location of specific genes. An illustration of the chromosome structure is provided below.

CHROMOSOME STRUCTURE

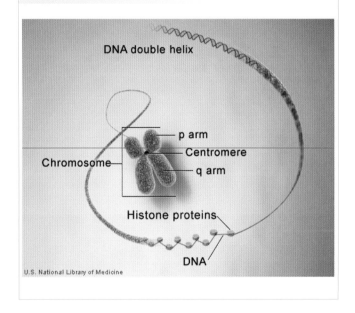

Each individual inherits one copy of his or her gene from each of the two parents. Every normal human cell (except reproductive cells) has 46 chromosomes, 22 paired chromosomes called *autosomes* that look the same in males and females and the 23rd chromosome, known as the sex chromosome, a pair of XX in the female and an X and a Y in the male. A person's individual set of 23 pairs of chromosomes is organized as a profile in what is known as a *karyotype*.

Chromosomes are arranged in the karyotype based on their size, with chromosome 1 as the largest spanning 249 million base pairs with chromosome 21 as the smallest spanning approximately 48 million base pairs (DNA building blocks). The location of a gene within a chromosome is identified using a diagram called an ideogram. Staining is performed to determine size, location, and banding patterns as done in the karyotype to look for abnormalities in the chromosome such as for Down's syndrome in chromosome 21. Staining is also used for the ideogram to describe each gene on the chromosome as seen in below illustration.

KARYOTYPE

Karyotype

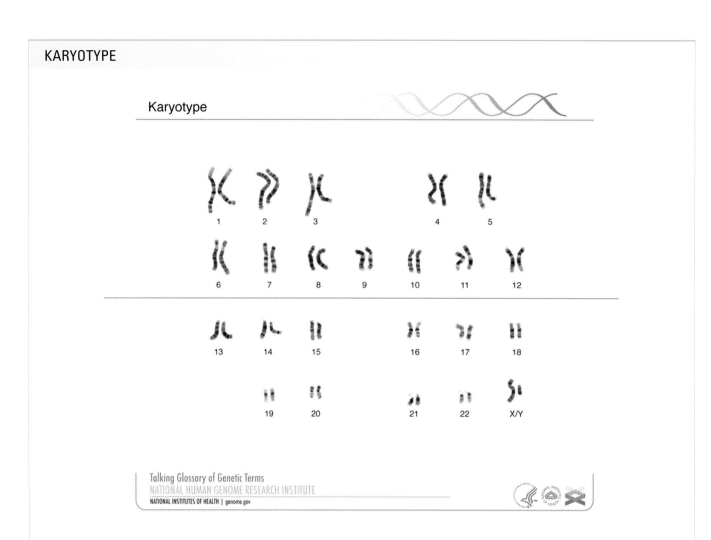

IDEOGRAM OF CHROMOSOME: SOURCE: https://www.ncbi.nlm.nih.gov/genome/tools/gdp

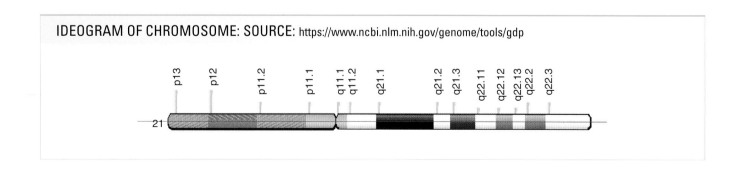

CHROMOSOME FORMATION

Chromosomal formation occurs through the processes of mitosis and meiosis as the two types of cell division. Chromosome formation occurs during mitosis and meiosis during cellular replication and division for autosomal and sex chromosomes.

Mitosis

Chromosomes divide and replicate through the process of mitosis. The cellular process of mitosis replicates chromosomes and prepares two identical nuclei as the fertilized ovum, known as the *zygote*, undergoes a kind of cell division. During this process, the double helix of DNA separates into two chains; each chain serves as a template for constructing a new chain. Individual DNA nucleotides are linked into new strands with bases complementary to those in the originals. In this way, two identical double helices are formed, each containing one of the original strands and a newly formed complementary strand. These double helices are duplicates of the original DNA chain.

Mitotic cell division occurs in five phases: *interphase, prophase, metaphase, anaphase,* and *telophase.* At interphase, one diploid cell of 46 chromosomes (2n) begins DNA replication of chromosomes as two sister chromatids attached at the centromere of the chromosome. At prophase, the nuclear membrane and nucleolus begin to break down as DNA condenses to form chromosomes while the mitotic proteins called microtubules form and attach to the kinetochores of each chromosome. In metaphase, DNA condenses the chromosomes that align at the center of the cell through the action of the microtubules fibers with DNA. At anaphase, the microtubules fibers shorten, pulling the chromatids of each chromosome to opposite poles of the cell while unattached fibers further elongate the cell. During telophase, the chromatids (called chromosomes) reach the poles of the cell as nuclear membranes reform as nucleoli,

as chromosomes relax and DNA unwinds. Cytokinesis then occurs as division of the cytoplasm forms two daughter cells with 46 (2n) chromosomes in each of these cells genetically identical to the original and to each other.

Meiosis

Meiosis is the process of formation of the egg cell found in the ovary for the female and for the sperm cell found in the testis for the male. As germ cells, these cells are diploid (2n) having two sets of chromosomes that will undergo meiosis to become a haploid cell (1n) or one set of chromosomes. During fertilization, haploid cells fuse to form a diploid offspring (female or male). Meiosis involves two divisions, as Meiosis I and Meiosis II, which result in four haploid cells (1n). In Meiosis I, beginning at Prophase I, identical sister chromatids are joined at their centromeres including two homologous chromosomes lined up next to each other that undergo crossing-over at the site of the centromere to exchange DNA. After crossing over, the sister chromatids of one chromosome are no longer identical to one another. In Metaphase I, homologous chromosomes line up randomly along the equator of the cell, known as the process of independent assortment where gametes have different combinations of parental chromosomes with spindle fibers that attach to each centromere. In Anaphase I, chromosomes move apart from one another along the spindle fibers to the opposite end of the cell, with each chromosome double-stranded with two sister chromatids while separating each homologous pair as haploid for the formation of two different new cells. In Telophase I, cytokinesis occurs with cell division to form two cells created with half the number of chromosomes of the original cell. Meiosis II starts similar to division in mitosis at Prophase II where two cells with two sets of chromosomes each include spindle fibers with formation at the poles of the cell. In Metaphase II, the chromosomes line up along the equator, as each cell has only one of each homologous chromosome. Then in Anaphase II, sister chromatids move away from each other. Cytokinesis occurs in Telophase II forming four genetically different (1n) haploid cells.

GENETIC VARIATIONS

Numerical Abnormalities from Nondisjunction

Nondisjunction occurs with chromosomes that fail to disjoin during mitosis or meiosis. There are three forms of nondisjunction that include failure of sister chromatids separating during mitosis, failure of a pair of homologous chromosomes to separate in Meiosis I, and failure of sister chromatids to separate in Anaphase II in Meiosis II. Monosomy refers to a nondisjunction in which an individual is missing one of a pair of chromosomes, as 2n − 1. An example of monosomy is Turner's syndrome where the female has only one X chromosome. Trisomy refers to a nondisjunction in which an individual has an extra chromosome, as 2n + 1. Down's syndrome, or trisomy 21, refers to an individual with 3 chromosomes found at chromosome 21 instead of having one pair of chromosomes.

Structural Abnormalities

Alteration of the structure of the chromosome can occur through a deletion, duplication, translocation (to another chromosome), inversion, or ring formation in the

MITOSIS

Interphase

1 Diploid cell
46 Chromosomes
(2n)

Chromosomes

Chromatin

DNA replication

4n

Prophase → Metaphase → Anaphase → Telophase

2n   2n

2 Diploid Cells
46 Chromosomes

2n   2n

Interphase

MITOSIS AND MEIOSIS COMPARED

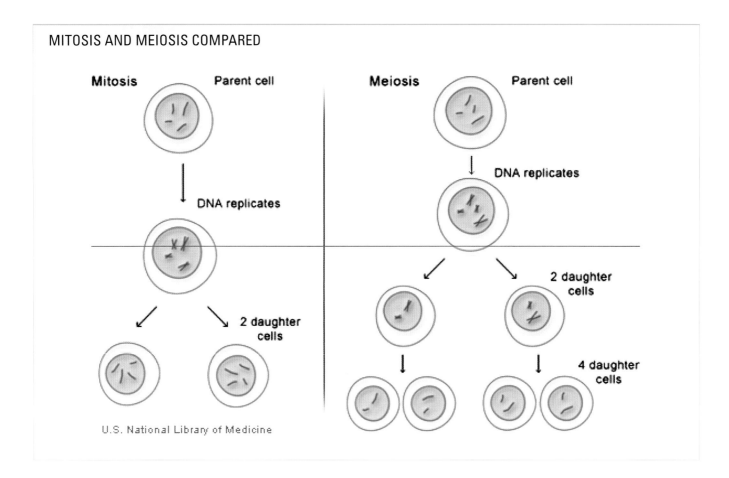

U.S. National Library of Medicine

chromosome. A de novo abnormality is a noninherited chromosomal condition, while maternal age and environment can also be factors for chromosomal abnormalities. Mosaicism is another abnormality referred to as an abnormal cell division in two or more cells creating different numbers of chromosomes.

Genetic Alterations

Genetic alterations related to cancer include aneuploidy, which refers to an abnormal chromosome number due to malignancy. Amplification occurs when overexpression of a gene results from an increase number of genes found in certain cancers. The four active stages in the cell cycle (G1, S, G2, and M) can also be altered when loss of checkpoints in one or more of these stages can also lead to genetic instability and cell damage.

DNA SEQUENCING

As mentioned previously, each of the two strands of DNA in a chromosome consists of thousands of combinations of four nucleotides: adenine (A), thymine (T), cytosine (C), and guanine (G), arranged in complementary triplet pairs (called *codons*), each of which represents an amino acid; a specific sequence of triplets represents a gene. The strands are held together loosely by chemical bonds between adenine and thymine or between cytosine and guanine. The looseness of the bonds allows the strands to separate easily during DNA

replication. The genes carry a code for each trait a person inherits, from blood type to eye color to body shape and a myriad of other traits.

DNA ultimately controls the formation of essential substances throughout the life of every cell in the body. It does this through the genetic code, the precise sequence of AT and CG pairs on the DNA molecule. Genes control not only hereditary traits, transmitted from parents to offspring, but also cell reproduction and the daily functions of all cells. Genes control cell function by controlling the structures and chemicals that are synthesized within the cell.

A multistep process occurs to encode genetic information. The first step involves transcription of DNA sequencing where proteins attach to the DNA strand to make copies of the DNA sequencing in the form of messenger RNA. The next step includes messenger RNA or mRNA, by a sequence of bases, transferring encoded genetic information across the cell nucleus to the outside of the cell. The genetic information is then used through the work of ribosomes to translate and synthesize proteins.

PATTERNS OF INHERITANCE

Autosomal disorders, sex-linked disorders, and multifactorial disorders result from changes to genes or chromosomes. Some defects arise spontaneously, whereas others may be caused by environmental agents, including mutagens, teratogens, and carcinogens.

Trait Predominance

Each parent contributes one set of chromosomes (and therefore one set of genes) so that every offspring has two genes for every locus on the autosomes. Some characteristics, or traits, such as eye color, are determined by one gene that may have many variants (alleles). Others, called *polygenic* traits, require the interaction of two or more genes. In addition, environmental factors may affect how genes are expressed.

Variations in a particular gene — such as brown, blue, or green eye color — are called *alleles*. A person who has identical genes on each member of the chromosome pair is *homozygous* for that gene; if the alleles are different, the person is said to be *heterozygous*.

Autosomal Inheritance

On autosomes, one allele may be more influential than another in determining a specific trait. The more powerful, or *dominant*, gene product is more likely to be exhibited in the offspring than the less influential, or *recessive*, gene product. Offspring will exhibit a dominant allele when one or both chromosomes in a pair carry it. A recessive allele will not be exhibited unless both chromosomes carry identical copies of the allele. For example, a child may receive a gene for brown eyes from one parent and a gene for blue eyes from the other parent. The gene for brown eyes is dominant, and the gene for blue eyes is recessive. Because the dominant allele is more likely to mask the recessive allele, the child is more likely to have brown eyes.

Sex-linked Inheritance

The X and Y chromosomes are not literally a pair because the X chromosome is much larger than the Y, with more genetic material. The male has only one copy of the gene on the X chromosome. Inheritance of those genes is called *X-linked*. A man will transmit one copy of each X-linked gene to his daughters and none to his sons. A woman will transmit one copy to each child, whether male or female.

Inheritance of genes on the X chromosome is different in another way. Females have two X chromosomes in each of their cells; however, only one X chromosome is active in each cell because of a process called *X inactivation*. X inactivation occurs during early embryogenesis in the female, and the X that is inactivated in each cell is random. In some cells, the X the female received from her mother is inactivated, while in other cells the X received from the father is inactivated. For this reason, at the cellular level, a heterozygous female will express the recessive gene in some cells and the dominant gene in others.

Multifactorial Inheritance

Multifactorial inheritance is inheritance that is determined by multiple factors, including genetic and possible non genetic (environmental), each with only a partial effect. The genetic factor may consist of variations for multiple genes: some that provide susceptibility and some that provide protection. Examples of environmental factors that may contribute to such a trait are nutrition, exposure to teratogens or carcinogens, viral infections, exposure to oxidants, and intake of antioxidants.

PATHOPHYSIOLOGIC CONCEPTS

Epigenetics

Epigenetics is the study of chemical alterations that activate or deactivate parts of the genome including environmental and lifestyle factors. The epigenome includes epigenetic chemical tags that "mark" the DNA and which shape the physical structure of the genome by instructing when, where, and what genes are expressed while relaxes genes to make them accessible. The epigenome can be influenced by natural sources (diet), environment teratogens (chemical toxins), and stress-related factors. These factors may modify information to be transcribed and translated in the genome thus influencing gene regulation while the process is still not fully understood.

Epigenetic factors appear to affect DNA methylation (biochemical methyl structure) and histone modification (formation of chromosome) processes that pack and wind DNA into chromosomes. Another factor involves RNA interference (RNA1) in special molecules of RNA that bind to messenger RNA, which may affect translation of DNA sequencing information.

Environmental Teratogens

Teratogens are environmental agents (infectious toxins, maternal systemic diseases, drugs, chemicals, and physical agents) that can harm the developing fetus by causing congenital, structural or functional defects. Teratogens may also cause spontaneous abortion, complications during labor and delivery, hidden defects in later development (such as cognitive or behavioral problems), or neoplastic transformations.

Environmental Mutagens and Carcinogens

A permanent change in genetic material is a *mutation*, which may occur spontaneously or after exposure of a cell to a mutagen, such as radiation, certain chemicals, or viruses. Mutations can occur at any location in the genome. Carcinogens are environmental agents, such as cigarette smoke or tobacco, indoor and outdoor air pollution, and preservatives in certain foods that may cause cancer.

Every cell has built-in defences against genetic damage. However, if a mutation is not identified or repaired, the mutation may produce a trait different from the original trait and may be transmitted to offspring. Mutations may have no effect; some may change expression of a trait, and others may change the way a cell functions. Many mutagens are also carcinogens because they alter cell function. Some mutations cause serious or fatal defects, such as congenital anomalies or cancer.

Autosomal Disorders

In single-gene disorders, an error occurs at a single gene site on the DNA strand. A mistake may occur in the copying and transcribing of a single codon through additions, deletions, or excessive repetitions.

Single-gene disorders are inherited in clearly identifiable patterns that are the same as those seen in inheritance of normal traits. Because every person has 22 pairs of autosomes and only one pair of sex chromosomes, most hereditary disorders are caused by autosomal defects.

Autosomal dominant transmission usually affects male and female offspring equally. Children of an affected parent have a 50% chance of being affected (see Figure). Autosomal recessive inheritance also usually affects male and female offspring equally. If both parents are affected, 100% of their offspring will be affected (see Figure). If both parents are unaffected but are heterozygous for the trait (carriers of the defective gene), a 25% chance exists that the child will be affected with each pregnancy. If only one parent is affected and the other parent is a noncarrier, the offspring are not affected but 100% are carriers for the defective gene. If one parent is affected and the other parent is a carrier, 50% of their children will be affected. Autosomal recessive disorders may occur when no family history of the disease exists.

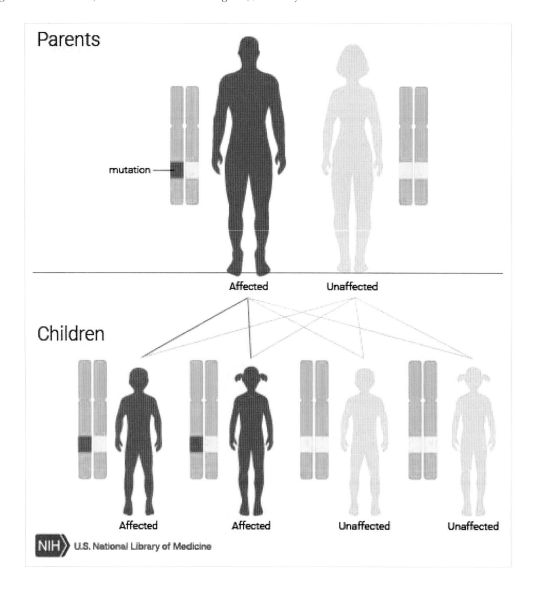

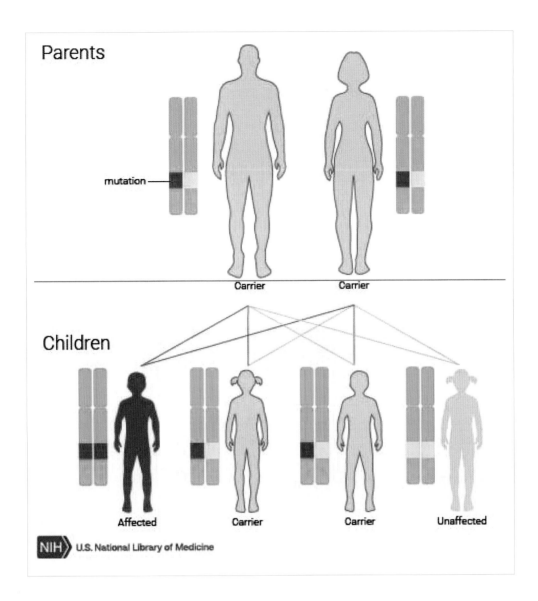

Parents

mutation —

Carrier   Carrier

Children

Affected   Carrier   Carrier   Unaffected

NIH⟩ U.S. National Library of Medicine

Sex-Linked Disorders

Genetic disorders caused by genes located on the sex chromosomes are termed *sex-linked disorders*. Most sex-linked disorders are controlled by genes located on the X chromosome, usually as recessive traits. Because males have only one X chromosome, a single X-linked recessive gene can cause disease to be exhibited in a male. Females receive two X chromosomes and thus can be homozygous for a disease allele, homozygous for a normal allele, or heterozygous.

Most people who express X-linked *recessive* traits are males with unaffected parents. In rare cases, the father is affected and the mother is a carrier. An affected father and an unaffected noncarrier mother will have daughters as 100% carriers and sons as 100% unaffected and noncarriers. An unaffected father and a mother who is a carrier will have a 50% chance of having an affected son and a 50% chance of having a daughter as a carrier of the trait. Fathers cannot pass X-linked traits to their sons. A pedigree figure of an X-linked recessive inheritance is illustrated below.

Characteristics of X-linked *dominant* inheritance include evidence of the inherited trait in the family history. A person with the abnormal trait must have one affected parent. If the father has an X-linked dominant disorder, 100% of his daughters will be affected while 100% of his sons will be unaffected. If a mother has an X-linked dominant disorder, each of her children has a 50% chance of being affected. A pedigree figure of an X-linked dominant inheritance is illustrated below.

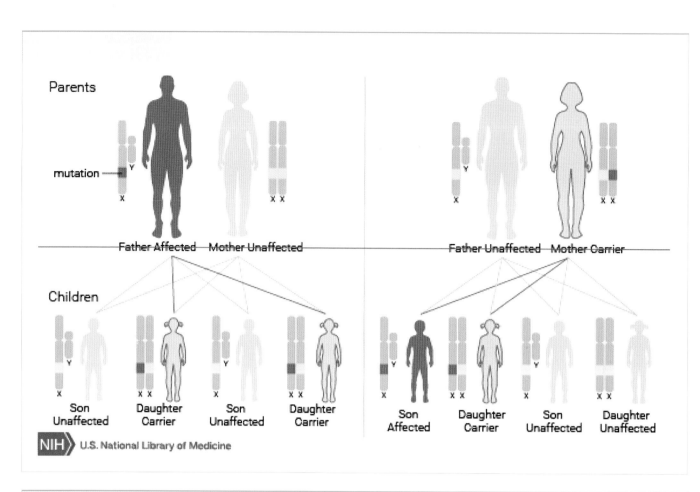

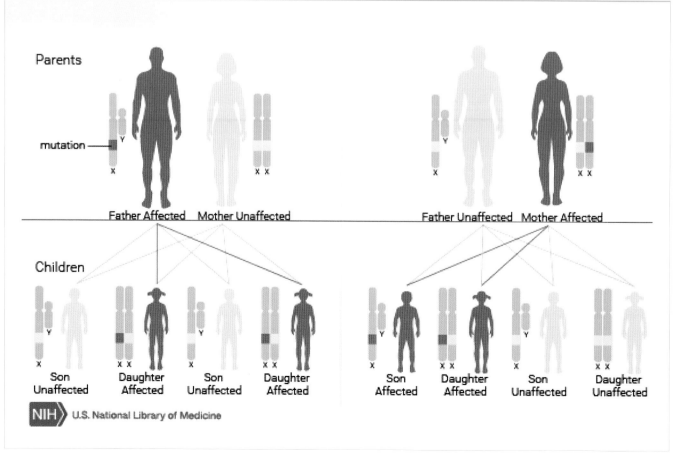

Multifactorial Disorders

Most multifactorial disorders result from the effects of several different genes and an environmental component. In *polygenic inheritance*, each gene has a small additive effect, and the effect of a combination of genetic errors in a person is unpredictable. Multifactorial disorders can result from a less-than-optimum expression of many different genes, not from a specific error.

Some multifactorial disorders are apparent at birth, such as cleft lip, cleft palate, congenital heart disease, anencephaly, clubfoot, and myelomeningocele. Others such disorders do not become apparent until later, such as type 2 diabetes mellitus, hypertension, hyperlipidemia, most autoimmune diseases, and many cancers. Multifactorial disorders that develop during adulthood are commonly believed to be strongly related to environmental factors, not only in incidence but also in the degree of expression.

GENETIC DISORDERS

Genetic disorders are commonly classified by pattern of inheritance, as shown in the accompanying chart. (See *Common genetic disorders.*) The Human Genome Project completed in 2003 has now mapped out the genes of the human individual while personalized and precision medicine is moving forward to better understand and study single and multifactorial causes of genetic disorders with the hope for future preventative and individualized therapies. The study of genomics, which includes all of the person's genes along with interactions with the environment, will be very important for future work in the genomic medicine era. Pharmacogenomics, the study of how genes affect an individual's response to drugs, is a rapidly growing field that continues to utilize these discoveries in genetic alterations to target ongoing drug therapies to also treat genetic disorders in individuals.

Common Genetic Disorders

DISORDER	PATHOPHYSIOLOGY	SIGNS AND SYMPTOMS
Autosomal recessive disorders		
Cystic fibrosis Inborn error in a cell-membrane transport protein. Dysfunction of the exocrine glands affects multiple organ systems. The disease affects males and females. It's the most common fatal genetic disease in white children.	Most cases arise from the mutation that affects the genetic coding for a single amino acid, resulting in a protein (cystic fibrosis transmembrane regulator [CFTR]) that doesn't function properly. This mutant CFTR resembles other transmembrane transport proteins, but it lacks the phenylalanine at position 508 in the protein produced by normal genes. This regulator interferes with cyclic adenosine monophosphate (cAMP)–regulated chloride channels and transport of other ions by preventing adenosine triphosphate from binding to the protein or by interfering with activation by protein kinase. The mutation affects volume-absorbing epithelia in the airways and intestines, salt-absorbing epithelia in sweat ducts, and volume-secretory epithelia in the pancreas. Mutations in CFTR lead to dehydration, which increases the viscosity of mucous gland secretions and consequently obstructs glandular ducts. Cystic fibrosis has varying effects on electrolyte and water transport.	• Chronic airway infections leading to bronchiectasis • Bronchiolectasis • Exocrine pancreatic insufficiency • Intestinal dysfunction • Abnormal sweat-gland function • Reproductive dysfunction
Phenylketonuria (PKU) Inborn error in metabolism of the amino acid phenylalanine. PKU has a low incidence among Blacks and Ashkenazic Jews and a high incidence among people of Irish and Scottish descent.	Patients with classic PKU have almost no activity of phenylalanine hydroxylase, an enzyme that helps convert phenylalanine to tyrosine. As a result, phenylalanine accumulates in the blood and urine, and tyrosine levels are low.	Treatment includes early diagnosis and avoidance of phenylalanine in the diet; however, if left untreated, these signs and symptoms can occur: • By age 4 months, signs of arrested brain development, including mental retardation • Personality disturbances • Seizures • Decreased IQ • Macrocephaly • Eczematous skin lesions or dry, rough skin • Hyperactivity • Irritability • Purposeless, repetitive motions • Awkward gait • Musty odor from skin and urine excretion of phenylacetic acid

(Continued)

DISORDER	PATHOPHYSIOLOGY	SIGNS AND SYMPTOMS
Sickle cell anemia Congenital hemolytic anemia resulting from defective hemoglobin molecules. In the United States, sickle cell anemia occurs primarily in persons of African and Mediterranean descent. It also affects populations in Puerto Rico, Turkey, India, and the Middle East.	Abnormal hemoglobin S in red blood cells becomes insoluble during hypoxia. As a result, these cells become rigid, rough, and elongated, forming a crescent or sickle shape. The sickling produces hemolysis. The altered cells also pile up in the capillaries and smaller blood vessels, making the blood more viscous. Normal circulation is impaired, causing pain, tissue infarctions, and swelling. Each patient with sickle cell anemia has a different hypoxic threshold and different factors that trigger a sickle cell crisis. Illness, exposure to cold, stress, acidotic states, or a pathophysiologic process that pulls water out of the sickle cells precipitates a crisis in most patients. The blockages then cause anoxic changes that lead to further sickling and obstruction.	• Symptoms of sickle cell anemia don't develop until after age 6 months because fetal hemoglobin protects infants for the first few months after birth • Chronic fatigue • Unexplained dyspnea on exertion • Joint swelling • Aching bones • Severe localized and generalized pain • Leg ulcers • Frequent infections • Priapism in males *In sickle cell crisis:* • Severe pain • Hematuria • Lethargy
Tay-Sachs disease Also known as *GM₂ gangliosidosis*, the most common lipid-storage disease. Tay-Sachs affects Ashkenazic Jews about 100 times more often than it does the general population.	The enzyme hexosaminidase A is absent or deficient. This enzyme is necessary to metabolize gangliosides, water-soluble glycolipids found primarily in the central nervous system (CNS). Without hexosaminidase A, lipid molecules accumulate, progressively destroying and demyelinating CNS cells.	• Exaggerated Moro's (startle) reflex at birth and apathy (response only to loud sounds) by age 3–6 mo • Inability to sit up, lift head, or grasp objects; difficulty turning over; progressive vision loss • Deafness, blindness, seizures, paralysis, spasticity, and continued neurologic deterioration (by age 18 mo) • Recurrent bronchopneumonia
Autosomal dominant disorders		
Marfan's syndrome Rare degenerative, generalized disease of the connective tissue that results from elastin and collagen defects. The syndrome occurs in 1 of 20,000 individuals, affecting males and females equally. Approximately 25% of cases represent new mutations.	Marfan's syndrome is caused by mutation in a single gene on chromosome 15, the gene that codes for fibrillin, a glycoprotein component of connective tissue. These small fibers are abundant in large blood vessels and the suspensory ligaments of the ocular lenses. The effect on connective tissue is variable and includes excessive bone growth, ocular disorders, and cardiac defects.	• Increased height, long extremities, and arachnodactyly (long, spiderlike fingers) • Defects of sternum (funnel chest or pigeon breast, for example), chest asymmetry, scoliosis, or kyphosis • Hypermobile joints • Myopia • Lens displacement • Valvular abnormalities (redundancy of leaflets, stretching of chordae tendineae, or dilation of valvulae anales) • Mitral valve prolapse • Aortic regurgitation

DISORDER	PATHOPHYSIOLOGY	SIGNS AND SYMPTOMS

X-linked recessive disorders

Fragile X syndrome

The most common inherited cause of mental retardation. Approximately 85% of males and 50% of females who inherit the fragile X mental retardation 1 (FMR1) mutation will demonstrate clinical features of the syndrome. It's estimated to occur in about 1 in 1,500 males and 1 in 2,500 females. It has been reported in almost all races and ethnic populations.

Fragile X syndrome is an X-linked condition that doesn't follow a simple X-linked inheritance pattern. The unique mutation that results consists of an expanding region of a specific triplet of nitrogenous bases: cytosine, guanine, and guanine (CGG) within the gene's DNA sequence. Normally, FMR1 contains 6–49 sequential copies of the CGG triplet. When the number of CGG triplets expands to the range of 50–200 and repeats, the region of DNA becomes unstable and is referred to as a premutation. A full mutation consists of more than 200 CGG triplet repeats. The full mutation typically causes abnormal methylation (methyl groups attach to components of the gene) of FMR1. Methylation inhibits gene transcription and, thus, protein production. The reduced or absent protein product is responsible for the clinical features of fragile X syndrome.

Postpubescent males with fragile X syndrome commonly have distinct physical features, behavioral difficulties, and cognitive impairment. Other signs and symptoms include:
- Prominent jaw and forehead and a head circumference exceeding the 90th percentile
- Long, narrow face with long or large ears that may be posteriorly rotated
- Connective tissue abnormalities, including hyperextension of the fingers, a floppy mitral valve (in 80% of adults), and mild to severe pectus excavatum
- Unusually large testes
- Average IQ of 30–70
- Hyperactivity, speech difficulties, language delay, and autisticlike behaviors

Females with fragile X syndrome tend to have more subtle symptoms, including:
- Learning disabilities
- IQ scores in the mental retardation range
- Excessive shyness or social anxiety
- Prominent ears and connective tissue manifestations

Hemophilia

Bleeding disorder; severity and prognosis vary with the degree of deficiency, or nonfunction, and the site of bleeding. Hemophilia occurs in 20 of 100,000 male births. Hemophilia A, or classic hemophilia, is a deficiency of clotting factor VIII; it's more common than is type B, affecting more than 80% of all hemophiliacs. Hemophilia B, or Christmas disease, affects 15% of all hemophiliacs and results from a deficiency of factor IX. There's no relationship between factor VIII and factor IX inherited defects.

Abnormal bleeding occurs because of specific clotting factor malfunction. Factors VIII and IX are components of the intrinsic clotting pathway; factor IX is an essential factor, and factor VIII is a critical cofactor. Factor VIII accelerates the activation of factor X by several thousand times. Excessive bleeding occurs when these clotting factors are reduced by more than 75%.

Hemophilia may be severe, moderate, or mild, depending on the degree of activation of clotting factors. A person with hemophilia forms a platelet plug at a bleeding site, but clotting factor deficiency impairs the ability to form a stable fibrin clot. Delayed bleeding is more common than is immediate hemorrhage.

- Spontaneous bleeding in severe hemophilia
- Excessive or continued bleeding or bruising
- Large subcutaneous and deep intramuscular hematomas
- Prolonged bleeding in mild hemophilia after major trauma or surgery, but no spontaneous bleeding after minor trauma
- Pain, swelling, and tenderness in joints
- Internal bleeding, commonly manifested as abdominal, chest, or flank pain
- Hematuria
- Hematemesis or tarry stools

Polygenic (multifactorial) disorders

Cleft lip and cleft palate

May occur separately or together. Cleft lip with or without cleft palate occurs twice as often in males as in females. Cleft palate without cleft lip is more common in females. Cleft lip deformities can occur unilaterally, bilaterally or, rarely, in the midline. Only the lip may be involved, or the defect may extend into the upper jaw or nasal cavity. Incidence is highest in children with a family history of cleft defects.

During the 2nd month of pregnancy, the front and sides of the face and the palatine shelves develop. Because of a chromosomal abnormality, exposure to teratogens, genetic abnormality, or environmental factors, the lip or palate fuses imperfectly. The deformity may range from a simple notch to a complete cleft.

A cleft palate may be partial or complete. A complete cleft includes the soft palate, the bones of the maxilla, and the alveolus on one or both sides of the premaxilla.

A double cleft is the most severe of the deformities. The cleft runs from the soft palate forward to either side of the nose. A double cleft separates the maxilla and premaxilla into freely moving segments. The tongue and other muscles can displace the segments, enlarging the cleft.

- Obvious cleft lip or cleft palate
- Feeding difficulties due to incomplete fusion of the palate

(Continued)

DISORDER	PATHOPHYSIOLOGY	SIGNS AND SYMPTOMS
Neural tube defects Serious birth defects that involve the spine or skull; they result from failure of the neural tube to close at ~28 d after conception. The most common forms of neural tube defects are spina bifida (50% of cases), anencephaly (40% of cases), and encephalocele (10% of cases). Spina bifida occulta is the most common and least severe spinal cord defect. The incidence of neural tube defects varies greatly among countries and by region in the United States. For example, the incidence is significantly higher in the British Isles and low southern China and Japan. In the United States, North and South Carolina have at least twice the incidence of neural tube defects as most other parts of the country. These birth defects are also less common in blacks than in whites.	Neural tube closure normally occurs at 24 d gestation in the cranial region and continues distally, with closure of the lumbar regions by 28 d. Spina bifida occulta is characterized by incomplete closure of one or more vertebrae without protrusion of the spinal cord or meninges. However, in more severe forms of spina bifida, incomplete closure of one or more vertebrae causes protrusion of the spinal contents in an external sac or cystic lesion (spina bifida cystica). Spina bifida cystica has two classifications: myelomeningocele (meningomyelocele) and meningocele. In myelomeningocele, the external sac contains meninges, cerebrospinal fluid (CSF), and a portion of the spinal cord or nerve roots distal to the conus medullaris. When the spinal nerve roots end at the sac, motor and sensory functions below the sac are terminated. In meningocele, less severe than myelomeningocele, the sac contains only meninges and CSF. Meningocele may produce no neurologic symptoms. In encephalocele, a saclike portion of the meninges and brain protrudes through a defective opening in the skull. Usually, it occurs in the occipital area, but it may also occur in the parietal, nasopharyngeal, or frontal area. In anencephaly, the most severe form of neural tube defect, the closure defect occurs at the cranial end of the neuroaxis and, as a result, part or the entire top of the skull is missing, severely damaging the brain. Portions of the brain stem and spinal cord may also be missing. No diagnostic or therapeutic efforts are helpful; this condition is invariably fatal.	Signs and symptoms depend on the type and severity of the neural tube defect: ● Possibly, a depression or dimple, tuft of hair, soft fatty deposits, port-wine nevi, or a combination of these abnormalities on the skin over the spinal defect (spina bifida occulta) ● Foot weakness or bowel and bladder disturbances, especially likely during rapid growth phases (spina bifida occulta) ● Saclike structure that protrudes over the spine (myelomeningocele, meningocele) ● Depending on the level of the defect, permanent neurologic dysfunction, such as flaccid or spastic paralysis and bowel and bladder incontinence (myelomeningocele)

Disorders of chromosome number

Down's syndrome (trisomy 21) Spontaneous chromosome abnormality that causes characteristic facial features, other distinctive physical abnormalities (cardiac defects in 60% of affected persons), and mental retardation. It occurs in 1 of 650–700 live births.	Nearly all cases of Down's syndrome result from trisomy 21 (three copies of chromosome 21). The result is a karyotype of 47 chromosomes instead of the usual 46. In 4% of patients, Down's syndrome results from an unbalanced translocation or chromosomal rearrangement in which the long arm of chromosome 21 breaks and attaches to another chromosome. Some affected persons and some asymptomatic parents may have chromosomal mosaicism, a mixture of two cell types, some with the normal 46 and some with an extra chromosome 21.	● Distinctive facial features (low nasal bridge, epicanthic folds, protruding tongue, and low-set ears); small open mouth and disproportionately large tongue ● Single transverse crease on the palm (simian crease) ● Small white spots on the iris (Brushfield's spots) ● Mental retardation (estimated IQ of 20–50) ● Developmental delay ● Congenital heart disease, mainly septal defects and especially of the endocardial cushion ● Impaired reflexes

DISORDER	PATHOPHYSIOLOGY	SIGNS AND SYMPTOMS
Trisomy 18 syndrome Also known as *Edwards' syndrome*, it's the second most common multiple malformation syndrome. Most affected infants have full trisomy 18, involving an extra (third) copy of chromosome 18 in each cell, but partial trisomy 18 (with varying phenotypes) and translocation types have also been reported. Full trisomy 18 syndrome is generally fatal or has an extremely poor prognosis. Most trisomic conceptions are spontaneously aborted; 30%–50% of infants die within the first 2 mo of life, and 90% die within the first year. Most surviving patients are profoundly mentally retarded. Incidence ranges from 1 in 3,000–8,000 neonates, with 3–4 females affected for every 1 male.	Most cases result from spontaneous nondisjunction meiotic, leading to an extra copy of chromosome 18 in each cell.	• Growth retardation, which begins in utero and remains significant after birth • Initial hypotonia that may soon cause hypertonia • Microcephaly and dolichocephaly • Micrognathia • Short and narrow nose with upturned nares • Unilateral or bilateral cleft lip and palate • Low-set, slightly pointed ears • Short neck • Conspicuous clenched hand with overlapping fingers (commonly seen on ultrasound in utero as well) • Cystic hygroma • Choroid plexus cysts (also seen in some normal infants)
Trisomy 13 syndrome Also known as *Patau's syndrome*, it's the third most common multiple malformation syndrome. Most affected infants have full trisomy 13 at birth; a few have the rare mosaic partial trisomy 13 syndrome (with varying phenotypes) or translocation types. Full trisomy 13 syndrome is fatal. Many trisomic zygotes are spontaneously aborted; 50%–70% of infants die within 1 month after birth, and 85% by the first year. Only isolated cases of survival beyond 5 years have been reported in full trisomy 13 patients. Incidence is estimated to be 1 in 4,000–10,000 neonates.	Approximately 75% of all cases result from chromosomal nondisjunction. About 20% result from chromosomal translocation, involving a rearrangement of chromosomes 13 and 14. About 5% of cases are estimated to be mosaics; the clinical effects in these cases may be less severe.	• Microcephaly • Varying degrees of holoprosencephaly • Sloping forehead with wide sutures and fontanelle • Scalp defect at the vertex • Bilateral cleft lip with associated cleft palate (in 45% of cases) • Flat and broad nose • Low-set ears and inner ear abnormalities • Polydactyly of the hands and feet • Club feet • Omphaloceles • Neural tube defects • Cystic hygroma • Genital abnormalities • Cystic kidneys • Hydronephrosis • Failure to thrive, seizures, apnea, and feeding difficulties

Suggested References

Genetics Science Learning Center. (2015, January 7). Your guide to understanding genetic conditions. Retrieved from http://learn.genetics.utah.edu/ on January 7, 2017.

McGraw Hill Global Education. (2017). Human anatomy. Retrieved from http://highered.mheducation.com/sites/0072495855/student_view0/chapter28/animation__how_meiosis_works.html

National Institute of Health. (2016). Genetics home reference. Retrieved from http://www.ghr.nlm.nih.gov on January 7, 2017.

U.S. National Library of Medicine. (2016a). Comprehensive one-stop genomic information center. Hosted by the National Biotechnology Information (NCBI). Retrieved on January 7, 2017.

U.S. National Library of Medicine. (2016b). Human genome resources. Retrieved from http:///www.ncbi.nlm.nih.gov/genome/guide/human on January 7, 2017.

FLUIDS AND ELECTROLYTES

The body is mostly liquid — various electrolytes dissolved in water. Electrolytes are ions (electrically charged versions) of essential elements — predominantly sodium (Na^+), chloride (Cl^-), oxygen (O_2), hydrogen (H^+), bicarbonate (HCO_3^-), calcium (Ca^{2+}), potassium (K^+), sulfate (SO_4^{2-}), and phosphate (PO_4^{3-}). Only ionic forms of elements can dissolve or combine with other elements. Electrolyte balance must remain in a narrow range for the body to function. The kidneys maintain chemical balance throughout the body by producing and eliminating urine. They regulate the volume, electrolyte concentration, and acid-base balance of body fluids; detoxify and eliminate wastes; and regulate blood pressure by regulating fluid volume. The skin and lungs also play a vital role in fluid and electrolyte balance. Sweating results in loss of sodium and water, and every breath contains water vapor.

FLUID BALANCE

The kidneys maintain fluid balance in the body by regulating the amount and components of fluid inside and around the cells.

Intracellular Fluid

The fluid inside each cell is called *intracellular fluid*. Each cell has its own mixture of components in the intracellular fluid, but the amounts of these substances are similar in every cell. Intracellular fluid contains large amounts of potassium, magnesium, and phosphate ions.

Extracellular Fluid

The fluid in the spaces outside the cells, called *extracellular fluid*, is constantly moving. Normally, extracellular fluid includes blood plasma and interstitial fluid. In some pathologic states, it accumulates in a so-called *third space*, the space around organs in the chest or abdomen.

Extracellular fluid is rapidly transported through the body by circulating blood and between blood and tissue fluids by fluid and electrolyte exchange across the capillary walls. It contains large amounts of sodium, chloride, and bicarbonate ions, plus such cell nutrients as oxygen, glucose, fatty acids, and amino acids. It also contains carbon dioxide (CO_2), transported from the cells to the lungs for excretion, and other cellular products, transported from the cells to the kidneys for excretion.

The kidneys maintain the volume and composition of extracellular fluid and, to a lesser extent, intracellular fluid by continually exchanging water and ionic solutes, such as hydrogen, sodium, potassium, chloride, bicarbonate, sulfate, and phosphate ions, across the cell membranes of the renal tubules.

Fluid Exchange

Four forces act to equalize concentrations of fluids, electrolytes, and proteins on both sides of the capillary wall by moving fluid between the vessels and the interstitial fluid. Forces that move fluid out of blood vessels are:

- hydrostatic pressure of blood
- osmotic pressure of interstitial fluid.

  Forces that move fluid into blood vessels are:

- oncotic pressure of plasma proteins
- hydrostatic pressure of interstitial fluid.

Hydrostatic pressure is higher at the arteriolar end of the capillary bed than at the venular end. Oncotic pressure of plasma increases slightly at the venular end as fluid is drawn into the blood vessel. When the endothelial barrier (capillary wall) is normal and intact, fluid escapes at the arteriolar end of the capillary bed and is returned at the venular end. The small amount of fluid lost from the capillaries into the interstitial tissue spaces is drained off through the lymphatic system and returned to the bloodstream.

Alterations in Tonicity

ALTERATIONS	PATHOPHYSIOLOGY	CAUSES
Isotonic	• Intracellular fluids and extracellular fluids have equal osmotic pressure, but there's a dramatic change in total body fluid volume. • No cellular swelling or shrinkage exists because osmosis doesn't occur.	• Blood loss from penetrating trauma • Expansion of fluid volume if a patient receives too much normal saline
Hypertonic	• Extracellular fluid is more concentrated than is intracellular fluid. • Water flows out of the cell through the semipermeable cell membrane, causing cell shrinkage.	• Administration of hypertonic (>0.9%) saline • Hypernatremia from severe dehydration • Sodium retention from renal disease
Hypotonic	• Decreased osmotic pressure forces some extracellular fluid into the cells, causing them to swell. • In extreme hypotonicity, cells may swell until they burst and die.	• Overhydration

Normal Electrolyte Values

SODIUM	CALCIUM
135–145 mEq/L	8.5–10.5 mg/dL
POTASSIUM	**MAGNESIUM**
3.5–5 mEq/L	1.8–2.5 mEq/L
CHLORIDE	**PHOSPHATE**
96–106 mEq/L	2.5–4.5 mg/dL

Acid-Base Balance

Regulation of the extracellular fluid environment involves the ratio of acid to base, measured clinically as pH. In physiology, all positively charged ions are acids and all negatively charged ions are bases. To regulate acid-base balance, the kidneys secrete hydrogen ions (acid), reabsorb sodium (acid) and bicarbonate ions (base), acidify phosphate salts, and produce ammonium ions (acid). This keeps the blood at its normal pH of 7.35 to 7.45. Important pH boundaries include:

- <6.8 incompatible with life
- <7.2 cell function seriously impaired
- <7.35 acidosis
- 7.35 to 7.45 normal
- >7.45 alkalosis
- >7.55 cell function seriously impaired
- >7.8 incompatible with life.

PATHOPHYSIOLOGIC CONCEPTS

The regulation of intracellular and extracellular electrolyte concentrations depends on these factors:

- balance between intake of substances containing electrolytes and output of electrolytes in urine, feces, and sweat
- transport of fluid and electrolytes between extracellular and intracellular fluid.

Fluid imbalance occurs when regulatory mechanisms can't compensate for abnormal intake and output at any level from the cell to the organism. Fluid and electrolyte imbalances include edema, isotonic alterations, hypertonic alterations, hypotonic alterations, and electrolyte imbalances. Disorders of fluid volume or osmolarity result. Many conditions also affect capillary exchange, resulting in fluid shifts.

Edema

Despite almost constant interchange through the endothelial barrier, the body maintains a steady state of extracellular water balance between the plasma and interstitial fluid. Increased fluid volume in the interstitial spaces is called *edema*. It's classified as localized or systemic. Obstruction of the veins or lymphatic system or increased vascular permeability usually causes localized edema in the affected area, such as the swelling around an injury. Systemic, or generalized, edema may be due to heart failure or renal disease. Massive systemic edema is called *anasarca*.

Edema results from abnormal expansion of the interstitial fluid or the accumulation of fluid in a third space, such as the

Major Electrolytes

ELECTROLYTE	CHARACTERISTICS
Sodium	• Major extracellular fluid cation • Maintains tonicity of extracellular fluid • Regulates acid-base balance by renal reabsorption of sodium ion (base) and excretion of hydrogen ion (acid) • Facilitates nerve conduction and neuromuscular function • Facilitates glandular secretion • Maintains water balance
Potassium	• Major intracellular fluid cation • Maintains cell electrical neutrality • Facilitates cardiac muscle contraction and electrical conductivity • Facilitates neuromuscular transmission of nerve impulses • Maintains acid-base balance
Chloride	• Mainly an extracellular fluid anion • Accounts for two-thirds of all serum anions • Secreted by the stomach mucosa as hydrochloric acid, providing an acid medium for digestion and enzyme activation • Helps maintain acid-base and water balances • Influences tonicity of extracellular fluid • Facilitates exchange of oxygen and carbon dioxide in red blood cells • Helps activate salivary amylase, which triggers the digestive process
Calcium	• Indispensable to cell permeability, bone and teeth formation, blood coagulation, nerve impulse transmission, and normal muscle contraction • Plays a vital role in cardiac action potential and is essential for cardiac pacemaker automaticity
Magnesium	• Present in small quantities, but physiologically as significant as the other major electrolytes • Enhances neuromuscular communication • Stimulates parathyroid hormone secretion, which regulates intracellular calcium • Activates many enzymes in carbohydrate and protein metabolism • Facilitates cell metabolism • Facilitates sodium, potassium, and calcium transport across cell membranes • Facilitates protein transport
Phosphate	• Involved in cellular metabolism as well as neuromuscular regulation and hematologic function • Phosphate reabsorption in the renal tubules inversely related to calcium levels (an increase in urinary phosphorous triggers calcium reabsorption and vice versa)

Disorders of Fluid Balance: Hypovolemia

CAUSES	PATHOPHYSIOLOGY	SIGNS AND SYMPTOMS	DIAGNOSTIC TEST RESULTS	TREATMENT
Hypovolemia is an isotonic disorder. Fluid volume deficit decreases capillary hydrostatic pressure and fluid transport. Cells are deprived of normal nutrients that serve as substrates for energy production, metabolism, and other cellular functions. Hypovolemia results from these causes: *Fluid loss* • Hemorrhage • Excessive perspiration • Renal failure with polyuria • Surgery • Vomiting or diarrhea • Nasogastric drainage • Diabetes mellitus with polyuria or diabetes insipidus • Fistulas • Excessive use of laxatives; diuretic therapy • Fever *Reduced fluid intake* • Dysphagia • Coma • Environmental conditions preventing fluid intake • Psychiatric illness *Fluid shift from extracellular fluid* • Burns (during the initial phase) • Acute intestinal obstruction • Acute peritonitis • Pancreatitis • Crushing injury • Pleural effusion • Hip fracture	Decreased renal blood flow triggers the renin-angiotensin system to increase sodium and water reabsorption. The cardiovascular system compensates by increasing heart rate, cardiac contractility, venous constriction, and systemic vascular resistance, thus increasing cardiac output and mean arterial pressure (MAP). Hypovolemia also triggers the thirst response, releasing more antidiuretic hormone and producing more aldosterone. When compensation fails, hypovolemic shock occurs in this sequence: • decreased intravascular fluid volume • diminished venous return, which reduces preload and decreases stroke volume • reduced cardiac output • decreased MAP • impaired tissue perfusion • decreased oxygen and nutrient delivery to cells • multiple organ dysfunction syndrome.	• Orthostatic hypotension **(in major blood or fluid loss)** • Tachycardia • Thirst • Flattened jugular veins • Sunken eyeballs • Dry mucous membranes • Diminished skin turgor • Rapid weight loss • Decreased urine output • Prolonged capillary refill time	• Increased blood urea nitrogen • Elevated serum creatinine level • Increased serum protein, hemoglobin, and hematocrit (unless caused by hemorrhage, when loss of blood elements causes subnormal values) • Rising blood glucose • Elevated serum osmolality (except in hyponatremia, where serum osmolality is low) • Serum electrolyte and arterial blood gas analysis may reflect associated clinical problems resulting from the underlying cause of hypovolemia or the treatment regimen • Urine specific gravity > 1.030 • Increased urine osmolality • Urine sodium level < 50 mEq/L	• Oral fluids • Parenteral fluids • Fluid resuscitation by rapid I.V. administration • Blood or blood products (with hemorrhage) • Antidiarrheals as needed • Antiemetics as needed • I.V. dopamine (Intropin) or norepinephrine (Levophed) to increase cardiac contractility and renal perfusion (if patient remains symptomatic after fluid replacement) • Autotransfusion (for some patients with hypovolemia caused by trauma)

peritoneum (ascites), pleural cavity (hydrothorax), or pericardial sac (pericardial effusion).

Tonicity

Many fluid and electrolyte disorders are classified according to how they affect osmotic pressure, or tonicity. (See *Alterations in Tonicity*.) *Tonicity* describes the relative concentrations of electrolytes (osmotic pressure) on both sides of a semipermeable membrane (the cell wall or the capillary wall). The word *normal* in this context refers to the usual electrolyte concentration of physiologic fluids. Normal saline solution has a sodium chloride concentration of 0.9%.

• *Isotonic* solutions have the same electrolyte concentration and therefore the same osmotic pressure as extracellular fluid.
• *Hypertonic* solutions have a greater than normal concentration of some essential electrolyte, usually sodium.
• *Hypotonic* solutions have a lower than normal concentration of some essential electrolyte, also usually sodium.

Electrolyte Balance

The major electrolytes are the cations sodium, potassium, calcium, and magnesium and the anions chloride, phosphate, and bicarbonate. The body continuously attempts to maintain intracellular and extracellular equilibrium of electrolytes. Too much

Disorders of Fluid Balance: Hypervolemia

CAUSES	PATHOPHYSIOLOGY	SIGNS AND SYMPTOMS	DIAGNOSTIC TEST RESULTS	TREATMENT
Hypervolemia is an abnormal increase in the volume of circulating fluid (plasma) in the body. It results from these causes: *Increased risk for sodium and water retention* • Heart failure • Hepatic cirrhosis • Nephrotic syndrome • Corticosteroid therapy • Low dietary protein intake • Renal failure *Excessive sodium and water intake* • Parenteral fluid replacement with normal saline or lactated Ringer's solution • Blood or plasma replacement • Excessive dietary intake of water, sodium chloride, or other salts *Fluid shift to extracellular fluid* • Remobilization of fluid after burn treatment • Intake of hypertonic fluids • Intake of colloid oncotic fluids	Increased extracellular fluid volume causes this sequence of events: • circulatory overload • increased cardiac contractility and mean arterial pressure (MAP) • increased capillary hydrostatic pressure • shift of fluid to the interstitial space • edema Elevated MAP inhibits secretion of antidiuretic hormone and aldosterone and consequent increased urinary elimination of water and sodium. These compensatory mechanisms usually restore normal intravascular volume. If hypervolemia is severe or prolonged or the patient has a history of cardiovascular dysfunction, compensatory mechanisms may fail, and heart failure and pulmonary edema may ensue.	• Rapid breathing • Dyspnea • Crackles • Rapid, bounding pulse • Hypertension • Jugular vein distention • Moist skin • Acute weight gain • Edema • S_3 gallop (**depending on cause**)	• Decreased serum potassium and blood urea nitrogen • Decreased hematocrit due to hemodilution • Normal or low serum sodium • Low urine sodium excretion • Increased hemodynamic values	• Treatment of underlying condition • Oxygen administration (if indicated) • Use of thromboembolic disease support hose to help mobilize edematous fluid • Bed rest • Restricted sodium and water intake • Preload reduction agents and afterload reduction agents • Hemodialysis or peritoneal dialysis • Continuous arteriovenous hemofiltration • Continuous venovenous hemofiltration

or too little of any electrolyte will affect most body systems. (See *Major Electrolytes*, page 39, and *Normal Electrolyte Values*, page 39.)

Electrolyte imbalances can affect all body systems. Too much or too little potassium or too little calcium or magnesium can increase the excitability of the cardiac muscle, causing arrhythmias. Multiple neurologic symptoms may result from electrolyte imbalance, ranging from disorientation or confusion to a completely depressed central nervous system. Too much or too little sodium or too much potassium can cause oliguria. Blood pressure may be increased or decreased. The GI tract is particularly susceptible to electrolyte imbalance:

- too much potassium — leads to abdominal cramps, nausea, and diarrhea
- too little potassium — leads to paralytic ileus
- too much magnesium — leads to nausea, vomiting, and diarrhea
- too much calcium — leads to nausea, vomiting, and constipation.

Acid-Base Imbalance

Acid-base balance is essential to life. Concepts related to imbalance include:

- *acidemia* — arterial blood pH less than 7.35, which reflects a relative excess of acid in the blood. The hydrogen ion content in extracellular fluid increases, and the hydrogen ions move to the intracellular fluid. To keep the intracellular fluid electrically neutral, an equal amount of potassium leaves the cell, creating a relative hyperkalemia.
- *alkalemia* — arterial blood pH greater than 7.45, which reflects a relative excess of base in the blood. In alkalemia, an excess of hydrogen ions in the intracellular fluid forces them into the extracellular fluid. To keep the intracellular fluid electrically neutral, potassium moves from the extracellular to the intracellular fluid, creating a relative hypokalemia.
- *acidosis* — a systemic increase in hydrogen ion concentration. If the lungs fail to eliminate CO_2 or if volatile (carbonic) or nonvolatile (lactic) acid products of metabolism accumulate, hydrogen ion concentration rises. Acidosis can also occur if persistent diarrhea causes loss of basic bicarbonate anions or the kidneys fail to reabsorb bicarbonate or secrete hydrogen ions.
- *alkalosis* — a bodywide decrease in hydrogen ion concentration. An excessive loss of CO_2 during hyperventilation, loss of nonvolatile acids during vomiting, or excessive ingestion of base may decrease hydrogen ion concentration.
- *compensation* — the lungs and kidneys, along with a number of chemical buffer systems in the intracellular and extracellular compartments, work together to maintain plasma pH in the range of 7.35 to 7.45.

Disorders of Electrolyte Balance

ELECTROLYTE IMBALANCE	SIGNS AND SYMPTOMS	DIAGNOSTIC TEST RESULTS
Hyponatremia	• Muscle twitching and weakness • Lethargy, confusion, seizures, and coma • Hypotension and tachycardia • Nausea, vomiting, and abdominal cramps • Oliguria or anuria	• Serum sodium < 135 mEq/L • Decreased urine specific gravity • Decreased serum osmolality • Urine sodium > 100 mEq/24 h • Increased red blood cell count
Hypernatremia	• Agitation, restlessness, fever, and decreased level of consciousness • Muscle irritability and convulsions • Hypertension, tachycardia, pitting edema, and excessive weight gain • Thirst, increased viscosity of saliva, and rough tongue • Dyspnea, respiratory arrest, and death	• Serum sodium > 145 mEq/L • Urine sodium < 40 mEq/24 h • High serum osmolality
Hypokalemia	• Dizziness, hypotension, arrhythmias, electrocardiogram (ECG) changes, and cardiac and respiratory arrest • Nausea, vomiting, anorexia, diarrhea, decreased peristalsis, abdominal distention, and paralytic ileus • Muscle weakness, fatigue, and leg cramps	• Serum potassium < 3.5 mEq/L • Coexisting low serum calcium and magnesium levels not responsive to treatment for hypokalemia usually suggest hypomagnesemia • Metabolic alkalosis • ECG changes, including flattened T waves, elevated U waves, and depressed ST segment
Hyperkalemia	• Tachycardia changing to bradycardia, ECG changes, and cardiac arrest • Nausea, diarrhea, and abdominal cramps • Muscle weakness and flaccid paralysis	• Serum potassium > 5 mEq/L • Metabolic acidosis • ECG changes, including tented and elevated T waves, widened QRS complex, prolonged PR interval, flattened or absent P waves, and depressed ST segment
Hypochloremia	• Muscle hyperexcitability and tetany • Shallow, depressed breathing • Usually associated with hyponatremia and its characteristic symptoms, such as muscle weakness and twitching	• Serum chloride < 96 mEq/L • Serum pH > 7.45, serum CO > 32 mEq/L (supportive values)
Hyperchloremia	• Deep, rapid breathing • Weakness • Lethargy, possibly leading to coma	• Serum chloride > 108 mEq/L • Serum pH < 7.35, serum CO < 22 mEq/L (supportive values)
Hypocalcemia	• Anxiety, irritability, twitching around the mouth, laryngospasm, seizures, positive Chvostek's and Trousseau's signs • Hypotension and arrhythmias due to decreased calcium influx	• Serum calcium < 8.5 mg/dL • Low platelet count • ECG changes: lengthened QT interval, prolonged ST segment, and arrhythmias
Hypercalcemia	• Drowsiness, lethargy, headaches, irritability, confusion, depression, apathy, tingling and numbness of fingers, muscle cramps, and convulsions • Weakness and muscle flaccidity • Bone pain and pathological fractures • Heart block • Anorexia, nausea, vomiting, constipation, dehydration, and abdominal cramps • Flank pain	• Serum calcium > 10.5 mg/dL • ECG changes: signs of heart block and shortened QT interval • Decreased parathyroid hormone level • Calcium stones in urine
Hypomagnesemia	• Nearly always coexists with hypokalemia and hypocalcemia • Hyperirritability, tetany, leg and foot cramps, positive Chvostek's and Trousseau's signs, confusion, delusions, and seizures • Arrhythmias, vasodilation, and hypotension	• Serum magnesium < 1.8 mEq/L • Coexisting low serum potassium and calcium levels

ELECTROLYTE IMBALANCE	SIGNS AND SYMPTOMS	DIAGNOSTIC TEST RESULTS
Hypermagnesemia	• Central nervous system depression, lethargy, and drowsiness • Diminished reflexes; muscle weakness to flaccid paralysis • Respiratory depression • Heart block, bradycardia, widened QRS, and prolonged QT interval • Hypotension	• Serum magnesium > 2.5 mEq/L • Coexisting elevated potassium and calcium levels
Hypophosphatemia	• Muscle weakness, tremor, and paresthesia • Tissue hypoxia • Bone pain, decreased reflexes, and seizures • Weak pulse • Hyperventilation • Dysphagia and anorexia	• Serum phosphate < 2.5 mg/dL • Urine phosphate > 1.3 g/2 h
Hyperphosphatemia	• Usually asymptomatic unless leading to hypocalcemia, then evidenced by tetany and seizures • Hyperreflexia, flaccid paralysis, and muscular weakness	• Serum phosphate > 4.5 mg/dL • Serum calcium < 8.5 mg/dL • Urine phosphorus < 0.9 g/24 h

Buffer Systems

A buffer system consists of a weak acid (one that doesn't readily release free hydrogen ions) and a corresponding base such as sodium bicarbonate. These buffers resist or minimize a change in pH when an acid or base is added to the buffered solution. Buffers work in seconds.

The four major buffers or buffer systems are:

- carbonic acid–bicarbonate system
- hemoglobin-oxyhemoglobin system
- other protein buffers
- phosphate system.

When primary disease processes alter either the acid or base component of the ratio, the lungs or kidneys (whichever isn't affected by the disease process) act to restore the ratio and normalize pH. Because the body's mechanisms that regulate pH occur in stepwise fashion over time, the body tolerates gradual changes in pH better than it does abrupt ones.

Renal Mechanisms

If a respiratory disorder causes acidosis or alkalosis, the kidneys respond by altering the processing of hydrogen and bicarbonate ions to return the pH to normal. Renal compensation begins hours to days after a respiratory alteration in pH. Despite this delay, renal compensation is powerful.

- *Acidemia* — Kidneys excrete excess hydrogen ions, which may combine with phosphate or ammonia to form titratable acids in the urine. The net effect is to *raise* the concentration of bicarbonate ions in the extracellular fluid and restore acid-base balance.

- *Alkalemia* — Kidneys excrete excess bicarbonate ions, usually with sodium ions. The net effect is to *reduce* the concentration of bicarbonate ions in the extracellular fluid and restore acid-base balance.

Pulmonary Mechanisms

If acidosis or alkalosis results from a metabolic or renal disorder, the respiratory system regulates the respiratory rate to return pH to normal. The partial pressure of carbon dioxide in arterial blood ($PaCO_2$) reflects CO_2 levels proportionate to blood pH. As the concentration of the gas increases, so does its partial pressure. Within minutes after the slightest change in $PaCO_2$, central chemoreceptors in the medulla that regulate the rate and depth of ventilation detect the change and respond as follows:

- *acidemia* — increased respiratory rate and depth to eliminate CO_2
- *alkalemia* — decreased respiratory rate and depth to retain CO_2.

DISORDERS

Fluid and electrolyte balance is essential for health. Many factors, such as illness, injury, surgery, and treatments, can disrupt fluid and electrolyte balances. (See *Disorders of Fluid Balance: Hypovolemia*, page 40; *Disorders of Fluid Balance: Hypervolemia*, page 41; and *Disorders of Electrolyte Balance*, pages 42–43.)

Acid-base disturbances can cause respiratory acidosis or alkalosis or metabolic acidosis or alkalosis. (See *Disorders of Acid-Base Balance*, pages 44–45.)

DISORDER AND CAUSES	PATHOPHYSIOLOGY	SIGNS AND SYMPTOMS	DIAGNOSTIC TEST RESULTS	TREATMENT
Respiratory acidosis				
• Airway obstruction or parenchymal lung disease • Mechanical ventilation • Chronic metabolic alkalosis as respiratory compensatory mechanisms try to normalize pH • Chronic bronchitis • Extensive pneumonia • Large pneumothorax • Pulmonary edema • Asthma • Chronic obstructive pulmonary disease (COPD) • Drugs • Cardiac arrest • Central nervous system (CNS) trauma • Neuromuscular diseases • Sleep apnea	When pulmonary ventilation decreases, partial pressure of carbon dioxide in arterial blood ($PaCO_2$) increases and carbon dioxide (CO_2) level rises. Retained CO_2 combines with water (H_2O) to form carbonic acid (H_2CO_3), which dissociates to release free hydrogen (H^+) and bicarbonate (HCO_3^-) ions. Increased $PaCO_2$ and free H^+ ions stimulate the medulla to increase respiratory drive and expel CO_2. As pH falls, 2,3-diphosphoglycerate (2,3-DPG) accumulates in red blood cells, where it alters hemoglobin (Hb) to release oxygen. The Hb picks up H^+ ions and CO_2 and removes them from the serum. As respiratory mechanisms fail, rising $PaCO_2$ stimulates the kidneys to retain HCO_3^- and sodium (Na^+) ions and excrete H^+ ions. As the H^+ ion concentration overwhelms compensatory mechanisms, H^+ ions move into cells and potassium (K^+) ions move out. Without enough oxygen, anaerobic metabolism produces lactic acid.	• Restlessness • Confusion • Apprehension • Somnolence • Asterixis • Headaches • Dyspnea and tachypnea • Papilledema (if secondary to increased intracranial pressure) • Depressed reflexes • Hypoxemia • Tachycardia • Hypertension/ hypotension • Atrial and ventricular arrhythmias • Coma	Arterial blood gas (ABG) analysis: $PaCO_2 > 45$ mm Hg; pH < 7.35–7.45; and normal HCO_3^- in the acute stage and elevated HCO_3^- in the chronic stage	*For pulmonary causes* • Removal of foreign body obstructing the airway • Mechanical ventilation • Bronchodilators • Antibiotics for pneumonia • Chest tubes for pneumothorax • Thrombolytics or anticoagulants for pulmonary emboli • Bronchoscopy to remove excess secretions *For COPD (may have chronic respiratory acidosis)* • Bronchodilators • Oxygen at low flow rates • Corticosteroids *For other causes* • Drug therapy • Dialysis or activated charcoal to remove toxins • Correction of metabolic alkalosis • I.V. sodium bicarbonate (only in specific cases)
Respiratory alkalosis				
• Acute hypoxemia, pneumonia, interstitial lung disease, pulmonary vascular disease, or acute asthma • Anxiety • Hypermetabolic states, such as fever and sepsis • Excessive mechanical ventilation • Salicylate toxicity • Metabolic acidosis • Hepatic failure • Pregnancy	As pulmonary ventilation increases, excessive CO_2 is exhaled. Resulting hypocapnia leads to reduction of H_2CO_3 excretion of H^+ and HCO_3^- ions, and rising serum pH. Against rising pH, the hydrogen-potassium buffer system pulls H^+ ions out of cells and into blood in exchange for K^+ ions. H^+ ions entering blood combine with HCO_3^- ions to form H_2CO_3, and pH falls. Hypocapnia causes an increase in heart rate, cerebral vasoconstriction, and decreased cerebral blood flow. After 6 h, kidneys secrete more HCO_3^- and less H^+. Continued low $PaCO_2$ and vasoconstriction increases cerebral and peripheral hypoxia. Severe alkalosis inhibits calcium (Ca^+) ionization, increasing nerve and muscle excitability.	• Deep, rapid breathing • Light-headedness or dizziness • Agitation • Circumoral and peripheral paresthesias • Carpopedal spasms, twitching, and muscle weakness	ABG analysis showing $PaCO_2 < 35$ mm Hg; elevated pH in proportion to decrease in $PaCO_2$ in the acute stage but decreasing toward normal in the chronic stage; normal HCO_3^- in the acute stage but less than normal in the chronic stage	• Removal of ingested toxins, such as salicylates, by inducing emesis or using gastric lavage • Treatment of fever or sepsis • Oxygen for acute hypoxemia • Treatment of CNS disease • Having patient breathe into a paper bag • Adjustments to mechanical ventilation to decrease minute ventilation

DISORDER AND CAUSES	PATHOPHYSIOLOGY	SIGNS AND SYMPTOMS	DIAGNOSTIC TEST RESULTS	TREATMENT
Metabolic acidosis				
• Excessive acid accumulation • Deficient HCO_3^- scores • Decreased acid excretion by the kidneys • Diabetic ketoacidosis • Chronic alcoholism • Malnutrition or a low-carbohydrate, high-fat diet • Anaerobic carbohydrate metabolism • Underexcretion of metabolized acids or inability to conserve base • Diarrhea, intestinal malabsorption, or loss of sodium bicarbonate from the intestines • Salicylate intoxication, exogenous poisoning or, less frequently, Addison's disease • Inhibited secretion of acid	As H^+ ions begin accumulating in the body, chemical buffers (plasma HCO_3^- and proteins) in cells and extracellular fluid bind them. Excess H^+ ions decrease blood pH and stimulate chemoreceptors in the medulla to increase respiration. Consequent fall of partial pressure of $PaCO_2$ frees H^+ ions to bind with HCO_3^- ions. Respiratory compensation occurs but isn't sufficient to correct acidosis. Healthy kidneys compensate, excreting excess H^+ ions, buffered by phosphate or ammonia. For each H^+ ion excreted, renal tubules reabsorb and return to blood one Na^+ ion and one HCO_3^- ion. Excess H^+ ions in extracellular fluid passively diffuse into cells. To maintain balance of charge across cell membrane, cells release K^+ ions. Excess H^+ ions change the normal balance of K^+, Na^+, and Ca^+ ions, impairing neural excitability.	• Headache and lethargy progressing to drowsiness, CNS depression, Kussmaul's respirations, hypotension, stupor, and coma and death • Associated GI distress leading to anorexia, nausea, vomiting, diarrhea, and possibly dehydration • Warm, flushed skin • Fruity-smelling breath	• Arterial blood pH < 7.35; $PaCO_2$ normal or <35 mm Hg as respiratory compensatory mechanisms take hold; HCO_3^- may be <22 mEq/L • Urine pH < 4.5 in the absence of renal disease • Elevated plasma lactic acid in lactic acidosis • Anion gap > 14 mEq/L in high anion gap metabolic acidosis, lactic acidosis, ketoacidosis, aspirin overdose, alcohol poisoning, renal failure, or any disorder caused by accumulation of organic acids, sulfates, or phosphates • Anion gap 12 mEq/L or less in normal anion gap metabolic acidosis from HCO_3^- loss, GI or renal loss, increased acid load, rapid I.V. saline administration, or other disorders characterized by HCO_3^- loss	• Sodium bicarbonate I.V. for severe high anion gap (in severe acidosis, usually <7.1) • I.V. lactated Ringer's solution (can exacerbate increase in lactate) • Evaluation and correction of electrolyte imbalances • Correction of underlying cause • Mechanical ventilation to maintain respiratory compensation, if needed • Antibiotic therapy to treat infection • Dialysis for patients with renal failure or certain drug toxicities • Antidiarrheal agents for diarrhea-induced HCO_3^- loss • Position patient to prevent aspiration • Seizure precautions
Metabolic alkalosis				
• Chronic vomiting • Nasogastric tube drainage or lavage without adequate electrolyte replacement • Fistulas • Use of steroids and certain diuretics (furosemide [Lasix], thiazides, and ethacrynic acid [Edecrin]) • Massive blood transfusions • Cushing's disease, primary hyperaldosteronism, and Bartter's syndrome • Excessive intake of bicarbonate of soda, other antacids, or absorbable alkali • Excessive amounts of I.V. fluids; high serum concentrations of bicarbonate or lactate • Respiratory insufficiency • Low serum chloride • Low serum potassium	Chemical buffers in extracellular and intracellular fluid bind HCO_3^- in the body. Excess unbound HCO_3^- raises blood pH, depressing chemoreceptors in the medulla, inhibiting respiration, and raising $PaCO_2$. CO_2 combines with H_2O to form H_2CO_3. Low oxygen limits respiratory compensation. When blood HCO_3^- rises to 28 mEq/L, the amount filtered by renal glomeruli exceeds reabsorptive capacity of the renal tubules. Excess HCO_3^- is excreted in urine, and H^+ ions are retained. To maintain electrochemical balance, Na^+ ions and water are excreted with HCO_3^- ions. When H^+ ion levels in extracellular fluid are low, H^+ ions diffuse passively out of cells and extracellular K^+ ions move into cells. As intracellular H^+ ion levels fall, calcium ionization decreases, and nerve cells become permeable to Na^+ ions. Na^+ ions moving into cells trigger neural impulses in the peripheral nervous system and the CNS.	• Irritability, picking at bedclothes (carphology), twitching, and confusion • Nausea, vomiting, and diarrhea • Cardiovascular abnormalities due to hypokalemia • Respiratory disturbances (such as cyanosis and apnea) and slow, shallow respirations • Possible carpopedal spasm in the hand caused by diminished peripheral blood flow during repeated blood pressure checks	• Arterial blood pH > 7.45; HCO_3^- > 26 mEq/L • Low potassium (<3.5 mEq/L), calcium (<8.9 mg/dL), and chloride (<98 mEq/L)	• Cautious use of ammonium chloride I.V. (rarely) or hydrochloride to restore extracellular fluid hydrogen and chloride levels • Potassium chloride (KCl) and normal saline solution (use very judiciously) • Discontinuation of diuretics and supplementary KCl • Oral or I.V. acetazolamide

Suggested References

Cline, D. M., Ma, J., Cydulka, R. K., Meckler, G. D., Thomas, S. H., & Handel, D. A. (2012). *Tintinalli's emergency medicine manual* (7th ed.). New York: McGraw-Hill. ISBN: 978-07-178184-8.

Kasper, D., Fauci, A., Hauser, S., Longo, D., Jameson, J. L., & Loscalzo, J. (2015). *Harrison's principles of internal medicine* (19th ed.). New York: McGraw-Hill. ISBN: 978-0-07-1802-154.

Kemp, W. L., Burns, D. K., & Brown, T. G. (2007). *Pathology: The big picture*. New York: McGraw-Hill. ISBN: 13-978-0071477482.

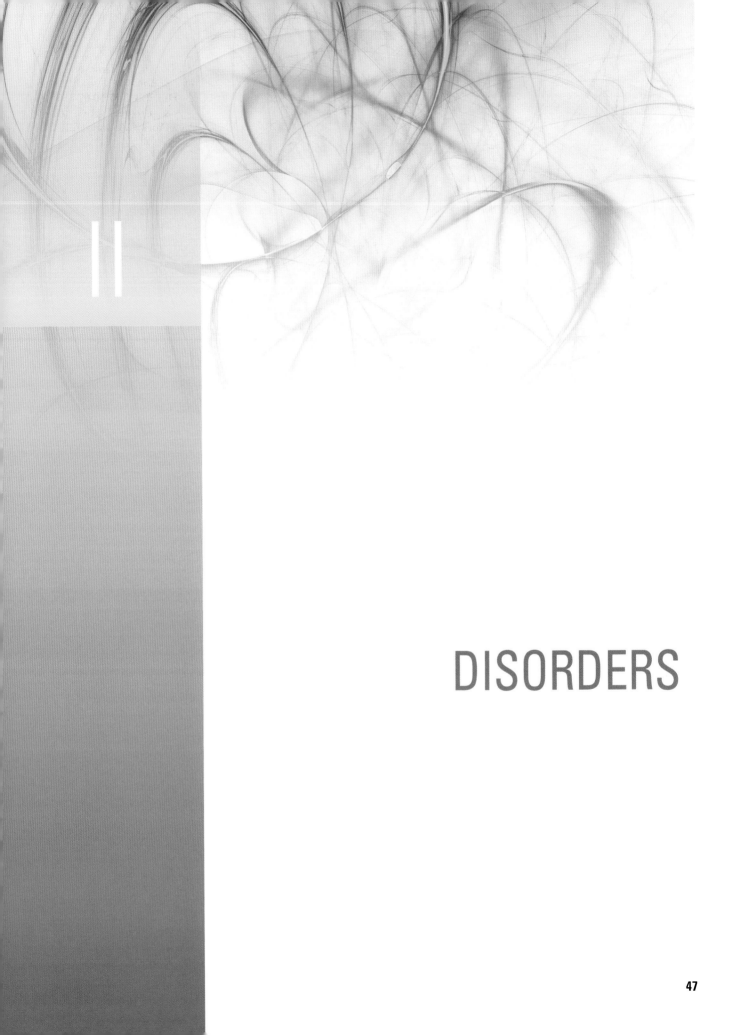

II

DISORDERS

AORTIC ANEURYSM

A thoracic aortic aneurysm is an abnormal widening of the ascending, transverse, or descending part of the aorta. Aneurysm of the ascending aorta is the most common type and has the highest mortality. An abdominal aneurysm generally occurs in the aorta between the renal arteries and the iliac branches.

Causes

Aneurysm commonly results from atherosclerosis, which weakens the aortic wall and gradually distends the lumen. The exact cause is unknown, but there are factors that contribute which are included here:

- age and family history
- fungal infection (mycotic aneurysms) of the aortic arch and descending segments
- bicuspid aortic valve
- congenital disorders, such as coarctation of the aorta or Marfan syndrome
- inflammatory disorders
- trauma
- syphilis
- hypertension (in dissecting aneurysm)
- tobacco use.

AGE ALERT

Ascending aortic aneurysms, the most common type, are usually seen in hypertensive men under age 60. Descending aortic aneurysms, usually found just below the origin of the subclavian artery, are most common in elderly men with hypertension. They may also occur in younger patients after traumatic chest injury or, less commonly, after infection.

Pathophysiology

First, degenerative changes create a focal weakness in the muscular layer of the aorta (tunica media), allowing the inner layer (tunica intima) and outer layer (tunica adventitia) to stretch outward. The outward bulge is the aneurysm. The pressure of blood pulsing through the aorta progressively weakens the vessel walls and enlarges the aneurysm. As the vessel dilates, wall tension increases. This increases arterial pressure and dilates the aneurysm further.

Aneurysms may be *dissecting*, a hemorrhagic separation in the aortic wall, usually within the medial layer; *saccular*, an outpouching of the arterial wall; or *fusiform*, a spindle-shaped enlargement encompassing the entire aortic circumference.

A false aneurysm occurs when the entire wall is injured, with blood contained in the surrounding tissue. A sac eventually forms and communicates with an artery or the heart.

COMPLICATIONS

- Cardiac tamponade if aneurysm ruptures
- Dissection
- Rupture

Signs and Symptoms

Ascending Aneurysm

- Pain, the most common symptom of thoracic aortic aneurysm
- Bradycardia
- Murmur of aortic insufficiency
- Pericardial friction rub (caused by a hemopericardium)
- Unequal intensities of the right carotid and left radial pulses
- Difference in blood pressure between the right and left arms
- Jugular vein distention

Descending Aneurysm

- Pain, usually starting suddenly between the shoulder blades; may radiate to the chest
- Hoarseness
- Dyspnea and stridor
- Dysphagia
- Dry cough

Abdominal Aneurysm

Although abdominal aneurysms usually don't produce symptoms, most are evident as a pulsating mass in the periumbilical area. Other signs include:

- systolic bruit over the aorta
- tenderness on deep palpation
- lumbar pain that radiates to the flank and groin.

CLINICAL TIP

Pain caused by a dissecting aortic aneurysm:

- may be described as "ripping" or "tearing"
- commonly radiates to the anterior chest, neck, back, or abdomen
- usually has an abrupt onset.

Diagnostic Test Results

- Echocardiography shows the aneurysm and its size.
- Anteroposterior and lateral abdominal X-rays show aortic calcifications present in abdominal aortic aneurysms; posteroanterior and oblique chest X-rays will show widening of the aorta and mediastinum in thoracic aortic aneurysms.
- Computed tomography scan shows the effects on nearby organs.
- Aortography shows the size and location of the aneurysm.
- Complete blood count reveals decreased hemoglobin levels.

- Abdominal ultrasound can detect and monitor the progression of AAA.

Treatment

A dissecting aortic aneurysm is an emergency that requires prompt surgery and stabilizing measures. Treatment includes:

- antihypertensives such as nitroprusside
- negative inotropic agents to decrease force of contractility
- beta-adrenergic blockers
- oxygen for respiratory distress
- opioids for pain
- I.V. fluids
- possibly, whole blood transfusions.

Treatment of stable AAA focuses on surveillance and tight BP control to prevent enlargement.

TYPES OF AORTIC ANEURYSMS

Dissecting aneurysm

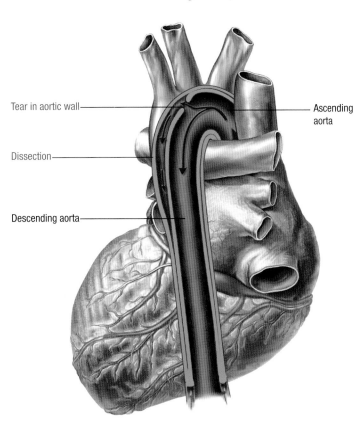

Tear in aortic wall

Dissection

Descending aorta

Ascending aorta

Fusiform aneurysm

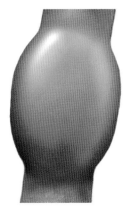

False aneurysm

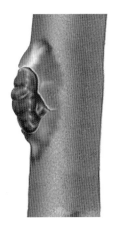

Saccular aneurysm

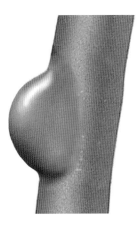

CARDIAC ARRHYTHMIAS

Abnormal electrical conduction or automaticity changes heart rate and rhythm. Arrhythmias vary in severity — from mild, producing no symptoms, and requiring no treatment (such as sinus arrhythmia, in which heart rate increases and decreases with respiration), to catastrophic ventricular fibrillation, which mandates immediate resuscitation. Arrhythmias are generally classified according to their origin (ventricular or supraventricular). Their effect on cardiac output and blood pressure, partially influenced by the site of origin, determines their clinical significance. (See the appendix "Types of cardiac arrhythmias.")

Causes

Each arrhythmia may have its own specific cause. Common causes include:

- congenital defects
- myocardial ischemia or infarction
- organic heart disease
- drug toxicity
- degeneration or obstruction of conductive tissue
- connective tissue disorders
- electrolyte imbalances
- hypertrophy of heart muscle
- acid-base imbalances
- emotional stress.

AGE ALERT
Electrocardiogram changes that occur with age include:

- longer PR, QRS, and QT intervals
- lower amplitude of QRS complex
- leftward shift of QRS axis.

Pathophysiology

Altered automaticity, reentry, or conduction disturbances may cause cardiac arrhythmias. Enhanced automaticity is the result of partial depolarization, which may increase the intrinsic rate of the sinoatrial node or latent pacemakers or may induce ectopic pacemakers to reach threshold and depolarize.

Ischemia or deformation causes an abnormal circuit to develop within conductive fibers. Although current flow is blocked in one direction within the circuit, the descending impulse can travel in the other direction. By the time the impulse completes the circuit, the previously depolarized tissue within the circuit is no longer refractory to stimulation; therefore, arrhythmias occur.

Conduction disturbances occur when impulses are conducted too quickly or too slowly.

COMPLICATIONS
- Impaired cardiac output
- Cardiac arrest in certain arrhythmias
- Stroke in prolonged atrial arrhythmias

Signs and Symptoms

Signs and symptoms of arrhythmias result from reduced cardiac output and altered perfusion to the organs and may include:

- dyspnea
- hypotension
- dizziness, syncope, and weakness
- chest pain
- cool, clammy skin
- altered level of consciousness
- reduced urinary output
- palpitations.

Diagnostic Test Results

- Electrocardiography (ECG) detects arrhythmias as well as ischemia and infarction by showing prolonged or shortened intervals, elevated or depressed T waves, premature contractions, or absence of waves.
- Blood tests reveal electrolyte abnormalities, such as hyperkalemia or hypokalemia and hypermagnesemia or hypomagnesemia, as well as drug toxicities.
- Arterial blood gas analysis reveals acid-base abnormalities, such as acidemia or alkalemia.
- Holter monitoring, event monitoring, and loop recording show the presence of an arrhythmia.
- Exercise testing detects exercise-induced arrhythmias.
- Electrophysiologic testing identifies the mechanism of an arrhythmia and the location of accessory pathways; it also assesses the effectiveness of antiarrhythmic drugs, radiofrequency ablation, and implantable cardioverter–defibrillators (ICDs).

Treatment

Follow the specific treatment guidelines or protocols for each arrhythmia. Treatment generally focuses on the underlying problem and may include:

- antiarrhythmic medications
- electrolyte correction
- oxygen
- correction of acid-base balance
- cardioversion
- radiofrequency ablation
- ICD
- pacemaker
- cardiopulmonary resuscitation.

Sinus node arrhythmias
- Sinoatrial block
- Sinus bradycardia
- Sinus tachycardia

Atrial arrhythmias
- Premature atrial contractions
- Atrial fibrillation
- Atrial flutter

Atrioventricular (AV) blocks
- First-degree AV block
- Second-degree AV block
- Third-degree AV block

Junctional arrhythmia
- Junctional rhythm

Ventricular arrhythmias
- Premature ventricular contractions
- Ventricular fibrillation
- Ventricular tachycardia

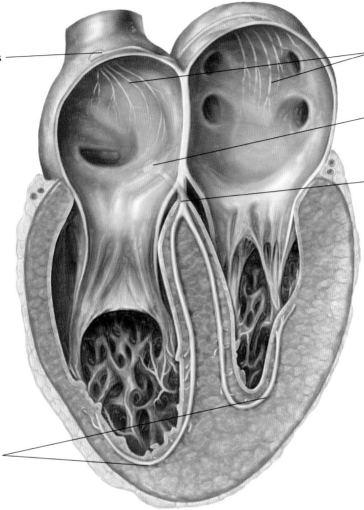

CARDIAC TAMPONADE

Cardiac tamponade is a rapid, unchecked rise in pressure in the pericardial sac that compresses the heart, impairs diastolic filling, and limits cardiac output. The rise in pressure usually results from blood or fluid accumulation in the pericardial sac (pericardial effusion). Even a small amount of fluid (50 to 100 mL) can cause a serious tamponade if it accumulates rapidly.

Causes

- Idiopathic
- Effusion (due to cancer, bacterial infections, tuberculosis, or, rarely, acute rheumatic fever)
- Traumatic or nontraumatic hemorrhage
- Viral or postirradiation pericarditis
- Chronic renal failure requiring dialysis
- Drug reaction (procainamide, hydralazine, minoxidil, isoniazid, penicillin, or daunorubicin)
- Heparin- or warfarin-induced tamponade
- Connective tissue disorders
- Postcardiac surgery
- Acute myocardial infarction (MI)
- Pericarditis

Pathophysiology

In cardiac tamponade, the progressive accumulation of fluid in the pericardial sac causes compression of the heart chambers. This compression obstructs filling of the ventricles and reduces the amount of blood that can be pumped out of the heart with each contraction.

Each time the ventricles contract, more fluid accumulates in the pericardial sac. This further limits the amount of blood that can fill the ventricular chambers, especially the left ventricle, during the next cardiac cycle.

The amount of fluid necessary to cause cardiac tamponade varies greatly; it may be as little as 50 to 100 mL when the fluid accumulates rapidly or more than 2,000 mL if the fluid accumulates slowly and the pericardium stretches to adapt. Prognosis is inversely proportional to the amount of fluid accumulated.

COMPLICATIONS
- Decreased cardiac output
- Cardiogenic shock
- Death if untreated

Signs and Symptoms

- Elevated central venous pressure (CVP) with jugular vein distention
- Muffled heart sounds
- Pulsus paradoxus (decreases systolic blood pressure with inspiration)
- Diaphoresis and cool, clammy skin
- Anxiety, restlessness, and syncope
- Cyanosis
- Weak, rapid pulse
- Cough, dyspnea, orthopnea, and tachypnea

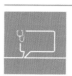

CLINICAL TIP
Cardiac tamponade has three classic features, known as Beck's triad, that include:

- elevated CVP with jugular vein distention
- muffled heart sounds
- pulsus paradoxus.

Diagnostic Test Results

- Chest X-rays show a slightly widened mediastinum and possible cardiomegaly. The cardiac silhouette may have a goblet-shaped appearance.
- ECG detects a low-amplitude QRS complex and electrical alternans, an alternating beat-to-beat change in amplitude of the P wave, QRS complex, and T wave. Generalized ST-segment elevation is noted in all leads.
- Pulmonary artery catheterization detects increased right atrial pressure, right ventricular diastolic pressure, and CVP.
- Echocardiography reveals pericardial effusion with signs of right ventricular and atrial compression.

Treatment

- Supplemental oxygen
- Continuous ECG and hemodynamic monitoring
- Pericardiocentesis
- Pericardectomy
- Resection of a portion or all of the pericardium (pericardial window)
- Trial volume loading with crystalloids
- Inotropic drugs, such as isoproterenol or dopamine
- Posttraumatic injury: blood transfusion, thoracotomy to drain reaccumulating fluid, or repair of bleeding sites may be needed
- Heparin-induced tamponade: heparin antagonist protamine sulfate to stop bleeding
- Warfarin-induced tamponade: vitamin K to stop bleeding

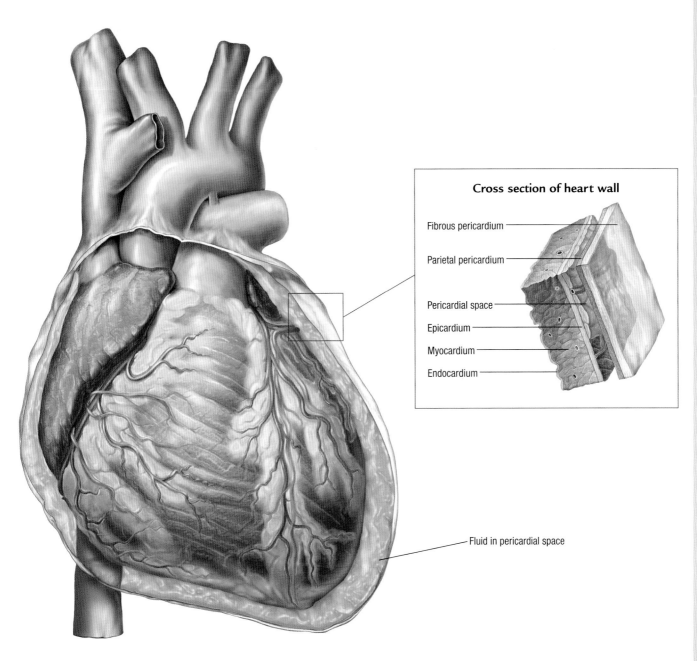

Cross section of heart wall

Fibrous pericardium

Parietal pericardium

Pericardial space

Epicardium

Myocardium

Endocardium

Fluid in pericardial space

CARDIOMYOPATHY

Cardiomyopathy is classified as dilated, hypertrophic, or restrictive.

Dilated cardiomyopathy (DCM) results from damage to cardiac muscle fibers; loss of muscle tone grossly dilates all four chambers of the heart, giving the heart a globular shape.

Hypertrophic cardiomyopathy (HCM) is characterized by disproportionate, asymmetrical thickening of the interventricular septum and left ventricular hypertrophy.

Restrictive cardiomyopathy (RCM) is characterized by restricted ventricular filling due to decreased ventricular compliance and endocardial fibrosis and thickening. If severe, it's irreversible.

Causes

Most patients with cardiomyopathy have idiopathic disease, but some are secondary to these possible causes:

- viral infection
- long-standing hypertension
- ischemic heart disease or valvular disease
- chemotherapy
- cardiotoxic effects of drugs or alcohol
- metabolic disease, such as diabetes or thyroid disease.

Pathophysiology

In DCM, extensive damage to cardiac muscle fibers reduces contractility in the left ventricle. As systolic function declines, stroke volume, ejection fraction, and cardiac output fall.

COMPLICATIONS
- Heart failure
- Emboli
- Syncope
- Sudden death

In HCM, hypertrophy of the left ventricle and interventricular septum obstruct left ventricular outflow. The heart compensates for the decreased cardiac output (caused by obstructed outflow) by increasing the rate and force of contractions. The hypertrophied ventricle becomes stiff and unable to relax and fill during diastole. As left ventricular volume diminishes and filling pressure rises, pulmonary venous pressure also rises, leading to venous congestion and dyspnea.

COMPLICATIONS
- Pulmonary hypertension
- Heart failure
- Sudden death

In RCM, left ventricular hypertrophy and endocardial fibrosis limit myocardial contraction and emptying during systole as well as ventricular relaxation and filling during diastole. As a result, cardiac output falls.

COMPLICATIONS
- Heart failure
- Arrhythmias
- Emboli
- Sudden death

Signs and Symptoms

- Shortness of breath
- Peripheral edema
- Fatigue
- Weight gain
- Cough and congestion
- Nausea
- Bloating
- Palpitations
- Syncope
- Chest pain
- Tachycardia

Diagnostic Test Results

- Chest X-rays show cardiomegaly and increase in heart size.
- Echocardiography reveals left ventricular dilation and dysfunction or left ventricular hypertrophy and a thick, asymmetrical intraventricular septum. It can also quantify the outlet left ventricular outflow gradient in HCM.
- Cardiac catheterization shows left ventricular dilation and dysfunction, elevated left ventricular and, commonly, right ventricular filling pressures, and diminished cardiac output.
- Thallium or cardiolite scan usually reveals myocardial perfusion defects.
- Cardiac catheterization reveals elevated left ventricular end-diastolic pressure and, possibly, mitral insufficiency.
- ECG usually shows left ventricular hypertrophy; ST-segment and T-wave abnormalities; Q waves in leads II, III, and aV_F, and in V_4 to V_6; left anterior hemiblock; left axis deviation; and ventricular and atrial arrhythmias.

Treatment

- Treatment of underlying cause
- Control of arrhythmias
- Angiotensin-converting enzyme inhibitors, diuretics, digoxin (not used in HCM), hydralazine, isosorbide dinitrate, beta-adrenergic blockers, antiarrhythmics, and anticoagulants
- Revascularization
- Valve repair or replacement
- Heart transplantation
- Lifestyle modifications, such as quitting smoking; avoiding alcohol; eating a low-fat, low-salt diet; and restricting fluids
- Ventricular myotomy or myectomy
- Mitral valve repair or replacement
- Defibrillator placement with or without biventricular pacing

Dilated

Hypertrophic

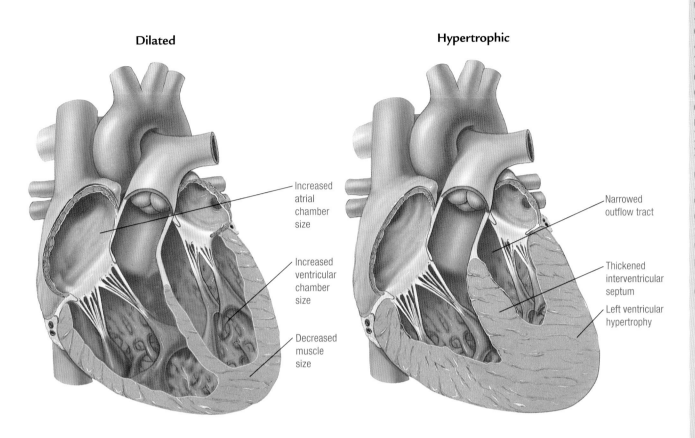

Increased atrial chamber size

Increased ventricular chamber size

Decreased muscle size

Narrowed outflow tract

Thickened interventricular septum

Left ventricular hypertrophy

Restrictive

Walls of ventricles become stiff but not necessarily thickened

CONGENITAL DEFECTS

The most common congenital defects of the heart are atrial septal defect (ASD), coarctation of the aorta, patent ductus arteriosus (PDA), tetralogy of Fallot, transposition of the great arteries, and ventricular septal defect (VSD). Causes of all six defects remain unknown, although some have specific clinical associations.

ATRIAL SEPTAL DEFECT

An opening between the left and right atria permits blood flow from the left atrium to the right atrium rather than from the left atrium to the left ventricle. ASD is associated with Down syndrome.

Pathophysiology

Blood shunts from the left atrium to the right atrium because left atrial pressure is normally slightly higher than right atrial pressure. This difference forces large amounts of blood through a defect that results in right heart volume overload, affecting the right atrium, right ventricle, and pulmonary arteries. Eventually, the right atrium enlarges, and the right ventricle dilates to accommodate the increased blood volume. If pulmonary artery hypertension develops, increased pulmonary vascular resistance and right ventricular hypertrophy follow.

COMPLICATIONS
- Right-sided heart failure
- Heart rhythm abnormalities
- Pulmonary hypertension

Signs and Symptoms

- Fatigue
- Early to midsystolic murmur and low-pitched diastolic murmur
- Fixed, widely split S_2
- Systolic click or late systolic murmur at the apex
- Clubbing of nails and cyanosis with a right-to-left shunt
- Palpable pulsation of the pulmonary artery

COARCTATION OF THE AORTA

Coarctation is a narrowing of the aorta, usually just below the left subclavian artery, near the site where the ligamentum arteriosum joins the pulmonary artery to the aorta. Coarctation of the aorta is associated with Turner's syndrome and congenital abnormalities of the aortic valve.

Pathophysiology

Coarctation of the aorta may develop as a result of spasm and constriction of the smooth muscle in the ductus arteriosus as it closes. Possibly, this contractile tissue extends into the aortic wall, causing narrowing. The obstructive process causes hypertension in the aortic branches above the constriction and diminished pressure in the vessel below the constriction.

Restricted blood flow through the narrowed aorta increases the pressure load on the left ventricle and causes dilation of the proximal aorta and ventricular hypertrophy.

As oxygenated blood leaves the left ventricle, a portion travels through the arteries that branch off the aorta proximal to the coarctation. If PDA is present, the remaining blood travels through the coarctation, mixes with deoxygenated blood from the PDA, and travels to the legs. If the ductus arteriosus is closed, the legs and lower portion of the body must rely solely on the blood that circulates through the coarctation.

COMPLICATIONS
- Rupture of the aorta
- Stroke
- Cerebral aneurysm

Signs and Symptoms

- Heart failure
- Claudication and hypertension
- Headache, vertigo, and epistaxis
- Blood pressure greater in upper than in lower extremities
- Pink upper extremities and cyanotic lower extremities
- Absent or diminished femoral pulses
- Possible murmur
- Possibly, chest and arms more developed than legs

PATENT DUCTUS ARTERIOSUS

The ductus arteriosus is a fetal blood vessel that connects the pulmonary artery to the descending aorta, just distal to the left subclavian artery. Normally, the ductus closes within days to weeks after birth. In PDA, the lumen of the ductus remains open after birth. This creates a left-to-right shunt of blood from the aorta to the pulmonary artery and results in recirculation of arterial blood through the lungs. PDA is associated with premature birth, rubella syndrome, coarctation of the aorta, VSD, and pulmonic and aortic stenosis.

Pathophysiology

The ductus arteriosus normally closes as the neonate takes his first breath but may take as long as 3 months in some infants.

In PDA, relative resistance in pulmonary and systemic vasculature and the size of the ductus determine the quantity of blood that's shunted from left to right. Because of increased aortic pressure, oxygenated blood is shunted from the aorta through the ductus arteriosus to the pulmonary artery. The blood returns to the left side of the heart and is pumped out to the aorta once more.

Increased pulmonary venous return causes increased filling pressure and workload on the left side of the heart as well as left ventricular hypertrophy and possibly heart failure.

COMPLICATIONS
- Chronic pulmonary hypertension
- Cyanosis
- Left-sided heart failure

Atrial septal defect

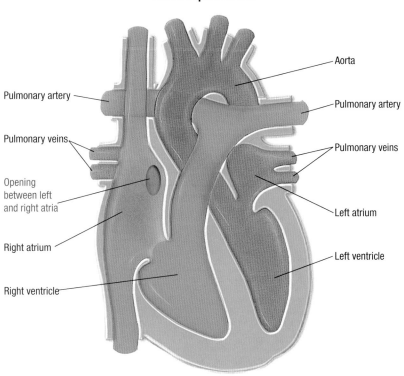

Pulmonary artery

Pulmonary veins

Opening between left and right atria

Right atrium

Right ventricle

Aorta

Pulmonary artery

Pulmonary veins

Left atrium

Left ventricle

Coarctation of the aorta

Narrowing of the aorta

Patent ductus arteriosus

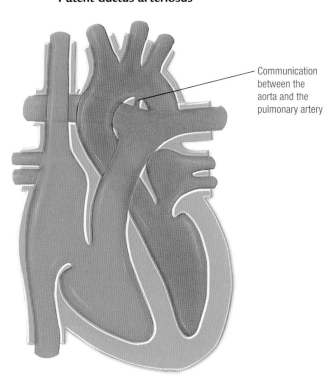

Communication between the aorta and the pulmonary artery

Signs and Symptoms

- Respiratory distress with signs of heart failure in infants
- Gibson murmur
- Thrill palpated at left sternal border
- Prominent left ventricular impulse
- Corrigan's pulse
- Wide pulse pressure
- Slow motor development and failure to thrive

TETRALOGY OF FALLOT

Tetralogy of Fallot is a combination of four cardiac defects: VSD, right ventricular outflow tract obstruction, right ventricular hypertrophy, and an aorta positioned above the VSD (overriding aorta). This defect is associated with fetal alcohol syndrome and Down syndrome.

Pathophysiology

Unoxygenated venous blood entering the right side of the heart may pass through the VSD to the left ventricle, bypassing the lungs, or it may enter the pulmonary artery, depending on the extent of the pulmonic stenosis. The VSD usually lies in the outflow tract of the right ventricle and is generally large enough to permit equalization of right and left ventricular pressures. However, the ratio of systemic vascular resistance to pulmonic stenosis affects the direction and magnitude of shunt flow across the VSD.

COMPLICATIONS
- Endocarditis
- Stroke

Signs and Symptoms

- Cyanosis or "blue" spells (Tet spells)
- Clubbing of digits, diminished exercise tolerance, dyspnea on exertion, growth retardation, and eating difficulties
- Squatting to reduce shortness of breath
- Loud systolic murmur and continuous murmur of the ductus
- Thrill at left sternal border
- Right ventricular impulse and prominent inferior sternum

TRANSPOSITION OF GREAT ARTERIES

The aorta rises from the right ventricle and the pulmonary artery from the left ventricle, producing two noncommunicating circulatory systems. This defect is associated with VSD, VSD with pulmonic stenosis, ASD, and PDA.

Pathophysiology

The transposed pulmonary artery carries oxygenated blood back to the lungs, rather than to the left side of the heart. The transposed aorta returns unoxygenated blood to the systemic circulation rather than to the lungs. Communication between the pulmonary and systemic circulations is necessary for survival. In infants with isolated transposition, blood mixes only at the patent foramen ovale and at the PDA, resulting in slight mixing of unoxygenated systemic blood and oxygenated pulmonary blood. In infants with concurrent cardiac defects, greater mixing of blood occurs.

COMPLICATIONS
- Heart failure
- Arrhythmias

Signs and Symptoms

- Hypoxemia, cyanosis, tachypnea, and dyspnea
- Gallop rhythm, tachycardia, hepatomegaly, and cardiomegaly
- Murmurs of ASD, VSD, or PDA; loud S_2
- Diminished exercise tolerance, fatigue, and clubbing

VENTRICULAR SEPTAL DEFECT

VSD is an opening in the septum between the ventricles that allows blood to shunt between the left and right ventricles. However, the defect is usually small and will close spontaneously. VSD is associated with Down syndrome and other autosomal trisomies, renal anomalies, prematurity, fetal alcohol syndrome, PDA, and coarctation of the aorta.

Pathophysiology

In neonates with a VSD, the ventricular septum fails to close completely by 8 weeks' gestation. VSDs are located in the membranous or muscular portion of the ventricular septum and vary in size. Some defects close spontaneously; in other defects, the septum is entirely absent, creating a single ventricle.

A VSD isn't readily apparent at birth because right and left pressures are approximately equal and pulmonary artery resistance is elevated. Alveoli aren't yet completely opened, so blood doesn't shunt through the defect. As the pulmonary vasculature gradually relaxes, between 4 and 8 weeks after birth, right ventricular pressure decreases, allowing blood to shunt from the left to the right ventricle. Initially, large VSD shunts cause left atrial and left ventricular hypertrophy.

COMPLICATIONS
- Right ventricular hypertrophy
- Heart failure
- Endocarditis

Signs and Symptoms

- Failure to thrive
- Loud, harsh systolic murmur (along the left sternal border at the third or fourth intercostal space) and palpable thrill
- Loud, widely split pulmonic component of S_2
- Displacement of point of maximal impulse to left or down
- Prominent anterior chest, cyanosis, and clubbing
- Liver, heart, and spleen enlargement
- Diaphoresis, tachycardia, and rapid, grunting respirations

Diagnostic Test Results

- Chest X-ray reveals cardiomegaly and ventricular and aortic enlargement.
- ECG may be normal or may reveal ventricular hypertrophy or axis deviation.
- Echocardiography detects the presence and size of a defect.
- Fetal echocardiogram can reveal a defect before birth.
- Cardiac catheterization confirms the diagnosis and damage.

- Arterial blood gas analysis reveals hypoxemia and acid-base disturbances.
- Atrial balloon septostomy (for transposition of the great arteries).

Treatment

- Surgery

- Medications, such as diuretics, angiotensin-converting enzyme inhibitors, indomethacin (for PDA), and prostaglandin
- Oxygen therapy
- Antibiotic prophylaxis
- Atrial balloon septostomy (for transposition of the great arteries)
- Treatment of complications

CONGENITAL HEART DEFECTS (continued)

Tetralogy of Fallot

Aorta

Pulmonary artery

Pulmonary artery

Pulmonary veins

Pulmonary veins

Right ventricular outflow tract obstruction

Left atrium

Right atrium

Overriding aorta

Right ventricle

Ventricular septal defect

Right ventricular hypertrophy

Left ventricle

Transposition of great arteries

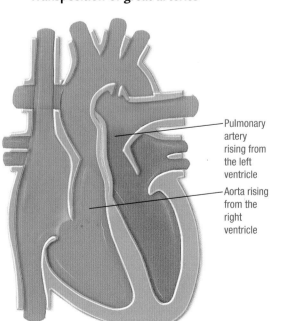

Pulmonary artery rising from the left ventricle

Aorta rising from the right ventricle

Ventricular septal defect

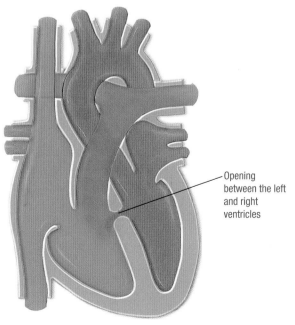

Opening between the left and right ventricles

CORONARY ARTERY DISEASE

Coronary artery disease (CAD) results from the narrowing of the coronary arteries over time because of atherosclerosis. The primary effect of CAD is a diminished supply of oxygen and nutrients to myocardial tissue because of decreased blood flow.

AGE ALERT
The lifetime risk of CAD after age 40 is 49% for men and 32% for women. As women age, their risk increases.

Causes

- Atherosclerosis (most common)
- Dissecting aneurysm
- Infectious vasculitis
- Syphilis
- Congenital abnormalities
- Radiation to the chest

Pathophysiology

Fatty, fibrous plaques progressively occlude the coronary arteries, reducing the volume of blood that can flow through them and leading to myocardial ischemia.

As atherosclerosis progresses, luminal narrowing is accompanied by vascular changes that impair the ability of the diseased vessel to dilate. The consequent precarious balance between myocardial oxygen supply and demand threatens the myocardium distal to the lesion. When oxygen demand exceeds what the diseased vessel can supply, the result is localized myocardial ischemia.

Myocardial cells become ischemic within 10 seconds after coronary artery occlusion. Transient ischemia causes reversible changes at the cellular and tissue levels, depressing myocardial function. Within several minutes, oxygen deprivation forces the myocardium to shift from aerobic to anaerobic metabolism, leading to accumulation of lactic acid and reduction of cellular pH. Without intervention, this sequence of events can lead to tissue injury or necrosis.

The combination of hypoxia, reduced energy availability, and acidosis rapidly impairs left ventricular function. As the fibers become unable to shorten normally, the force of contractions and velocity of blood flow in the affected myocardial region become inadequate. Moreover, wall motion in the ischemic area becomes abnormal and each contraction ejects less blood from the heart. Restoring blood flow through the coronary arteries restores aerobic metabolism and contractility.

COMPLICATIONS
- Angina pectoris
- Myocardial infarction
- Cardiac arrest

Signs and Symptoms

- Angina (pain may be described as burning, squeezing, or tightness that radiates to the left arm, neck, jaw, or shoulder blade)
- Nausea and vomiting
- Cool extremities and pallor
- Diaphoresis caused by sympathetic stimulation
- Fatigue and dyspnea
- Xanthelasma (fat deposits on the eyelids)

AGE ALERT
The older adult with CAD may be asymptomatic because the sympathetic response to ischemia is impaired. In an active older adult, dyspnea and fatigue are two key signals of ischemia.

Diagnostic Test Results

- ECG shows ischemic changes during anginal episode.
- Stress testing detects ST-segment changes during exercise or pharmacologic stress.
- Coronary angiography reveals the location and degree of coronary artery stenosis or obstruction, collateral circulation, and the condition of the artery beyond the narrowing.
- Myocardial perfusion imaging with thallium 201 or technetium 99m (Cardiolite) may be performed during treadmill exercise to detect ischemic areas of the myocardium.
- Stress echocardiography shows abnormal wall motion in ischemic areas.
- Electron beam computed tomography identifies calcium deposits in coronary arteries.
- Cardiac catheterization reveals blockage in the coronary arteries.
- Lipid profile shows elevated cholesterol levels.

CLINICAL TIP
The lipid profile consists of these components:

- low-density lipoprotein (LDL) — "bad" lipoprotein; carries most of the cholesterol molecules
- high-density lipoprotein (HDL) — "good" lipoprotein; removes lipids from cells
- apolipoprotein B — major component of LDL
- apolipoprotein A-1 — major component of HDL
- lipoprotein a — one of the most atherogenic lipoproteins.

Treatment

- Drug therapy: angiotensin-converting enzyme inhibitors, thrombolytics, diuretics, glycoprotein IIb/IIIa inhibitors, nitrates, and beta-adrenergic or calcium channel blockers; antiplatelet, antilipemic, and antihypertensive drugs
- Coronary artery bypass graft (CABG) surgery
- "Keyhole" or minimally invasive surgery, an alternative to traditional CABG
- Angioplasty and stent placement
- Atherectomy
- Lifestyle modifications to limit progression of CAD: stopping smoking, exercising regularly, maintaining ideal body weight, and eating a low-fat, low-sodium diet

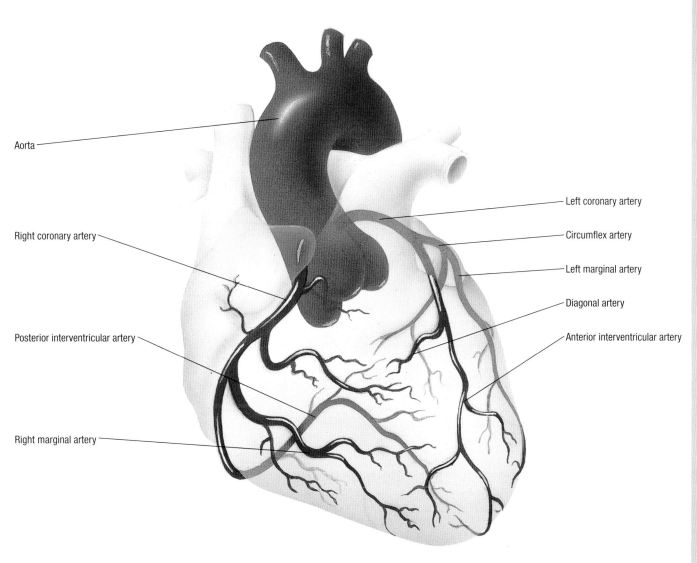

Aorta

Right coronary artery

Posterior interventricular artery

Right marginal artery

Left coronary artery

Circumflex artery

Left marginal artery

Diagonal artery

Anterior interventricular artery

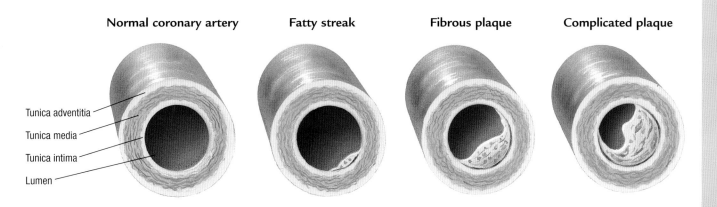

Normal coronary artery

Fatty streak

Fibrous plaque

Complicated plaque

Tunica adventitia

Tunica media

Tunica intima

Lumen

DEEP VEIN THROMBOSIS

An acute condition characterized by inflammation and thrombus formation, deep vein thrombosis (DVT) mainly refers to thrombosis in the deep veins of the legs. Without treatment, this disorder is typically progressive and can lead to potentially lethal pulmonary embolism. DVT commonly begins with localized inflammation alone (phlebitis), which rapidly provokes thrombus formation. Rarely, venous thrombosis develops without associated inflammation of the vein.

Causes

- Idiopathic
- Endothelial damage
- Accelerated blood clotting
- Reduced blood flow, stasis
- Virchow's triad

Predisposing Risk Factors

- Prolonged bed rest
- Trauma, especially hip fracture
- Surgery, especially hip, knee, or gynecologic surgery
- Childbirth
- Hormonal contraceptives such as estrogens
- Age over 40
- Obesity
- Cancer

Pathophysiology

A thrombus forms when an alteration in the epithelial lining causes platelet aggregation and consequent fibrin entrapment of red and white blood cells and additional platelets. Thrombus formation is more rapid in areas where blood flow is slower, because contact between platelets increases and thrombin accumulates. The rapidly expanding thrombus initiates a chemical inflammatory process in the vessel epithelium, which leads to fibrosis (narrowing of the blood vessel). The enlarging clot may occlude the vessel lumen partially or totally, or it may detach and embolize to lodge elsewhere in the systemic circulation.

COMPLICATIONS
- Pulmonary embolism
- Chronic venous insufficiency

Signs and Symptoms

- Vary with site and length of the affected vein (may produce no symptoms)
- Pain or tenderness
- Fever and chills
- Malaise
- Edema (unilateral edema is most common sign and may be only sign of DVT)
- Redness and warmth over the affected area
- Palpable vein
- Surface veins more visible
- Lymphadenitis

CLINICAL TIP
Some patients may display signs of inflammation.

Diagnostic Test Results

- Duplex Doppler ultrasonography reveals sluggish blood flow.
- Impedance plethysmography shows a difference in blood pressure between the arms and the legs.
- Impedance phlebography shows decreased blood flow.
- Coagulation studies reveal an elevated prothrombin time in the presence of a hypercoagulable state.
- Clotting factor deficiencies can be identified on blood work.
- CT scan is more accurate in identifying presence of DVT.

Treatment

The goals of treatment are to control thrombus development, prevent complications, relieve pain, and prevent recurrence of the disorder. Treatment includes:

- bed rest with elevation of the affected arm or leg
- warm, moist soaks over the affected area
- analgesics
- antiembolism stockings
- anticoagulants (initially, heparin; later, warfarin) — this is most important
- streptokinase
- simple ligation to vein plication, or clipping
- embolectomy and insertion of a vena caval umbrella or filter.

Deep veins of leg

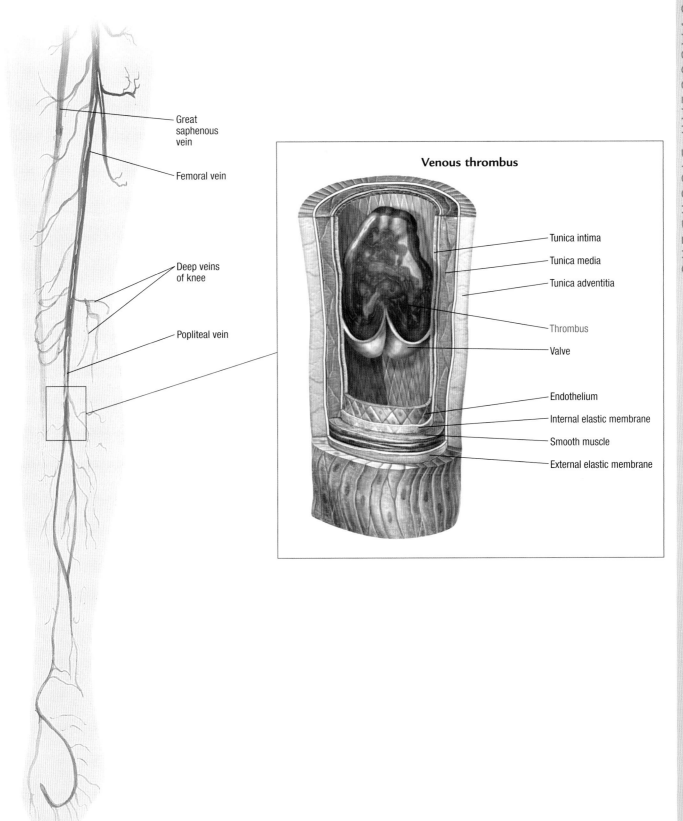

Great
saphenous
vein

Femoral vein

Deep veins
of knee

Popliteal vein

Venous thrombus

Tunica intima

Tunica media

Tunica adventitia

Thrombus

Valve

Endothelium

Internal elastic membrane

Smooth muscle

External elastic membrane

ENDOCARDITIS

Endocarditis, also known as *infective* or *bacterial endocarditis*, is an infection of the endocardium, heart valves, or cardiac prosthesis resulting from bacterial or fungal invasion.

Causes

- I.V. drug abuse
- Prosthetic heart valves
- Mitral valve prolapse
- Rheumatic heart disease

Other Predisposing Conditions

- Congenital abnormalities — coarctation of aorta and tetralogy of Fallot
- Subaortic and valvular aortic stenosis
- Ventricular septal defects
- Pulmonary stenosis
- Marfan syndrome
- Degenerative heart disease
- Syphilis
- Prior history of endocarditis
- Pregnancy
- Arteriovenous dialysis catheters

Native Valve Endocarditis (Non-I.V. Drug Abusers)

- Streptococci, especially *Streptococcus viridans*
- Staphylococci
- Enterococci
- Fungi (rare)

I.V. Drug Abusers

- *Staphylococcus aureus*
- Streptococci
- Enterococci
- Gram-negative bacilli
- Fungi

Prosthetic Valve Endocarditis (Within 60 Days of Insertion)

- Staphylococcal infection
- Gram-negative aerobic organisms
- Fungi
- Streptococci
- Enterococci
- Diphtheroids

Pathophysiology

In endocarditis, bacteremia — even transient bacteremia following dental or urogenital procedures — introduces the pathogen into the bloodstream. This infection causes fibrin and platelets to aggregate on the heart valve tissue and engulf circulating bacteria or fungi that flourish and form friable, wartlike vegetative growths on the valves, the endocardial lining of a heart chamber, or the epithelium of a blood vessel.

COMPLICATIONS

- Left-sided heart failure
- Valvular stenosis
- Myocardial erosion
- Vascular insufficiency
- Embolic events (CVA, arterial thrombosis) from embolism of vegetations

Signs and Symptoms

- Malaise, weakness, and fatigue
- Weight loss and anorexia
- Arthralgia
- Intermittent fever, night sweats, and chills
- Valvular insufficiency
- Loud, regurgitant murmur
- Suddenly changing murmur or new murmur in the presence of fever
- Splenic infarction — left upper quadrant pain radiating to left shoulder and abdominal rigidity
- Renal infarction — hematuria, pyuria, flank pain, and decreased urine output
- Cerebral infarction — hemiparesis, aphasia, and other neurologic deficits
- Pulmonary infarction — cough, pleuritic pain, pleural friction rub, dyspnea, and hemoptysis
- Peripheral vascular occlusion — numbness and tingling in an arm, leg, finger, or toe

Diagnostic Test Results

- Positive blood cultures identify the causative organism.

CLINICAL TIP

Three or more blood cultures in a 24- to 48-hour period (each from a separate venipuncture) identify the causative organism in up to 90% of patients. Blood cultures should be drawn from three different sites with at least 1 to 3 hours between each draw.

- Complete blood count shows normal or elevated white blood cell counts.
- Blood smear shows abnormal histiocytes (macrophages).
- Erythrocyte sedimentation rate is elevated.
- Anemia panel reveals normocytic, normochromic anemia.
- Urinalysis shows proteinuria and microscopic hematuria.
- Serum rheumatoid factor is positive in about one-half of all patients after endocarditis is present for 6 weeks.
- Echocardiography (particularly transesophageal) identifies valvular damage.
- Electrocardiogram shows atrial fibrillation or other arrhythmias.
- Chest X-ray shows the presence of pulmonic emboli.

Treatment

- Penicillin and an aminoglycoside, usually gentamicin

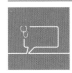

CLINICAL TIP

Any patient who's susceptible to endocarditis, such as those with valvular defects or another predisposing factor, should have prophylactic antibiotics prior to dental or other invasive procedures.

- Bed rest
- NSAIDs or acetaminophen for fever and aches
- Sufficient fluid intake
- Corrective surgery, if refractory heart failure develops or if damage to heart structures occurs
- Replacement of an infected prosthetic valve

TISSUE CHANGES IN ENDOCARDITIS

Normal heart wall

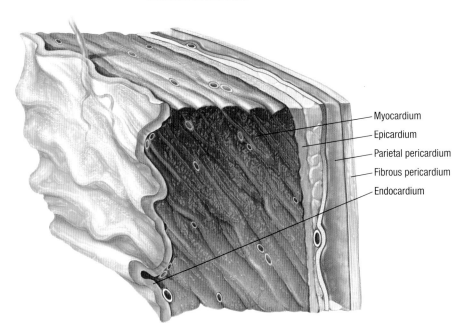

- Myocardium
- Epicardium
- Parietal pericardium
- Fibrous pericardium
- Endocardium

Endocarditis

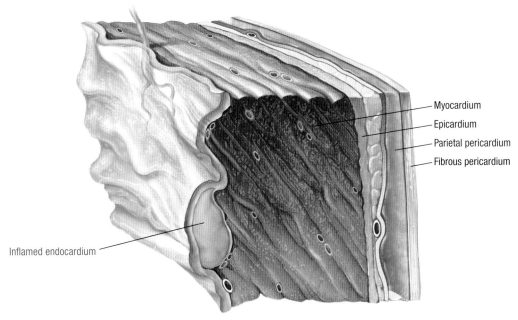

- Myocardium
- Epicardium
- Parietal pericardium
- Fibrous pericardium

Inflamed endocardium

HEART FAILURE

A syndrome rather than a disease, heart failure occurs when the heart can't pump enough blood to meet the metabolic needs of the body. Heart failure results in intravascular and interstitial volume overload and poor tissue perfusion.

Causes

Abnormal Cardiac Muscle Function

- Myocardial infarction (MI)
- Cardiomyopathy

Abnormal Left Ventricular Volume

- Valvular insufficiency
- High-output states: chronic anemia, arteriovenous fistula, thyrotoxicosis, pregnancy, septicemia, and hypervolemia

Abnormal Left Ventricular Pressure

- Hypertension
- Pulmonary hypertension
- Chronic obstructive pulmonary disease
- Aortic or pulmonic valve stenosis

Abnormal Left Ventricular Filling

- Mitral valve stenosis
- Tricuspid valve stenosis
- Constrictive pericarditis
- Atrial fibrillation
- Hypertension

Pathophysiology

Heart failure may be classified according to the side of the heart affected or by the cardiac cycle involved.

- *Left-sided heart failure:* decreased left ventricular contractile function. Cardiac output falls, and blood backs up into the left atrium and then into the lungs.
- *Right-sided heart failure:* ineffective right ventricular contractile function. Blood backs up into the right atrium and into the peripheral circulation.
- *Systolic dysfunction:* left ventricle can't pump enough blood out to the systemic circulation during systole; the ejection fraction falls. Blood backs up into the pulmonary circulation, pressure rises in the pulmonary venous system, and cardiac output falls.
- *Diastolic dysfunction:* left ventricle can't relax and fill during diastole. The stroke volume falls.

All causes of heart failure eventually reduce cardiac output and trigger compensatory mechanisms that improve cardiac output at the expense of increased ventricular work.

- Increased sympathetic activity enhances peripheral vascular resistance, contractility, heart rate, and venous return. It also restricts blood flow to the kidneys, causing them to secrete renin, which, in turn, converts angiotensinogen to angiotensin I to angiotensin II — a potent vasoconstrictor.
- Angiotensin causes the adrenal cortex to release aldosterone, leading to sodium and water retention and an increase in circulating blood volume. If the renal mechanism persists unchecked, it can aggravate heart failure.

- The increase in end-diastolic ventricular volume causes increased stroke work and volume during contraction, stretching cardiac muscle fibers. The muscle becomes stretched beyond optimum limits and contractility declines.

In heart failure, the body produces counterregulatory substances (prostaglandins, atrial natriuretic factor, and brain natriuretic peptide [BNP]) to reduce the negative effects of volume overload and vasoconstriction.

When blood volume increases in the ventricles, the heart makes these compensations:

- *Short-term:* as the end-diastolic fiber length increases, the ventricular muscle dilates and increases the force of contraction
- *Long-term:* ventricular hypertrophy increases the heart muscles' ability to contract and push its volume of blood into the circulation.

With heart failure, compensation may occur for a long time before signs and symptoms develop.

COMPLICATIONS
- Pulmonary edema
- MI
- Decreased perfusion to major organs

Signs and Symptoms

Left-Sided Heart Failure

- Dyspnea, orthopnea, and paroxysmal nocturnal dyspnea
- Nonproductive cough and crackles
- Hemoptysis
- Tachycardia; S_3 and S_4 heart sounds
- Cool, pale skin

Right-Sided Heart Failure

- Jugular vein distention
- Hepatojugular reflux and hepatomegaly
- Right upper quadrant pain
- Anorexia, fullness, and nausea
- Weight gain, edema, ascites, or anasarca
- Dyspnea, orthopnea, and paroxysmal nocturnal dyspnea

Diagnostic Test Results

- Chest X-rays show increased pulmonary vascular markings, interstitial edema, or pleural effusion and cardiomegaly.
- ECG shows hypertrophy, ischemic changes, or infarction and may also reveal tachycardia and extrasystoles.
- BNP assay, a blood test, may show elevated levels.
- Echocardiography reveals left ventricular hypertrophy, dilation, and abnormal contractility. Echo can also show valvular abnormalities and inability to relax (diastolic dysfunction).
- Pulmonary artery monitoring typically shows elevated pulmonary artery and pulmonary artery wedge pressures (PAWP), left ventricular end-diastolic pressure in left-sided failure, and right atrial pressure or CVP in right-sided failure.

- Radionuclide ventriculography reveals an ejection fraction less than 40%; in diastolic dysfunction, the ejection fraction may be normal.

Treatment

- Treatment of the underlying cause, if known
- Angiotensin-converting enzyme inhibitors or ARBs (for patients with left ventricular dysfunction), specific beta-adrenergic blockers (for patients with left ventricular dysfunction), diuretics, digoxin, nitrates, morphine, or oxygen
- Dobutamine, milrinone, and nesiritide (for refractory HF)
- Lifestyle modifications to reduce risk factors
- Coronary artery bypass surgery (if caused by CAD), angioplasty, or heart transplantation
- Placement of prophylactic ICD (with or without Bivent pacing) for patients with low EF

TYPES OF HEART FAILURE

Right-sided heart failure

Ineffective right ventricular contractility

⬇

Failure of right ventricular pumping ability

⬇

Decreased cardiac output to lungs

⬇

Blood backup into right atrium and peripheral circulation

⬇

Weight gain, peripheral edema, engorgement of liver and other organs

Left-sided heart failure

Ineffective left ventricular contractility

⬇

Failure of left ventricular pumping ability

⬇

Decreased cardiac output to body

⬇

Blood backup into left atrium and lungs

⬇

Pulmonary congestion, dyspnea, activity intolerance

⬇

Pulmonary edema and right-sided heart failure

NORMAL CARDIAC CIRCULATION

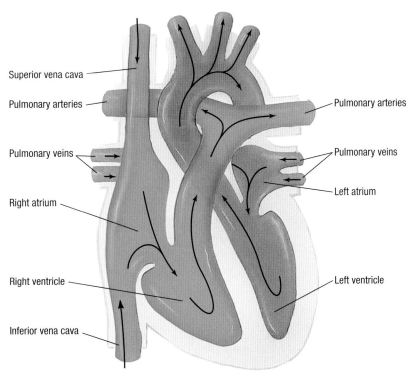

Superior vena cava

Pulmonary arteries

Pulmonary veins

Right atrium

Right ventricle

Inferior vena cava

Pulmonary arteries

Pulmonary veins

Left atrium

Left ventricle

HYPERTENSION

Hypertension, an elevation in diastolic or systolic blood pressure, occurs as two major types: *primary* (idiopathic), which is the most common, and *secondary*, which results from renal disease or another identifiable cause. Malignant hypertension is a severe, fulminant form of either type.

Causes

Risk Factors for Primary Hypertension

- Family history
- Advancing age
- Race (most common in blacks)
- Obesity
- Tobacco use
- High intake of sodium or saturated fat
- Excessive alcohol consumption
- Sedentary lifestyle and stress

Causes of Secondary Hypertension

- Excess renin
- Mineral deficiencies (calcium, potassium, and magnesium)
- Diabetes mellitus
- Coarctation of the aorta
- Renal artery stenosis or parenchymal disease
- Brain tumor, quadriplegia, and head injury
- Pheochromocytoma, Cushing's syndrome, and hyperaldosteronism
- Thyroid, pituitary, or parathyroid dysfunction
- Hormonal contraceptives, cocaine, epoetin alfa, sympathetic stimulants, monoamine oxidase inhibitors taken with tyramine, estrogen replacement therapy, and nonsteroidal anti-inflammatory drugs
- Pregnancy

Pathophysiology

Arterial blood pressure is a product of total peripheral resistance and cardiac output. Cardiac output is increased by conditions that increase heart rate or stroke volume, or both. Peripheral resistance is increased by factors that increase blood viscosity or reduce the lumen size of vessels.

Several mechanisms may lead to hypertension, including:

Cause of primary hypertension is largely unknown but several mechanisms that may lead to HTN are identified below:

- changes in the arteriolar bed causing increased peripheral vascular resistance
- abnormally increased tone in the sympathetic nervous system that originates in the vasomotor system centers, causing increased peripheral vascular resistance
- increased blood volume resulting from renal or hormonal dysfunction
- arteriolar thickening caused by genetic factors, leading to increased peripheral vascular resistance
- abnormal renin release, resulting in the formation of angiotensin II and aldosterone, which constricts the arteriole and increases blood volume.

Prolonged hypertension increases the workload of the heart as resistance to left ventricular ejection increases. To increase contractile force, the left ventricle hypertrophies, raising the oxygen demand and workload of the heart.

The pathophysiology of secondary hypertension is related to the underlying disease or medication.

COMPLICATIONS
- Stroke
- Myocardial infarction
- Heart failure
- Arrhythmias
- Retinopathy
- Encephalopathy
- Renal failure

Signs and Symptoms

- Generally produces no symptoms
- Serial blood pressure readings classify hypertension:
  - Prehypertension: Systolic blood pressure greater than 120 mm Hg but less than 140 mm Hg or diastolic blood pressure greater than 80 mm Hg but less than 90 mm Hg
  - Stage 1 hypertension: Systolic blood pressure greater than 139 mm Hg but less than 160 mm Hg or diastolic blood pressure greater than 89 mm Hg but less than 100 mm Hg
  - Stage 2 hypertension: Systolic blood pressure greater than 159 mm Hg or diastolic blood pressure greater than 99 mm Hg

Treatment for HTN should begin based on the following guidelines (JNC-8 guidelines):

General population greater than 140/90 mm Hg

Population greater than 60 years old greater than 150/90 mm Hg

Diabetics regardless of age greater than 140/90 mm Hg

- Occipital headache
- Epistaxis possibly due to vascular involvement
- Bruits (renal artery bruits present if renal artery stenosis is the cause)
- Dizziness, confusion, and fatigue
- Blurry vision
- Nocturia
- Edema

Diagnostic Test Results

- Serial blood pressure measurements show elevation. Must be elevated on two separate visits for diagnosis of HTN.
- Urinalysis shows protein, casts, red blood cells, or white blood cells, suggesting renal disease; presence of catecholamines associated with pheochromocytoma; or glucose, suggesting diabetes.
- Blood chemistry reveals elevated blood urea nitrogen and serum creatinine levels suggestive of renal disease or hypokalemia indicating adrenal dysfunction.
- Excretory urography may reveal renal atrophy, indicating chronic renal disease.
- ECG detects left ventricular hypertrophy or ischemia.
- Chest X-rays show cardiomegaly.
- Echocardiography reveals left ventricular hypertrophy, which indicates target organ damage.
- Renal ultrasound identifies renal artery stenosis.

Treatment

Goal is to avoid target organ damage and complications.

- Treatment of underlying cause if secondary HTN
- Lifestyle modifications to reduce risk factors

- Diuretics
- Angiotensin-converting enzyme inhibitors
- Alpha-receptor agonists
- Beta-adrenergic blockers

BLOOD VESSEL DAMAGE IN HYPERTENSION

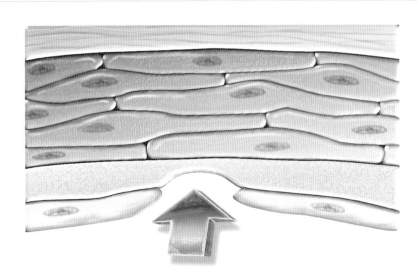

Increased intra-arterial pressure damages the endothelium.

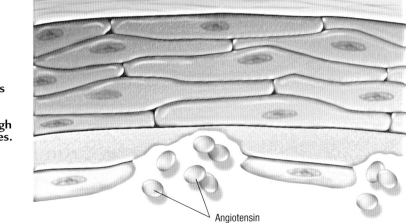

Angiotensin II induces endothelial wall contraction, allowing plasma to leak through interendothelial spaces.

Angiotensin

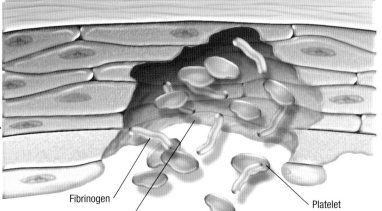

Plasma constituents deposited in the vessel wall cause medial necrosis.

Fibrinogen

Medial necrosis

Platelet

MITRAL VALVE PROLAPSE

Mitral valve prolapse is also called *systolic click-murmur syndrome* and *floppy mitral valve syndrome*. It's probably a congenital abnormality.

Causes

- Autosomal dominant inheritance
- Inherited connective tissue disorders, such as Marfan syndrome, Ehlers-Danlos syndrome, and osteogenesis imperfecta
- Genetic or environmental interruption of valve development during week 5 or 6 of gestation

Pathophysiology

The cusps of the mitral valve are enlarged, thickened, and scalloped, possibly secondary to collagen abnormalities. The chordae tendineae may be longer than usual, allowing the cusps to stretch upward.

COMPLICATIONS

- Mitral regurgitation
- Infective endocarditis
- Arrhythmias

Signs and Symptoms

- Commonly produces no symptoms
- Late systolic regurgitant murmur
- Midsystolic click
- Palpitations, arrhythmias, and tachycardia
- Light-headedness or syncope
- Fatigue, especially in the morning; lethargy; weakness
- Dyspnea and hyperventilation
- Chest tightness and atypical chest pain
- Anxiety, panic attacks, and depression

CLINICAL TIP

The high incidence of mitral valve prolapse (3% to 8% of adults) suggests that it may be a normal variant. It occurs more often in women than in men. Although severe sequelae may occur (such as ruptured chordae tendineae, ventricular failure, emboli, bacterial endocarditis, and sudden death), mortality and morbidity are low. Most affected persons experience no physical limitations. The psychological effects of the diagnosis may be more disabling than the disease process itself.

Diagnostic Test Results

- Echocardiography reveals mitral valve prolapse with or without mitral insufficiency.
- ECG (resting and exercise) is usually normal but may show atrial or ventricular arrhythmia.
- Holter monitor detects arrhythmias.

Treatment

- Corresponds to degree of mitral regurgitation
- In the presence of regurgitation, antibiotic prophylaxis before invasive procedures to prevent infective endocarditis (considered moderate risk for SBE)
- Beta-adrenergic blockers
- Measures to prevent hypovolemia, such as avoidance of diuretics, because hypervolemia can decrease ventricular volume, thereby increasing stress on the prolapsed mitral valve
- Surgical repair or valve replacement with severe mitral regurgitation

Cross section of left ventricle

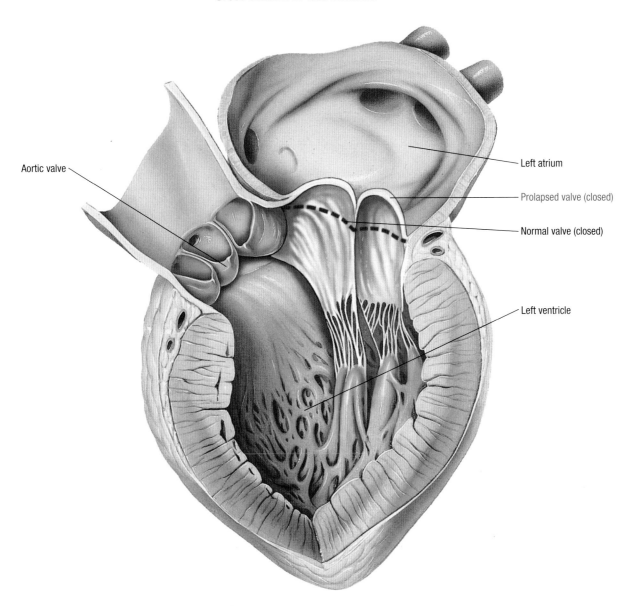

Aortic valve

Left atrium

Prolapsed valve (closed)

Normal valve (closed)

Left ventricle

MYOCARDIAL INFARCTION

In MI, a form of acute coronary syndrome, reduced blood flow through one or more coronary arteries initiates myocardial ischemia and necrosis. (See also "Coronary artery disease," page 60.)

Causes

- Thrombosis
- Coronary artery stenosis or spasm

Predisposing Risk Factors

- Family history of heart disease
- Atherosclerosis, hypertension, diabetes mellitus, and obesity
- Elevated serum triglyceride, total cholesterol, and LDL levels
- Excessive intake of saturated fats, carbohydrates, or salt
- Sedentary lifestyle and tobacco smoking
- Drug use, especially cocaine and amphetamines

Pathophysiology

If coronary artery occlusion causes prolonged ischemia, lasting longer than 30 to 45 minutes, irreversible myocardial cell damage and muscle death occur. Nonocclusive coronary atheromas can rupture and cause thrombus or emboli causing complete occlusion of coronary artery and infarct.

Occlusion of the circumflex branch of the left coronary artery causes a lateral wall infarction; occlusion of the anterior descending branch of the left coronary artery, an anterior wall infarction. True posterior or inferior wall infarctions generally result from occlusion of the right coronary artery or one of its branches.

Right ventricular infarctions can also result from right coronary artery occlusion, can accompany inferior infarctions, and may cause right-sided heart failure. In ST-elevation (transmural) MI, tissue damage extends through all myocardial layers; in non–ST-elevation (subendocardial) MI, damage occurs only in the innermost and, possibly, the middle layers.

All infarcts have a central area of necrosis surrounded by an area of potentially viable hypoxic injury, which may be salvaged if circulation is restored or may progress to necrosis. The zone of injury is surrounded by viable ischemic tissue.

The infarcted myocardial cells release cardiac enzymes and proteins. Within 24 hours, the infarcted muscle becomes edematous and cyanotic. During the next several days, leukocytes infiltrate the necrotic area and begin to remove necrotic cells, thinning the ventricular wall. Scar formation begins by the 3rd week after MI; by the 6th week, scar tissue is well established.

The scar tissue that forms on the necrotic area inhibits contractility. Compensatory mechanisms try to maintain cardiac output. Ventricular dilation may also occur in a process called *remodeling*. MI may cause reduced contractility with abnormal wall motion, altered left ventricular compliance, reduced stroke volume, reduced ejection fraction, and elevated left ventricular end-diastolic pressure.

COMPLICATIONS
- Arrhythmias
- Cardiogenic shock
- Heart failure
- Valve problems

Signs and Symptoms

- Persistent, crushing substernal chest pain that may radiate to the left arm, jaw, neck, or shoulder blades
- Cool extremities, perspiration, anxiety, and restlessness
- Shortness of breath
- Fatigue and weakness
- Nausea and vomiting
- Jugular vein distention

CLINICAL TIP
Signs and symptoms of MI in women may be different or less noticeable than MI in men and may include abdominal pain or "heartburn," back pain, jaw or teeth discomfort, shortness of breath, clammy skin, light-headedness, and unusual or unexplained fatigue.

Diagnostic Test Results

- Serial 12-lead ECG may reveal ST-segment depression or elevation. An ECG also identifies the location of MI, arrhythmias, hypertrophy, and pericarditis. (Non–Q-wave MIs may not have any ECG changes.)
- Serial cardiac enzymes and proteins show a characteristic rise and fall — specifically, CK-MB, the proteins troponin T and I, and myoglobin. Troponin is the most sensitive to cardiac damage.
- Complete blood count and other blood tests show elevated white blood cell count, C-reactive protein level, and erythrocyte sedimentation rate due to inflammation.
- Blood chemistry shows increased glucose levels following the release of catecholamines.
- Echocardiography shows ventricular wall motion abnormalities and detects septal or papillary muscle rupture.
- Chest X-rays show left-sided heart failure or cardiomegaly.
- Nuclear imaging scanning identifies areas of infarction and viable muscle cells.
- Cardiac catheterization identifies the involved coronary artery and provides information on ventricular function and volumes within the heart.

Treatment

Goal of treatment is to intervene to prevent permanent damage to myocardium. Time is muscle.

- Assessment of patients with chest pain in the emergency department within 10 minutes of symptom onset
- Oxygen
- Nitroglycerin
- Morphine
- Aspirin
- Continuous cardiac monitoring
- I.V. fibrinolytic therapy if primary coronary intervention not available
- Glycoprotein IIb/IIIa receptor blockers
- I.V. heparin

- Percutaneous transluminal coronary angioplasty with or without stent placement
- Atropine, lidocaine, transcutaneous pacing patches or a transvenous pacemaker, a defibrillator, and epinephrine
- Beta-adrenergic blockers, angiotensin-converting enzyme inhibitors, and magnesium sulfate

TISSUE DESTRUCTION IN MYOCARDIAL INFARCTION

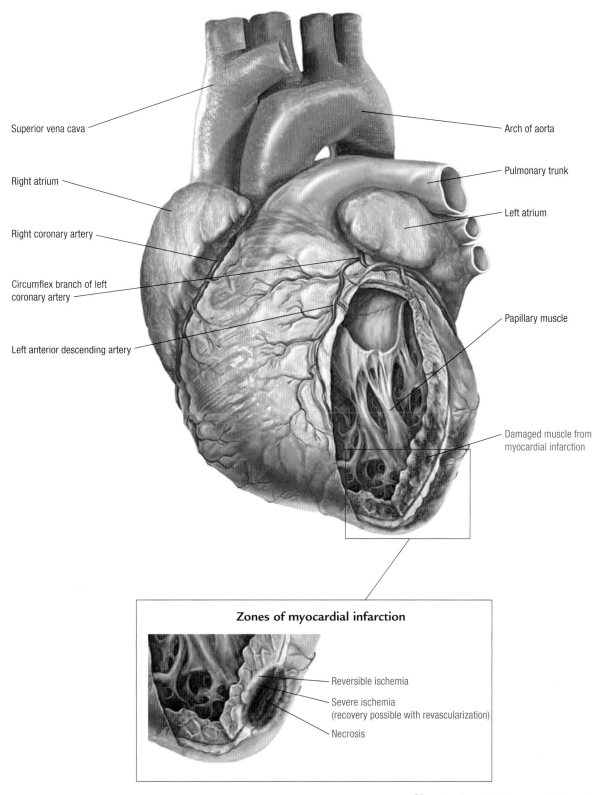

Superior vena cava

Right atrium

Right coronary artery

Circumflex branch of left coronary artery

Left anterior descending artery

Arch of aorta

Pulmonary trunk

Left atrium

Papillary muscle

Damaged muscle from myocardial infarction

Zones of myocardial infarction

Reversible ischemia

Severe ischemia (recovery possible with revascularization)

Necrosis

MYOCARDITIS

Myocarditis is focal or diffuse inflammation of the cardiac muscle (myocardium). It may be acute or chronic and can occur at any age. In many cases, myocarditis causes neither specific cardiovascular symptoms nor electrocardiogram abnormalities, and recovery is usually spontaneous without residual defects.

Causes

- Infections: viral, bacterial, parasitic-protozoan, fungal, or helminthic (such as trichinosis)
- Hypersensitive immune reactions, such as acute rheumatic fever or postcardiotomy syndrome
- Radiation therapy or chemotherapeutic agents
- Toxins, such as lead, chemicals, or cocaine
- Chronic alcoholism
- Systemic autoimmune disorders, such as systemic lupus erythematosus and sarcoidosis

Pathophysiology

Damage to the myocardium occurs when an infectious organism triggers an autoimmune, cellular, or humoral reaction; noninfectious causes can lead to toxic inflammation. In either case, the resulting inflammation may lead to hypertrophy, fibrosis, and inflammatory changes of the myocardium and conduction system. The heart muscle weakens, and contractility is reduced. The heart muscle becomes flabby and dilated, and pinpoint hemorrhages may develop.

COMPLICATIONS
- Left-sided heart failure (occasionally)
- Cardiomyopathy (rare)
- Recurrence of myocarditis
- Chronic valvulitis
- Arrhythmias
- Thromboembolism

Signs and Symptoms

- Fatigue, dyspnea, and palpitations
- Fever
- Chest pain or mild, continuous pressure or soreness in the chest
- Tachycardia and S_3 and S_4 gallops
- Murmur of mitral insufficiency and pericardial friction rub
- Right-sided and left-sided heart failure (jugular vein distention, dyspnea, edema, pulmonary congestion, persistent fever with resting or exertional tachycardia disproportionate to the degree of fever, and supraventricular and ventricular arrhythmias)

CLINICAL TIP
To auscultate for a pericardial friction rub, have the patient sit upright, lean forward, and exhale. Listen over the third intercostal space on the left side of the chest. A pericardial rub has a scratchy, rubbing quality. If you suspect a rub and have difficulty hearing one, have the patient hold his breath.

Diagnostic Test Results

- Blood testing shows elevated levels of creatine kinase (CK), CK-MB, troponin I, troponin T, aspartate aminotransferase, and lactate dehydrogenase. Also, inflammation and infection cause elevated white blood cell count and erythrocyte sedimentation rate.
- Antibody titers are elevated, such as antistreptolysin-O titer, in rheumatic fever.
- Electrocardiogram illustrates diffuse ST-segment and T-wave abnormalities, conduction defects (prolonged PR interval, bundle-branch block, or complete heart block), supraventricular arrhythmias, and ventricular extrasystoles.
- Chest X-rays show an enlarged heart and pulmonary vascular congestion.
- Echocardiography demonstrates some left ventricular dysfunction.
- Radionuclide scanning identifies inflammatory and necrotic changes characteristic of myocarditis.
- Laboratory cultures of stool, throat, and other body fluids identify bacterial or viral causes of infection.
- Endomyocardial biopsy shows damaged myocardial tissue and inflammation.

Treatment

- No treatment for benign self-limiting disease
- Antibiotics
- Antipyretics
- Restricted activity
- Supplemental oxygen therapy
- Sodium restriction and diuretics
- Angiotensin-converting enzyme inhibitors
- Beta-adrenergic blockers
- Digoxin
- Antiarrhythmic drugs, such as quinidine or procainamide
- Temporary pacemaker
- Anticoagulants
- Corticosteroids and immunosuppressants
- Cardiac assist devices or heart transplantation

Normal heart wall

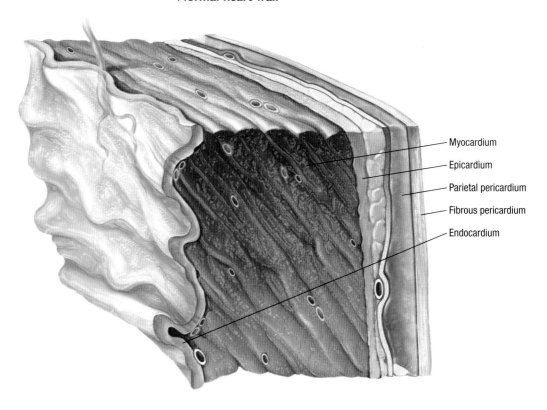

Myocardium
Epicardium
Parietal pericardium
Fibrous pericardium
Endocardium

Myocarditis

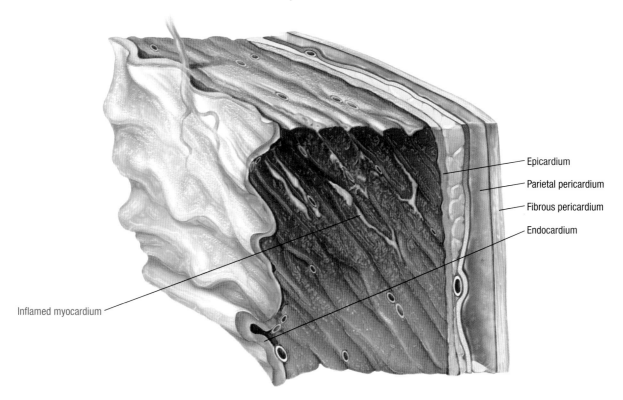

Epicardium
Parietal pericardium
Fibrous pericardium
Endocardium

Inflamed myocardium

PERICARDITIS

Pericarditis is inflammation of the pericardium — the fibro-serous sac that envelops, supports, and protects the heart. Acute pericarditis can be fibrinous or effusive, with purulent, serous, or hemorrhagic exudate. Chronic constrictive pericarditis is characterized by dense fibrous pericardial thickening. The prognosis depends on the underlying cause but is generally good in acute pericarditis, unless constriction occurs.

Causes

- Bacterial, fungal, or viral infection
- Neoplasm
- High-dose radiation to the chest
- Uremia
- Hypersensitivity or autoimmune disease
- Previous cardiac injury, such as MI, trauma, or surgery (postcardiotomy syndrome)
- Drugs, such as hydralazine or procainamide
- Idiopathic factors
- Aortic aneurysm
- Myxedema

AGE ALERT
Pericarditis most commonly affects men ages 20 to 50, generally following respiratory illness. It can also occur in children.

Pathophysiology

Pericardial tissue damaged by bacteria or other substances releases chemical mediators of inflammation (prostaglandins, histamines, bradykinins, and serotonin) into the surrounding tissue, thereby initiating the inflammatory process. Friction occurs as the inflamed pericardial layers rub against each other. Histamines and other chemical mediators dilate vessels and increase vessel permeability. Vessel walls then leak fluids and protein (including fibrinogen) into tissues, causing extracellular edema. Macrophages already present in the tissue begin to phagocytize the invading bacteria and are joined by neutrophils and monocytes. After several days, the area fills with an exudate composed of necrotic tissue and dead and dying bacteria, neutrophils, and macrophages. If the cause of pericarditis isn't infection, the exudate may be serous (as with autoimmune disease) or hemorrhagic (as seen with trauma or surgery). Eventually, the contents of the cavity autolyze and are gradually reabsorbed into healthy tissue.

Chronic constrictive pericarditis develops if the chronic or recurrent pericarditis makes the pericardium thick and stiff, encasing the heart in a stiff shell and preventing proper filling during diastole. Consequently, left- and right-side filling pressures rise as stroke volume and cardiac output fall.

COMPLICATIONS
- Pericardial effusion
- Cardiac tamponade
- Shock
- Cardiovascular collapse

Signs and Symptoms

- Pericardial friction rub
- Sharp and (commonly) sudden pain, usually starting over the sternum and radiating to the neck, shoulders, back, and arms
- Shallow, rapid respirations
- Mild fever
- Dyspnea, orthopnea, and tachycardia
- Heart failure
- Muffled, distant heart sounds (if effusion present)
- Pallor, clammy skin, hypotension, pulsus paradoxus, jugular vein distention — indicates tamponade
- Possible progression to cardiovascular collapse
- Fluid retention, ascites, and hepatomegaly
- Pericardial knock in early diastole along the left sternal border produced by restricted ventricular filling
- Kussmaul's sign (increased jugular vein distention on inspiration caused by restricted right-sided filling)

CLINICAL TIP
The pain in pericarditis is commonly pleuritic, increasing with deep inspiration and decreasing when the patient sits up and leans forward, pulling the heart away from the diaphragmatic pleurae of the lungs.

Diagnostic Test Results

- Twelve-lead ECG reveals diffuse ST-segment elevation in the limb leads and most precordial leads that reflect the inflammatory process. Downsloping PR segments and upright T waves are present in most leads. QRS segments may be diminished when pericardial effusion exists. Arrhythmias, such as atrial fibrillation and sinus arrhythmias, may occur. In chronic constrictive pericarditis, there may be low-voltage QRS complexes, T-wave inversion or flattening, and P mitral (wide P waves) in leads I, II, and V_6.
- Blood testing reveals an elevated erythrocyte sedimentation rate as a result of the inflammatory process and a normal or elevated white blood cell count, especially in infectious pericarditis. C-reactive protein may be elevated.
- Blood cultures identify an infectious cause.
- Antistreptolysin-O titers are positive if pericarditis is caused by rheumatic fever.
- Purified protein derivative skin tests are positive if pericarditis is caused by tuberculosis.
- Echocardiography shows an echo-free space between the ventricular wall and the pericardium and reduced pumping action of the heart.
- Chest X-rays show an enlarged cardiac silhouette with a water bottle shape caused by fluid accumulation if pleural effusion is present.
- Chest or heart magnetic resonance imaging shows enlargement of the heart and signs of inflammation.

Treatment

- Bed rest as long as fever and pain persist
- Treatment of the underlying cause, if it can be identified

- Nonsteroidal anti-inflammatory drugs and corticosteroids
- Antibacterial, antifungal, or antiviral therapy
- Partial or total pericardectomy
- Diuretics
- Pericardiocentesis

TISSUE CHANGES IN PERICARDITIS

Normal heart wall

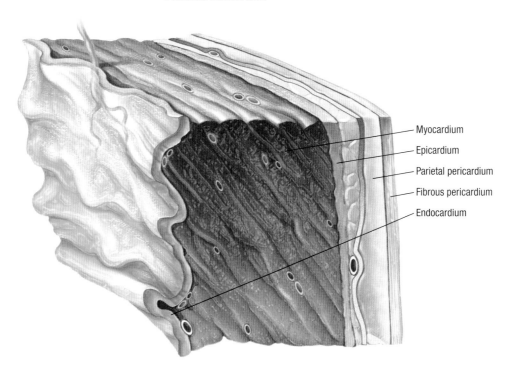

Myocardium
Epicardium
Parietal pericardium
Fibrous pericardium
Endocardium

Pericarditis

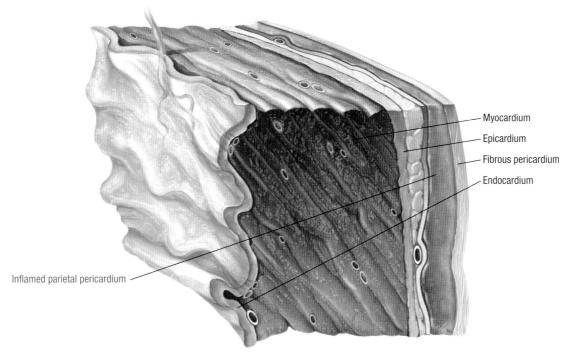

Myocardium
Epicardium
Fibrous pericardium
Endocardium

Inflamed parietal pericardium

Chapter 6 • Cardiovascular Disorders **77**

RAYNAUD'S DISEASE

Raynaud's disease is one of several primary disorders characterized by episodic spasms of the small peripheral arteries and arterioles, precipitated by exposure to cold or stress. This condition occurs bilaterally and usually affects the hands or, less often, the feet. It's benign, requires no specific treatment, and has no serious sequelae. Raynaud's *phenomenon*, however, is secondary to any of several connective disorders — such as scleroderma, systemic lupus erythematosus, or polymyositis — and progresses to ischemia, gangrene, and amputation. Distinguishing between the two disorders is difficult because some patients experience mild symptoms of Raynaud's disease for several years and then develop overt connective tissue disease, especially scleroderma.

AGE ALERT
Raynaud's disease is most prevalent in females, particularly between puberty and age 40.

Causes

Raynaud's Disease

- Unknown; family history is a risk factor

Raynaud's Phenomenon

- Connective tissue disorders, such as scleroderma, rheumatoid arthritis, systemic lupus erythematosus, or polymyositis
- Pulmonary hypertension
- Thoracic outlet syndrome
- Arterial occlusive disease
- Myxedema
- Trauma
- Serum sickness
- Exposure to heavy metals
- Long-term exposure to cold, vibrating machinery (such as operating a jackhammer), or pressure to the fingertips (as in typists and pianists)

Pathophysiology

Raynaud's disease is a syndrome of episodic constriction of the arterioles and arteries of the extremities, resulting in pallor and cyanosis of the fingers and toes. Several mechanisms may account for the reduced digital blood flow, including:

- intrinsic vascular wall hyperactivity to cold
- increased vasomotor tone due to sympathetic stimulation

- antigen-antibody immune response (most likely because abnormal immunologic test results accompany Raynaud's phenomenon).

COMPLICATIONS
- Ischemia
- Gangrene
- Amputation

Signs and Symptoms

- Bilateral blanching (pallor) of the fingers after exposure to cold or stress:
  - Vasoconstriction or vasospasm reduces blood flow.
  - Cyanosis caused by increased oxygen extraction results from sluggish blood flow.
  - Spasm resolves, and fingers turn red (rubor) as blood rushes back into the arterioles.
- Cold and numbness
- Throbbing, aching pain, swelling, and tingling
- Trophic changes (as a result of ischemia), such as sclerodactyly, ulcerations, or chronic paronychia

Diagnostic Test Results

- Antinuclear antibody (ANA) titer identifies autoimmune disease as an underlying cause of Raynaud's phenomenon; further tests must be performed if the ANA titer is positive.
- Doppler ultrasonography shows reduced blood flow if the symptoms result from arterial occlusive disease.

Treatment

- Avoiding triggers, such as cold, and mechanical or chemical injury
- Smoking cessation and avoidance of decongestants and caffeine to reduce vasoconstriction
- Calcium channel blockers, such as nifedipine, diltiazem, and nicardipine
- Alpha-adrenergic blockers, such as phenoxybenzamine or reserpine
- Biofeedback and relaxation exercises to reduce stress and improve circulation
- Sympathectomy or amputation

Pallor due to decreased or absent blood flow

Cyanosis due to capillary dilation

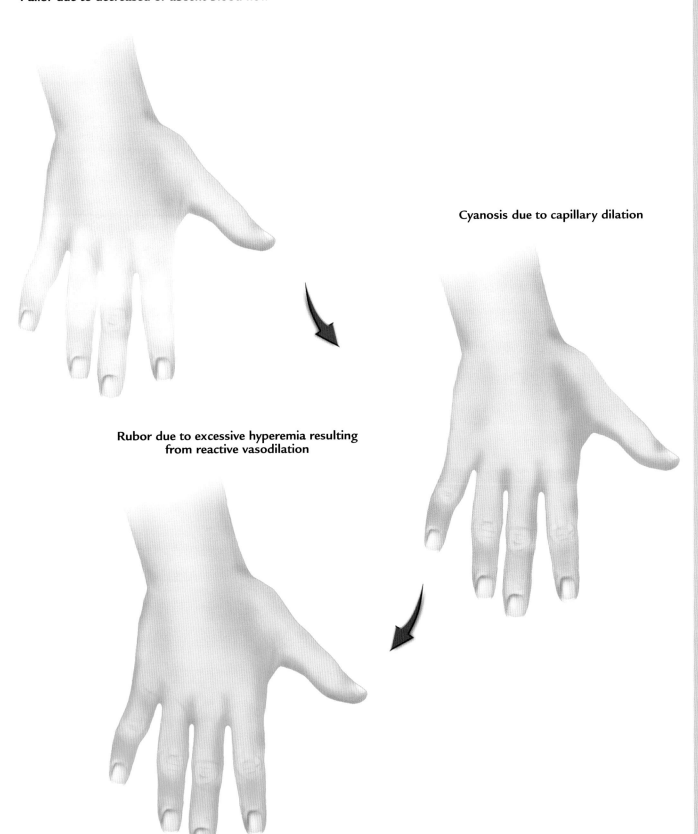

Rubor due to excessive hyperemia resulting from reactive vasodilation

RHEUMATIC HEART DISEASE

A systemic inflammatory disease of childhood, acute rheumatic fever develops after infection of the upper respiratory tract with group A beta-hemolytic streptococci. It mainly involves the heart, joints, central nervous system, skin, and subcutaneous tissues and commonly recurs. Rheumatic heart disease refers to the cardiac manifestations of rheumatic fever and includes pancarditis during the early acute phase and chronic valvular disease later. Cardiac involvement develops in up to 50% of patients.

Rheumatic fever tends to run in families, lending support to the existence of genetic predisposition. Environmental factors also seem to be significant in the development of the disorder.

Causes

Rheumatic fever is caused by group A beta-hemolytic streptococcal pharyngitis.

Rheumatic fever appears to be a hypersensitivity reaction to a group A beta-hemolytic streptococcal infection. Because few persons (3%) with streptococcal infections contract rheumatic fever, altered host resistance must be involved in its development or recurrence.

Pathophysiology

The antigens of group A streptococci bind to receptors in the heart, muscle, brain, and synovial joints, causing an autoimmune response. Because the antigens of the streptococcus are similar to some antigens of the body's own cells, antibodies may attack healthy body cells.

Carditis may affect the endocardium, myocardium, or pericardium during the early acute phase.

COMPLICATIONS
- Chronic valvular disease
- Pericarditis
- Pericardial effusion

Signs and Symptoms

- Polyarthritis or migratory joint pain
- Erythema marginatum
- Subcutaneous nodules
- Chorea
- Streptococcal infection a few days to 6 weeks before onset of symptoms
- Fever
- New or worsening mitral or aortic murmur
- Pericardial friction rub
- Chest pain, commonly pleuritic
- Dyspnea, tachypnea, nonproductive cough, bibasilar crackles, and edema

Diagnostic Test Results

- During the acute phase, complete blood count reveals an elevated white blood cell count and an elevated erythrocyte sedimentation rate.
- Hemoglobin and hematocrit are decreased because of suppressed erythropoiesis during inflammation.
- C-reactive protein is positive, especially during the acute phase.

- Cardiac enzyme levels are increased in severe carditis.
- Antistreptolysin-O titer is elevated in 95% of patients within 2 months of onset.
- Throat cultures show the presence of group A beta-hemolytic streptococci; however, they usually occur in small numbers.
- ECG shows a prolonged PR interval.
- Chest X-rays show normal heart size or cardiomegaly, pericardial effusion, or heart failure.
- Echocardiography detects valvular damage and pericardial effusion, measures chamber size, and provides information on ventricular function.
- Cardiac catheterization provides information on valvular damage and left ventricular function.

CLINICAL TIP
Jones Criteria for diagnosis require either two major criteria or one major criterion and two minor, plus evidence of a previous group A streptococcal infection.

Major Criteria

- Carditis
- Migratory joint pain
- Sydenham's chorea
- Subcutaneous nodules, usually near tendons or bony prominences of joints, especially the elbows, knuckles, wrists, and knees
- Erythema marginatum

Minor Criteria

- Fever
- Arthralgia
- Elevated acute phase reactants
- Prolonged PR interval

Treatment

- Prompt treatment of all group A beta-hemolytic streptococcal pharyngitis with oral penicillin V or I.M. benzathine penicillin G; erythromycin for patients with penicillin hypersensitivity
- Salicylates
- Corticosteroids
- Strict bed rest for about 5 weeks
- Sodium restriction, angiotensin-converting enzyme inhibitors, digoxin, and diuretics
- Corrective surgery, such as commissurotomy, valvuloplasty, or valve replacement for severe mitral or aortic valvular dysfunction that causes persistent heart failure
- Secondary prevention of rheumatic fever, which begins after the acute phase subsides:
  - monthly I.M. injections of penicillin G benzathine or daily doses of oral penicillin V or sulfadiazine
  - continued treatment, usually for at least 5 years or until age 21, whichever is longer
- Prophylactic antibiotics for dental work and other invasive or surgical procedures (in the presence of valve disorders only. Rheumatic fever without valve disease does increase the risk of SBE beyond the general population

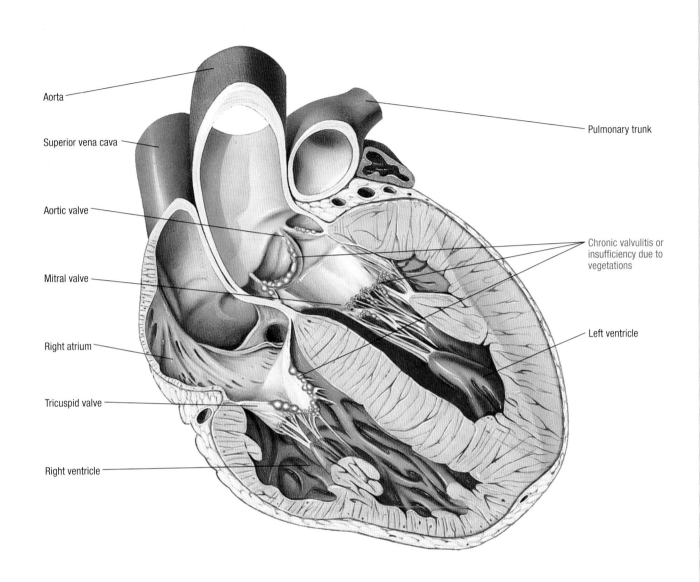

Aorta

Superior vena cava

Aortic valve

Mitral valve

Right atrium

Tricuspid valve

Right ventricle

Pulmonary trunk

Chronic valvulitis or insufficiency due to vegetations

Left ventricle

SHOCK

Shock is a clinical syndrome that leads to reduced perfusion of tissues and organs and organ failure. Shock can be classified into three categories: distributive (neurogenic and septic), cardiogenic, and hypovolemic.

Causes

Neurogenic Shock

- Spinal cord injury and spinal anesthesia
- Vasomotor center depression
- Severe pain
- Medications
- Hypoglycemia

Septic Shock

- Gram-negative bacteria and gram-positive bacteria
- Viruses, fungi, rickettsiae, parasites, yeast, protozoa, and mycobacteria

Cardiogenic Shock

- MI, most common cause
- Heart failure and cardiomyopathy
- Pericardial tamponade
- Pulmonary embolism

Hypovolemic Shock

- Blood loss (most common cause)
- GI fluid loss, renal loss, and fluid shifts causing severe dehydration
- Burns

Pathophysiology

Each type of shock has three stages.

Compensatory stage: When arterial pressure and tissue perfusion fall, compensatory mechanisms are activated to maintain cardiac output and perfusion to the heart and brain. As the baroreceptors in the carotid sinus and aortic arch sense a drop in blood pressure, epinephrine and norepinephrine are secreted to increase peripheral resistance, blood pressure, and myocardial contractility. Reduced blood flow to the kidney activates the renin-angiotensin-aldosterone system, causing vasoconstriction and sodium and water retention.

Progressive stage: When compensatory mechanisms can't maintain cardiac output, tissues become hypoxic. Cells switch to anaerobic metabolism and lactic acid accumulates, producing metabolic acidosis. Tissue hypoxia promotes the release of endothelial mediators, leading to venous pooling and increased capillary permeability. Sluggish blood flow increases the risk of disseminated intravascular coagulation (DIC).

Irreversible (refractory) stage: Inadequate perfusion damages cell membranes, lysosomal enzymes are released, and energy stores are depleted, leading to cell death. Lactic acid continues to accumulate, increasing capillary permeability and the movement of fluid out of the vascular space, further contributing to hypotension. Perfusion to the coronary arteries is reduced, causing myocardial depression and a further reduction in cardiac output. Circulatory failure and respiratory failure occur.

COMPLICATIONS

- Kidney or brain damage (cardiogenic and hypovolemic)
- Liver damage (cardiogenic)
- Respiratory or cardiac failure (septic) in all types of shock

Signs and Symptoms

Compensatory Stage

- Tachycardia, bounding pulse, and tachypnea
- Reduced urinary output
- Cool, pale skin (or warm, dry skin in septic shock)

Progressive Stage

- Hypotension
- Narrowed pulse pressure; weak, rapid, thready pulse
- Cold, clammy skin; cyanosis and shallow respirations

Irreversible Stage

- Unconsciousness and absent reflexes
- Rapidly falling blood pressure; weak pulse
- Slow, shallow, or Cheyne-Stokes respirations

Diagnostic Test Results

- Hematocrit is reduced in hemorrhage or elevated in other types of shock caused by hypovolemia.
- Blood, urine, and sputum cultures identify the organism responsible for septic shock.
- Coagulation studies may detect coagulopathy from DIC.
- Complete blood count reveals increased white blood cell count and erythrocyte sedimentation rate.
- Blood chemistry reveals elevated blood urea nitrogen and creatinine levels and elevated serum glucose (in early stages).
- Serum lactate increases secondary to anaerobic metabolism.
- Elevated cardiac enzymes and proteins indicate MI as a cause of cardiogenic shock.
- Arterial blood gas analysis reveals respiratory alkalosis.
- Urine specific gravity will be elevated in response to the effects of antidiuretic hormone.
- Chest X-rays will be normal in early stages; pulmonary congestion may be seen in later stages.
- ECG may show arrhythmias, ischemic changes, and an MI.
- Echocardiography reveals valvular abnormalities.

Treatment

- Identification and treatment of the underlying cause
- Maintaining a patent airway, oxygen and mechanical ventilation, and continuous cardiac monitoring
- I.V. fluids, crystalloids, colloids, or blood products

Neurogenic Shock

- Vasopressor drugs

Septic Shock

- Treatment with drotrecogin alfa (Xigris) antibiotics and inotropic and vasopressor drugs

Cardiogenic Shock

- Inotropic drugs, vasodilators, and diuretics
- Intra-aortic balloon pump therapy
- Thrombolytic therapy or coronary artery revascularization

- Ventricular assist device
- Heart transplantation

Hypovolemic Shock

- Pneumatic antishock garment

MULTIORGAN SYSTEM EFFECTS OF SHOCK

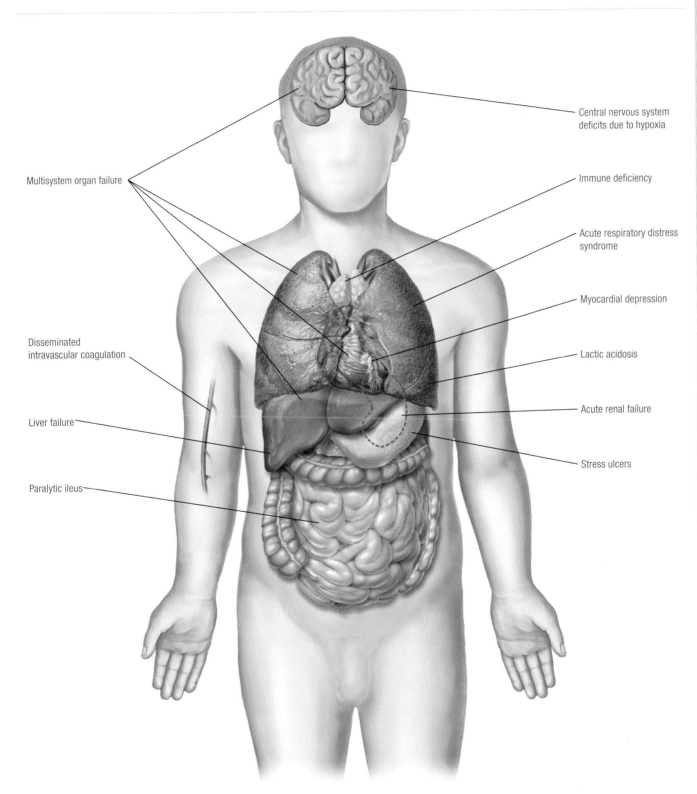

Multisystem organ failure

Central nervous system deficits due to hypoxia

Immune deficiency

Acute respiratory distress syndrome

Myocardial depression

Disseminated intravascular coagulation

Lactic acidosis

Acute renal failure

Liver failure

Stress ulcers

Paralytic ileus

VALVULAR HEART DISEASE

In valvular heart disease, three types of mechanical disruptions can occur: stenosis, or narrowing, of the valve opening (called insufficiency, incompetence, or regurgitation); incomplete closure of the valve; or prolapse of the valve.

Causes

The causes of valvular heart disease are varied and differ for each type of valve disorder.

Mitral Stenosis

- Rheumatic fever
- Congenital anomalies

Mitral Insufficiency

- Rheumatic fever
- Mitral valve prolapse
- Myocardial infarction
- Severe left ventricular failure
- Ruptured chordae tendineae
- Marfan syndrome

Aortic Insufficiency

- Rheumatic fever
- Syphilis
- Hypertension
- Endocarditis
- Marfan syndrome

Aortic Stenosis

- Congenital
- Bicuspid aortic valve
- Rheumatic fever
- Atherosclerosis

Pulmonic Stenosis

- Congenital
- Rheumatic fever (rare)

Pathophysiology

Pathophysiology of valvular heart disease varies according to the valve and the disorder.

Mitral stenosis: Structural abnormality, fibrosis, or calcification obstructs blood flow from the left atrium to the left ventricle. Left atrial volume and pressure rise, and the chamber dilates. Greater resistance to blood flow causes pulmonary hypertension, right ventricular hypertrophy, and right-sided heart failure. Inadequate filling of the left ventricle causes low cardiac output.

COMPLICATIONS
- Pulmonary edema
- Atrial fibrillation
- Pulmonary hypertension
- Right-sided heart failure
- Emboli
- Stroke

Mitral insufficiency: An abnormality of the mitral leaflets, mitral annulus, chordae tendineae, papillary muscles, left atrium, or left ventricle can lead to mitral regurgitation. Blood from the left ventricle flows back into the left atrium during systole, and the atrium enlarges to accommodate the backflow. The left ventricle also dilates to accommodate the increased volume of blood from the atrium and to compensate for diminishing cardiac output. Ventricular hypertrophy and increased end-diastolic pressure raise pulmonary artery pressure.

COMPLICATIONS
- Endocarditis
- Heart failure
- Emboli
- Stroke
- Arrhythmias

Aortic insufficiency: Blood flows back into the left ventricle during diastole, causing fluid overload in the ventricle, which dilates and hypertrophies. The excess volume causes fluid overload in the left atrium and, finally, the pulmonary system.

COMPLICATIONS
- Left-sided heart failure
- Pulmonary edema

Aortic stenosis: Over time, left ventricular pressure rises to overcome the resistance of the narrowed valvular opening. The added workload increases the demand for oxygen, and diminished cardiac output causes poor coronary artery perfusion.

COMPLICATIONS
- Ischemia of left ventricle
- Left-sided heart failure
- Arrhythmias
- Endocarditis

Pulmonic stenosis: Obstructed right ventricular outflow causes right ventricular hypertrophy, resulting in right-sided heart failure.

COMPLICATIONS
- Heart failure
- Right ventricular hypertrophy

Signs and Symptoms

The clinical manifestations vary according to valvular defects and the severity of the defect. The patient may be asymptomatic.

Common to All Valvular Disorders

- Dyspnea, weakness, and fatigue

Mitral Stenosis

- Orthopnea
- Palpitations, right-sided heart failure, crackles, and jugular vein distention
- Atrial fibrillation
- Diastolic thrill, loud S_1, and opening snap-diastolic murmur

Mitral Insufficiency

- Palpitations, angina, and tachycardia
- Left-sided heart failure, pulmonary edema, and crackles
- Split S_2; S_3; holosystolic murmur at apex
- Apical thrill

Aortic Insufficiency

- Palpitations, angina, and syncope
- Cough
- Pulmonary congestion and left-sided heart failure
- Quincke's sign
- Pulsus bisferiens and visible apical pulse
- S_3 and blowing diastolic murmur at left sternal border

Aortic Stenosis

- Palpitations, angina, and arrhythmias
- Dyspnea
- Syncope
- Pulmonary congestion and left-sided heart failure
- Diminished carotid pulses and systolic thrill (carotid)
- Decreased cardiac output
- Systolic ejection murmur that radiates to neck and S_4

Pulmonic Stenosis

- Commonly produces no symptoms
- Syncope, chest pain, and right-sided heart failure
- Systolic murmur at left sternal border and S_2 split

Diagnostic Test Results

Diagnostic test results vary with the type of valvular disease that's present. Cardiac catheterization, chest X-ray, echocardiography, and ECG are the standard diagnostic tools used to detect valvular heart disease.

Mitral Stenosis

- Cardiac catheterization reveals diastolic pressure gradient across the valve; elevated left atrial and PAWP with severe pulmonary hypertension; elevated right-sided heart pressure with decreased cardiac output; and abnormal contraction of the left ventricle.
- Chest X-ray shows left atrial and ventricular enlargement, enlarged pulmonary arteries, and mitral valve calcification.
- Echocardiography reveals left atrial and ventricular enlargement, enlarged pulmonary arteries, and mitral valve calcification.
- ECG detects left atrial hypertrophy, atrial fibrillation, right ventricular hypertrophy, and right axis deviation.

Mitral Insufficiency

- Cardiac catheterization reveals mitral regurgitation with increased left ventricular end-diastolic volume and pressure, increased atrial pressure and PAWP, and decreased cardiac output.
- Chest X-ray shows left atrial and ventricular enlargement and pulmonary venous congestion.
- Echocardiography shows abnormal valve leaflet motion and left atrial enlargement.
- ECG may show left atrial and ventricular hypertrophy, sinus tachycardia, and atrial fibrillation.

Aortic Insufficiency

- Cardiac catheterization reveals reduction in arterial diastolic pressure, aortic regurgitation, other valvular abnormalities, and increased left ventricular end-diastolic pressure.
- Chest X-ray shows left ventricular enlargement and pulmonary vein congestion.
- Echocardiography shows left ventricular enlargement, alteration in mitral valve movement, and mitral valve thickening.
- ECG shows sinus tachycardia, left ventricular hypertrophy, and left atrial hypertrophy in severe disease.

Aortic Stenosis

- Cardiac catheterization reveals pressure gradient across valve and increased left ventricular end-diastolic pressures.
- Chest X-ray shows valvular calcification, left ventricular enlargement, and pulmonary vein congestion.
- Echocardiography shows thickened aortic valve and left ventricular wall, possibly coexisting with mitral valve stenosis.
- ECG shows left ventricular hypertrophy.

Pulmonic Stenosis

- Cardiac catheterization reveals increased right ventricular pressure, decreased pulmonary artery pressure, and abnormal valve orifice.
- ECG shows right ventricular hypertrophy, right axis deviation, right atrial hypertrophy, and atrial fibrillation.

Treatment

- Digoxin, anticoagulants, nitroglycerin, beta-adrenergic blockers, diuretics, vasodilators, and angiotensin-converting enzyme inhibitors
- Low-sodium diet
- Oxygen
- Prophylactic antibiotics for invasive procedures, such as dental cleanings, endoscopies, and other procedures where the risk of introducing bacteria into the bloodstream is present. Not indicated for all valvular dysfunctions. See SBE guidelines
- Cardioversion
- Open or closed commissurotomy
- Annuloplasty or valvuloplasty
- Prosthetic valve for mitral or aortic valve disease

VARICOSE VEINS

Varicose veins are dilated, tortuous veins, engorged with blood and resulting from poor venous valve function. They can be primary, originating in the superficial veins, or secondary, occurring in the deep veins.

Causes

Primary Varicose Veins

- Congenital weakness of valves or vein wall
- Prolonged venous stasis or increased intra-abdominal pressure, as in pregnancy, obesity, constipation, or wearing tight clothes
- Standing for an extended period of time
- Family history

Secondary Varicose Veins

- Deep vein thrombosis
- Venous malformation
- Arteriovenous fistulas
- Venous trauma
- Occlusion

Pathophysiology

Veins are thin-walled, distensible vessels with valves that keep blood flowing in one direction. Any condition that weakens, destroys, or distends these valves allows the backflow of blood to the previous valve. If a valve can't hold the pooling blood, it can become incompetent, allowing even more blood to flow backward. The increasing volume of blood in the vein raises pressure and distends the vein. As the veins are stretched, their walls weaken and lose their elasticity, and they become lumpy and tortuous. Rising hydrostatic pressure forces plasma into the surrounding tissues, resulting in edema.

People who stand for prolonged periods may also develop venous pooling because there's no muscular contraction in the legs, forcing blood back up to the heart. If the valves in the veins are too weak to hold the pooling blood, they begin to leak, allowing blood to flow backward.

COMPLICATIONS
- Phlebitis
- Leg ulcers

Signs and Symptoms

- Dilated, tortuous, purplish, ropelike veins, particularly in the calves
- Edema of the calves and ankles
- Leg heaviness that worsens in the evening and in warm weather
- Dull aching in the legs after prolonged standing or walking
- Aching during menses

AGE ALERT
As a person ages, veins dilate and stretch, increasing susceptibility to varicose veins and chronic venous insufficiency. Because the skin becomes friable and can easily break down, ulcers caused by chronic venous insufficiency may take longer to heal.

Diagnostic Test Results

CLINICAL TIP
Manual compression test detects a palpable impulse when the vein is firmly occluded at least 8 inches (20.3 cm) above the point of palpation, indicating incompetent valves in the vein.

Trendelenburg's test (retrograde filling test) detects incompetent valves when the vein is occluded with the patient in the supine position and the leg is elevated 90 degrees. When the person stands (still with the vein occluded), the saphenous veins should fill slowly from below in about 30 seconds.

- Photoplethysmography characterizes venous blood flow by noting changes in the skin's circulation.
- Doppler ultrasonography detects the presence or absence of venous backflow in deep or superficial veins.
- Venous outflow and reflux plethysmography detects deep vein occlusion; this test is invasive and not routinely used.
- Ascending and descending venography demonstrate venous occlusion and patterns of collateral flow.

Treatment

- Treatment of underlying cause (if possible), such as abdominal tumor or obesity
- Antiembolism stockings or elastic bandages
- Regular exercise
- Injection of a sclerosing agent into small- to medium-sized varicosities
- Surgical stripping and ligation of severe varicose veins
- Phlebectomy (removing the varicose vein through small incisions in the skin)

Normal veins

Varicose veins

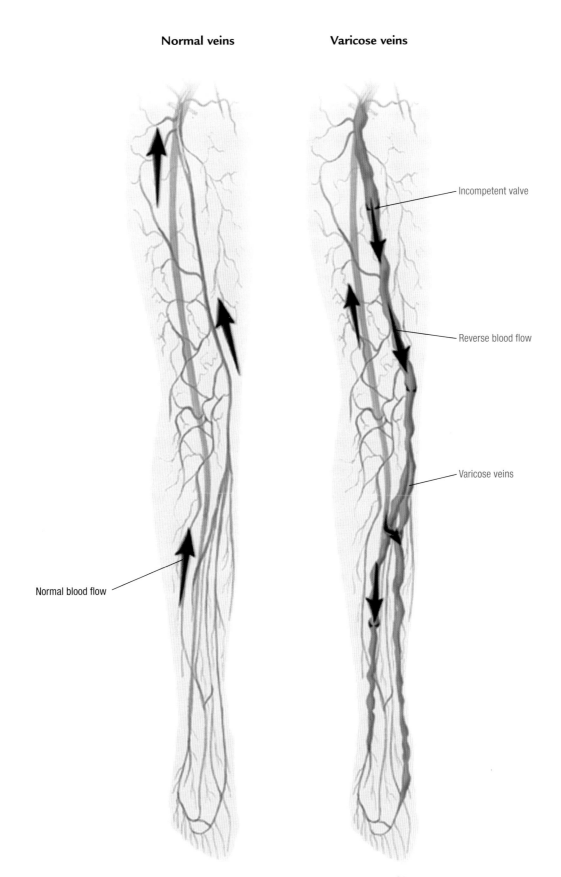

Incompetent valve

Reverse blood flow

Varicose veins

Normal blood flow

RESPIRATORY DISORDERS

ACUTE RESPIRATORY DISTRESS SYNDROME

Acute respiratory distress syndrome (ARDS) is characterized by pulmonary edema and refractory hypoxemia. ARDS can lead to multiple organ failure and has a high rate of mortality. Increased capillary permeability is the hallmark of ARDS. Diagnosis is often difficult, and death can occur within 48 hours of onset if ARDS is not promptly diagnosed and appropriately treated.

Causes

The most common cause of ARDS is sepsis. Infection, including severe sepsis and pneumonia, is the leading predisposing factor for ARDS.

- Injury to the lung from trauma
- Sepsis
- Trauma-related factors, such as fat emboli, sepsis, shock, pulmonary contusions, and multiple transfusions
- Aspiration of gastric contents, viral pneumonia
- Anaphylaxis
- Drug overdose
- Idiosyncratic drug reaction to ampicillin or hydrochlorothiazide
- Inhalation of noxious gases (nitrous oxide, ammonia, chlorine)
- Near drowning
- Oxygen toxicity
- Coronary artery bypass grafting
- Hemodialysis
- Leukemia
- Acute miliary tuberculosis
- Pancreatitis
- Thrombotic thrombocytopenic purpura
- Uremia
- Venous air embolism

Pathophysiology

ARDS is a heterogeneous syndrome that involves lung injury, which may develop as a result of endothelial and epithelial cell injury. Symptoms present from direct injury, including aspiration of gastric contents or inhalation of noxious gases, or indirect sources, such as chemical mediators released in response to systemic disease. Injury in ARDS involves both the alveolar and the pulmonary capillary epithelium. The causative agent triggers a cascade of cellular and biochemical changes.

Acute Phase: Sloughing of the Bronchial and Alveolar Epithelial Cells

In the acute phase of ARDS, protein-rich hyaline membranes form on the denuded basement membrane. Neutrophils adhere to the injured capillary endothelium and marginate through the interstitium into the air space filled with protein-rich edema fluid.

After it is initiated, the causative agent triggers neutrophils, macrophages, monocytes, and lymphocytes to produce various cytokines — which promote cellular activation, chemotaxis, and adhesion — and inflammatory mediators, including oxidants, proteases, kinins, growth factors, and neuropeptides, which initiate the complement cascade, intravascular coagulation, and fibrinolysis.

These cellular events increase vascular permeability to proteins, increasing the hydrostatic pressure gradient of the capillary. Elevated capillary pressure, such as results from fluid overload or cardiac dysfunction, greatly increases interstitial and alveolar edema, which is evident on chest X-rays as whitened areas in the lower lung. Alveolar closing pressure then exceeds pulmonary pressures, and the alveoli begin to collapse.

Exudative Phase

The exudative phase, or phase 1, usually occurs the first 2 to 4 days after onset of injury and involves inflammatory cells that have entered the air spaces from the alveolar capillaries.

During the exudative phase, fluid accumulates in the lung interstitium, alveolar spaces, and small airways. This causes the lungs to stiffen, impairing ventilation and reducing oxygenation of the pulmonary capillary blood, which results in reduced blood flow to the lungs. Platelets begin to aggregate and release substances (serotonin, bradykinin, and histamine), which attract and activate neutrophils.

Proliferative Phase

The proliferative phase, or phase 2, begins 1 to 2 weeks after the initial lung injury. There is an influx of neutrophils, monocytes, lymphocytes, and fibroblast proliferation. This is a part of the inflammatory response.

During the proliferative phase, the released substances inflame and damage the alveolar membrane and later increase capillary permeability. Additional chemotactic factors released include endotoxins, tumor necrosis factor, and interleukin-1. The activated neutrophils release several inflammatory mediators and platelet aggravating factors that damage the alveolar capillary membrane and increase capillary permeability, allowing fluids to move into the interstitial space.

Next, as capillary permeability increases, proteins, blood cells, and more fluid leak out, increasing interstitial osmotic pressure and causing pulmonary edema.

The resulting pulmonary edema and hemorrhage significantly reduce lung compliance and impair alveolar ventilation.

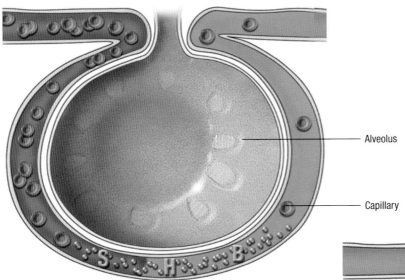

Alveolus

Capillary

Phase 1. Injury reduces normal blood flow to the lungs. Platelets aggregate and release histamine (H), serotonin (S), and bradykinin (B).

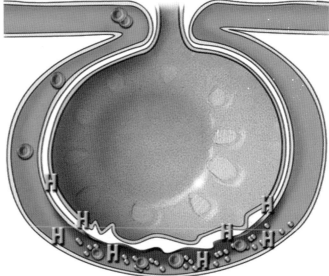

Phase 2. Those substances, especially histamine, inflame and damage the alveolocapillary membrane, increasing capillary permeability. Fluids then shift into the interstitial space.

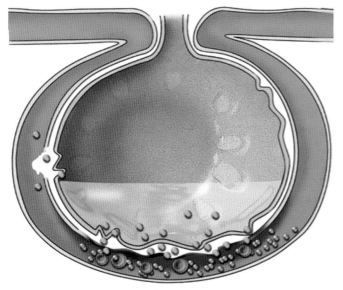

Phase 3. As capillary permeability increases, proteins and fluids leak out, increasing interstitial osmotic pressure and causing pulmonary edema.

Then, mediators released by neutrophils and macrophages also cause varying degrees of pulmonary vasoconstriction, resulting in pulmonary hypertension. The result of these changes is a mismatch in the ventilation-perfusion ratio. Although the patient responds with an increased respiratory rate, sufficient oxygen cannot cross the alveolar capillary membrane. Carbon dioxide continues to cross easily and is lost with every exhalation.

Finally, pulmonary edema worsens and hyaline membranes form. Inflammation leads to fibrosis, which further impedes gas exchange. Fibrosis progressively obliterates alveoli, respiratory bronchioles, and the interstitium. Functional residual capacity decreases, and shunting becomes more serious. Hypoxemia leads to metabolic acidosis. At this final stage, the patient develops increasing partial pressure of arterial carbon dioxide ($PaCO_2$), decreasing pH and partial pressure of arterial oxygen (PaO_2), decreasing bicarbonate levels, and mental confusion. The end result is respiratory failure.

COMPLICATIONS
- Metabolic and respiratory acidosis
- Cardiac arrest
- Pneumothorax
- Pulmonary fibrosis
- Abnormal lung functions
- Pulmonary embolism
- Infection

Signs and Symptoms

- Rapid, shallow breathing and dyspnea
- Increased rate of ventilation
- Intercostal and suprasternal retractions
- Crackles and rhonchi
- Restlessness, apprehension, and mental sluggishness
- Motor dysfunction
- Tachycardia
- Respiratory acidosis
- Metabolic acidosis

Diagnostic Test Results

- Arterial blood gas (ABG) analysis with the patient breathing room air initially reveals a reduced PaO_2 (less than 60 mm Hg) and a decreased $PaCO_2$ (less than 35 mm Hg). Hypoxemia, despite increased supplemental oxygen, is the hallmark of ARDS. The resulting blood pH reflects respiratory alkalosis.

As ARDS progresses and the work of breathing increases, the partial pressure of carbon dioxide (PCO_2) begins to rise and PaO_2 decreases, despite oxygen therapy.

CLINICAL TIP
It is important to understand how ARDS differs from acute lung injury. Both have an acute onset, and patients have bilateral infiltrates on frontal chest radiograph and pulmonary artery wedge pressure (PAWP) less than or equal to 18 mm Hg or no clinical evidence of left atrial hypertension. The difference with ARDS is that the PaO_2 is less than or equal to 200 mm Hg regardless of positive end-expiratory pressure (PEEP) level; with ALI, the PaO_2 is less than or equal to 300 mm Hg regardless of PEEP level.

- Pulmonary artery catheterization may show a PAWP of 12 to 18 mm Hg, and pulmonary artery pressure may show decreased cardiac output.
- Serial chest X-rays in early stages show bilateral infiltrates and in later stages, long fields with a ground-glass appearance and "white outs" of both lung fields. Note: ARDS is defined by the presence of bilateral pulmonary infiltrates.
- Chest computed tomography reveals bilateral opacities, pleural effusions, and decreased lung volume.
- Sputum analysis, including Gram stain and culture and sensitivity, identifies causative organisms.
- Blood cultures identify infectious organisms.
- Toxicology testing reveals possible drug ingestion.

Treatment

Therapy is focused on correcting the causes of ARDS and preventing progression of hypoxemia and respiratory acidosis.
Treatment may include:

- intubation and mechanical ventilation
- humidified oxygen
- PEEP
- pressure-controlled inverse ratio ventilation
- high-frequency ventilation
- airway pressure release ventilation
- liquid ventilation
- inhaled nitric oxide
- permissive hypercapnia
- sedatives, opioids, and neuromuscular blockers
- high-dose corticosteroids
- sodium bicarbonate
- I.V. fluid administration or fluid restrictions
- vasopressors
- antimicrobial drugs
- diuretics
- correction of electrolyte and acid-base imbalances
- prone positioning
- extracorporeal membrane oxygenation
- surfactant administration.

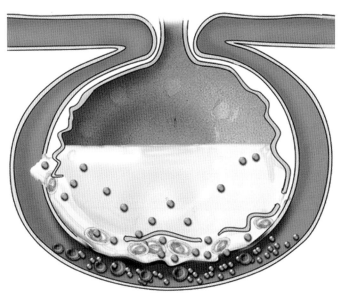

Phase 4. Decreased blood flow and fluids in the alveoli damage surfactant and impair the cell's ability to produce more. As a result, alveoli collapse, impeding gas exchange and decreasing lung compliance.

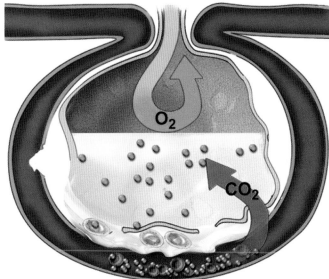

Phase 5. Sufficient oxygen can't cross the alveolocapillary membrane, but carbon dioxide (CO_2) can and is lost with every exhalation. Oxygen (O_2) and CO_2 levels decrease in the blood.

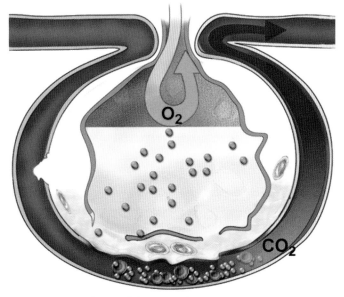

Phase 6. Pulmonary edema worsens, inflammation leads to fibrosis, and gas exchange is further impeded.

ASTHMA

Asthma is a complex disorder of the airways that is characterized by variable and recurring symptoms, airflow obstruction, bronchial hyperresponsiveness, and an underlying inflammation. Airflow limitation is caused by changes in the airway, causing bronchoconstriction, airway edema, and mucus hypersecretion. The National Heart Lung and Blood Institute, National Asthma Education and Prevention Program. Expert Panel Report 3 (EPR-3) recommends monitoring of clinically relevant aspects of care and the importance of planned primary care and providing patients practical tools for self-management.

Causes

The development of asthma involves interaction between genetics and environmental exposures (EPR-3, 2007; GINA, 2017). Patients who are at high risk for asthma-related death require special attention.

- Viral infections (one of the most important causes of asthma)
- Pollen, air pollution
- Animal dander
- House dust or mold
- Kapok or feather pillows
- Food additives, including sulfites and some dyes
- Noxious fumes, tobacco smoke

Patients with intrinsic, or nonatopic, asthma react to internal, nonallergenic factors.

- Irritants
- Emotional stress and anxiety
- Respiratory infections
- Endocrine changes
- Temperature or humidity variations
- Coughing or laughing
- Genetic factors

Pathophysiology

Airway inflammation contributes to airway hyperresponsiveness, airflow limitation, respiratory symptoms, and disease chronicity (see the EPR-3 guidelines for pathophysiology).

In asthma, bronchial linings overreact to various stimuli, causing inflammation and smooth muscle spasms — contraction that severely constrict the airways. When the hypersensitive patient inhales a triggering substance, abnormal antibodies stimulate mast cells in the lung interstitium to release histamine and leukotriene. Histamine attaches to receptor sites in the larger bronchi, where it causes swelling in smooth muscles. Leukotriene attaches to receptor sites in the smaller bronchi and causes swelling of smooth muscle there. It also causes fatty acids called prostaglandins to travel by way of the bloodstream to the lungs, where they enhance histamine's effects.

Histamine stimulates the mucous membranes to secrete excessive mucus, further narrowing the bronchial lumen. On inhalation, the narrowed bronchial lumen can still expand slightly, allowing air to reach the alveoli. On exhalation, increased intrathoracic pressure closes the bronchial lumen completely. Mucus fills the lung bases, inhibiting alveolar

ventilation. Blood, shunted to alveoli in other lung parts, still cannot compensate for diminished ventilation.

COMPLICATIONS
- Status asthmaticus
- Respiratory failure

CLINICAL TIP
Asthma symptoms typically vary in frequency and intensity and contribute to the burden of asthma for the patient. Poor symptom control is also strongly associated with an increased risk of asthma exacerbations (GINA, 2017). Pharmacologic therapy for asthma is the cornerstone of its management.

Status asthmaticus is an acute exacerbation of asthma that remains unresponsive to treatment, despite appropriate medical treatment regimens. When status asthmaticus occurs, hypoxia worsens, expiratory flow slows, and expiratory volumes decrease. If treatment is not initiated promptly, the patient begins to tire. Acidosis develops as arterial carbon dioxide increases. The situation becomes life threatening when no air movement is audible on auscultation (a silent chest) and partial pressure of arterial carbon dioxide ($PaCO_2$) rises to over 70 mm Hg.

Identify:

- Usual prodromal signs or symptoms
- Rapidity of onset
- Associated illnesses and/or comorbid conditions
- Emergency department visits, hospitalizations, ICU admissions, intubations
- Usual prodromal signs or symptoms
- Limitations with exercise
- Missed days from work or school.

Signs and Symptoms

- Sudden dyspnea, wheezing, and tightness in the chest
- Coughing that produces thick, clear, or yellow sputum
- Tachypnea, along with use of accessory respiratory muscles
- Rapid pulse
- Profuse perspiration
- Hyperresonant lung fields
- Diminished breath sounds

Diagnostic Test Results

Be careful not to confuse diagnostic criteria with contributing information. Diagnostic criteria include the following:

- Episodic symptoms of airflow obstruction are present.
- Airflow obstruction or symptoms are at least partially reversible.
- Exclusion of alternative diagnoses.
- Pulmonary function tests reveal low-normal or decreased vital capacity, increased total lung and residual capacities, and decreased FEV1.

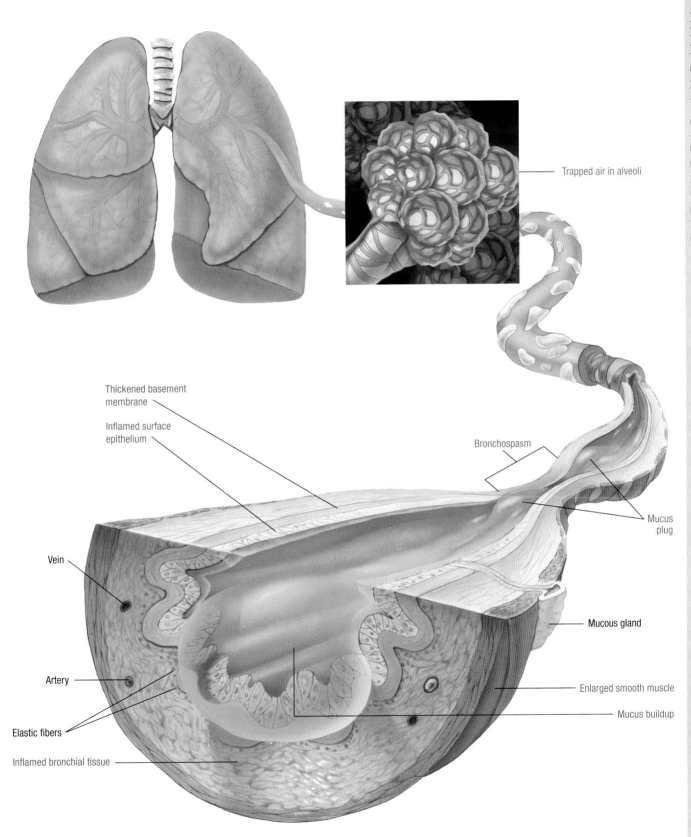

Trapped air in alveoli

Thickened basement membrane

Inflamed surface epithelium

Bronchospasm

Mucus plug

Vein

Mucous gland

Artery

Enlarged smooth muscle

Mucus buildup

Elastic fibers

Inflamed bronchial tissue

- Serum immunoglobulin E levels may increase from an allergic reaction. This is not diagnostic of asthma.
- Complete blood count with differential reveals an increased eosinophil count.
- Chest X-rays may show hyperinflation with areas of atelectasis.
- With ABG analysis, partial pressure of arterial oxygen and $PaCO_2$ are usually decreased, except in severe asthma, when $PaCO_2$ may be normal or increased, indicating severe bronchial obstruction.
- Skin testing identifies specific allergens but is not diagnostic of asthma. Skin testing to aeroallergens identifies contributing factors.
- Pulmonary function testing includes pre- and postbronchodilator. A bronchial challenge could be considered a methacholine challenge, which would absolutely be contraindicated in a patient with diagnosed asthma.
- Electrocardiography shows sinus tachycardia exacerbation or right axis deviation and peaked P waves (indicating cor pulmonale during a severe attack that resolves after the attack).

Exercise-induced bronchospasm (EIB) is a phenomenon of airway narrowing that occurs during or after exercise or physical exertion. EIB controlled by a short-acting β-adrenergic agonist 15 minutes before exercise or physical exertion.

Asthma Control

The National Asthma Education and Prevention Program Expert Panel Report 3, (EPR-3) define asthma control as "the degree to which the manifestations of asthma symptoms, functional impairments, and risks of untoward events are minimized and the goals of therapy are met." Every patient with asthma should be able to recognize symptoms that suggest inadequate asthma control. Written action plans detailing medications and environmental control strategies tailored for each patient are recommended for all patients with asthma.

Monitoring asthma control is the goal for asthma therapy and distinguishing between classifying asthma severity and monitoring asthma control.

Distinguishing between classifying asthma severity and monitoring asthma control.

Severity: the intrinsic intensity of the disease process. Assess asthma severity to initiate therapy.

Control: the degree to which the manifestations of asthma are minimized by therapeutic interventions and the goals of therapy are met. Assess and monitor asthma control to adjust therapy.

Impairment and Risk of Asthma:

The two key domains of severity and control are impairment and risk. The domains represent different manifestations of asthma, they may not correlate with each other, and they may respond differentially to treatment.

Impairment: frequency and intensity of symptoms and functional limitations the patient is experiencing currently or has recently experienced.

Risk: the likelihood of either asthma exacerbations, progressive decline in lung function (or, for children, lung growth), or risk of adverse effects from medication.

Treatment

Quick-relief medicines are taken at the first sign of symptoms for immediate relief:

- Short-acting inhaled beta2 agonists
- Anticholinergics.

Long-term control medicines are taken every day to prevent symptoms and attacks:

- Inhaled corticosteroids: the most effective long-term maintenance medications for chronic asthma
- Inhaled corticosteroids and long-acting inhaled beta2-agonists
- Long-acting beta2agonist are ALWAYS administered and inhaled corticosteroid
- Antileukotrienes or leukotriene modifiers — montelukast sodium
- Cromolyn sodium
- Methylxanthines
- Oral corticosteroids
- Immunomodulators
- Identification and avoidance of precipitating factors
- Desensitization to specific antigens
- Low-flow humidified oxygen (supplemental oxygen is rarely prescribed at home for patients with asthma)
- Mechanical ventilation
- Relaxation exercises controlled breathing exercises.

Assessing Asthma Control

Asthma questionnaire tools assess asthma control and identify patients at risk for an asthma exacerbation. The Asthma Control Test (ACT) is an example of one of the asthma assessment tools. The ACT is a short, simple, patient-based tool for assessing asthma control, including identifying patients with poorly controlled asthma. The ACT is reliable, valid, and responsive to changes in asthma control over time. A cutoff score of 19 or less identifies patients with poorly controlled asthma.

The 2007 National Asthma Education and Prevention Expert Panel Report 3 guidelines classify asthma severity:

Intermittent asthma is characterized as follows:

- Symptoms of cough, wheezing, chest tightness, or difficulty breathing less than twice a week.
- Flare-ups are brief, but intensity may vary.

- Nighttime symptoms less than twice a month.
- No symptoms between flare-ups.
- Lung function test FEV1 is 80% or more above normal values.
- Peak flow has less than 20% variability am to am or am to pm, day to day.

Mild persistent asthma is characterized as follows:

- Symptoms of cough, wheezing, chest tightness, or difficulty breathing 3 to 6 times a week.
- Flare-ups may affect activity level.
- Nighttime symptoms 3 to 4 times a month.
- Lung function test FEV1 is 80% or more above normal values.
- Peak flow has less than 20% to 30% variability.

Moderate persistent asthma is characterized as follows:

- Symptoms of cough, wheezing, chest tightness, or difficulty breathing daily.
- Flare-ups may affect activity level.
- Nighttime symptoms 5 or more times a month.
- Lung function test FEV1 is above 60% but below 80% of normal values.
- Peak flow has more than 30% variability.

Severe persistent asthma is characterized as follows:

- Symptoms of cough, wheezing, chest tightness, or difficulty breathing that are continual.
- Frequent nighttime symptoms.
- Lung function test FEV1 is 60% or less of normal values.
- Peak flow has more than 30% variability.

ACUTE BRONCHITIS

Acute bronchitis is a common, self-limiting, respiratory tract infection characterized primarily by a cough generally lasting 1 to 3 weeks. The distinguishing characteristic of bronchitis is obstruction of airflow and an inflammatory response within the epithelium of the bronchi causing airway hyperresponsiveness and increased mucus production. The inflammation occurs as a result of an airway infection or environmental triggers. The causative pathogen for bronchitis is rarely identified, although viral infections accounting for an estimated 89% to 95% cases (Tackett & Atkins, 2012). The most common viral pathogens include adenovirus, coronavirus, influenza A and B, metapneumovirus, parainfluenza virus, respiratory syncytial virus, and rhinovirus (Albert, 2010). Bacteria may cause bronchitis in people with underlying respiratory disease. *Mycoplasma pneumoniae* and *Chlamydia pneumoniae* are bacterial pathogens that primarily affect young adults. *Bordetella pertussis* can also lead to acute bronchitis especially in unvaccinated patients (Albert, 2010). Testing for pertussis may be warranted. Chest radiographs are indicated when acute bronchitis cannot be clinically distinguished from pneumonia. Inflammation in acute bronchitis is usually transient and resolves after the infection has subsided.

The management of acute bronchitis is primarily supportive and is focused on controlling cough. Antibiotic therapy has a minor role in acute bronchitis (Hart, 2014). Inappropriate use of antibiotics for viral respiratory infections contribute to antibiotic resistance and possible adverse events. Inhaled beta agonists should be reserved for patients with underlying pulmonary disease. Over-the-counter medications, such as dextromethorphan or guaifenesin, administered as directed in the appropriate age group may be efficacious, despite lack of substantial evidence. Antitussive therapy may be helpful for sleep distribution contributed to nocturnal cough.

Expectorants have been shown to be ineffective in the treatment of acute bronchitis (Albert, 2010). Patient education must address etiology and symptomatology, rationale for duration of cough, and appropriate medical interventions.

CHRONIC OBSTRUCTIVE PULMONARY DISEASE

Chronic obstructive pulmonary disease (COPD) is a common yet preventable disease characterized by persistent respiratory symptoms and airflow limitation due to airway and/or alveolar abnormalities (GOLD, 2017). This disorder leads to airway obstruction, hyperinflation, and abnormal gas exchange causing dyspnea and functional limitation. Overlap is present between COPD and the other disorders that cause airflow limitation, such as asthma emphysema, chronic bronchitis, bronchiectasis, and bronchiolitis. Spirometry is required to make the diagnosis of COPD. The primary risk factor for COPD is cigarette smoking.

COPD should be considered in any patient who has dyspnea, chronic cough or sputum, and/or a history of exposure to risk factors for the disease (GOLD, 2017). Management for stable COPD is based on the individualized assessment of symptoms and future risk of exacerbations (GOLD, 2017).

Diagnosis

The formal diagnosis of COPD is made with spirometry; when the ratio of forced expiratory volume in 1 second over forced vital capacity (FEV1/FVC) is less than 70% of that predicted for a matched control, it is diagnostic for a significant obstructive defect. Criteria for assessing the severity of airflow obstruction (based on the percent predicted post bronchodilator FEV1) are as follows:

- Stage I (mild): FEV1 80% or greater of predicted
- Stage II (moderate): FEV1 50% to 79% of predicted
- Stage III (severe): FEV1 30% to 49% of predicted
- Stage IV (very severe): FEV1 less than 30% of predicted or FEV1 less than 50% and chronic respiratory failure.

Causes

- Cigarette smoking
- Exposure to irritants
- Genetic predisposition
- Exposure to organic or inorganic dusts
- Exposure to noxious gases
- Respiratory tract infection

Pathophysiology

COPD is characterized by increased numbers of neutrophils, macrophages, and T lymphocytes (CD8 more than CD4) in the lungs.

The irritants inflame the tracheobronchial tree, leading to increased mucus production and a narrowed or blocked airway. As the inflammation continues, changes in the cells lining the respiratory tract increase resistance in the small airways, and severe imbalance in the ventilation-perfusion ($\dot{V}/\dot{Q}$) ratio decreases arterial oxygenation.

Additional effects include narrowing and widespread inflammation within the airways. Bronchial walls become inflamed and thickened from edema and accumulation of inflammatory cells, and smooth muscle bronchospasm further narrows the lumen. Initially, only large bronchi are involved, but eventually, all airways are affected. Airways become obstructed and close, especially on expiration, trapping the gas in the distal portion of the lung. Consequent hypoventilation leads to a $\dot{V}/\dot{Q}$ mismatch and resultant hypoxemia and hypercapnia.

CHRONIC BRONCHITIS

Chronic bronchitis is defined clinically as the presence of a chronic productive cough for 3 months during each of 2 consecutive years with other causes of cough being excluded (GOLD, 2017). Chronic bronchitis is caused by the overproduction and hypersecretion of mucus by goblet cells. Mechanisms responsible for excessive mucus in COPD are overproduction and hypersecretion by goblet cells and decreased elimination of mucus. Chronic bronchitis leads to decreased airflow obstruction by luminal obstruction of small airways, epithelial remodeling, and decreased airway surface tension.

Chronic bronchitis causes hypertrophy of airway smooth muscle and hyperplasia of the mucous glands, increased numbers of goblet cells, ciliary damage, squamous metaplasia of the columnar epithelium, and chronic leukocytic and lymphocytic infiltration of bronchial walls. Hypersecretion of the goblet cells blocks the free movement of the cilia, which normally sweep dust, irritants, and mucus away from the airways. Accumulating mucus and debris impair the defenses and increase the likelihood of respiratory tract infections.

COMPLICATIONS
- Pneumonia
- Lung cancer

Signs and Symptoms

- Copious gray, white, or yellow sputum
- Dyspnea and tachypnea
- Cyanosis
- Use of accessory muscles
- Pedal edema
- Jugular vein distention
- Weight gain due to edema or weight loss due to difficulty eating and increased metabolic rate
- Wheezing, prolonged expiratory time, and rhonchi
- Pulmonary hypertension

Diagnostic Test Results: Chronic Bronchitis

- Chest X-rays show hyperinflation and increased bronchovascular markings.
- Pulmonary function studies indicate increased residual volume, decreased vital capacity and forced expiratory flow, and normal static compliance and diffusing capacity.
- ABG analysis reveals decreased partial pressure of arterial oxygen and normal or increased partial pressure of arterial carbon dioxide. ABGs provide the best evidence as to acuteness and severity of disease exacerbation.
- Sputum analysis reveals many microorganisms and neutrophils.
- Electrocardiography shows atrial arrhythmias; peaked P waves in leads II, III, and aV_F and, occasionally, right ventricular hypertrophy.

Treatment

- Beta2 agonists (bronchodilators)
- Short-acting beta agonist (SABA)
- Long-acting beta agonist (LABA)
- Corticosteroids
- Long-acting muscarinic agonist (LAMA)
- LAMA-LABA combination
- Phosphodiesterase inhibitors
- Antibiotics
- Mucolytic agents
- Oxygen therapy

Vaccination according to the Center of Disease Control and Prevention (CDC) is a safe and effective modality to reduce infection. Infections lead to exacerbations of COPD (GOLD, 2017).

- Smoking cessation
- Avoidance of air pollutants
- Adequate hydration

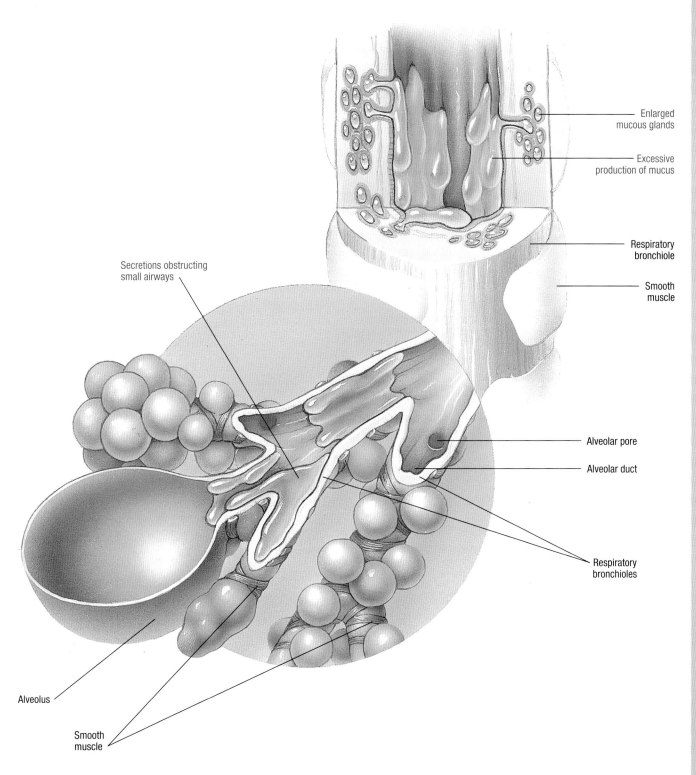

Enlarged
mucous glands

Excessive
production of mucus

Respiratory
bronchiole

Smooth
muscle

Secretions obstructing
small airways

Alveolar pore

Alveolar duct

Respiratory
bronchioles

Alveolus

Smooth
muscle

EMPHYSEMA

Emphysema is pathologically defined as an abnormal permanent enlargement of air spaces distal to the terminal bronchioles, accompanied by the destruction of alveolar walls (GOLD, 2017). Airflow limitation in emphysema is due to loss of elastic recoil and decrease in airway tethering. A permanent enlargement of air spaces distal to the terminal bronchioles, emphysema leads to a significant decline in the alveolar surface area available for gas exchange. Loss of individual alveoli with septal wall destruction leads to airflow limitation. The various subtypes of emphysema include proximal acinar, panacinar, or distal acinar.

Physical examination thoracic examination reveals diminished breath sounds, diffuse or focal wheezing, diffusely, hyperresonance upon percussion, prolonged expiration, and classically a 2:1 increase in anterior to posterior diameter.

The Global Initiative for Chronic Obstructive Lung Disease (GOLD, 2017) guidelines recommend various instruments to assess severity of symptoms, risk of exacerbations, and the presence of comorbidities, which are important to the patient's experience of the disease and prognosis. The most widely used research tool, the St. George's Respiratory Questionnaire (SGRQ), is a 76-item questionnaire that includes three component scores (i.e., symptoms, activity, and impact on daily life) and a total score. The GOLD guidelines suggest using the COPD Assessment Tool (CAT) or the modified Medical Research Council (mMRC) dyspnea scale.

AGE ALERT
Aging is a risk factor for emphysema. Senile emphysema results from degenerative changes that cause stretching without destruction of the smooth muscle. Connective tissue is not usually affected.

COMPLICATIONS
- Respiratory failure
- Cor pulmonale

Signs and Symptoms

- Tachypnea
- Dyspnea
- Barrel chest
- Prolonged expiration and grunting
- Crackles and wheezing on inspiration
- Decreased breath sounds
- Hyperresonance
- Clubbed fingers and toes
- Decreased tactile fremitus
- Decreased chest expansion
- Chronic cough with or without sputum production
- Accessory muscle use
- Mental status changes, if carbon dioxide retention worsens
- Anorexia and cachexia

Diagnostic Test Results

- Chest X-rays in advanced disease show a flattened diaphragm, reduced vascular markings at the lung periphery, overaeration of the lungs, a vertical heart, enlarged anteroposterior chest diameter, and a large retrosternal air space.
- Pulmonary function studies indicate increased residual volume and total lung capacity, reduced diffusing capacity, increased inspiratory flow, and decreased FEV1/FVC.
- ABG analysis usually reveals reduced partial pressure of arterial oxygen and a normal partial pressure of arterial carbon dioxide until late in the disease process. ABGs provide the best evidence as to acuteness and severity of disease exacerbation.
- Electrocardiography shows tall, symmetrical P waves in leads II, III, and aV$_F$; a vertical QRS axis and signs of right ventricular hypertrophy are seen late in the disease.
- Complete blood count usually reveals an increased hemoglobin level late in the disease when the patient has persistent, severe hypoxia.

Treatment

CLINICAL TIP
Pneumococcal conjugate vaccine is recommended for all babies and children younger than 2 years of age, all adults 65 years or older, and people 2 through 64 years old with certain medical conditions. Pneumococcal polysaccharide vaccine is recommended for all adults 65 years or older, people 2 through 64 years old who are at increased risk for disease due to certain medical conditions, and adults 19 through 64 years old who smoke cigarettes (CDC, 2016, pneumococcal vaccination).

- Adequate hydration
- Chest physiotherapy
- Oxygen therapy
- Mucolytics
- Aerosolized or systemic corticosteroids
- Lung volume reduction surgery
- Lung transplantation

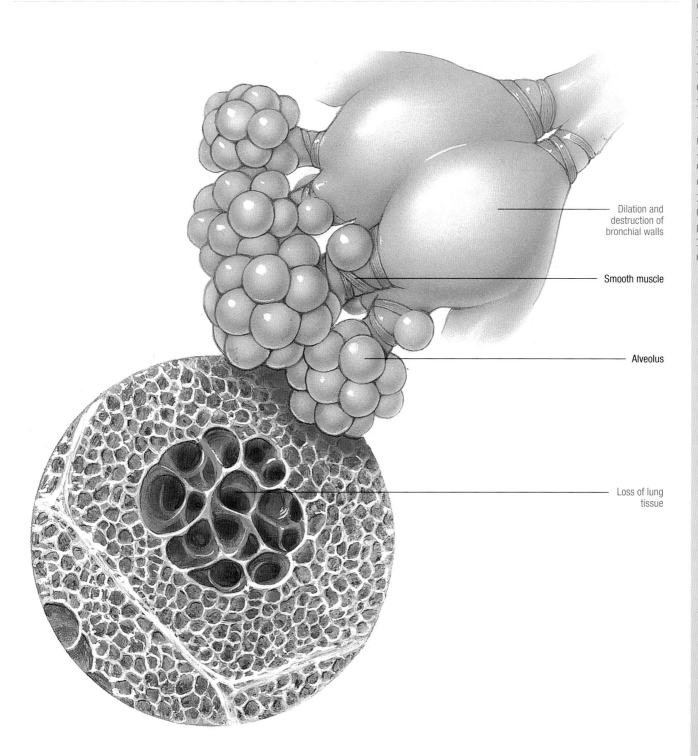

Dilation and destruction of bronchial walls

Smooth muscle

Alveolus

Loss of lung tissue

CYSTIC FIBROSIS

Cystic fibrosis is a hereditary disorder affecting the exocrine gland and causing severe damage to multiple organ systems. Chronic progressive lung disease is the most prominent cause of morbidity and death in patients with cystic fibrosis.

Cystic fibrosis is accompanied by many complications and has a median survival rate of 31 years. The disease affects males and females and is the most common fatal genetic disease in children of European ancestry. There are more than 30,000 patients with cystic fibrosis in the United States (Cystic Fibrosis Foundation, 2017).

Cause

Inherited as an autosomal recessive trait, the responsible gene, on chromosome 7q, encodes a membrane-associated protein called the cystic fibrosis transmembrane regulator (CFTR). The exact function of CFTR remains unknown, but it appears to help regulate chloride and sodium transport across epithelial membranes.

Pathophysiology

Most cases of cystic fibrosis arise from the mutation that affects the genetic coding for a single amino acid, resulting in a protein (CFTR) that doesn't function properly. CFTR resembles other transmembrane transport proteins, but it lacks the phenylalanine in the protein produced by normal genes. This regulator interferes with chloride channels regulated by cyclic adenosine monophosphate, and with other ions, by preventing adenosine triphosphate from binding to the protein or by interfering with activation by protein kinase.

The mutation affects volume-absorbing epithelia (in the airways and intestines), salt-absorbing epithelia (in sweat ducts), and volume-secretory epithelia (in the pancreas). Lack of phenylalanine leads to dehydration, which increases the viscosity of mucous gland secretions and leads to obstruction of glandular ducts. Cystic fibrosis has a variable effect on electrolyte and water transport.

COMPLICATIONS
- Nasal polyps
- Cor pulmonale
- Cholecystitis
- Pneumothorax
- Rectal prolapse
- Bowel obstruction

Signs and Symptoms

- Thick, sticky secretions and dehydration
- Chronic infections
- Dyspnea and paroxysmal cough
- Failure to thrive: poor weight gain, poor growth, distended abdomen, thin extremities, and poor skin turgor
- Crackles and wheezes
- Bulky, greasy stools
- Obstruction of small and large intestines; biliary cirrhosis

Diagnostic Test Results

All states screen newborns for CF using a genetic test or a blood test.

The Cystic Fibrosis Foundation has developed certain criteria for definitive diagnosis:

- Two sweat tests (to detect elevated sodium chloride levels) using a pilocarpine solution (a sweat inducer) and presence of an obstructive pulmonary disease, confirmed pancreatic insufficiency or failure to thrive, or a family history of cystic fibrosis.

AGE ALERT
The sweat test may be inaccurate in very young infants because they may not produce enough sweat for a valid test.

- Chest X-rays show an enlarged chest cavity and decreased lung markings, reflecting destruction of lung tissue.
- Stool specimen analysis indicates the absence of trypsin, suggesting pancreatic insufficiency.

These test results may support the diagnosis:

- DNA testing can locate the presence of the Delta F508 deletion (found in about 70% of patients with cystic fibrosis, although the disease can cause more than 100 other mutations). It allows prenatal diagnosis in families with a previously affected child.
- Pulmonary function tests reveal decreased vital capacity, elevated residual volume due to air entrapments, and decreased forced expiratory volume in 1 second. The severity of lung disease and rate of lung function decline are widely variable.
- Liver enzyme tests reveal hepatic insufficiency.
- Sputum culture reveals organisms that cystic fibrosis patients typically and chronically colonize, such as *Staphylococcus* and *Pseudomonas*.
- Serum albumin measurement helps assess nutritional status.
- Electrolyte analysis assesses hydration status.

Treatment

- High-frequency chest compression vest
- Diet with increased fat and sodium or salt supplements
- Pancreatic enzyme replacement
- Breathing exercises, chest percussion, and postural drainage
- Inhaled bronchodilators
- Antibiotics such as azithromycin
- Transplantation of heart or lungs
- Mucus-thinning drugs such as dornase alfa
- Positive expiratory pressure devices
- Flutter valves

Treatment goals include:

- Bronchial hygiene and mobilizing mucus
- Preventing and controlling infections
- Providing adequate nutrition
- Treating and preventing adverse complications

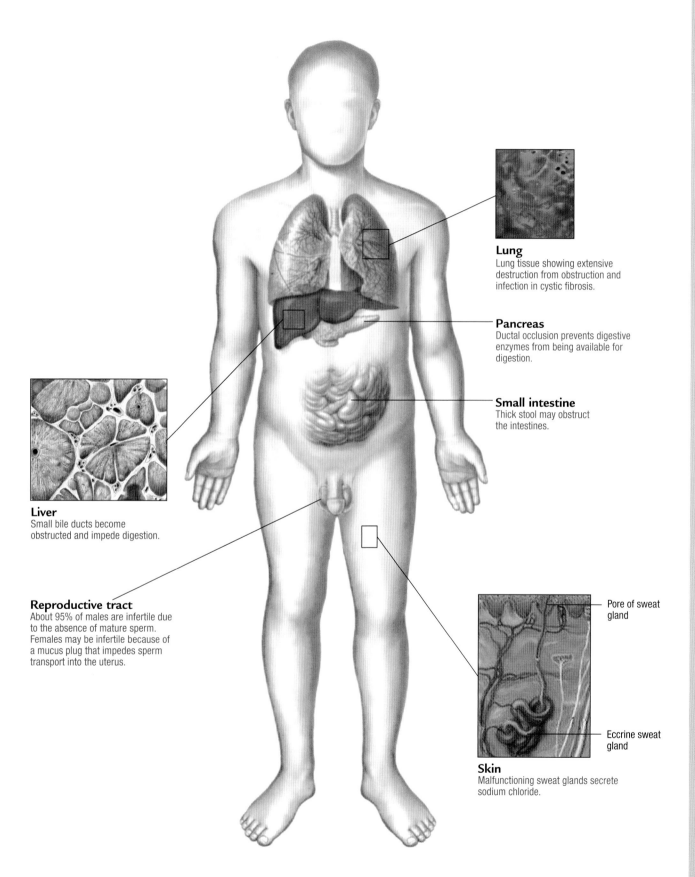

Lung
Lung tissue showing extensive destruction from obstruction and infection in cystic fibrosis.

Pancreas
Ductal occlusion prevents digestive enzymes from being available for digestion.

Small intestine
Thick stool may obstruct the intestines.

Liver
Small bile ducts become obstructed and impede digestion.

Reproductive tract
About 95% of males are infertile due to the absence of mature sperm. Females may be infertile because of a mucus plug that impedes sperm transport into the uterus.

Pore of sweat gland

Eccrine sweat gland

Skin
Malfunctioning sweat glands secrete sodium chloride.

FAT EMBOLISM SYNDROME

Fat embolism syndrome is a rare but potentially fatal problem. The syndrome involves pulmonary, cerebral, and cutaneous manifestations and occurs 24 to 48 hours postinjury.

AGE ALERT
Young men with fractures are at an increased risk for developing fat embolism syndrome.

Causes

- Fractures of the pelvis, femur, tibia, or ribs
- Orthopedic surgery

Pathophysiology

Bone marrow from a fractured bone or other injured adipose tissue releases fatty globules that enter the systemic circulation through torn veins at the injury site. These fatty globules travel to the lungs, where they form an embolus that blocks pulmonary circulation. Lipase breaks down the trapped fat emboli into free fatty acids.

This process causes a local toxic effect that damages the epithelium, increases capillary permeability, and inactivates lung surfactant. The increased capillary permeability allows protein-rich fluid to leak into the interstitial space and alveoli, increasing the workload of the right side of the heart and causing pulmonary edema. The decreased surfactant causes alveolar collapse, a decrease in functional reserve capacity, and ventilation-perfusion mismatch, leading to hypoxemia. Platelet aggregation on fat, normal injury-related platelet consumption, and platelet dilution through I.V. crystalloid administration all contribute to thrombocytopenia, petechiae, and, possibly, disseminated intravascular coagulation.

COMPLICATIONS
- Respiratory distress

Signs and Symptoms

- Petechiae
- Increased respiratory rate
- Dyspnea
- Accessory muscle use
- Mental status changes
- Jaundice
- Fever

Diagnostic Test Results

CLINICAL TIP
Gurd's criteria are used to diagnose fat embolism syndrome. At least one major and three minor criteria are required for diagnosis. Major criteria include:

- petechiae in a "vest" distribution
- hypoxia, with a partial pressure of arterial oxygen (PaO_2) less than 60 mm Hg
- pulmonary edema
- change in level of consciousness.

Minor criteria include:

- tachycardia, with a heart rate greater than 110 beats/min
- pyrexia, with a temperature higher than 103°F (39.4°C)
- retinal changes
- fat in urine or sputum
- unexplained drop in hematocrit or platelet count
- increasing erythrocyte sedimentation rate
- jaundice
- renal changes.

- ABG analysis reveals PaO_2 less than 60 mm Hg; partial pressure of arterial carbon dioxide initially decreases and later increases.
- Chest X-ray is normal initially but later shows patchy areas of consolidation to complete "white out," if the condition progresses.
- Complete blood count shows decreased platelets and decreased hemoglobin levels.

Treatment

- Supplemental oxygen
- Endotracheal intubation and mechanical ventilation
- I.V. fluids such as crystalloids (avoid colloids)
- Coughing and deep breathing

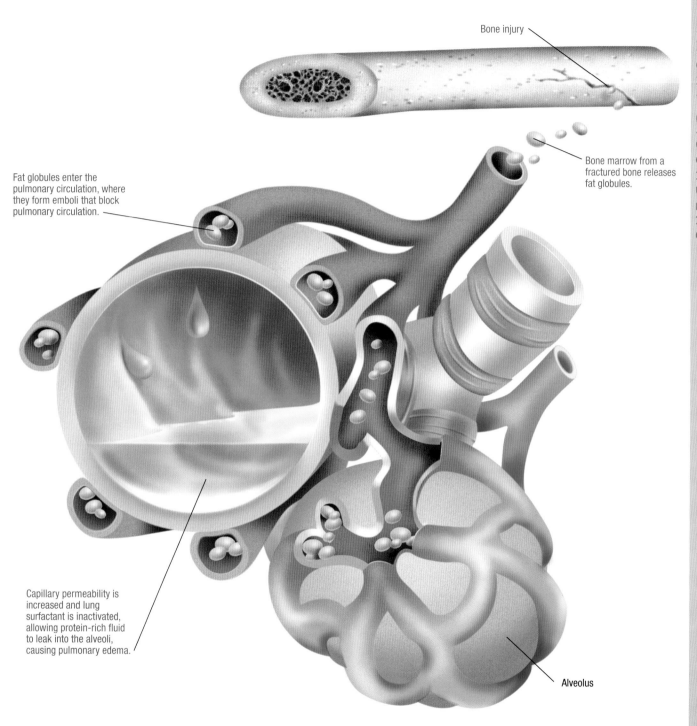

Bone injury

Bone marrow from a fractured bone releases fat globules.

Fat globules enter the pulmonary circulation, where they form emboli that block pulmonary circulation.

Capillary permeability is increased and lung surfactant is inactivated, allowing protein-rich fluid to leak into the alveoli, causing pulmonary edema.

Alveolus

IDIOPATHIC PULMONARY FIBROSIS

Idiopathic pulmonary fibrosis is a chronic and usually fatal interstitial pulmonary disease. Once thought to be a rare condition, it is now diagnosed with much greater frequency. Despite successful development of new therapies, survival has not been convincingly improved. Survival is estimated at 3 to 5 years after diagnosis.

The American Thoracic Society and the European Respiratory Society define idiopathic pulmonary fibrosis as "a specific form of chronic, progressive fibrosing interstitial pneumonia of unknown cause, occurring primarily in older adults, and limited to the lungs" (Oldham & Noth, 2014).

AGE ALERT
Idiopathic pulmonary fibrosis occurs most commonly in people between ages 50 and 70.

Causes

Unknown

Pathophysiology

Idiopathic pulmonary fibrosis reflects the accumulation of excessive fibrous or connective tissue in the lung parenchyma. It is the result of a cascade of inflammatory, immune, and fibrotic processes in the lung. Despite many studies, the stimulus that begins the progression remains unknown. Speculation has revolved around viral and genetic causes, but no evidence has been found to support either theory. However, it is clear that chronic inflammation plays an important role. Inflammation develops the injury and the fibrosis that ultimately distorts and impairs the structure and function of the alveolocapillary gas exchange surface. The lungs become stiff and difficult to ventilate, and the diffusion capacity of the alveolocapillary membrane decreases, leading to hypoxemia.

Idiopathic pulmonary fibrosis is characterized by progressive worsening of dyspnea and lung function. Underlying lesions may be more fibrotic than inflammatory.

COMPLICATIONS
- Respiratory failure
- Heart failure
- Pulmonary embolism
- Pneumonia
- Lung cancer

Signs and Symptoms

- Dyspnea and rapid, shallow breathing. Dyspnea is the most frequently reported symptom in lung cancer patients
- Dry, hacking cough
- Fatigue

- End-expiratory crackles and bronchial breath sounds
- Clubbed fingers and toes
- Cyanosis
- Pulmonary hypertension
- Profound hypoxemia and severe, debilitating dyspnea in advanced disease
- Chest pain

Diagnostic Test Results

Diagnosis begins with a thorough patient history to exclude any of the more common causes of interstitial lung disease, such as:

- environmental or occupational exposure — coal dust, asbestos, silica, beryllium
- connective tissue diseases — scleroderma, rheumatoid arthritis
- drug use — amiodarone, tocainide, crack cocaine.

Tests that help to confirm the diagnosis include:

- lung biopsy — shows mixed areas of normal tissue, interstitial inflammation, fibrosis, and honeycombing
- chest X-ray and high-resolution computed tomography — show a pattern of diffuse interstitial lung disease, with fibrosis and honeycombing
- pulmonary function tests — reveal decreased total lung volumes.

Treatment

- Oxygen therapy
- Corticosteroids
- Immunosuppressants, such as cyclophosphamide and azathioprine
- Colchicine
- Pulmonary rehabilitation
- Lung transplantation (therapeutic option)

Because idiopathic pulmonary fibrosis generally responds poorly to treatment and drug therapies cause many adverse reactions, research studies are currently aimed at learning which factors may improve the patient's response to treatment. The chances of a positive response to therapy and extended survival seem to be best for young female patients with less-than-average dyspnea and hypoxemia, more normal lung function, and no history of smoking. Evidence of inflammation (lymphocytes in bronchoalveolar lavage fluid, circulating immune complexes, and positive response to corticosteroids) also seems to predict a better outcome. Indicators of a poor prognosis are irreversible lung destruction and fibrosis (severe hypoxemia, decreased diffusing capacity for carbon monoxide, and neutrophils and eosinophils in bronchoalveolar lavage fluid).

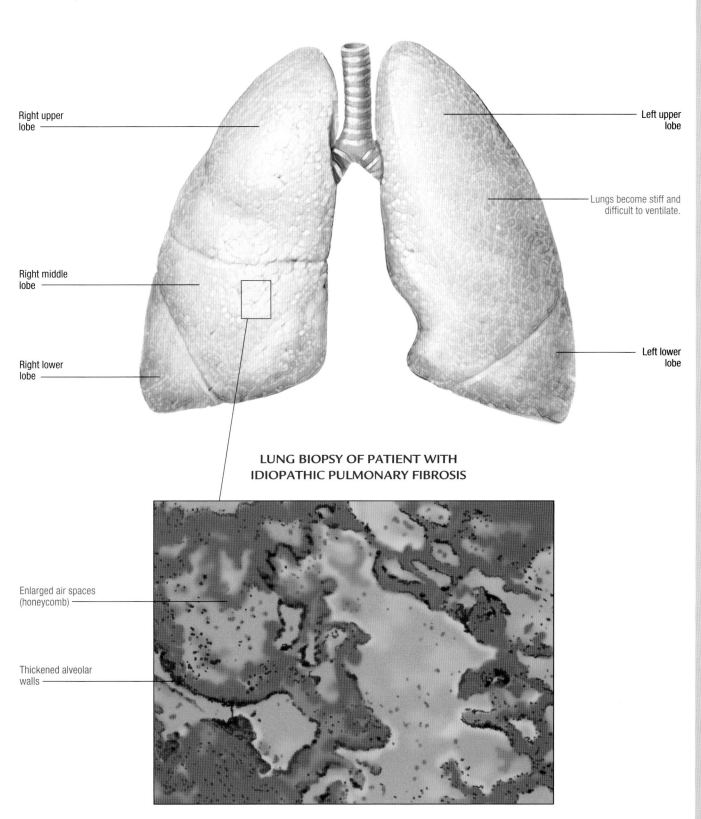

Right upper lobe

Left upper lobe

Lungs become stiff and difficult to ventilate.

Right middle lobe

Right lower lobe

Left lower lobe

LUNG BIOPSY OF PATIENT WITH IDIOPATHIC PULMONARY FIBROSIS

Enlarged air spaces (honeycomb)

Thickened alveolar walls

LUNG CANCER

Lung cancer is the leading cause of cancer death among men and women (National Cancer Institute, 2017).

AGE ALERT
Lung cancer is fairly rare in people younger than age 40. The average age at diagnosis is 60.

The two main types of lung cancer are small-cell lung cancer (SCLC) and non–small-cell lung cancer (NSCLC). If the cancer has features of both, it's called *mixed small-cell/large-cell cancer.*

About 20% of all lung cancers are SCLC. Although the cancer cells are small, they can multiply quickly and form large tumors that spread to the lymph nodes and to other organs, such as the brain, liver, and bones. Therefore, treatment must include drugs that kill this widespread disease. SCLC is extremely rare in someone who has never smoked.

Recommend including → Smoking remains the predominant risk factor for lung cancer.

The remaining 80% of lung cancers are NSCLC, which includes three subtypes. The cells in these subtypes differ in size, shape, and chemical makeup. They include:

- *squamous cell carcinoma*, which is commonly linked to a history of smoking and tends to be found centrally, near a bronchus
- *adenocarcinoma*, which is usually found in the outer region of the lung
- *large-cell undifferentiated carcinoma*, which can appear in any part of the lung and tends to grow and spread quickly. (This type of cancer has a poor prognosis.)

Causes

- Tobacco smoke
- Carcinogenic industrial and air pollutants (asbestos, uranium, arsenic, nickel, iron oxides, chromium, radioactive dust, coal dust, radon)

Pathophysiology

Lung cancer begins with the transformation of one epithelial cell of the airway. The bronchi, and certain portions of the bronchi, such as the segmental bifurcations and sites of mucus production, are thought to be more vulnerable to injury from carcinogens.

As a lung tumor grows, it can partially or completely obstruct the airway, resulting in lobar collapse distal to the tumor. A lung tumor can also hemorrhage, causing hemoptysis. Early metastasis may occur to other thoracic structures, such as hilar lymph nodes or the mediastinum. Distant metastasis can occur to the brain, liver, bone, and adrenal glands.

COMPLICATIONS
- Phrenic nerve paralysis
- Tracheal obstruction
- Esophageal compression
- Pleural effusion

Signs and Symptoms

- Cough, hoarseness, wheezing, dyspnea, hemoptysis, and chest pain
- Fever, weight loss, weakness, and anorexia
- Bone and joint pain
- Cushing's syndrome
- Hypercalcemia
- Hemoptysis, atelectasis, pneumonitis, and dyspnea
- Shoulder pain and unilateral paralysis of diaphragm
- Dysphagia
- Jugular vein distention and facial, neck, and chest edema
- Piercing chest pain, increasing dyspnea, and severe arm pain

Diagnostic Test Results

- Chest X-ray shows an advanced lesion, including size and location.
- Sputum cytology reveals possible cell type.
- Computed tomography (CT) scan of the chest delineates tumor size and relationship to surrounding structures.
- Bronchoscopy locates tumor; washings reveal malignant cell type.
- Needle lung biopsy confirms cell type.
- Mediastinal and supraclavicular node biopsies reveal possible metastasis.
- Thoracentesis shows malignant cells in pleural fluid.
- Bone scan, bone marrow biopsy, and CT scan of the brain and abdomen reveal metastasis.

Treatment

- Lobectomy, wedge resection, or pneumonectomy
- Video-assisted chest surgery
- Laser surgery
- Radiation
- Chemotherapy

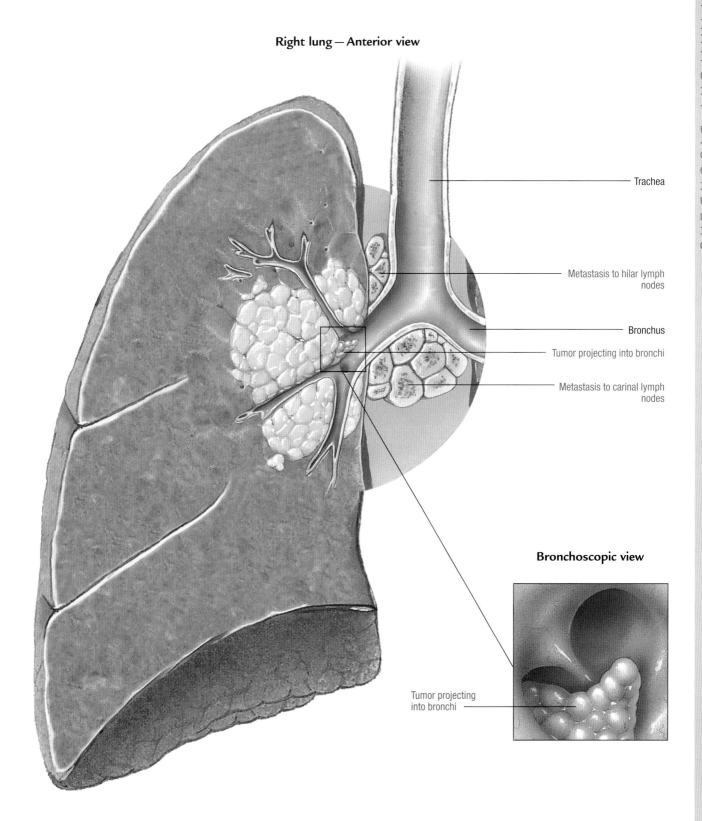

Right lung — Anterior view

Trachea

Metastasis to hilar lymph nodes

Bronchus

Tumor projecting into bronchi

Metastasis to carinal lymph nodes

Bronchoscopic view

Tumor projecting into bronchi

PLEURAL EFFUSION

Pleural effusion is an excess of fluid in the pleural space. Normally, this space contains a small amount of extracellular fluid that lubricates the pleural surfaces. Increased production or inadequate removal of this fluid results in transudative or exudative pleural effusion. Empyema is the accumulation of pus and necrotic tissue in the pleural space. The most common associated symptoms are cough, progressive dyspnea, and pleuritic chest pain.

Causes

Transudative Pleural Effusion

- Heart failure
- Hepatic disease with ascites
- Peritoneal dialysis
- Hypoalbuminemia
- Disorders causing expanded intravascular volume

Exudative Pleural Effusion

- Tuberculosis (TB)
- Subphrenic abscess
- Pancreatitis
- Bacterial or fungal pneumonitis or empyema
- Malignancy
- Pulmonary embolism with or without infarction
- Collagen disease such as systemic lupus erythematosus
- Myxedema
- Chest trauma

Empyema

- Idiopathic infection
- Pneumonitis
- Carcinoma
- Perforation
- Esophageal rupture

Pathophysiology

The balance of osmotic and hydrostatic pressures in parietal pleural capillaries normally results in fluid movement into the pleural space. Balanced pressures in visceral pleural capillaries promote reabsorption of this fluid. Excessive hydrostatic pressure or decreased osmotic pressure can cause excessive amounts of fluid to pass across intact capillaries. The result is a *transudative pleural effusion*, an ultrafiltrate of plasma containing low concentrations of protein.

Exudative pleural effusion results when capillary permeability increases with or without changes in hydrostatic and colloid osmotic pressures, allowing protein-rich fluid to leak into the pleural space.

Empyema is usually associated with infection in the pleural space.

COMPLICATIONS
- Atelectasis
- Infection
- Hypoxemia

Signs and Symptoms

- Characteristically related to underlying pathologic condition and how quickly effusion develops
- Dyspnea
- Pleuritic chest pain
- Fever
- Malaise
- Displaced point of maximum impulse, based on size of effusion
- Decreased breath sounds
- Dullness over the effused areas (doesn't change with breathing)

Diagnostic Test Results

- Chest X-ray shows radiopaque fluid in dependent regions.
- Computed tomography scan will show the location of the pleural effusions.

Diagnosis also requires other tests to distinguish transudative from exudative effusions and to help pinpoint the underlying disorder. The most useful test is thoracentesis, in which analysis of aspirated pleural fluid shows:

- transudative effusions — lactate dehydrogenase (LD) levels less than 200 International Units and protein levels less than 3 g/dL
- exudative effusions — ratio of protein in pleural fluid to serum of 0.5 or more, LD in pleural fluid of 200 International Units or more, and ratio of LD in pleural fluid to LD in serum of 0.6 or more
- empyema — acute inflammatory white blood cells and microorganisms
- empyema or rheumatoid arthritis — extremely decreased pleural fluid glucose levels.

In addition, if a pleural effusion results from esophageal rupture or pancreatitis, fluid amylase levels are usually higher than serum levels. Aspirated fluid may be tested for lupus erythematosus cells, antinuclear antibodies, and neoplastic cells. It may also be analyzed for color and consistency; acid-fast bacillus, fungal, and bacterial cultures; and triglycerides (in chylothorax). Cell analysis shows leukocytosis in empyema. A negative tuberculin skin test strongly rules against TB as the cause. In exudative pleural effusions in which thoracentesis isn't definitive, pleural biopsy may be done. It is particularly useful for confirming TB or malignancy.

Treatment

- Thoracentesis
- Chest tube insertion
- Pleurodesis (injection of a sclerosing agent such as talc)
- Decortication
- Rib resection
- Parenteral antibiotics
- Oxygen therapy
- Pleuroperitoneal shunt
- PleurX catheter

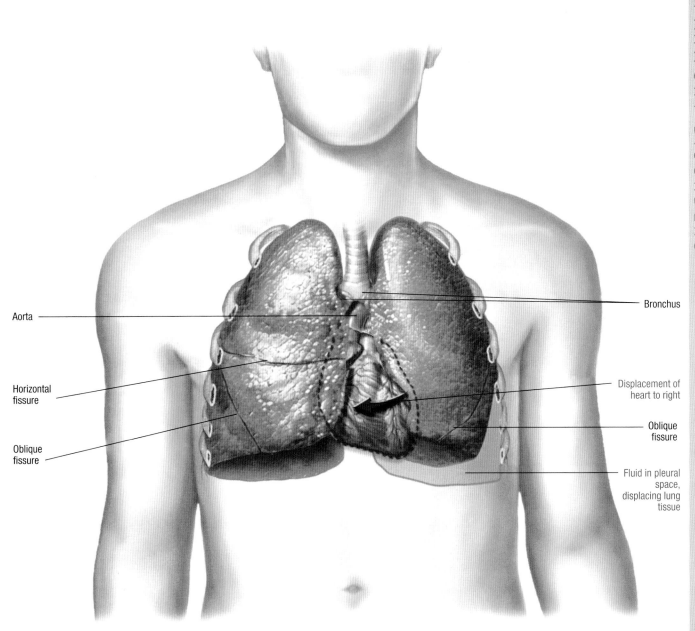

Aorta

Horizontal
fissure

Oblique
fissure

Bronchus

Displacement of
heart to right

Oblique
fissure

Fluid in pleural
space,
displacing lung
tissue

PNEUMONIA

Pneumonia is an acute infection of the lung parenchyma that commonly impairs gas exchange. The prognosis is generally good for people who have normal lungs and adequate host defenses before the onset of pneumonia.

Pneumonia is commonly classified according to location: *bronchopneumonia* involves distal airways and alveoli; *lobular pneumonia*, part of a lobe; and *lobar pneumonia*, an entire lobe. It can also be classified according to the causative agent, such as gram negative or gram positive, viral, bacterial, or the specific organ responsible such as pneumococcal pneumonia. Nosocomial pneumonia occurs during hospitalization for another condition.

AGE ALERT
Older patients and very young patients are at greater risk for pneumonia.

Other patients at greater risk are those who are immunocompromised, malnourished, or hospitalized in an intensive care unit; smokers or alcohol abusers; and those with a chronic condition such as cardiovascular disease.

Causes

Primary

- Inhalation or aspiration of a pathogen, including pneumococcal, viral, and mycoplasmal pneumonia

CLINICAL TIP
Streptococcus pneumoniae is the most common cause of bacterial pneumonia in children.
    Haemophilus influenzae type b (Hib) is the second most common cause of bacterial pneumonia.
    Respiratory syncytial virus is the most common viral cause of pneumonia.

Secondary

- After initial damage from a noxious chemical or other insult (superinfection)
- Hematogenous spread of bacteria from a distant focus

Pathophysiology

In bacterial pneumonia, an infection initially triggers alveolar inflammation and edema. This produces an area of low ventilation with normal perfusion. Capillaries become engorged with blood, causing stasis. As the alveolocapillary membrane breaks down, alveoli fill with blood and exudate, resulting in atelectasis.

In viral pneumonia, the virus first attacks bronchiolar epithelial cells. This causes interstitial inflammation and desquamation. The virus also invades bronchial mucous glands and goblet cells. It then spreads to the alveoli, which fill with blood and fluid. In advanced infection, a hyaline membrane may form.

In aspiration pneumonia, inhalation of gastric juices or hydrocarbons triggers inflammatory changes and inactivates surfactant over a large area. Decreased surfactant leads to alveolar collapse. Acidic gastric juices may damage the airways and alveoli. Particles containing aspirated gastric juices may obstruct the airways and reduce airflow, leading to secondary bacterial pneumonia.

COMPLICATIONS
- Septic shock
- Hypoxemia
- Respiratory failure
- Empyema or lung abscess
- Bacteremia
- Endocarditis
- Pericarditis
- Meningitis

Signs and Symptoms

- Coughing
- Sputum production
- Pleuritic chest pain
- Shaking chills
- Fever
- Wide range of physical signs, from diffuse, fine crackles to signs of localized or extensive consolidation and pleural effusion
- Dyspnea
- Tachypnea
- Malaise
- Decreased breath sounds

Diagnostic Test Results

- Chest X-rays identify infiltrates that confirm the diagnosis.
- Sputum specimen, Gram stain, and culture and sensitivity tests differentiate the type of infection.
- White blood cell (WBC) count indicates leukocytosis in bacterial pneumonia, and a normal or low WBC count in viral or mycoplasmal pneumonia.
- Blood cultures reflect bacteremia and are used to determine the causative organism.
- ABG levels vary, depending on the severity of pneumonia and the underlying lung state.
- Bronchoscopy or transtracheal aspiration allows the collection of material for culture.
- Pulse oximetry shows a reduced oxygen saturation level.

Treatment

- Antimicrobial therapy (varies with causative agent)
- Humidified oxygen therapy
- Mechanical ventilation
- High-calorie diet and adequate fluid intake
- Bed rest
- Analgesics
- PEEP to facilitate adequate oxygenation in patients on mechanical ventilation for severe pneumonia

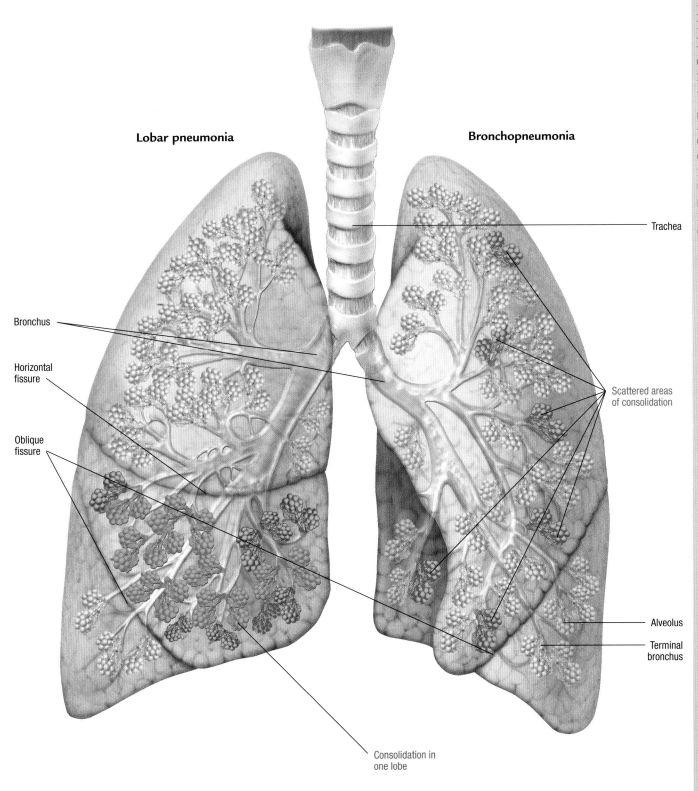

Lobar pneumonia

Bronchopneumonia

Trachea

Bronchus

Horizontal
fissure

Oblique
fissure

Scattered areas
of consolidation

Alveolus

Terminal
bronchus

Consolidation in
one lobe

PNEUMOTHORAX

Pneumothorax is an accumulation of air in the pleural cavity that leads to partial or complete lung collapse. When the air between the visceral and parietal pleurae collects and accumulates, increasing tension in the pleural cavity can cause the lung to progressively collapse. The amount of air trapped in the intrapleural space determines the degree of lung collapse. Venous return to the heart may be impeded to cause a life-threatening condition called *tension pneumothorax*. Pneumothoraces are usually classified as primary spontaneous, secondary spontaneous, traumatic, or tension.

Causes

Primary Spontaneous Pneumothorax

- Unknown
- Rupture of a bleb or a bulla

AGE ALERT
Primary spontaneous pneumothorax most commonly affects tall, thin men between ages 20 and 40.

Secondary Spontaneous Pneumothorax

- Chronic obstructive pulmonary disease
- Asthma
- Cystic fibrosis
- Tuberculosis
- Whooping cough

Traumatic Pneumothorax

- Traumatic chest injury
- Penetrating chest trauma (stab wound, gunshot)
- Blunt chest trauma (blow from a motor vehicle accident)
- Iatrogenic chest trauma, resulting from puncture of the lung during needle aspiration lung biopsy, thoracentesis, or central venous catheter placement

Tension Pneumothorax

- Lung collapse forced by excessive pressure

Pathophysiology

A rupture in the visceral or parietal pleura and chest wall causes air to accumulate and separate the visceral and parietal pleurae. Negative pressure is destroyed, and the elastic recoil forces are affected. The lung recoils by collapsing toward the hilus.

Open pneumothorax results when atmospheric air (positive pressure) flows directly into the pleural cavity (negative pressure). As the air pressure in the pleural cavity becomes positive, the lung collapses on the affected side, resulting in decreased total lung capacity, vital capacity, and lung compliance. Imbalances in the ventilation-perfusion ratio lead to hypoxia.

Closed pneumothorax occurs when air enters the pleural space from within the lung, causing increased pleural pressure, which prevents lung expansion during normal inspiration.

Tension pneumothorax results when air in the pleural space is under higher pressure than air in the adjacent lung. The air enters the pleural space from the site of pleural rupture, which acts as a one-way valve. Air is allowed to enter into the pleural space on inspiration but can't escape as the rupture site closes on expiration. More air enters on inspiration, and air pressure begins to exceed barometric pressure. Increasing air pressure pushes against the recoiled lung, causing compression atelectasis. Air also presses against the mediastinum, compressing and displacing the heart and great vessels. The air can't escape, and the accumulating pressure causes the lung to collapse. As air continues to accumulate and intrapleural pressures rise, the mediastinum shifts away from the affected side and decreases venous return. This leads to decreased cardiac output, which causes hypotension.

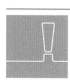

COMPLICATIONS

- Fatal pulmonary and circulatory impairment

Signs and Symptoms

- Sudden, sharp pleuritic pain exacerbated by chest movement, breathing, or coughing
- Asymmetrical chest wall movement
- Shortness of breath and respiratory distress
- Hypotension
- Cyanosis
- Decreased vocal fremitus
- Absent breath sounds and chest rigidity on the affected side
- Tachycardia
- Subcutaneous emphysema

Tension pneumothorax produces the most severe respiratory symptoms, including:

- decreased cardiac output, hypotension, and compensatory tachycardia
- tachypnea
- lung collapse
- mediastinal shift and tracheal deviation to the opposite side
- distended jugular veins.

Diagnostic Test Results

- Chest X-rays confirm the diagnosis by revealing air in the pleural space and, possibly, a mediastinal shift.
- ABG analysis may reveal hypoxemia, possibly with respiratory acidosis and hypercapnia. Partial pressure of arterial oxygen levels may decrease at first but typically returns to normal within 24 hours.

Treatment

- Bed rest
- Observation
- Oxygen
- Chest tube insertion
- Thoracostomy
- Analgesics
- Surgery

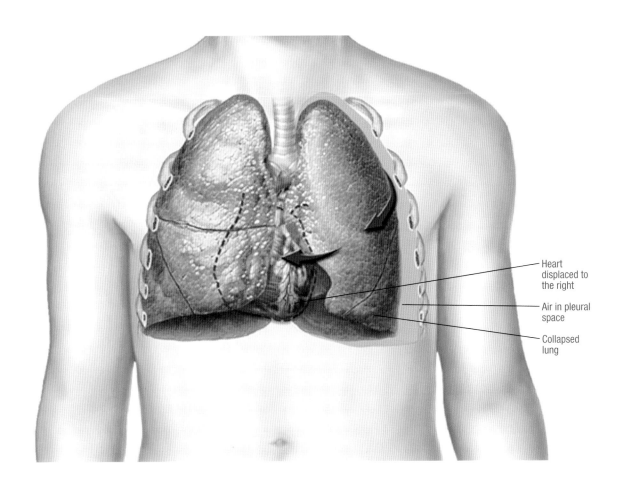

Heart displaced to the right

Air in pleural space

Collapsed lung

TENSION PNEUMOTHORAX

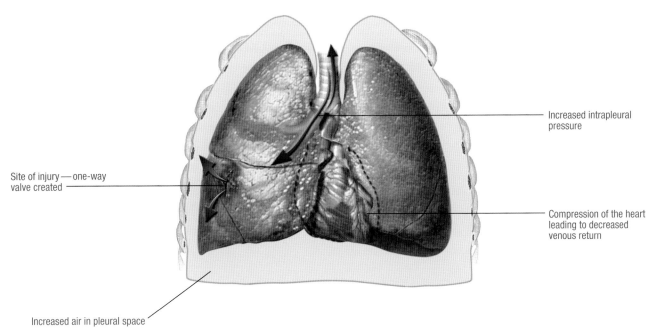

Site of injury — one-way valve created

Increased intrapleural pressure

Compression of the heart leading to decreased venous return

Increased air in pleural space

PULMONARY EDEMA

Pulmonary edema is an accumulation of fluid in the extra-vascular spaces of the lungs due to the movement of excess fluid into the alveoli. It is a common complication of cardiac disorders and may occur as a chronic condition or may develop quickly and rapidly become fatal.

Causes

Left-Sided Heart Failure

- Arteriosclerosis
- Cardiomyopathy
- Hypertension
- Valvular heart disease

Predisposing Factors

- Barbiturate or opiate poisoning
- Cardiac failure
- Excessive volume or too-rapid infusion of I.V. fluids
- Impaired pulmonary lymphatic drainage
- Inhalation of irritating gases
- Mitral stenosis and left atrial myxoma
- Pneumonia
- Pulmonary veno-occlusive disease

Pathophysiology

Normally, pulmonary capillary hydrostatic pressure, capillary oncotic pressure, capillary permeability, and lymphatic drainage are in balance. When this balance changes, or when the lymphatic drainage system is obstructed, fluid infiltrates into the lung and pulmonary edema results. If pulmonary capillary hydrostatic pressure increases, the compromised left ventricle requires increased filling pressures to maintain adequate cardiac output. These pressures are transmitted to the left atrium, pulmonary veins, and pulmonary capillary bed, forcing fluids and solutes from the intravascular compartment into the interstitium of the lungs. As the interstitium overloads with fluid, the fluid floods the peripheral alveoli and impairs gas exchange.

If colloid osmotic pressure decreases, the hydrostatic force that regulates intravascular fluids (the natural pulling force) is lost because there's no opposition. Fluid flows freely into the interstitium and alveoli, impairing gas exchange and leading to pulmonary edema.

Lymphatic vessels may be blocked by edema or tumor fibrotic tissue or by increased systemic venous pressure. Hydrostatic pressure in the large pulmonary veins rises, the pulmonary lymphatic system cannot drain into the pulmonary veins, and excess fluid moves into the interstitial space. Pulmonary edema then results from the accumulation of fluid.

Capillary injury and consequent increased permeability may occur in ARDS or after inhalation of toxic gases. Plasma proteins and water leak out of the injured capillary and into the interstitium, increasing the interstitial oncotic pressure, which is normally low. As interstitial oncotic pressure begins to equal capillary oncotic pressure, the water begins to move out of the capillary and into the lungs, resulting in pulmonary edema.

COMPLICATIONS

- Respiratory and metabolic acidosis
- Cardiac or respiratory arrest

Signs and Symptoms

Early Stage

- Dyspnea on exertion, paroxysmal nocturnal dyspnea, and orthopnea
- Cough
- Mild tachypnea
- Increased blood pressure
- Dependent crackles
- Jugular vein distention
- Tachycardia

Later Stages

- Labored, rapid respiration
- More diffuse crackles
- Cough producing frothy, bloody sputum
- Increased tachycardia, arrhythmias, and thready pulse
- Cold, clammy skin and diaphoresis
- Cyanosis
- Hypotension

Diagnostic Test Results

- ABG analysis usually reveals hypoxia with variable partial pressure of arterial carbon dioxide, depending on the patient's degree of fatigue. Respiratory acidosis may occur.
- Chest X-rays show diffuse haziness of the lung fields and, usually, cardiomegaly and pleural effusion.
- Pulse oximetry reveals decreasing arterial oxygen saturation levels.
- Pulmonary artery catheterization identifies left-sided heart failure and helps rule out ARDS.
- Electrocardiography shows previous or current myocardial infarction.

Treatment

- High concentrations of oxygen
- Diuretics, such as furosemide or bumetanide
- Positive inotropic agents, such as digoxin or inamrinone
- Vasopressors
- Arterial vasodilators such as nitroprusside
- Antiarrhythmics
- Morphine
- Mechanical ventilation
- Noninvasive ventilation using continuous positive airway pressure, bilevel positive airway pressure, and PEEP

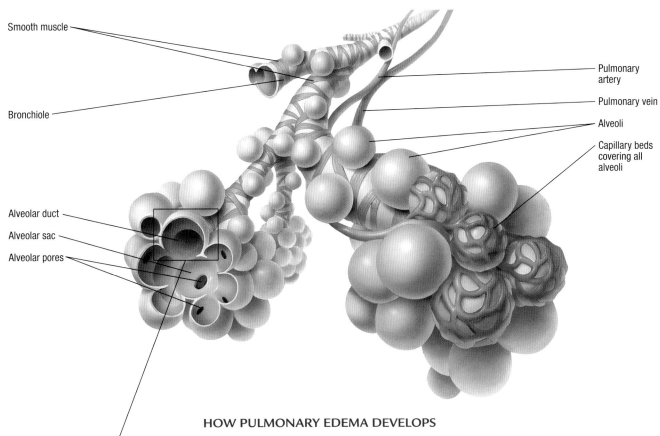

Smooth muscle

Bronchiole

Alveolar duct

Alveolar sac

Alveolar pores

Pulmonary artery

Pulmonary vein

Alveoli

Capillary beds covering all alveoli

HOW PULMONARY EDEMA DEVELOPS

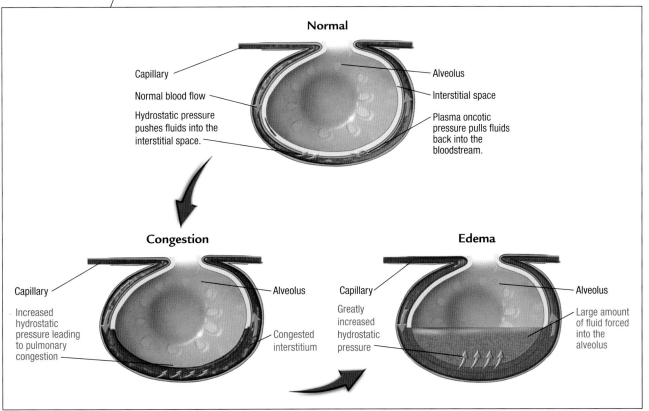

Normal

Capillary

Normal blood flow

Hydrostatic pressure pushes fluids into the interstitial space.

Alveolus

Interstitial space

Plasma oncotic pressure pulls fluids back into the bloodstream.

Congestion

Capillary

Increased hydrostatic pressure leading to pulmonary congestion

Alveolus

Congested interstitium

Edema

Capillary

Greatly increased hydrostatic pressure

Alveolus

Large amount of fluid forced into the alveolus

PULMONARY EMBOLISM

Pulmonary embolism is an obstruction of the pulmonary arterial bed by a dislodged thrombus, heart valve vegetation, or foreign substance. It frequently arises from thrombi that originate in the deep venous system of the lower extremities. It strikes about 6 million adults each year in the United States, resulting in 100,000 deaths.

Causes

- Dislodged thrombi, originating in leg veins (most common)
- Conditions that cause increased blood coagulability, such as cancer and hormonal contraceptives
- Surgery
- Long periods of inactivity
- Some medical conditions, such as stroke and myocardial infarction
- Injury to the vein

Predisposing Factors

- Obesity
- Some cancers, such as pancreatic, ovarian, and lung
- Smoking
- Pregnancy and childbirth
- Vascular injury and I.V. drug abuse

CLINICAL TIP

A triad of deep vein thrombosis (DVT) formation is stasis, endothelial injury, and hypercoagulability. Risk factors include long car or plane trips, cancer, pregnancy, hypercoagulability, and prior DVT or pulmonary emboli.

Pathophysiology

Thrombus formation results directly from vascular wall damage, venostasis, or hypercoagulability of the blood. Trauma, clot dissolution, sudden muscle spasm, intravascular pressure changes, or a change in peripheral blood flow can cause the thrombus to loosen or fragmentize. Then the thrombus — now called an embolus — floats to the heart's right side and enters the lung through the pulmonary artery. There, the embolus may dissolve, continue to fragmentize, or grow.

If the embolus occludes the pulmonary artery, it prevents alveoli from producing enough surfactant to maintain alveolar integrity. As a result, alveoli collapse and atelectasis develops. If the embolus enlarges, it may clog most or all of the pulmonary vessels and cause death.

Rarely, the emboli contain air, fat, bacteria, amniotic fluid, talc, or tumor cells.

COMPLICATIONS

- Pulmonary hypertension
- Cor pulmonale

Signs and Symptoms

Total occlusion of the main pulmonary artery is rapidly fatal; smaller or fragmented emboli produce symptoms that vary with the size, number, and location, as follows:

- dyspnea
- anxiety
- pleuritic chest pain
- tachycardia
- productive cough (sputum may be blood-tinged)
- low-grade fever
- pleural effusion.

Less common signs include the following:

- massive hemoptysis
- splinting of the chest
- leg edema and pain
- cyanosis, syncope, and distended jugular veins
- pleural friction rub
- signs of circulatory collapse (weak, rapid pulse and hypotension)
- signs of hypoxia (restlessness and anxiety)
- right ventricular S_3 gallop and increased intensity of a pulmonic component of S_2
- crackles and a pleural rub may be heard at the embolism site.

Diagnostic Test Results

- Chest X-ray may show areas of atelectasis, elevated diaphragm and pleural effusion, prominent pulmonary artery, and, occasionally, the characteristic wedge-shaped infiltrate suggestive of pulmonary infarction.
- Lung scan shows perfusion defects in areas beyond occluded vessels.
- Pulmonary angiography reveals the location of the emboli.
- Electrocardiography may show right axis deviation (extensive embolism); tall, peaked P waves (right bundle branch block); depression of ST segments and T-wave inversions (indicative of right-sided heart strain); and supraventricular tachyarrhythmias. A pattern sometimes observed is S_1, Q_3, and T_3 (S wave in lead I, Q wave in lead III, and inverted T wave in lead III).
- ABG measurements may show decreased partial pressure of arterial oxygen and partial pressure of arterial carbon dioxide.
- If pleural effusion is present, thoracentesis may rule out empyema, which indicates pneumonia.

Treatment

Treatment is designed to maintain adequate cardiovascular and pulmonary function during resolution of the obstruction and to prevent recurrence of embolic episodes. Because most emboli resolve within 10 to 14 days, treatment may consist of:

- oxygen therapy and fibrinolytic therapy
- anticoagulation with heparin
- embolectomy
- vasopressors and antibiotics
- vena caval ligation, plication, or insertion of a device to filter blood returning to the heart and lungs, to prevent future pulmonary emboli.

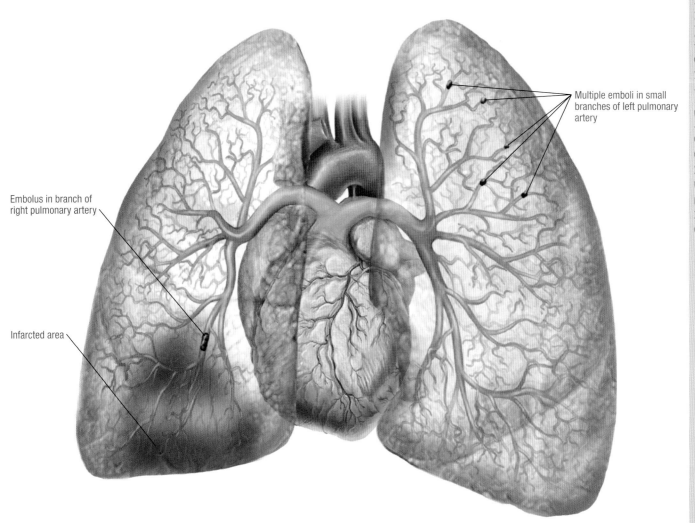

Multiple emboli in small branches of left pulmonary artery

Embolus in branch of right pulmonary artery

Infarcted area

PULMONARY HYPERTENSION

Pulmonary hypertension is a mean systolic pulmonary artery pressure (PAP) above 25 mm Hg at rest and 30 mm Hg during exercise. Primary or idiopathic pulmonary hypertension is characterized by increased PAP and increased pulmonary vascular resistance.

Mean pulmonary artery pressure (MPAP) greater than 25 mm Hg at rest with pulmonary capillary wedge pressure ≤ 15 mm Hg

Severity by MPAP:

26 to 35	Mild
36 to 45	Moderate
46 to 55	Severe
>55	Systemic

AGE ALERT
Primary pulmonary hypertension is most common in women ages 20 to 40 and is usually fatal within 3 to 4 years.

Pulmonary hypertension is a progressive disease that preferentially affects women of child-bearing age. It is characterized by an elevated pulmonary vascular resistance often leading to right ventricular failure and death if untreated.

Secondary pulmonary hypertension results from existing cardiac (patent ductus arteriosus or atrial or septal defect) or pulmonary disease (rheumatic valvular disease or mitral stenosis) or both. The prognosis in secondary pulmonary hypertension depends on the severity of the underlying disorder.

Causes

Primary Pulmonary Hypertension

- Unknown, but may include:
  - hereditary factors
  - altered immune mechanisms.

Secondary Pulmonary Hypertension

- Conditions causing alveolar hypoventilation include:
  - chronic obstructive pulmonary disease
  - sarcoidosis
  - diffuse interstitial pneumonia
  - malignant metastases
  - scleroderma
  - obesity
  - kyphoscoliosis.
- Conditions causing vascular obstruction include:
  - pulmonary embolism
  - vasculitis
  - left atrial myxoma
  - idiopathic veno-occlusive disease
  - fibrosing mediastinitis
  - mediastinal neoplasm.

Pathophysiology

In primary pulmonary hypertension, the smooth muscle in the pulmonary artery wall hypertrophies for no known reason, narrowing or obliterating the artery or arteriole. Fibrous lesions form around the vessels, impairing distensibility and increasing vascular resistance. Pressures in the left ventricle, which receives blood from the lungs, remain normal. However, the increased pressures generated in the lungs are transmitted to the right ventricle, which supplies the pulmonary artery. Progressive pulmonary hypertension may lead to right ventricular hypertrophy and eventually cor pulmonale.

Alveolar hypoventilation can result from diseases caused by alveolar destruction or from disorders that prevent the chest wall from expanding to allow air into the alveoli. The resulting decreased ventilation increases pulmonary vascular resistance. Hypoxemia resulting from this ventilation-perfusion mismatch also causes vasoconstriction, further increasing vascular resistance and resulting in pulmonary hypertension.

COMPLICATIONS
- Cor pulmonale
- Cardiac arrest

Signs and Symptoms

- Shortness of breath
- Increasing dyspnea on exertion
- Fatigue and weakness
- Chest pain
- Cough and hemoptysis
- Cyanosis, Raynaud's phenomenon, and syncope
- Ascites
- Jugular vein distention and reduced carotid pulse
- Restlessness and agitation, decreased level of consciousness, confusion, and memory loss
- Decreased diaphragmatic excursion and respiration
- Possible displacement of point of maximal impulse
- Peripheral edema
- Easily palpable right ventricular lift
- Palpable and tender liver
- Tachycardia
- Systolic ejection murmur
- Split S_2; presence of S_3 and S_4 sounds
- Decreased or loud, tubular breath sounds

Diagnostic Test Results

- ABG analysis reveals hypoxemia.
- Chest X-ray shows enlargement of main and hilar pulmonary arteries, narrowing of peripheral arteries, and enlargement of right atrium and ventricle.
- A chest computed tomography scan may show abnormal lung vessels or blood clots.
- Electrocardiography in right ventricular hypertrophy shows right axis deviation and tall or peaked P waves in inferior leads.
- Cardiac catheterization reveals MPAP above 25 mm Hg or an increased PAWP if the underlying cause is left atrial myxoma, mitral stenosis, or left-sided heart failure.
- Pulmonary angiography detects filling defects in pulmonary vasculature.

- Pulmonary function studies show decreased flow rates and increased residual volume (underlying obstructive disease) or reduced total lung capacity (underlying restrictive disease).
- Radionuclide imaging detects abnormalities in right and left ventricular functioning.
- Open lung biopsy determines the type of disorder.
- Echocardiography shows ventricular wall motion and possible valvular dysfunction, right ventricular enlargement, abnormal septal configuration consistent with right ventricular pressure overload, and reduction in left ventricular cavity size.
- Perfusion lung scanning shows multiple patchy and diffuse filling defects.

Treatment

- Treatment of the underlying cause
- Oxygen therapy
- Fluid restriction
- Digoxin, diuretics, vasodilators, pulmonary vasodilators, calcium channel blockers, β-adrenergic blockers, bronchodilators, and anticoagulants; endothelin receptor antagonists such as bosentan
- Pulmonary thromboendarterectomy
- Lung or heart-lung transplantation

NORMAL PULMONARY ARTERY

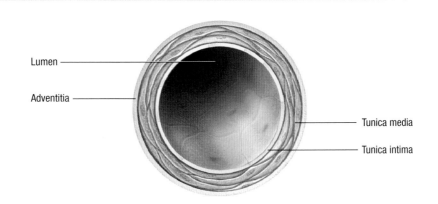

EARLY PULMONARY HYPERTENSION

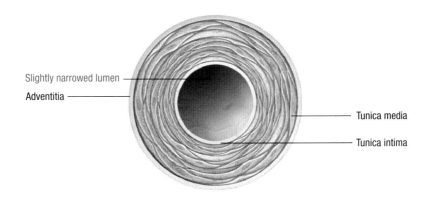

LATE PULMONARY HYPERTENSION

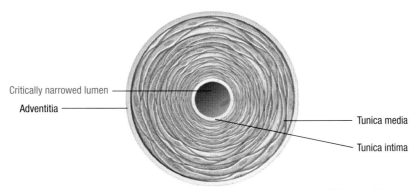

SARCOIDOSIS

Sarcoidosis is a multisystem, granulomatous disorder that characteristically produces lymphadenopathy, pulmonary infiltration, and skeletal, liver, eye, or skin lesions.

AGE ALERT
Sarcoidosis affects twice as many women as men. Onset usually occurs between ages 30 and 50.

Causes

Exact cause unknown

Possible Contributing Factors

- *Hypersensitivity response* (possibly from T-cell imbalance) to such agents as atypical mycobacteria, fungi, and pine pollen
- *Genetic predisposition* (suggested by a slightly higher incidence of sarcoidosis within the same family)
- *Chemicals*, such as zirconium and beryllium, which can lead to illnesses resembling sarcoidosis, suggesting an extrinsic cause for this disease

Pathophysiology

- Sarcoid inflammation is characterized by nonnecrotizing granulomas.
- T cells play a central role in the development of sarcoidosis, as they likely propagate an excessive cellular immune reaction.
- The condition is frequently characterized by a CD4+/CD8+ ratio of at least 3.5 in bronchoalveolar lavage fluid.
- Tumor necrosis factor (TNF) and TNF receptors are increased in this disease.

An excessive inflammatory process is initiated in the alveoli, bronchioles, and blood vessels of the lungs. Monocyte-macrophages accumulate in the target tissue, where they induce the inflammatory process. CD4+ T lymphocytes and sensitized immune cells form a ring around the inflamed area. Fibroblasts, mast cells, collagen fibers, and proteoglycans encase the inflammatory and immune cells, causing granuloma formation. Organ dysfunction results from the accumulation of T lymphocytes, mononuclear phagocytes, and nonsecreting epithelial granulomas, which distort normal tissue architecture, causing alveolitis.

COMPLICATIONS
- Pulmonary fibrosis
- Pulmonary hypertension
- Cor pulmonale

Signs and Symptoms

Initial symptoms of sarcoidosis include arthralgia (in the wrists, ankles, and elbows), fatigue, malaise, and weight loss. Sarcoidosis is characterized by formation of granulomatous tissue leading to pulmonary fibrosis. Other clinical features vary according to the extent and location of the fibrosis:

- *respiratory* — breathlessness, cough (usually nonproductive), and substernal pain; wheezing; pulmonary hypertension and cor pulmonale (in advanced pulmonary disease)
- *cutaneous* — erythema nodosum, subcutaneous skin nodules with maculopapular eruptions, and extensive nasal mucosal lesions
- *ophthalmic* — anterior uveitis (common) and glaucoma
- *lymphatic* — bilateral hilar and right paratracheal lymphadenopathy and splenomegaly
- *musculoskeletal* — muscle weakness, polyarthralgia, pain, and punched-out lesions on phalanges
- *hepatic* — granulomatous hepatitis (usually asymptomatic)
- *genitourinary* — hypercalciuria
- *cardiovascular* — arrhythmias and, rarely, cardiomyopathy
- *central nervous system (CNS)* — cranial or peripheral nerve palsies, basilar meningitis, seizures, and pituitary and hypothalamic lesions producing diabetes insipidus.

Diagnostic Test Results

- ABG analysis shows a decreased partial pressure of arterial oxygen.
- Chest X-rays show bilateral hilar and right paratracheal adenopathy, with or without diffuse interstitial infiltrates.
- Lymph node, skin, or lung biopsy shows noncaseating granulomas with negative cultures for mycobacteria and fungi.
- Pulmonary function tests show decreased total lung capacity and compliance and reduced diffusing capacity.

CLINICAL TIP
A positive Kveim-Siltzbach skin test supports the diagnosis. In this test, the patient receives an intradermal injection of an antigen prepared from human sarcoidal spleen or lymph nodes from patients with sarcoidosis. If the patient has active sarcoidosis, a granuloma develops at the injection site in 2 to 6 weeks.

Treatment

- No treatment for asymptomatic sarcoidosis
- With ophthalmic, respiratory, CNS, cardiovascular, or systemic symptoms or destructive skin lesions: systemic or topical steroids, usually for 1 to 2 years, but possibly lifelong
- With hypercalcemia: low-calcium diet and avoidance of direct exposure to sunlight

Normal lungs and alveoli

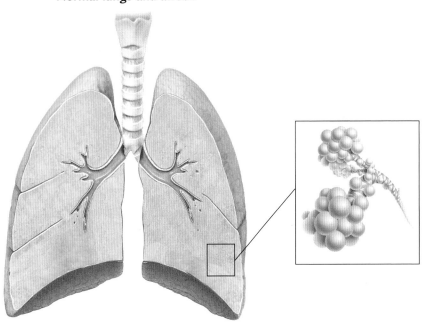

Granulomatous tissue formation   **Alveolitis**

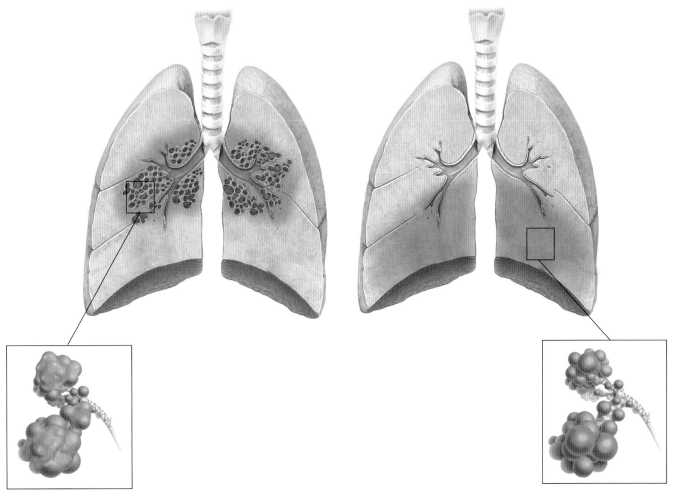

SEVERE ACUTE RESPIRATORY SYNDROME

Severe acute respiratory syndrome (SARS) is a serious form of pneumonia, resulting in acute respiratory distress and, in some cases, death. In February 2003, the World Health Organization (WHO) identified SARS as a global health threat and issued an unprecedented travel advisory. Over the next few months, the illness spread to more than two dozen countries in North America, South America, Europe, and Asia before the outbreak was contained.

Causes

- A member of the Coronaviridae family (the same family causing the common cold)

Pathophysiology

The virus spreads primarily by close human contact. Droplets containing SARS-associated coronavirus (SARS-CoV) can be released into the air when an infected person coughs or sneezes. Some specific medical procedures performed on SARS patients can also release virus-containing droplets into the air. Touching a SARS-CoV–infected surface and subsequently touching the eyes, nose, or mouth may also lead to infection.

In general, coronaviruses are a group of viruses that have a halo or crownlike (corona) appearance when viewed under a microscope. These viruses are a common cause of mild to moderate upper respiratory illness in humans and are associated with respiratory, GI, liver, and neurologic disease in animals.

COMPLICATIONS
- Respiratory failure
- Liver failure
- Heart failure
- Myelodysplastic syndromes
- Death

Signs and Symptoms

Stage 1: A flulike syndrome begins 2 to 7 days after incubation, lasting 3 to 7 days, and is characterized by:

- fever (greater than 100.4°F [38°C])
- fatigue
- headaches
- chills
- myalgias
- malaise
- anorexia
- diarrhea (in some cases).

Stage 2: The lower respiratory phase begins 3 or more days after incubation and is characterized by:

- dry cough
- dyspnea
- progressive hypoxemia
- respiratory failure (requiring mechanical ventilation).

Diagnostic Test Results

The SARS virus may be detected in a patient's nasopharyngeal or oropharyngeal secretions, blood serum, or stool. The WHO has developed three types of diagnostic tests for SARS:

- A reverse transcription polymerase chain reaction test to detect ribonucleic acid of SARS-CoV. Two tests on two different specimens must be positive.
- Serum tests to detect antibodies immunoglobulin (Ig) M and IgG.
- A cell culture test.

Additional testing may include the following:

- ABG analysis, which reveals hypoxemia.
- chest X-ray or chest computed tomography (CT) scan, which identifies the presence of pneumonia or acute respiratory distress syndrome but may also reveal no abnormalities; X-ray and CT scan frequently show focal interstitial infiltrates that may progress to a more patchy, generalized distribution.
- complete blood count, which reveals a low white blood cell count, low lymphocyte count, and low platelet count.
- serum chemistries, which typically show elevated lactate dehydrogenase, alanine aminotransferase, and creatine kinase. Sodium and potassium levels may be low.

Treatment

- Respiratory isolation
- Antibiotics
- Steroids
- Supplemental oxygen
- Mechanical ventilation
- Chest physiotherapy

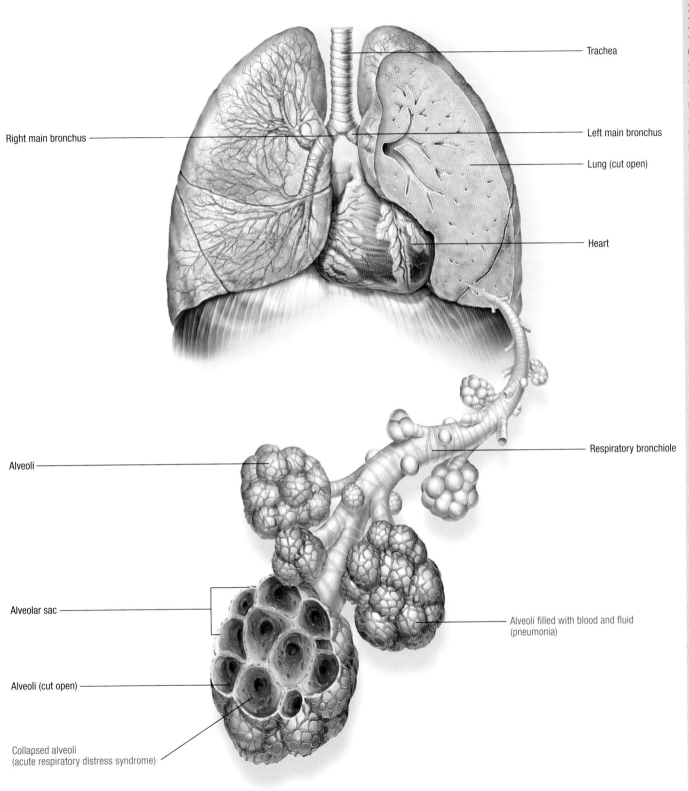

Trachea

Right main bronchus

Left main bronchus

Lung (cut open)

Heart

Respiratory bronchiole

Alveoli

Alveolar sac

Alveoli filled with blood and fluid
(pneumonia)

Alveoli (cut open)

Collapsed alveoli
(acute respiratory distress syndrome)

TUBERCULOSIS

Tuberculosis is an infectious disease caused by the bacterium *Mycobacterium tuberculosis*. TB is characterized by pulmonary infiltrates, formation of granulomas with caseation, fibrosis, and cavitation. Stages include latency, primary disease, primary progressive disease, and extrapulmonary disease. After exposure to *M. tuberculosis*, roughly 5% of infected people develop active TB within 1 year; in the remainder, microorganisms cause a latent infection.

People who live in crowded, poorly ventilated conditions and those who are immunocompromised are most likely to become infected. In patients with strains that are sensitive to the usual antitubercular agents, the prognosis is excellent with correct treatment. However, in those with strains that are resistant to two or more of the major antitubercular agents, mortality is 50%. The incidence of TB has been increasing in the United States secondary to homelessness, drug abuse, and human immunodeficiency virus (HIV) infection. Globally, TB is the leading infectious cause of morbidity and mortality, generating 8 to 10 million new cases each year.

Causes

Mycobacterium tuberculosis is spread by small airborne droplets, produced by the coughing, sneezing, or talking of a person with pulmonary or laryngeal TB. Although the primary infection site is the lungs, mycobacteria commonly exist in other parts of the body. A number of factors increase the risk of infection, including:

- gastrectomy
- uncontrolled diabetes mellitus
- Hodgkin's disease
- leukemia
- silicosis
- HIV infection
- treatment with corticosteroids or immunosuppressants.

Pathophysiology

Transmission of active disease is by droplet nuclei produced when infected persons cough or sneeze. The host's immune system usually controls the tubercle bacillus by killing it or walling it up in a tiny nodule (tubercle). However, the bacillus may lie dormant within the tubercle for years and later reactivate and spread. Persons with a cavitary lesion (large, granulomatous lesion) are particularly infectious because their sputum usually contains 1 million to 100 million bacilli per milliliter. If an inhaled tubercle bacillus settles in an alveolus, infection occurs, with alveolocapillary dilation and endothelial cell swelling. Alveolitis results, with replication of tubercle bacilli and influx of polymorphonuclear leukocytes. These organisms spread through the lymph system to the circulatory system and then throughout the body.

Cell-mediated immunity to the mycobacteria, which develops 3 to 6 weeks later, usually contains the infection and arrests the disease. If the infection reactivates, the body's response characteristically leads to caseation — the conversion of necrotic tissue to a cheeselike material. The caseum may localize,

undergo fibrosis, or excavate and form cavities, the walls of which are studded with multiplying tubercle bacilli. If this happens, infected caseous debris may spread throughout the lungs by the tracheobronchial tree. Sites of extrapulmonary TB include the pleurae, meninges, joints, lymph nodes, peritoneum, genitourinary tract, and bowel.

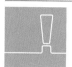

COMPLICATIONS
- Respiratory failure
- Pneumothorax
- Hemorrhage
- Pleural effusion
- Pneumonia
- Liver involvement from drug therapy

Signs and Symptoms

After an incubation period of 4 to 8 weeks, TB usually produces no symptoms in primary infection but may produce nonspecific symptoms, such as:

- fatigue and weakness
- anorexia, weight loss
- night sweats
- low-grade fever
- adenopathy
- malaise
- anxiety.

Physical examination may reveal crackles, decreased breath sounds, and clubbing of the fingers and toes.

In reactivation, symptoms may include a cough that produces mucopurulent sputum, occasional hemoptysis, and chest pain.

Diagnostic Test Results

- Chest X-ray shows nodular lesions, patchy infiltrates (mainly in upper lobes), cavity formation, scar tissue, and calcium deposits.
- Tuberculin skin test reveals infection at some point but doesn't indicate active disease.
- Stains and cultures of sputum, cerebrospinal fluid, urine, drainage from abscesses, or pleural fluid show heat-sensitive, nonmotile, aerobic, acid-fast bacilli.
- Computed tomography scan or magnetic resonance imaging allows the evaluation of lung damage and may confirm the diagnosis.
- Bronchoscopy shows inflammation and altered lung tissue. It may also be performed to obtain sputum if the patient can't produce an adequate sputum specimen.

Treatment

Antitubercular therapy is the main treatment. Daily doses of multiple drugs may include combinations of rifampin, isoniazid, pyrazinamide, and ethambutol. After 2 to 3 weeks of continuous medication, the disease generally is no longer infectious, and the patient can resume his normal lifestyle while continuing the medication.

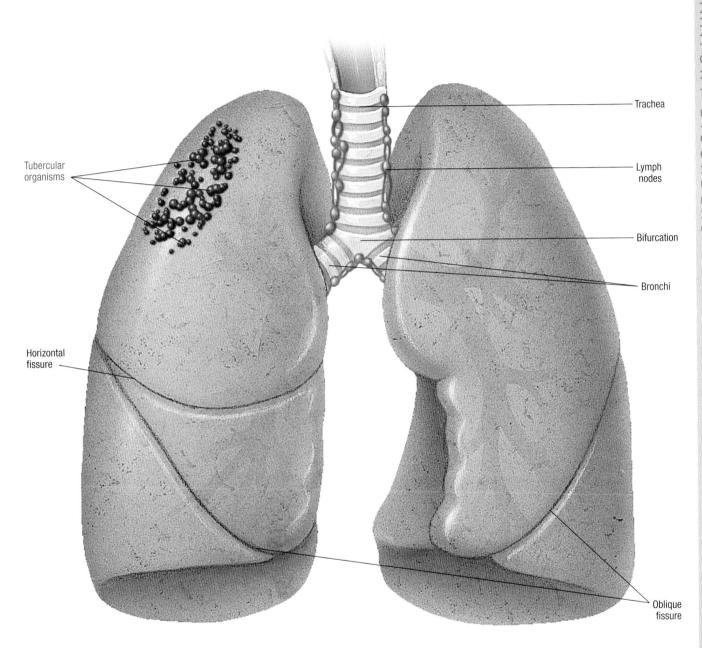

Trachea

Lymph nodes

Bifurcation

Bronchi

Tubercular organisms

Horizontal fissure

Oblique fissure

UPPER RESPIRATORY TRACT INFECTION

Upper respiratory tract infection (also known as the *common cold* or *acute coryza*) (URI) is an acute, usually afebrile viral infection that causes inflammation of the upper respiratory tract. Although a cold is benign and self-limiting, it can lead to secondary bacterial infections. The common cold is a benign self-limited syndrome representing a group of diseases caused by members of several families of viruses.

URI is a nonspecific term used to describe acute infections involving the nose, paranasal sinuses, pharynx, larynx, trachea, and bronchi. The prototype is the illness known as the common cold, which is discussed here, in addition to pharyngitis, sinusitis, and tracheobronchitis. Influenza is a systemic illness that involves the upper respiratory tract and should be differentiated from other URIs.

Viruses cause most upper respiratory infections. Rhinovirus, parainfluenza virus, coronavirus, adenovirus, respiratory syncytial virus, coxsackievirus, human metapneumovirus, and influenza virus account for most cases (CDC, 2017; Kistler, Avila, & Rouskin, 2007).

Causes

Over 100 viruses can cause the common cold. Major offenders include:

- rhinoviruses
- coronaviruses
- myxoviruses
- adenoviruses
- coxsackieviruses
- echoviruses.

Pathophysiology

Infection occurs when the offending organism gains entry into the upper respiratory tract, proliferates, and begins an inflammatory reaction. Acute inflammation of the upper airway structures, including the sinuses, nasopharynx, pharynx, larynx, and trachea, is seen. The presence of the pathogen triggers infiltration of the mucous membranes by inflammatory and infection-fighting cells. Mucosal swelling and secretion of a serous or mucopurulent exudate result.

COMPLICATIONS
- Otitis media
- Sinusitis
- Secondary infections (pneumonia, streptococcal pharyngitis, bronchitis, croup)

Signs and Symptoms

After a 1- to 4-day incubation period, the common cold produces:

- pharyngitis
- nasal congestion
- coryza
- sneezing
- headache
- burning, watery eyes.

Additional effects may include:

- fever
- chills
- myalgia
- arthralgia
- malaise
- lethargy
- hacking, nonproductive, or nocturnal cough.

As the cold progresses, clinical features develop more fully. After a day, symptoms include a feeling of fullness with a copious nasal discharge that commonly irritates the nose, adding to discomfort.

Diagnostic Test Results

No explicit diagnostic test exists to isolate the specific organism responsible for the common cold. Consequently, diagnosis rests on the typically mild, localized, and afebrile upper respiratory symptoms. Diagnosis must rule out allergic rhinitis, measles, rubella, and other disorders that produce similar early symptoms.

Treatment

The primary treatments — aspirin or acetaminophen, fluids, and rest — are purely symptomatic because the common cold has no cure.

Other treatments may include:

- decongestants
- throat lozenges
- steam.

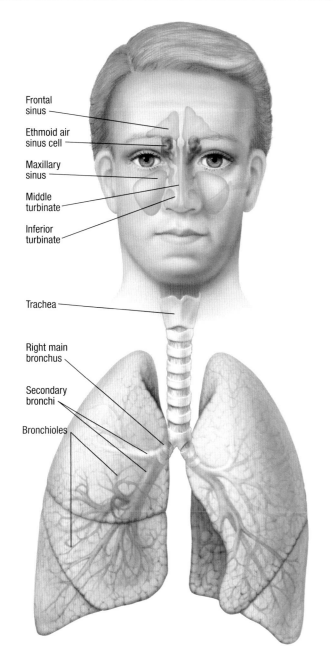

Frontal sinus
Ethmoid air sinus cell
Maxillary sinus
Middle turbinate
Inferior turbinate
Trachea
Right main bronchus
Secondary bronchi
Bronchioles

Sinusitis

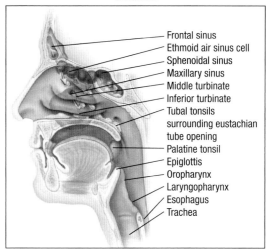

Frontal sinus
Ethmoid air sinus cell
Sphenoidal sinus
Maxillary sinus
Middle turbinate
Inferior turbinate
Tubal tonsils surrounding eustachian tube opening
Palatine tonsil
Epiglottis
Oropharynx
Laryngopharynx
Esophagus
Trachea

Rhinitis

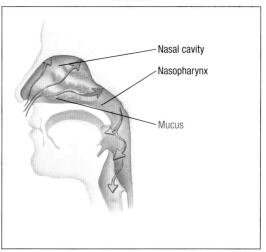

Nasal cavity
Nasopharynx
Mucus

Bronchitis

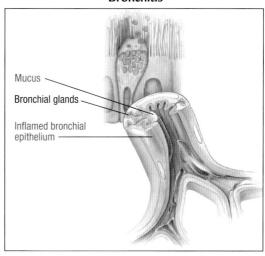

Mucus
Bronchial glands
Inflamed bronchial epithelium

Otitis media with effusion

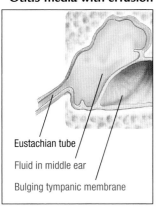

Eustachian tube
Fluid in middle ear
Bulging tympanic membrane

Acute otitis media

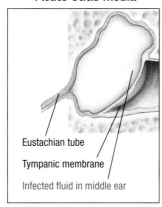

Eustachian tube
Tympanic membrane
Infected fluid in middle ear

Suggested References

Albert, R. H. (2010). Diagnosis and treatment of acute bronchitis. *American Family Physician*, 82(11), 1345–1350.

Bahmer T, Kirsten AM, Waschki B. et al. Prognosis and longitudinal changes of physical activity in idiopathic pulmonary fibrosis BMC Pulm Med. 2017; 17: 104. Published online 2017 Jul 25. doi: 10.1186/s12890-017-0444-0 PMCID: PMC5526311

Cystic Fibrosis Foundation. (2017). *About cystic fibrosis*. Retrieved from http://www.cff.org

Centers for Disease Control and Prevention. (2017). *Common cold*. Retrieved from https://www.cdc.gov

Global Initiative for Chronic Obstructive Lung Disease (GOLD). (2017). *Global strategy for the diagnosis, management and prevention of COPD*. Available from http://goldcopd.org

Hart, A. M. (2014). Evidence-based diagnosis and management of acute bronchitis. *The Nurse Practitioner*, 39(9), 32–39.

Kistler, A., Avila, P. C., Rouskin, S., Wang, D., Ward, T., Yagi, S., … Boushey, H. A. (2007). Pan-viral screening of respiratory tract infections in adults with and without asthma reveals unexpected human coronavirus and human rhinovirus diversity. *The Journal of Infectious Diseases* 196:817–825.

National Cancer Institute. (2017). *Cancer statistics*. Retrieved from https://www.cancer.gov/about-cancer/understanding/statistics

Oldham, J. M., & Noth, I. (2014). Idiopathic pulmonary fibrosis: Early detection and referral. *Respiratory Medicine*, 108(6):819–829.

Tackett, K. L., & Atkins, A. (2012). Evidence-based acute bronchitis therapy. *Journal of Pharmacy Practice*, 25(6), 586–590.

U.S. Department of Health and Human Services, National Institutes of Health, National Heart, Lung, and Blood Institute, National Asthma Education and Prevention Program. (2007). *Expert Panel Report 3 (EPR-3): Guidelines for the Diagnosis and Management of Asthma*. NIH Publication No. 07-40511-440. Bethesda, MD: U.S. Department of Health and Human Services, National Institutes of Health, National Heart, Lung, and Blood Institute. https://www.nhlbi.nih.gov/files/docs/guidelines/asthgdln.pdf

NEUROLOGIC DISORDERS

ACCELERATION-DECELERATION INJURIES

Acceleration-deceleration cervical injuries (commonly known as *whiplash*) result from sharp hyperextension and flexion of the neck that damages muscles, ligaments, disks, and nerve tissue. The prognosis for this type of injury is usually excellent; symptoms usually subside with treatment of symptoms.

Causes

- Motor vehicle and other transportation accidents
- Falls
- Sports-related accidents
- Crimes and assaults

Pathophysiology

The brain is shielded by the cranial vault (hair, skin, bone, meninges, and cerebrospinal fluid [CSF]), which intercepts the force of a physical blow. Below a certain level of force (the absorption capacity), the cranial vault prevents energy from affecting the brain. The degree of traumatic head injury usually is proportional to the amount of force reaching the cranial tissues. Furthermore, unless ruled out, neck injuries should be presumed present in patients with traumatic head injury.

In acceleration-deceleration cervical injuries, the head is propelled in a forward and downward motion in hyperflexion. A wedge-shaped deformity of the bone may be created if the anterior portions of the vertebrae are crushed. Intervertebral disks may be damaged; they may bulge or rupture, irritating spinal nerves. Then the head is forced backward. A tear in the anterior ligament may pull pieces of bone from cervical vertebrae. Spinous processes of the vertebrae may be fractured. Intervertebral disks may be compressed posteriorly and torn anteriorly. Vertebral arteries may be stretched, pinched, or torn, causing reduced blood flow to the brain. Nerves of the cervical sympathetic chain may also be injured.

A complex arrangement of ligaments holds the vertebrae in place. Some of the ligaments are barely a centimeter long, and all are only a few millimeters thick. In a whiplash injury, ligaments may be badly stretched, partially torn, or completely ruptured (arrows). Injuries of neck muscles may range from minor strains and microhemorrhages to severe tears. The anterior longitudinal ligament, running vertically along the anterior surface of the vertebrae, may be injured during hyperextension. The posterior longitudinal ligament, running on the posterior surface of the vertebral bodies, may be injured in hyperflexion. The broad ligamentum nuchae may also be stretched or torn.

Closed trauma is typically caused by a sudden acceleration-deceleration or *coup/contrecoup* injury. In coup/contrecoup, the head hits a relatively stationary object, injuring cranial tissues near the point of impact (coup); then the remaining force pushes the brain against the opposite side of the skull, causing a second impact and injury (contrecoup). Contusions and lacerations may also occur during contrecoup as the brain's soft tissues slide over the rough bone of the cranial cavity. In addition, rotational shear forces on the cerebrum may damage the upper midbrain and areas of the frontal, temporal, and occipital lobes.

COMPLICATIONS
- Nerve damage
- Numbness, tingling, or weakness

Signs and Symptoms

Although symptoms may develop immediately, they may be delayed 12 to 24 hours if the injury is mild. Whiplash produces moderate to severe anterior and posterior neck pain. Within several days, the anterior pain diminishes, but the posterior pain persists or even intensifies, causing patients to seek medical attention.

Whiplash may also cause:

- dizziness and gait disturbances
- vomiting
- headache, nuchal rigidity, and neck muscle asymmetry
- rigidity or numbness in the arms.

Diagnostic Test Results

- X-ray of the cervical spine will determine that vertebral injury hasn't occurred.

CLINICAL TIP
In all suspected spinal injuries, assume that the spine is injured until proven otherwise. Any patient with suspected whiplash or other injuries requires careful transportation from the accident scene. To do this, place the patient in a supine position on a spine board and immobilize the neck with tape and a hard cervical collar or sandbags. New literature suggests a hard board is not necessary.

Until an X-ray rules out a cervical fracture, move the patient as little as possible. Before the X-ray is taken, carefully remove any ear and neck jewelry. Don't undress the patient; cut clothes away, if necessary. Warn the patient against movements that could injure the spine. Patients need to be medically evaluated by trained clinicians prior to removal of collar.

Treatment

- Immobilization with a soft, padded cervical collar for several days or weeks
- Ice or cool compresses to the neck for the first 24 hours, followed by moist, warm heat thereafter
- Over-the-counter analgesics, such as acetaminophen or ibuprofen
- Muscle relaxants
- In severe muscle spasms, consider referral to physical therapy

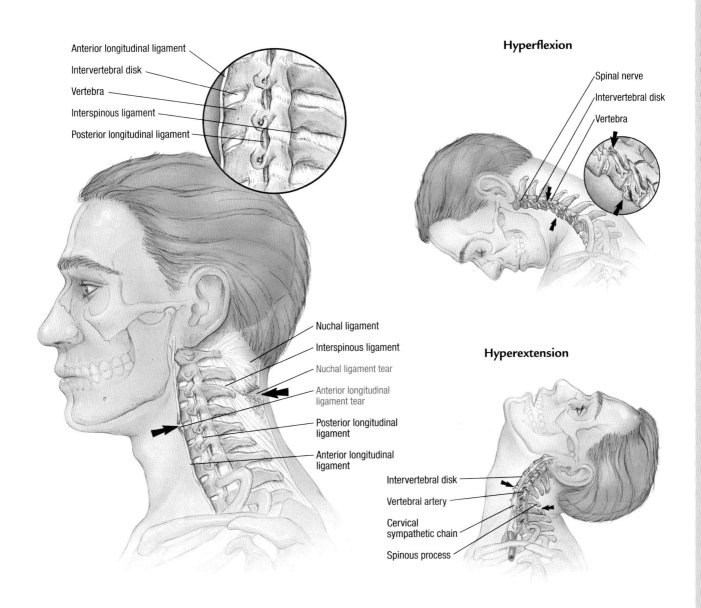

Anterior longitudinal ligament
Intervertebral disk
Vertebra
Interspinous ligament
Posterior longitudinal ligament

Nuchal ligament
Interspinous ligament
Nuchal ligament tear
Anterior longitudinal ligament tear
Posterior longitudinal ligament
Anterior longitudinal ligament

Hyperflexion

Spinal nerve
Intervertebral disk
Vertebra

Hyperextension

Intervertebral disk
Vertebral artery
Cervical sympathetic chain
Spinous process

Muscle injury

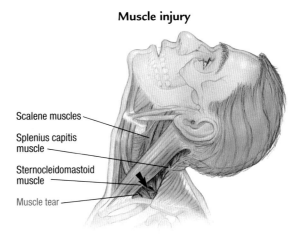

Scalene muscles
Splenius capitis muscle
Sternocleidomastoid muscle
Muscle tear

ALZHEIMER'S DISEASE

Alzheimer's disease is a progressive degenerative disorder of the cerebral cortex, especially the frontal lobe. It affects approximately 5 million Americans; by 2030, that figure may reach 7.7 million. It's the seventh-leading cause of death in the United states.

AGE ALERT
Alzheimer's disease typically affects adults older than age 65, but some cases have been reported in individuals as young as in their late 30s.

The disease has a poor prognosis. Typically, the duration of illness is 8 years, and patients die 2 to 5 years after the onset of debilitating brain symptoms.

Causes

- Exact cause unknown

Possible Contributing Factors

- Genetic patterns
- Beta-amyloid plaque development
- Inflammatory and oxidative stress processes
- The role of estrogen in the brain

Pathophysiology

The brain of a patient with Alzheimer's disease has three characteristic features: *neurofibrillary tangles* (fibrous proteins), *neuritic plaques* (composed of degenerating axons and dendrites), and *neuronal loss* (degeneration).

Neurofibrillary tangles are bundles of filaments found inside neurons that abnormally twist around one another. Abnormally phosphorylated tau proteins accumulate in the neurons as characteristic tangles and ultimately cause neuronal death. In a healthy brain, tau provides structural support for neurons, but in patients with Alzheimer's disease, this structural support collapses.

Neuritic plaques (senile plaques) form outside the neurons in the adjacent brain tissue. Plaques contain a core of beta-amyloid protein surrounded by abnormal nerve endings or neurites. Overproduction or decreased metabolism of beta-amyloid peptide leads to a toxic state causing degeneration of neuronal processes, neuritic plaque formation, and eventually neuronal loss and clinical dementia.

Tangles and plaques cause neurons in the brain of the patient with Alzheimer's disease to shrink and eventually die, first in the memory and language centers and finally throughout the entire brain. This widespread neuron degeneration leaves gaps in the brain's messaging network that may interfere with communication between cells, causing some of the symptoms of Alzheimer's disease.

COMPLICATIONS
- Injury from wandering, violent behavior, or unsupervised activity
- Pneumonia
- Malnutrition and dehydration
- Aspiration

Signs and Symptoms

Mild

- Disorientation to date
- Impaired recall
- Diminished insight
- Irritability
- Apathy

Moderate

- Increased disorientation (time and place)
- Fluent aphasia
- Difficulties with comprehension
- Impaired recognition
- Poor judgment
- Trouble performing activities of daily living (ADLs)
- Aggression
- Restlessness
- Psychosis
- Sleep disturbances
- Dysphoria

Severe

- Unable to use language appropriately
- Memory only to the moment
- Needs assistance with all ADLs
- Urinary and fecal incontinence

Diagnostic Test Results

- Neuropsychologic evaluation shows deficits in memory, reasoning, vision-motor coordination, and language function.
- Magnetic resonance imaging or computed tomography scan reveals brain atrophy at later stages of the disease.
- Positron emission tomography scanning shows decreased brain activity.
- EEG shows evidence of slowed brain waves at later stages of the disease.

Treatment

- Cholinesterase inhibitors, such as tacrine, donepezil, rivastigmine, and galantamine
- Memantine (Namenda) and *N*-methyl-D-aspartate receptor antagonists
- Behavioral therapy
- Nonsteroidal anti-inflammatory drugs
- Cholesterol-lowering drugs
- Estrogen

TISSUE CHANGES IN ALZHEIMER'S DISEASE

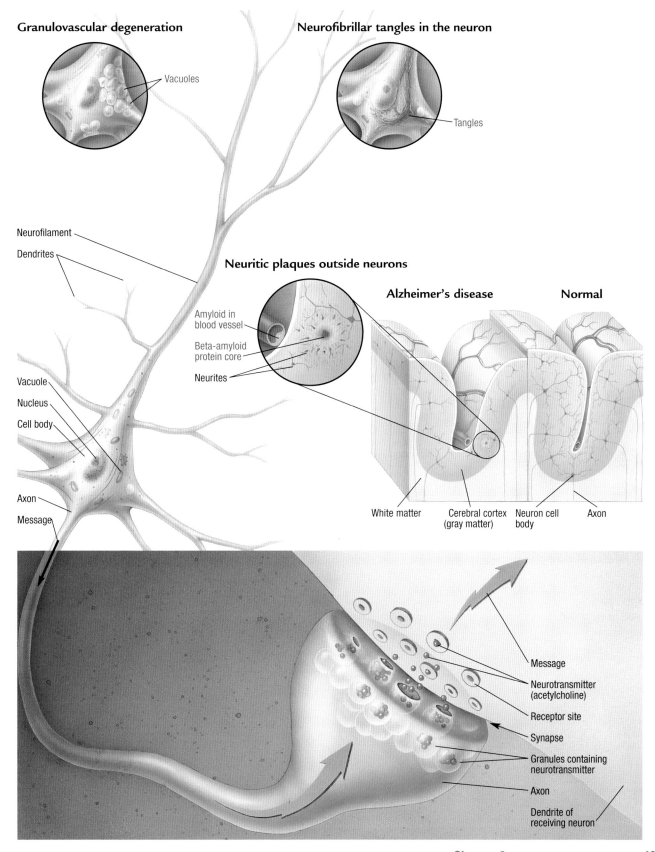

Granulovascular degeneration

Vacuoles

Neurofibrillar tangles in the neuron

Tangles

Neurofilament

Dendrites

Neuritic plaques outside neurons

Amyloid in
blood vessel

Beta-amyloid
protein core

Neurites

Alzheimer's disease

Normal

Vacuole

Nucleus

Cell body

Axon

Message

White matter   Cerebral cortex   Neuron cell   Axon
                (gray matter)   body

Message

Neurotransmitter
(acetylcholine)

Receptor site

Synapse

Granules containing
neurotransmitter

Axon

Dendrite of
receiving neuron

AMYOTROPHIC LATERAL SCLEROSIS

Commonly called *Lou Gehrig's disease*, after the New York Yankees first baseman who died of this disorder, amyotrophic lateral sclerosis (ALS) is the most common of the motor neuron diseases causing muscular atrophy. A chronic, progressively debilitating disease, ALS may be fatal in less than 1 year or continue for 10 years or more, depending on the muscles affected. More than 30,000 Americans have ALS; the disease affects three times as many men as women.

AGE ALERT
The average age of ALS onset is mid-50s but can range from the late teen years to the 80s.

Causes

The exact cause is unknown. A genetic (familial ALS "FALS") link is seen in 10% of all ALS cases. A specific gene mutation in an enzyme known as *superoxide dismutase 1* has been identified in about 20% of FALS cases. Over 90% of cases of ALS occur randomly with no identifiable cause and no risk factors and are referred to as sporadic ALS. Several theories have been proposed that explain why motor neurons die, including:

- glutamate excitotoxicity
- oxidative injury
- protein aggregates
- axonal strangulation
- autoimmune-induced calcium influx
- viral infections
- deficiency of nerve growth factor
- apoptosis (programmed cell death)
- trauma
- environmental toxins.

Pathophysiology

Current research suggests an excess accumulation of glutamate (an excitatory neurotransmitter) in the synaptic cleft. The affected motor units are no longer innervated, and progressive degeneration of axons causes loss of myelin. Some nearby motor nerves may sprout axons in an attempt to maintain function, but, ultimately, nonfunctional scar tissue replaces normal neuronal tissue.

COMPLICATIONS
- Pneumonia
- Pressure ulcers
- Weight loss
- Acute respiratory distress syndrome

Signs and Symptoms

- Fasciculations, spasticity, atrophy, weakness, and loss of functioning motor units (especially in forearms and hands)
- Impaired speech, chewing, and swallowing; choking; drooling
- Difficulty breathing, especially if the brain stem is affected
- Muscle atrophy
- Reactive depression

Diagnostic Test Results

- Electromyography shows abnormalities of electrical activity in involved muscles.
- Muscle biopsy shows atrophic fibers interspersed between normal fibers.
- CSF analysis by lumbar puncture reveals elevated protein levels.
- Nerve conduction studies show normal results.

Treatment

- Riluzole
- Baclofen or diazepam
- Trihexyphenidyl or amitriptyline
- Physical therapy
- Percutaneous feeding tubes
- Tracheostomy
- Speech therapy

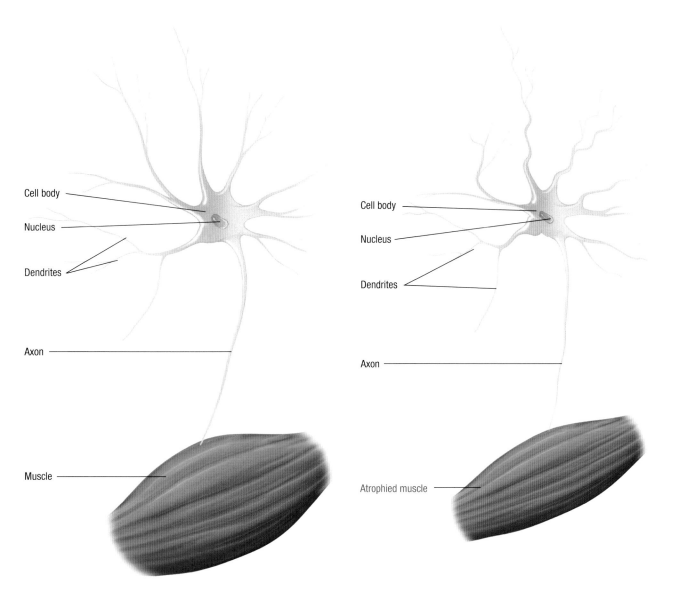

Normal nerve cell and muscle

Cell body

Nucleus

Dendrites

Axon

Muscle

Amyotrophic lateral sclerosis–affected nerve cell and muscle

Cell body

Nucleus

Dendrites

Axon

Atrophied muscle

ARTERIOVENOUS MALFORMATION

Arteriovenous malformations (AVMs) are tangled masses of thin-walled, dilated blood vessels between arteries and veins that aren't connected by capillaries. AVMs are common in the brain, primarily in the posterior portion of the cerebral hemispheres. Abnormal channels between the arterial and venous system mix oxygenated and unoxygenated blood and thereby prevent adequate perfusion of brain tissue.

AVMs range in size from a few millimeters to large malformations extending from the cerebral cortex to the ventricles. Usually, more than one AVM is present. Males and females are equally affected. Some evidence exists that AVMs occur run in families.

AGE ALERT
Most AVMs are present at birth; however, symptoms may occur at any time. Two-thirds of all cases occur before age 40.

Causes

- Congenital: hereditary defect
- Acquired: trauma such as penetrating injuries

Pathophysiology

AVMs lack the typical structural characteristics of the blood vessels. The vessel walls of an AVM are very thin; one or more arteries feed into the AVM, causing it to appear dilated and torturous. The typically high-pressured arterial flow moves into the venous system through the connecting channels to increase venous pressure, engorging and dilating the venous structures. An aneurysm may develop. If the AVM is large enough, the shunting can deprive the surrounding tissue of adequate blood flow. Additionally, the thin-walled vessels may ooze small amounts of blood or actually rupture, causing hemorrhage into the brain or subarachnoid space.

COMPLICATIONS
- Aneurysm and subsequent rupture
- Hemorrhage (intracranial, subarachnoid, subdural)
- Hydrocephalus

Signs and Symptoms

Typically, few or none.

If AVM Is Large, Leaks, or Ruptures

- Chronic headache and confusion
- Seizures
- Systolic bruit over carotid artery, mastoid process, or orbit
- Focal neurologic deficits (depending on the location of the AVM)
- Hydrocephalus
- Paralysis
- Loss of speech, memory, or vision

CLINICAL TIP
Symptoms of intracranial hemorrhage, indicating AVM rupture, include sudden severe headache, seizures, confusion, lethargy, and meningeal irritation.

Diagnostic Test Results

- Cerebral arteriogram confirms the presence of AVMs and evaluates blood flow.
- Doppler ultrasonography of the cerebrovascular system indicates abnormal, turbulent blood flow.

Treatment

- Supportive measures, including aneurysm precautions
- Surgery, including block dissection, laser, or ligation
- Embolization or radiation therapy
- Radiosurgery

Cerebral cortex — Sagittal section

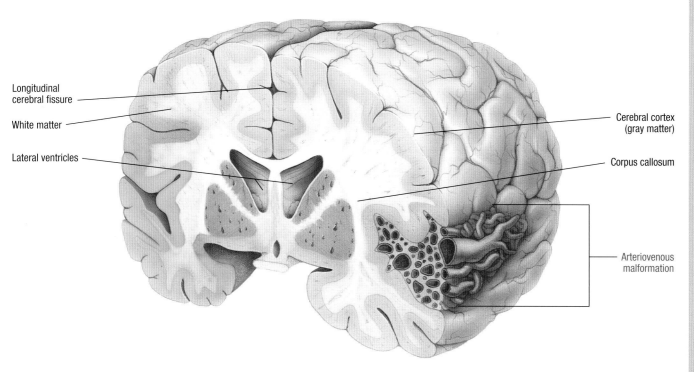

Longitudinal
cerebral fissure

White matter

Lateral ventricles

Cerebral cortex
(gray matter)

Corpus callosum

Arteriovenous
malformation

BELL'S PALSY

Bell's palsy is a disease of the facial nerve (cranial nerve VII) that produces unilateral or bilateral facial weakness. Onset is rapid. In 80% to 90% of patients, it subsides spontaneously and recovery is complete in 1 to 8 weeks. If recovery is partial, contractures may develop on the paralyzed side of the face. Bell's palsy may recur on the same or opposite side of the face.

AGE ALERT
Although Bell's palsy affects all age-groups, it occurs most commonly in people between ages 20 and 60. Recovery may be slower in elderly patients.

Causes

- Infection such as herpes simplex virus
- Tumor
- Meningitis
- Local trauma
- Lyme disease
- Hypertension
- Sarcoidosis

Pathophysiology

Bell's palsy reflects an inflammatory reaction around the seventh cranial nerve, usually at the internal auditory meatus where the nerve leaves bony tissue. The characteristic unilateral or bilateral facial weakness results from the lack of appropriate neural stimulation to the muscle by the motor fibers of the facial nerve.

COMPLICATIONS
- Corneal ulceration and blindness
- Impaired nutrition
- Psychosocial problems due to altered body image

Signs and Symptoms

- Unilateral face weakness
- Aching at jaw angle
- Drooping mouth
- Distorted taste or loss of taste
- Impaired ability to fully close the eye on the affected side
- Tinnitus
- Excessive or insufficient eye tearing on the affected side
- Hypersensitivity to sound on the affected side
- Headache

CLINICAL TIP
When the patient attempts to close the affected eye, it rolls upward (Bell's phenomenon) and shows excessive tearing.

Diagnostic Test Results

Diagnosis is based on clinical presentation. (See *Diagnosing Bell's Palsy.*) Other studies include:

- nerve conduction studies and electromyography to determine the extent of nerve damage
- blood tests to establish the presence of sarcoidosis or Lyme disease.

Treatment

- Oral corticosteroids such as prednisone
- Antivirals
- Analgesics
- Lubricating eyedrops or eye ointments
- Electrotherapy
- Antibiotics
- Surgery

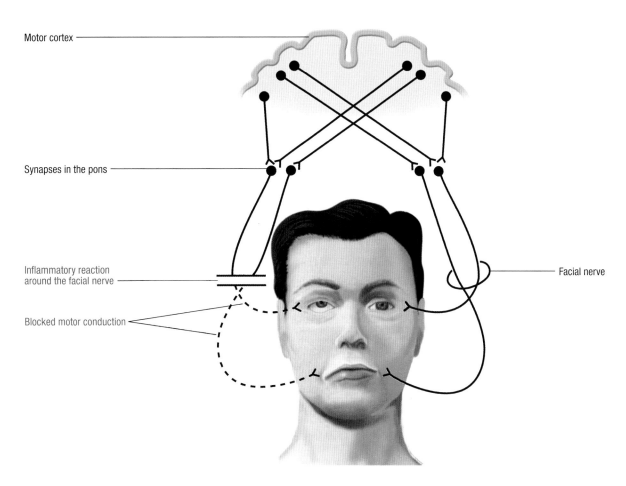

Motor cortex

Synapses in the pons

Inflammatory reaction around the facial nerve

Blocked motor conduction

Facial nerve

CLINICAL TIP

DIAGNOSING BELL'S PALSY

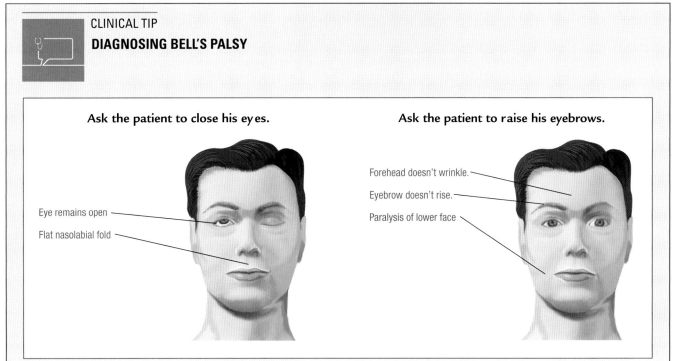

Ask the patient to close his eyes.

Eye remains open

Flat nasolabial fold

Ask the patient to raise his eyebrows.

Forehead doesn't wrinkle.

Eyebrow doesn't rise.

Paralysis of lower face

BRAIN TUMORS

Brain tumors are abnormal growths that develop after transformation of cells within the brain, cerebral vasculature, or meninges. They're usually referred to as *benign* or *malignant*. Malignancy in the brain is graded on the degree of cellularity, endothelial proliferation, nuclear atypia, and necrosis. Highly malignant brain tumors are aggressive tumors that grow and multiply rapidly. Survival and prognosis are directly related to tumor grade. However, even though benign tumors lack aggressiveness, they can be as devastating neurologically depending on their size and location. The most common types of primary brain tumors are gliomas, meningiomas, and pituitary adenomas.

AGE ALERT
Brain tumors are found in all age-groups, with peaks of incidence occurring in early childhood as well as in people ages 50 to 80.

Causes

- Unknown in most cases
- A genetic loss or mutation
- Prior cranial radiation exposure

Pathophysiology

At the level of the cell nucleus, both positive and negative regulators of growth are necessary for normal control of cell proliferation. The positive regulators, protooncogenes, have products that function as growth factors, growth factor receptors, and signaling enzymes. Excessive production may occur that converts protooncogenes into oncogenes, resulting in significant neoplastic growth.

Negative regulators of cell growth are called tumor suppressor genes. Suppressor genes inhibit cellular proliferation at the level of the nucleus. The loss of tumor suppressor genes by mutation, deletion, or reduced expression aids in the conversion of normal cells to malignant phenotypes. The excessive stimulation of proto-oncogenes and the lack of inhibition of tumor suppressor genes ultimately lead to neoplastic proliferation. As the tumor grows, edema develops in surrounding tissues and intracranial pressure (ICP) increases. As the tumor continues to grow, it may interfere with the normal flow and drainage of CSF, causing an increase in ICP.

The brain compensates for increases by regulating the volume of the three substances in the following ways: limiting blood flow to the head, displacing CSF into the spinal canal, and increasing absorption or decreasing production of CSF.

COMPLICATIONS
- Coma
- Respiratory or cardiac arrest
- Brain herniation

Signs and Symptoms

- Headache
- Decreased motor strength and coordination
- Seizures
- Altered vital signs
- Nausea and vomiting
- Increased ICP
- Neurologic deficits
- Diplopia
- Papilledema

Diagnostic Test Results

- Skull CT or bone scan confirms the presence of the tumor.
- Computed tomography (CT) and magnetic resonance imaging (MRI) show changes in brain tissue density.
- Magnetic resonance spectroscopy evaluates the neurochemical changes in the bed of the tumor. Elevation in choline is noted in high-grade gliomas, as compared with elevated lactate levels in intracranial abscess.
- Positron emission tomography evaluates the blood flow patterns in the brain and the tumor and differentiates normal brain tissue from the tumor.
- The MRI or CT angiogram evaluates the arterial and venous structures surrounding the tumor.
- Tissue biopsy confirms the presence of the tumor.
- Lumbar puncture shows increased CSF pressure, which reflects ICP, increased protein levels, decreased glucose levels, and, occasionally, tumor cells in CSF.

Treatment

- Surgery
- Radiation
- Chemotherapy
- Corticosteroids such as dexamethasone
- Anticonvulsants such as phenytoin
- Ranitidine or famotidine
- Analgesics

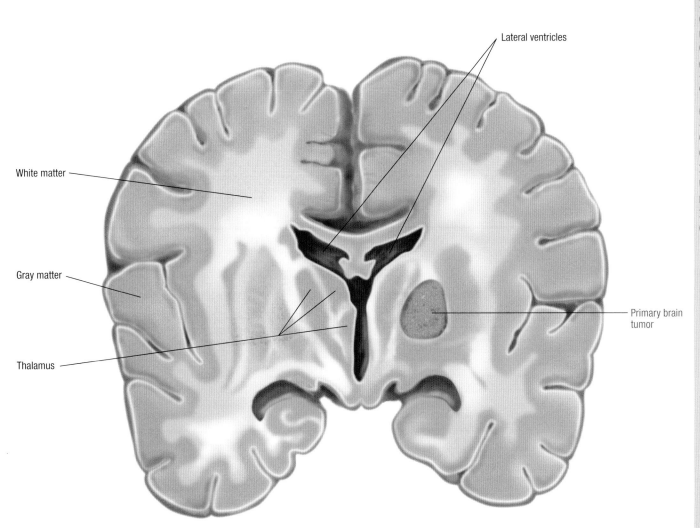

Lateral ventricles

White matter

Gray matter

Thalamus

Primary brain tumor

CEREBRAL ANEURYSM

In an intracranial, or cerebral, aneurysm, a weakness in the wall of a cerebral artery causes localized dilation. Cerebral aneurysms usually arise at an arterial junction in the circle of Willis, the circular anastomosis connecting the major cerebral arteries at the base of the brain. Many cerebral aneurysms rupture and cause subarachnoid hemorrhage.

AGE ALERT
Incidence is slightly higher in women than in men, especially those in their late 40s or early to mid-50s, but a cerebral aneurysm may occur at any age in either sex.

Causes

- Congenital defect
- Degenerative process such as atherosclerosis
- Hypertension
- Trauma
- Infection

Pathophysiology

Prolonged hemodynamic stress and local arterial degeneration at vessel bifurcations are believed to be a major contributing factor to the development and ultimate rupture of cerebral aneurysms. Bleeding spreads rapidly into the subarachnoid space and commonly into the intraventricular spaces and brain tissue, producing localized changes in the cerebral cortex and focal irritation of the cranial nerves and arteries. Increased ICP occurs, causing disruption of cerebral autoregulation and alterations in cerebral blood flow. Expanding intracranial hematomas may act as space-occupying lesions compressing or displacing brain tissue. Blockage of the ventricular system or decreased CSF absorption can result in hydrocephalus. Cerebral artery vasospasm occurs in the surrounding arteries and can further compromise cerebral blood flow, leading to cerebral ischemia and cerebral infarction.

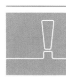

COMPLICATIONS
- Subarachnoid hemorrhage
- Brain tissue infarction
- Cerebral vasospasm
- Hydrocephalus
- Rebleeding
- Meningeal irritation from blood in the subarachnoid space

Signs and Symptoms

Cerebral aneurysms are generally asymptomatic until they rupture. Signs and symptoms of subarachnoid hemorrhage include:

- change in level of consciousness
- sudden-onset severe headache
- photophobia
- nuchal rigidity
- lower back pain
- nausea and vomiting
- fever
- positive Kernig's sign
- positive Brudzinski's sign
- seizure
- cranial nerve deficits
- motor weakness.

Diagnostic Test Results

- Cerebral arteriogram shows the presence of a cerebral aneurysm.
- Head Computed Tomography (CT) scan reveals subarachnoid hemorrhage.
- Transcranial Doppler ultrasound study shows increased blood flow if vasospasm occurs.
- Examination of CSF confirms bleeding.
- Electrocardiogram changes reveal bradycardia, atrioventricular blocks, and premature ventricular contractions.
- Complete blood count shows elevated white blood cell count.

Treatment

- Bed rest in a quiet, darkened room with minimal stimulation
- Surgical repair by clipping, ligation, or wrapping
- Endovascular coiling
- Triple H therapy (hypervolemia, hypertension, hemodilution)
- Calcium channel blockers such as nimodipine
- Avoidance of caffeine or other stimulants; avoidance of aspirin
- Codeine or another analgesic as needed
- Antihypertensives
- Anticonvulsants
- Sedatives

Circle of Willis

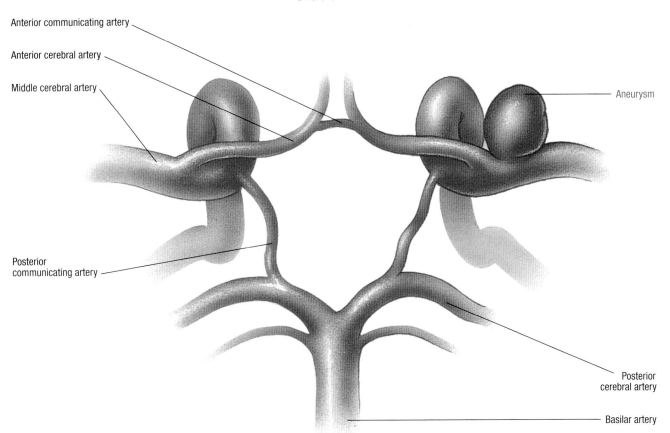

Anterior communicating artery

Anterior cerebral artery

Middle cerebral artery

Posterior communicating artery

Aneurysm

Posterior cerebral artery

Basilar artery

Vessels of the brain — Inferior view

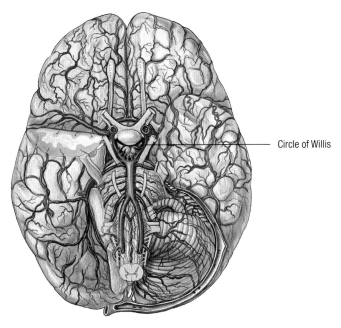

Circle of Willis

DEPRESSION

Depression is a chronic and recurrent mood disorder. Although many people may feel depressed at one time or another, clinical depression is defined when the symptoms interfere with everyday life for an extended period. It affects women twice as often as men, and it's reported to be significantly underdiagnosed and usually inadequately treated.

Forms of depression include major depression, dysthymia, postpartum depression, premenstrual dysphoric disorder, and seasonal affective disorder.

AGE ALERT
The peak age of depression onset is between 20 and 40.

Causes

Some people may have a genetic predisposition to developing depression.

Possible Contributing Factors

- Disappointment at home, work, or school
- Death of a friend or relative
- Prolonged pain or having a major illness
- Medical conditions, such as hypothyroidism, cancer, or hepatitis
- Drugs, such as sedatives and antihypertensives
- Alcohol or drug abuse
- Chronic stress
- Abuse or neglect
- Social isolation
- Nutritional deficiencies (such as folate and omega-3 fatty acids)
- Sleeping problems

Pathophysiology

An imbalance of the neurotransmitters is thought to be the underlying mechanism in depression. In a person with normal levels of neurotransmitters, serotonin and norepinephrine are released from one neuron and travel to another one, activating receptors. After the receptors are activated, the neurotransmitters are taken up by the presynaptic neuron. A patient with depression has inadequate levels of serotonin or norepinephrine, thus not allowing this smooth transmission of impulses.

COMPLICATIONS
- Suicide
- Altered social, family, and occupational functioning

Signs and Symptoms

- Persistent sad, anxious, or "empty" mood
- Feelings of hopelessness and pessimism
- Feelings of guilt, worthlessness, and helplessness
- Loss of interest or pleasure in hobbies and activities that were once enjoyed
- Loss of energy or fatigue
- Unexplained pain
- GI symptoms
- Headache
- Insomnia
- Dizziness
- Palpitations
- Heartburn
- Numbness
- Loss of appetite
- Premenstrual syndrome

AGE ALERT
In children, symptoms of depression include hyperactivity, poor school performance, somatic complaints, sleeping and eating disturbances, lack of playfulness, and suicidal ideation or actions.

Diagnostic Test Results

Several screening questionnaires are used to detect depressive symptoms. They include:

- Beck Depression Inventory
- Center for Epidemiological Studies Depression Scale
- Zung Self-Rating Depression Scale.

CLINICAL TIP
To screen for depression, ask your patient these two questions:

- Have you felt down, depressed, or hopeless for most of the past 2 weeks?
- Have you felt little interest or pleasure in performing activities for most of the past 2 weeks? If the patient answers yes to either question, further assessment is warranted.

Treatment

- Selective serotonin reuptake inhibitors, such as fluoxetine and sertraline
- Tricyclic antidepressants, such as nortriptyline and desipramine
- Venlafaxine
- Nefazodone
- Bupropion
- Monoamine oxidase inhibitors
- Psychotherapy
- Electroconvulsive therapy
- Exercise
- Support groups
- Self-help literature
- Light therapy

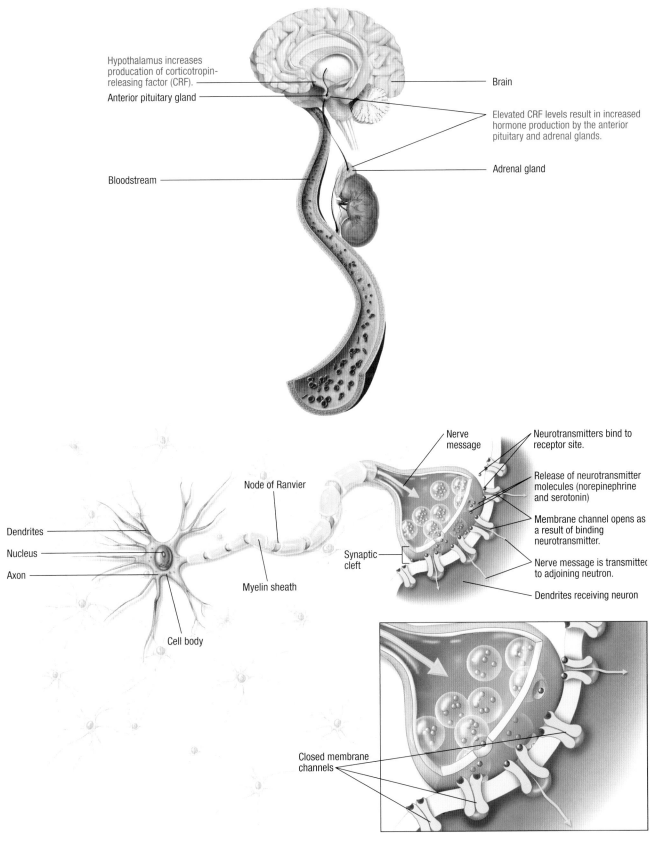

Hypothalamus increases production of corticotropin-releasing factor (CRF).

Anterior pituitary gland

Brain

Elevated CRF levels result in increased hormone production by the anterior pituitary and adrenal glands.

Adrenal gland

Bloodstream

Nerve message

Neurotransmitters bind to receptor site.

Release of neurotransmitter molecules (norepinephrine and serotonin)

Membrane channel opens as a result of binding neurotransmitter.

Nerve message is transmitted to adjoining neutron.

Dendrites receiving neuron

Node of Ranvier

Dendrites

Nucleus

Axon

Myelin sheath

Synaptic cleft

Cell body

Closed membrane channels

EPILEPSY

Epilepsy is a condition of the brain characterized by susceptibility to recurrent seizures — paroxysmal events associated with abnormal electrical discharges of neurons in the brain.

Generalized seizures originate from multiple areas of the brain simultaneously. Partial seizures originate from a single focus but can spread or be generalized.

Causes

- Half of all cases are idiopathic
- Birth trauma
- Anoxia
- Perinatal infection
- Genetic abnormalities, such as tuberous sclerosis and phenylketonuria
- Perinatal injuries
- Metabolic abnormalities, such as hypoglycemia, pyridoxine deficiency, or hypoparathyroidism
- Brain tumors or other space-occupying lesions
- Meningitis, encephalitis, or brain abscess
- Traumatic injury
- Ingestion of toxins, such as mercury, lead, or carbon monoxide
- Stroke
- Apparent familial incidence in some seizure disorders

Pathophysiology

Some neurons in the brain may depolarize easily or be hyperexcitable; this *epileptogenic focus* fires more readily than normal when stimulated. In these neurons, the membrane potential at rest is less negative or inhibitory connections are missing, possibly because of decreased gamma-aminobutyric acid activity or localized shifts in electrolytes.

On stimulation, the epileptogenic focus fires and spreads electrical current toward the synapse and surrounding cells. These cells fire in turn, and the impulse cascades to one side of the brain (a partial seizure), both sides of the brain (a generalized seizure), or cortical, subcortical, or brain stem areas.

The brain's metabolic demand for oxygen increases dramatically during a seizure. If this demand isn't met, hypoxia and brain damage ensue. Firing of inhibitory neurons causes the excitatory neurons to slow their firing and eventually stop.

If this inhibitory action doesn't occur, the result is status epilepticus: one prolonged seizure or one seizure occurring right after another and another. Without treatment, this may be fatal.

COMPLICATIONS
- Anoxia
- Traumatic injury
- Death from status epilepticus

Signs and Symptoms

Generalized Tonic-Clonic Seizures

- Altered consciousness
- Tonic stiffening followed by clonic muscular contractions
- Tongue biting

- Incontinence
- Labored breathing
- Apnea
- Cyanosis

Absence Seizures

- Change in level of awareness
- Blank stare
- Automatisms (purposeless motor activity)

Atonic Seizures

- Sudden loss of postural tone
- Temporary loss of alertness

Myoclonic Seizures

- Brief muscle contractions that appear as jerks or twitching

Diagnostic Test Results

- EEG reveals paroxysmal abnormalities to confirm the diagnosis and provide evidence of the continuing tendency to have seizures. In tonic-clonic seizures, high, fast voltage spikes are present in all leads; in absence seizures, rounded spike wave complexes are diagnostic. A negative EEG doesn't rule out epilepsy because the abnormalities occur intermittently.
- Computed tomography scan and magnetic resonance imaging show abnormalities in internal structures.
- Skull X-ray shows evidence of fractures or shifting of the pineal gland, bony erosion, or separated sutures.
- Brain scan reveals malignant lesions when X-ray findings are normal or questionable.
- Cerebral angiography shows cerebrovascular abnormalities, such as aneurysm or tumor.
- Serum chemistry blood studies show hypoglycemia, electrolyte imbalances, elevated liver enzymes, and elevated alcohol levels, providing clues to underlying conditions that increase the risk of seizure activity.

Treatment

- Drug therapy specific to the type of seizure, including phenytoin, carbamazepine, phenobarbital, gabapentin, and primidone for generalized tonic-clonic seizures and complex partial seizures
- Valproic acid, clonazepam, and ethosuximide for absence seizures
- Gabapentin and felbamate and other anticonvulsant drugs
- Surgical removal of a demonstrated focal lesion, if drug therapy is ineffective
- Surgery to remove the underlying cause, such as a tumor, abscess, or vascular problem
- Vagus nerve stimulator implant
- I.V. diazepam, lorazepam, phenytoin, or phenobarbital for status epilepticus
- Administration of dextrose (when seizures are secondary to hypoglycemia) or thiamine (in chronic alcoholism or withdrawal)

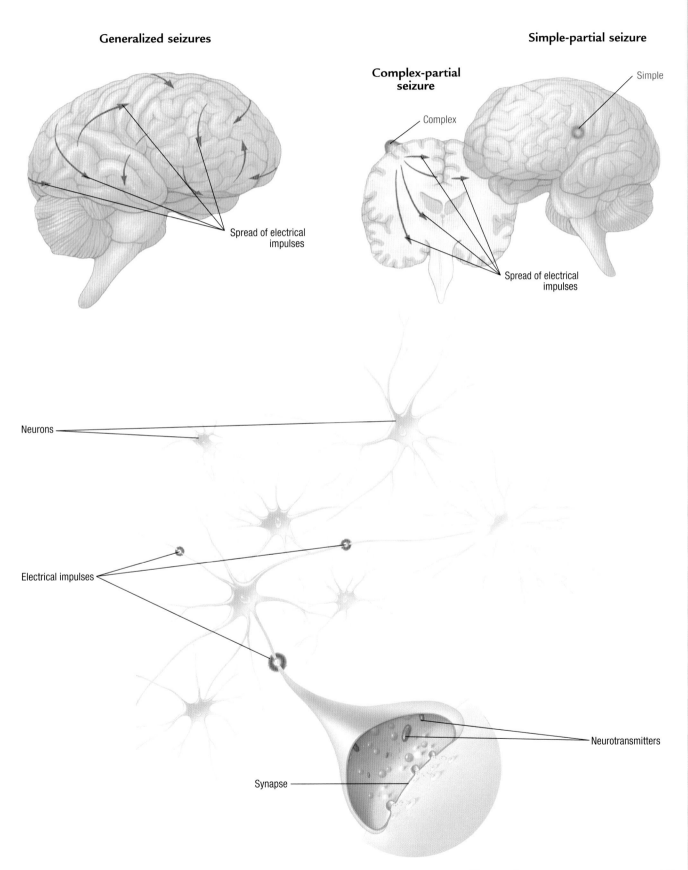

Generalized seizures

Spread of electrical impulses

Complex-partial seizure

Simple-partial seizure

Simple

Complex

Spread of electrical impulses

Neurons

Electrical impulses

Neurotransmitters

Synapse

GUILLAIN-BARRÉ SYNDROME

Also known as *infectious polyneuritis, Landry-Guillain-Barré syndrome,* or *acute idiopathic polyneuritis,* Guillain-Barré syndrome is a rapidly progressive and potentially fatal motor neuropathy of uncertain cause. Generally, the syndrome reaches its peak progress within 7 days to 4 weeks. Recovery occurs over weeks to months with approximately 10% to 25% of the population suffering with permanent weakness and disability.

AGE ALERT
The average age of onset of Guillain-Barré syndrome is 40.

Causes

An exact cause is unknown; however, in many cases, the syndrome is preceded by a viral infection that produces a cell-mediated immune reaction. The most common infection is *Campylobacter jejuni,* occurring in about 30% to 40% of the cases. Epstein-Barr virus, cytomegalovirus, human immunodeficiency virus, coxsackievirus, herpes simplex, hepatitis A virus, and *Mycoplasma* pneumonia have also been implicated.

Other Precipitating Factors

- Hematologic malignancies
- Hyperthyroidism
- Collagen vascular diseases
- Sarcoidosis
- Pregnancy
- Surgical procedures
- Transplants
- Immunizations (swine flu)
- Certain drugs (heroin)

Pathophysiology

Guillain-Barré syndrome is triggered by an autoimmune response in which the body's immune system starts to destroy the myelin sheath that surrounds the axons of many peripheral nerves or even the axons themselves. It's possible that the virus changes the nature of the cells in the nervous system so that the immune system treats them as foreign cells. It's also possible that the virus makes the immune itself less discriminating about what cells it recognizes, thereby allowing some of the immune cells, such as certain kinds of lymphocytes and macrophages, to attack the myelin. Sensitized T lymphocytes cooperate with B lymphocytes to produce antibodies against components of the myelin sheath and may contribute to destruction of the myelin as well.

Myelin destruction causes segmental demyelination of the peripheral nerves, preventing normal transmission of electrical impulses. Inflammation and degenerative changes in both the posterior (sensory) and anterior (motor) nerve roots result in signs of sensory and motor losses simultaneously. The autonomic nervous system may also be impaired.

COMPLICATIONS
- Thrombophlebitis
- Pressure ulcers
- Contractures and muscle wasting
- Aspiration
- Respiratory tract infections
- Life-threatening respiratory and cardiac failure
- Paralysis

Signs and Symptoms

- Symmetrical muscle weakness (major neurologic sign) appearing in the legs first (ascending type) and then extending to the arms and facial nerves within 24 to 72 hours
- Muscle weakness developing in the arms first (descending type) or in the arms and legs simultaneously
- Absent deep tendon reflexes
- Paresthesia, sometimes preceding muscle weakness but vanishing quickly
- Diplegia, possibly with ophthalmoplegia
- Dysphagia and dysarthria
- Hypotonia and areflexia

Diagnostic Test Results

- CSF analysis by lumbar puncture reveals elevated protein levels, peaking in 4 to 6 weeks, probably as a result of widespread inflammation of the nerve roots; the CSF white blood cell count remains normal, but in severe disease, CSF pressure may rise above normal.
- Complete blood count shows leukocytosis with immature forms early in the illness and then quickly returns to normal.
- Electromyography possibly shows repeated firing of the same motor unit instead of widespread sectional stimulation.
- Nerve conduction velocities show slowing soon after paralysis develops.
- Serum immunoglobulin measurements reveal elevated levels from inflammatory response.

Treatment

- Endotracheal intubation or tracheotomy, as indicated to clear secretions
- Plasmapheresis
- Continuous electrocardiogram monitoring
- I.V. immunoglobulin
- Pain management, with anti-inflammatories and opioids
- Rehabilitation

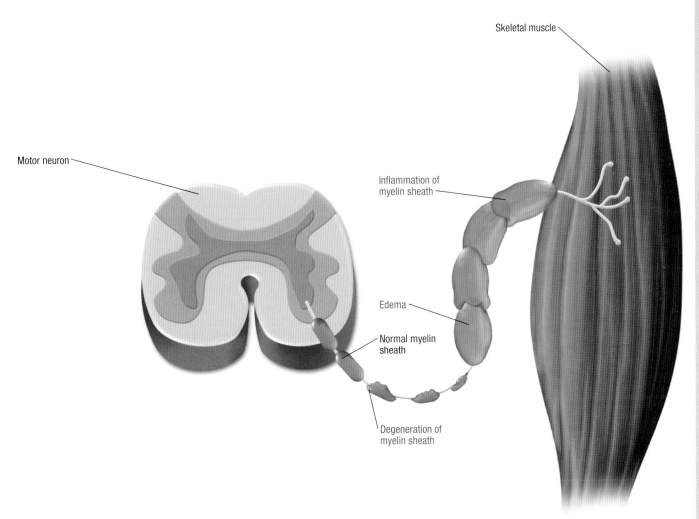

Skeletal muscle

Motor neuron

Inflammation of
myelin sheath

Edema

Normal myelin
sheath

Degeneration of
myelin sheath

HEADACHE

Headache, although usually benign, can be a serious and commonly disabling disorder. The International Headache Society identified a comprehensive classification system that includes more than 100 types of headaches, which are divided into 13 categories. Various processes may cause headache, and they range from benign to life threatening.

Causes

Primary headaches are classified based on their symptom profiles and account for 90% to 98% of headaches. Primary headaches include migraines, tension type, and cluster.

Acute and progressive, secondary headaches are the result of an identifiable structural or physiologic cause, including:

- head trauma
- vascular disorders
- nonvascular intracranial disorders
- substance abuse and substance withdrawal
- infections
- metabolic disorders
- disorders of the face and neck
- cranial neuralgias.

Pathophysiology

Primary headaches occur when pain-sensitive structures of the head, including the cerebral vasculature, musculature, and cranial or cervical nerves, are irritated.

Vascular changes occur as follows:

- Stimulation of the trigeminal ganglion located in the midbrain releases substance P and calcitonin gene-related peptide.
- The release of substance P causes degranulation of mast cells. Mast cells release histamine, and platelets release serotonin.
- Inflammation and release of substance P cause distention of cranial arteries and headache pain.
- Vasodilation, plasma extravasation, and inflammation occur.
- Triggers either directly act on the vasomotor tone or mediate the neurochemical release of vasoactive substances.
- Vasoconstriction, platelet changes, and neurochemical mediators initiate cerebral ischemia and activate the trigeminal-vascular system.

COMPLICATIONS
- Rebound headaches
- Serotonin syndrome

Signs and Symptoms

Migraine

- Commonly preceded by temporary focal neurologic signs known as *auras* (Auras are usually visual — scotomata, zigzag, flashing lights and colors, geometric shapes, jagged lines.)
- Unilateral in onset but may become generalized
- Begins as a dull ache that progressively worsens and develops into throbbing, pulsating pain
- Commonly associated with photophobia, nausea and vomiting, phonophobia, and paresthesia

Tension-Type

- Gradual onset of bilateral bandlike pressure or tightening of mild to moderate intensity; usually doesn't prohibit daily activities
- Not aggravated by physical activity or accompanied by associated symptoms; may have phonophobia or photophobia
- May be triggered by stress, fatigue, loud noises, heat, or bright lights
- Chronic form possibly resembles depression or fibromyalgia syndrome

Cluster

- Acute onset of excruciating severe unilateral orbital pain lasting 15 to 180 minutes
- Episodic clusters; one every other day to eight per day; commonly nocturnal
- Accompanied by ipsilateral lacrimation, conjunctival injection, rhinorrhea, miosis, ptosis, and nasal congestion

CLINICAL TIP
The presence of one or more of these factors is an indication for further evaluation:

- first-onset headache that begins after age 50
- sudden-onset headache
- accelerating pattern of headaches
- new-onset headache in a patient with cancer or human immunodeficiency virus
- headache with systemic illness (fever, stiff neck, or rash)
- presence of focal neurologic symptoms (not typical aura)
- papilledema.

Diagnostic Test Results

- Skull X-rays identify skull fracture.
- Computed tomography scan shows tumor or subarachnoid hemorrhage or other intracranial pathology; sinus CT reveals pathology of sinuses.
- Lumbar puncture shows increased ICP suggesting tumor, edema, or hemorrhage.
- EEG shows alterations in the brain's electrical activity, suggesting intracranial lesion, head injury, meningitis, or encephalitis.
- Sinus X-rays show sinusitis (not routinely performed).

Treatment

Migraines

- Beta-adrenergic blockers and calcium channel blockers to reduce frequency and severity of migraines
- Analgesics or combination analgesics
- Ergotamine tartrate, dihydroergotamine, butalbital combinations, and opiates

- Serotonin agonists, such as sumatriptan, naratriptan, rizatriptan, and zolmitriptan
- Antiemetics
- Tricyclic antidepressants (migraine)
- Antiseizure drugs (divalproex and topiramate) for migraine

Tension Headaches

- Analgesics
- Rest
- Stress reduction

VASCULAR CHANGES IN HEADACHE

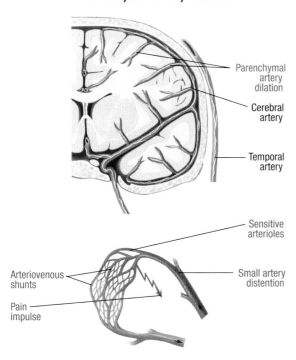

Normal

- Parenchymal artery
- Cerebral artery
- Temporal artery
- Extracranial artery
- Lumen
- Intima
- Muscle
- Outer coat
- Autonomic nerve

Parenchymal artery dilation

- Parenchymal artery dilation
- Cerebral artery
- Temporal artery
- Sensitive arterioles
- Arteriovenous shunts
- Small artery distention
- Pain impulse

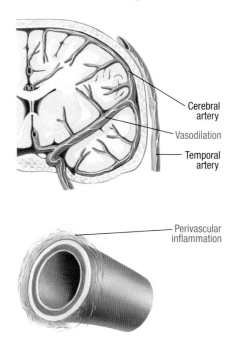

Vasoconstriction (aura) phase

- Vasoconstriction of cerebral arteries
- Temporal artery
- Platelet aggregation and release of serotonin granules

Vasodilation (headache) phase

- Cerebral artery
- Vasodilation
- Temporal artery
- Perivascular inflammation

A herniated disk, also called a *ruptured* or *slipped disk* or a *herniated nucleus pulposus (HNP)*, occurs when all or part of the *nucleus pulposus* — the soft, gelatinous, central portion of an intervertebral disk — protrudes through the disk's weakened or torn outer ring (*anulus fibrosus*).

Herniated disks usually occur in adults (mostly men) older than age 45. About 90% of herniated disks are lumbar or lumbosacral; 8%, cervical; and 1% to 2%, thoracic. Patients with a congenitally small lumbar spinal canal or with osteophyte formation along the vertebrae may be more susceptible to nerve root compression and more likely to have neurologic symptoms.

AGE ALERT
A herniated disk occurs more frequently in middle-aged and older men.

Causes

- Severe trauma or strain
- Intervertebral joint degeneration

AGE ALERT
In older patients whose vertebral disks have begun to degenerate, even minor trauma may cause herniation.

Pathophysiology

An intervertebral disk has two parts: the soft center called the *nucleus pulposus* and the tough, fibrous surrounding ring called the *anulus fibrosus*. The nucleus pulposus acts as a shock absorber, distributing the mechanical stress applied to the spine when the body moves.

Physical stress, usually a twisting motion, can tear or rupture the anulus fibrosus so that the nucleus pulposus herniates into the spinal canal. The vertebrae move closer together and in turn exert pressure on the nerve roots as they exit between the vertebrae.

Herniation occurs in three steps:

- *protrusion* — the nucleus pulposus presses against the anulus fibrosus
- *extrusion* — the nucleus pulposus bulges forcibly though the anulus fibrosus, pushing against the nerve root
- *sequestration* — the anulus gives way as the disk's core bursts and presses against the nerve root.

COMPLICATIONS
- Neurologic deficits
- Loss of bowel and bladder function

Signs and Symptoms

- Severe lower back pain to the buttocks, legs, and feet; can be unilaterally or bilaterally
- Sudden pain after trauma, subsiding in a few days, and then recurring at shorter intervals and with progressive intensity
- Sciatic pain following trauma, beginning as a dull pain in the buttocks (Valsalva's maneuver, coughing, sneezing, and bending intensify the pain, which is commonly accompanied by muscle spasms)
- Sensory and motor loss in the area innervated by the compressed spinal nerve root and, in later stages, weakness and atrophy of leg muscles

Diagnostic Test Results

- Straight-leg raising test is positive only if the patient has posterior leg (sciatic) pain, not back pain.
- Cross-straight leg is positive when raising the contralateral leg elicits pain.
- Lasègue's test reveals resistance and pain as well as loss of ankle or knee-jerk reflex, indicating spinal root compression.
- Rectal exam to check for weak or loss sphincter tone
- Myelogram, computed tomography scan, and magnetic resonance imaging show spinal canal compression as evidenced by herniated disk material.

Treatment

- Heat applications
- Physical Therapy
- Exercise program
- Nonsteroidal anti-inflammatory drugs such as ibuprofen, naproxen, or aspirin
- Corticosteroids such as dexamethasone
- Muscle relaxants, such as diazepam, methocarbamol, or cyclobenzaprine
- Surgery, including laminectomy to remove the protruding disk, spinal fusion to overcome segmental instability, or both to stabilize the spine

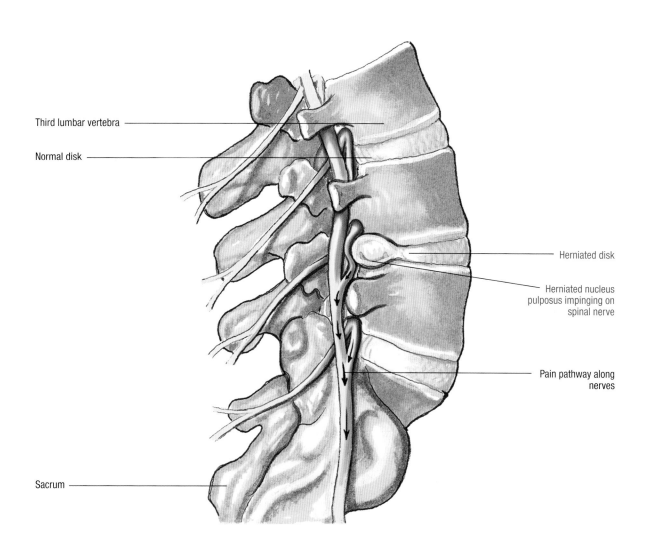

Third lumbar vertebra

Normal disk

Herniated disk

Herniated nucleus pulposus impinging on spinal nerve

Pain pathway along nerves

Sacrum

HYDROCEPHALUS

Hydrocephalus is a condition that results from an excessive accumulation of CSF in the brain. It results in an increase in ICP with corresponding enlargement of the ventricular system. The condition is congenital or acquired, and communicating or noncommunicating (obstructive).

AGE ALERT
Hydrocephalus occurs most commonly in children but may also occur in adults and elderly people.

Causes

- Genetic inheritance (aqueductal stenosis)
- Developmental disorders such as those associated with neural tube defects (NTDs), including spina bifida and encephalocele
- Complications of premature birth such as intraventricular hemorrhage
- Diseases (such as meningitis), tumors, traumatic head injury, or subarachnoid hemorrhage blocking the exit from the ventricles to the cisterns, thereby eliminating the cisterns

Pathophysiology

Ventricular dilation produces an increase in CSF pressure and volume, resulting in an increase in ICP. Compression of adjacent brain structures and cerebral blood vessels may lead to ischemia and, eventually, cell death.

COMPLICATIONS
- Mental retardation
- Impaired motor function
- Vision loss
- Death from increased ICP
- Death from infection and malnutrition (infants)

Signs and Symptoms

In Infants

- Rapid increase in head circumference or an unusually large head size
- Vomiting
- Sleepiness
- Irritability
- Downward deviation of the eyes (also called *sunsetting*)
- Seizures

In Older Children and Adults

- Headache
- Vomiting
- Nausea
- Papilledema (swelling of the optic disk that's part of the optic nerve)
- Blurred vision
- Diplopia (double vision)
- Sunsetting of the eyes
- Problems with balance
- Poor coordination
- Gait disturbance
- Urinary incontinence
- Slowing or loss of development
- Lethargy
- Drowsiness
- Irritability
- Other changes in personality or cognition, including memory loss

Diagnostic Test Results

- Skull X-rays show thinning of the skull with separation of the sutures and widening of the fontanels.
- Angiography shows vessel abnormalities due to stretching.
- Computed tomography scan and magnetic resonance imaging reveal variations in tissue density and fluid in the ventricular system.
- Lumbar puncture reveals increased fluid pressure from communicating hydrocephalus.
- Ventriculography shows ventricular dilation with excess fluid.

CLINICAL TIP
In infants, abnormally large head size for the patient's age strongly suggests hydrocephalus. Measurement of the head circumference is the most important diagnostic technique.

Treatment

- Surgical correction by insertion of a ventriculoperitoneal or ventriculoatrial shunt
- Antibiotics
- Serial lumbar puncture
- Endoscopic third ventriculostomy

Normal brain — Lateral view

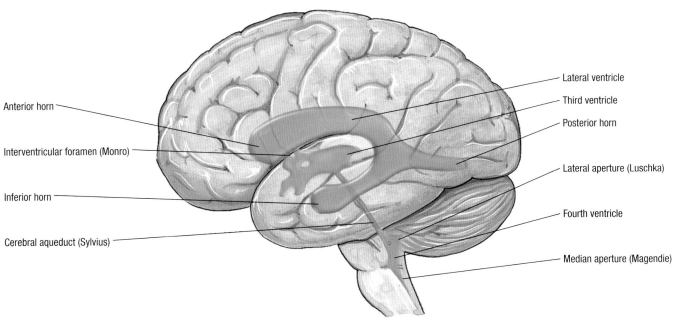

Anterior horn

Interventricular foramen (Monro)

Inferior horn

Cerebral aqueduct (Sylvius)

Lateral ventricle

Third ventricle

Posterior horn

Lateral aperture (Luschka)

Fourth ventricle

Median aperture (Magendie)

Ventricular enlargement

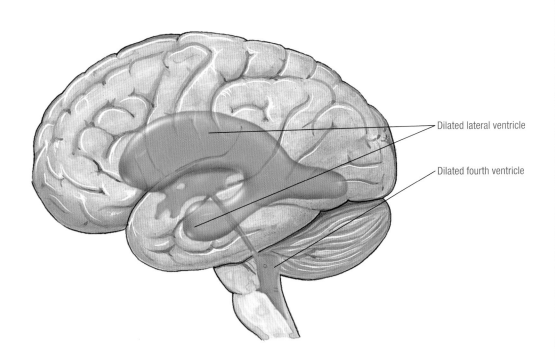

Dilated lateral ventricle

Dilated fourth ventricle

MENINGITIS

In meningitis, the brain and the spinal cord meninges become inflamed, usually because of bacterial infection. Such inflammation may involve all three meningeal membranes — the dura mater, arachnoid, and pia mater.

Causes

Meningitis is usually a complication of bacteremia, especially due to:

- pneumonia
- empyema
- osteomyelitis
- endocarditis.

Other infections associated with the development of meningitis include:

- sinusitis
- otitis media
- encephalitis
- myelitis
- brain abscess, usually caused by *Neisseria meningitidis*, *Haemophilus influenzae*, *Streptococcus pneumoniae*, and *Escherichia coli.*

Meningitis may follow trauma or invasive procedures, including:

- skull fracture
- penetrating head wound
- lumbar puncture
- ventricular shunting.

Aseptic meningitis may result from a virus or other organism. Sometimes no causative organism can be found.

Pathophysiology

Meningitis commonly begins as an inflammation of the pia-arachnoid, which may progress to congestion of adjacent tissues and destroy some nerve cells. The microorganism typically enters the central nervous system by way of blood. Other sources include direct communication between CSF and the environment (trauma); along cranial or peripheral nerves; or through the mouth or nose. Microorganisms can reach a fetus through the intrauterine environment.

The invading organism triggers an inflammatory response in the meninges. In an attempt to ward off the invasion, neutrophils gather in the area and produce an exudate in the subarachnoid space, causing the CSF to thicken. The thickened CSF flows less readily around the brain and spinal cord, and it can block the arachnoid villi, causing hydrocephalus.

The exudate also:

- exacerbates the inflammatory response, increasing the pressure in the brain
- can extend to the cranial and peripheral nerves, triggering additional inflammation
- irritates the meninges, disrupting their cell membranes and causing edema.

The consequences are elevated ICP, engorged blood vessels, disrupted cerebral blood supply, possible thrombosis or rupture,

and, if ICP isn't reduced, cerebral infarction. Encephalitis may also ensue as a secondary infection of the brain tissue.

In aseptic meningitis, lymphocytes infiltrate the pia-arachnoid layers, but usually not as severely as in bacterial meningitis, and no exudate is formed. Thus, aseptic meningitis is self-limiting.

COMPLICATIONS
- Blindness
- Loss of speech
- Brain damage
- Deafness
- Paralysis

Signs and Symptoms

- Fever, chills, and malaise
- Headache, vomiting and, rarely, papilledema
- Signs of meningeal irritation, including nuchal rigidity, positive Brudzinski's and Kernig's signs, exaggerated and symmetrical deep tendon reflexes, and opisthotonos (neck spasm)
- Irritability, delirium, deep stupor, coma, and photophobia, diplopia, or other vision problems

Diagnostic Test Results

- Lumbar puncture shows elevated CSF pressure (from obstructed CSF outflow at the arachnoid villi), cloudy or milky-white CSF, high protein level, positive Gram stain and culture (unless a virus is responsible), and decreased glucose concentration.
- Cultures of blood, urine, and nose and throat secretions reveal the offending organism.
- Chest X-ray reveals pneumonitis or lung abscess, tubercular lesions, or granulomas secondary to a fungal infection.
- Sinus and skull X-rays identify cranial osteomyelitis or paranasal sinusitis as the underlying infectious process, or skull fracture as the mechanism for entrance of the microorganism.
- White blood cell count reveals leukocytosis.
- Computed tomography scan reveals hydrocephalus, cerebral hematoma, hemorrhage, or tumor.
- Electrocardiogram reveals sinus arrhythmia.

Treatment

- I.V. antibiotics for at least 2 weeks, followed by oral antibiotics selected by culture and sensitivity testing
- I.V. fluids
- Agents to control arrhythmias
- Mannitol
- Anticonvulsant (usually given I.V.) or a sedative
- Aspirin or acetaminophen

CLINICAL TIP
Health care workers should take droplet precautions (in addition to standard precautions) for meningitis caused by *H. influenzae* or *N. meningitidis*, until 24 hours after the start of effective therapy.

MENINGES AND CEREBROSPINAL FLUID FLOW

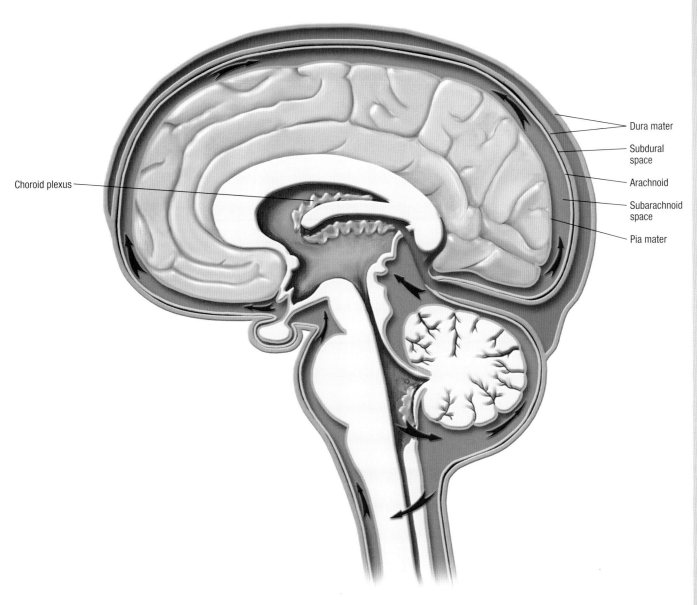

Choroid plexus

Dura mater

Subdural space

Arachnoid

Subarachnoid space

Pia mater

NORMAL MENINGES

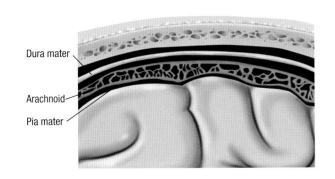

Dura mater

Arachnoid

Pia mater

INFLAMMATION IN MENINGITIS

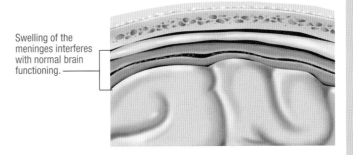

Swelling of the meninges interferes with normal brain functioning.

MULTIPLE SCLEROSIS

Multiple sclerosis (MS) causes demyelination of the white matter of the brain and spinal cord and damage to nerve fibers and their targets. Characterized by exacerbations and remissions, MS is a major cause of chronic disability in young adults and its prognosis varies. MS may progress rapidly, disabling the patient by early adulthood or causing death within months of onset. However, 70% of patients lead active, productive lives with prolonged remissions.

AGE ALERT
MS usually produces symptoms between ages 20 and 40 (the average age of onset is 27).

Types of MS include:

- *elapsing-remitting* — clear relapses (or acute attacks or exacerbations) with full recovery or partial recovery and lasting disability (The disease doesn't worsen between the attacks.)
- *primary progressive* — steady progression from the onset with minor recovery or plateaus (This form is uncommon and may involve different brain and spinal cord damage than other forms.)
- *secondary progressive* — begins as a pattern of clear-cut relapses and recovery (This form becomes steadily progressive and worsens between acute attacks.)
- *progressive relapsing* — steadily progressive from the onset, but also has clear acute attacks. (This form is rare.)

Causes

- Exact cause unknown

Possible Causes

- Autoimmune response to a slow-acting or latent viral infection
- Environmental or genetic factors

Pathophysiology

Evidence suggests that activation of T lymphocytes against the myelin antigens, axons, and oligodendrocytes triggers an immunologic cascade. Recruitment of inflammatory cells and local release of lymphokines and cytokines results in injury to the myelin and the underlying axon. Axon demyelination and nerve fiber loss occur in patches throughout the central nervous system. The damaged myelin sheath can't conduct normally, and the partial loss or dispersion of the action potential causes neurologic dysfunction.

COMPLICATIONS
- Injuries from falls
- Urinary tract infections (UTIs)
- Constipation
- Joint contractures
- Pressure ulcers
- Rectal distention
- Pneumonia

Signs and Symptoms

- Optic neuritis, diplopia, ophthalmoplegia, blurred vision, and nystagmus
- Sensory impairment, such as burning, pins and needles, and electrical sensations
- Fatigue (usually the most debilitating symptom)
- Weakness, paralysis ranging from monoplegia to quadriplegia, spasticity, hyperreflexia, intention tremor, and ataxia
- Incontinence, frequency, urgency, and frequent UTIs
- Involuntary evacuation or constipation
- Poorly articulated or scanning speech (syllables separated by pauses)
- Dysphagia

Diagnostic Test Results

Diagnosis of MS requires evidence of two or more neurologic attacks. These tests may also be useful:

- Magnetic resonance imaging reveals MS plaque or scarring.
- Lumbar puncture shows the elevation of certain immune system proteins (immunoglobulin [Ig] and IgG) and the presence of oligoclonal bands seen in 90% to 95% of people with MS.
- Evoked potential studies (visual, brain stem, auditory, and somatosensory) reveal slowed conduction of nerve impulses in most patients.
- Blood tests rule out other conditions.

Treatment

The aim of treatment is threefold: treat the acute exacerbation, treat the disease process, and treat the related signs and symptoms.

- I.V. methylprednisolone followed by oral therapy
- Interferon beta-1b and beta-1a or glatiramer
- Stretching and range-of-motion exercises, coupled with correct positioning, adaptive devices, and physical therapy
- Muscle relaxants, such as baclofen and tizanidine
- Frequent rest periods
- Natalizumab
- Speech and vision therapy
- Mitoxantrone

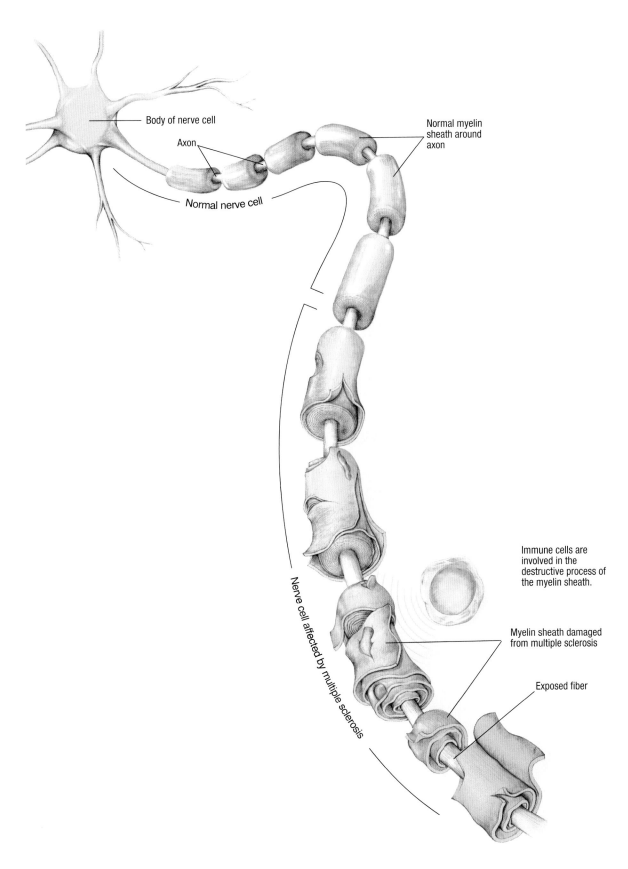

Body of nerve cell

Axon

Normal myelin sheath around axon

Normal nerve cell

Nerve cell affected by multiple sclerosis

Immune cells are involved in the destructive process of the myelin sheath.

Myelin sheath damaged from multiple sclerosis

Exposed fiber

MYASTHENIA GRAVIS

Myasthenia gravis is an autoimmune disorder that causes sporadic but progressive weakness and abnormal fatigability of striated (skeletal) muscles. Muscle weakness is exacerbated by continuing activity and repeated movement and is relieved by rest.

Myasthenia gravis follows an unpredictable course of periodic exacerbations and remissions. There's no known cure. Drug treatment has improved the prognosis and allows patients to lead relatively normal lives, except during exacerbations. When the disease involves the respiratory system, it may be life threatening.

AGE ALERT
Women are most commonly affected in their 20s and 30s, while men are usually affected in their 60s and 70s.

Causes

- Exact cause unknown

Possible Causes

- Autoimmune response
- Ineffective acetylcholine release
- Inadequate muscle-fiber response to acetylcholine

Pathophysiology

Myasthenia gravis is an autoimmune disease of the neuromuscular junction resulting from the production of antibodies against the acetylcholine receptor protein of skeletal muscles. Musclelike (myoid) cells in the thymus gland bear surface acetylcholine receptors, and a break in immune regulation interferes with tolerance and initiates antibody production. The site of action is the postsynaptic membrane. The antibodies reduce the number of acetylcholine receptors available at each neuromuscular junction and thereby impair muscle depolarization necessary for movement.

Scientists believe the thymus gland may give incorrect instructions to developing immune cells, ultimately resulting in autoimmunity and the production of the acetylcholine receptor antibodies and thereby allowing for the attack on neuromuscular transmission.

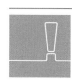

COMPLICATIONS
- Respiratory distress
- Pneumonia
- Chewing and swallowing difficulties leading to choking and food aspiration

Signs and Symptoms

- Weak eye closure, ptosis, and diplopia
- Skeletal muscle weakness and fatigue, increasing through the day but decreasing with rest (in the early stages, easy fatigability of certain muscles may appear with no other findings; later, it may be severe enough to cause paralysis)
- Progressive muscle weakness and accompanying loss of function depending on the muscle group affected; becoming more intense during menses and after emotional stress, prolonged exposure to sunlight or cold, or infections
- Blank, expressionless facial appearance and nasal vocal tones
- Frequent nasal regurgitation of fluids; difficulty chewing and swallowing
- Weak neck muscles (may become too weak to support the head without bobbing); patient must tilt head back to see
- Weak respiratory muscles; low tidal volume and vital capacity

CLINICAL TIP
Respiratory muscle weakness seen in myasthenic crisis may be severe enough to require emergency intubation and mechanical ventilation.

Diagnostic Test Results

- Tensilon test confirms diagnosis — temporarily improved muscle function within 30 to 60 seconds after I.V. injection of edrophonium or neostigmine and lasting up to 30 minutes.
- Electromyography with repeated neural stimulation shows progressive decrease in muscle-fiber contraction.
- Blood chemistry studies reveal elevated serum antiacetylcholine antibody titer.
- Chest X-ray reveals thymoma (in about 15% of patients).

Treatment

- Anticholinesterase drugs, such as neostigmine and pyridostigmine
- Immunosuppressant therapy with corticosteroids, azathioprine, cyclosporine, and cyclophosphamide used in a progressive fashion
- Immunoglobulin G during acute relapses or plasmapheresis in severe exacerbations
- Plasmapheresis
- Thymectomy
- Tracheotomy, positive-pressure ventilation, and vigorous suctioning
- Discontinuation of anticholinesterase drugs in myasthenic crisis until respiratory function improves

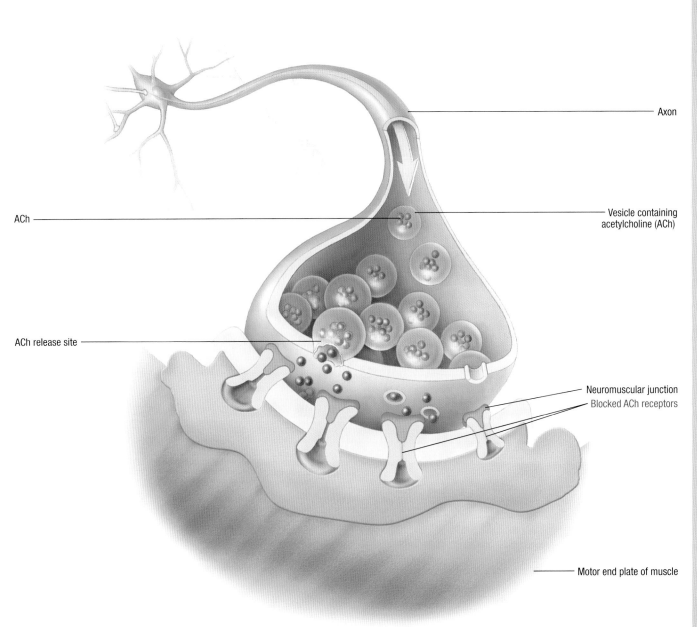

Axon

ACh

Vesicle containing
acetylcholine (ACh)

ACh release site

Neuromuscular junction

Blocked ACh receptors

Motor end plate of muscle

PARKINSON'S DISEASE

Parkinson's disease is a neurodegenerative disorder of the extrapyramidal system. It characteristically produces progressive muscle rigidity, akinesia, and involuntary tremor. Death may result from complications, such as aspiration pneumonia or other infection.

AGE ALERT
Parkinson's disease is one of the most common crippling diseases in the United States. It strikes 1 in every 100 people over age 60 and affects men more often than women.

Causes

Exact cause unknown

Possible Contributing Factors

- Advanced age
- Genetics
- Environment (rural residence with exposure to well water, herbicides, and pesticides)
- Industrial chemicals (such metals as manganese, iron, and steel alloys)

Pathophysiology

Parkinson's disease is a degenerative process involving the dopaminergic neurons in the substantia nigra (the area of the basal ganglia that produces and stores the neurotransmitter dopamine). This area plays an important role in the extrapyramidal system, which controls posture and coordination of voluntary motor movements.

Normally, stimulation of the basal ganglia results in refined motor movement because acetylcholine (excitatory) and dopamine (inhibitory) release is balanced. Degeneration of the dopaminergic neurons and loss of available dopamine lead to an excess of excitatory acetylcholine at the synapse and consequent rigidity, tremors, and bradykinesia. Other nondopaminergic neurons may be affected, possibly contributing to depression and the other nonmotor symptoms associated with this disease. Also, the basal ganglia are interconnected to the hypothalamus, potentially affecting autonomic and endocrine function as well.

Current research on the pathogenesis of Parkinson's disease focuses on damage to the substantia nigra from oxidative stress. Oxidative stress is believed to diminish brain iron content, impair mitochondrial function, inhibit antioxidant and protective systems, reduce glutathione secretion, and damage lipids, proteins, and deoxyribonucleic acid. Brain cells are less capable of repairing oxidative damage than are other tissues.

COMPLICATIONS
- Injury from falls
- Food aspiration
- Urinary tract infections
- Skin breakdown

Signs and Symptoms

- Muscle rigidity, akinesia, and an insidious tremor beginning in the fingers (unilateral pill-roll tremor) that increases during stress or anxiety and decreases with purposeful movement and sleep
- Resistance to passive muscle stretching, which may be uniform (lead-pipe rigidity) or jerky (cogwheel rigidity)
- Akinesia causing difficulty walking (gait lacks normal parallel motion and may be retropulsive or propulsive)
- Loss of posture control
- Drooling and excessive sweating
- Masklike facial expression
- Dysarthria, dysphagia, or both
- Oculogyric crises or blepharospasm
- Decreased motility of GI and genitourinary smooth muscle
- Orthostatic hypotension
- Oily skin

Diagnostic Test Results

Generally, diagnostic tests are of little value in identifying Parkinson's disease. Diagnosis is based on the patient's age and history and on the characteristic clinical picture. However, urinalysis may support the diagnosis by revealing decreased dopamine levels.

A conclusive diagnosis is possible only after ruling out other causes of tremor, involutional depression, cerebral arteriosclerosis, intracranial tumors, Wilson's disease, or phenothiazine or other drug toxicity.

Treatment

- Levodopa, a dopamine replacement most effective during early stages and given in increasing doses until symptoms are relieved or adverse effects appear
- Drugs that enhance the therapeutic effect of levodopa — anticholinergics such as trihexyphenidyl; antihistamines such as diphenhydramine; amantidine, an antiviral agent; selegiline, an enzyme-inhibiting agent
- Deep brain stimulation surgery
- Physical therapy, including active and passive range-of-motion exercises, routine daily activities, walking, baths, and massage

Brain — Coronal section

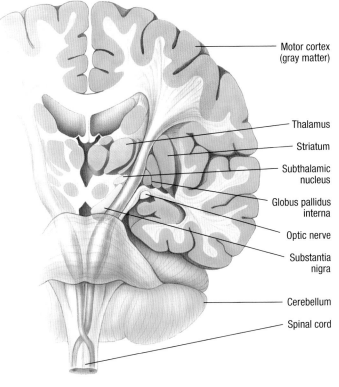

Motor cortex
(gray matter)

Thalamus

Striatum

Subthalamic
nucleus

Globus pallidus
interna

Optic nerve

Substantia
nigra

Cerebellum

Spinal cord

Brain — Lateral view

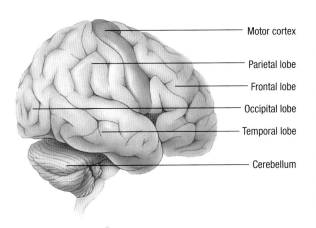

Motor cortex

Parietal lobe

Frontal lobe

Occipital lobe

Temporal lobe

Cerebellum

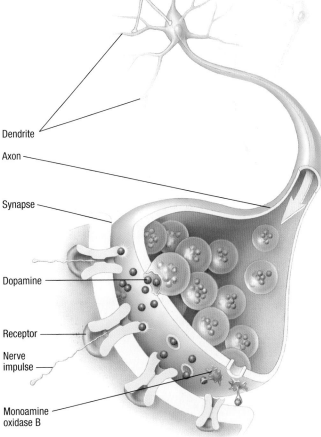

Dendrite

Axon

Synapse

Dopamine

Receptor

Nerve
impulse

Monoamine
oxidase B

Dopamine levels

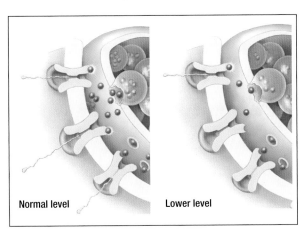

Normal level

Lower level

SPINA BIFIDA

Spina bifida and other NTDs are serious birth defects that involve the spine and spinal cord. In spina bifida, the neural tube fails to close at approximately 28 days after conception.

Causes

Exact cause and most of the specific environmental triggers unknown.

Possible Causes

- Maternal folic acid deficiency
- Fetal exposure to a teratogen such as valproic acid
- Multiple malformation syndrome (for example, chromosomal abnormalities such as trisomy 18 or 13 syndrome)
- Isolated NTDs (not due to a specific teratogen or associated with other malformations) believed to be caused by a combination of genetic and environmental factors

Pathophysiology

Spina bifida occulta is the most common and least severe spinal cord defect. It's characterized by incomplete closure of one or more vertebrae without protrusion of the spinal cord or meninges.

However, in more severe forms of spina bifida, the spinal contents protrude in an external sac or cystic lesion (spina bifida cystica). *Spina bifida cystica* has two forms: *myelomeningocele (meningomyelocele)* and *meningocele.* In myelomeningocele, the external sac contains meninges, CSF, and a portion of the spinal cord or nerve roots distal to the conus medullaris. When the spinal nerve roots end at the sac, motor and sensory function below the sac is abolished. Arnold-Chiari syndrome is a form of meningomyelocele in which part of the brain protrudes into the spinal canal. Meningocele, in which the sac contains only meninges and CSF, is less severe and may not produce symptoms.

COMPLICATIONS
- Hydrocephalus
- Infection
- Paralysis
- Physical and mental disabilities

Signs and Symptoms

Spina Bifida Occulta

- Depression or dimple, tuft of hair, soft fatty deposits, portwine nevi, or a combination of these abnormalities on the skin over the spinal defect
- Occasionally associated with foot weakness or bowel and bladder disturbances

Meningocele

- Saclike structure protrudes over the spine
- Seldom causes neurologic deficit

Myelomeningocele (Meningomyelocele)

- Saclike protrusion containing nerve tissue
- Depending on the level of the defect, causes permanent neurologic dysfunction

Associated Disorders

- Trophic skin disturbances (ulcerations, cyanosis), clubfoot, knee contractures, curvature of the spine, hydrocephalus (in about 90% of patients), and, possibly, mental retardation

Diagnostic Test Results

- Amniocentesis detects elevated alpha fetoprotein (AFP) levels in amniotic fluid, which indicates the presence of an open NTD.
- Fetal karyotype detects chromosomal abnormalities.
- Maternal serum AFP screening is used in combination with other serum markers, such as human chorionic gonadotropin (HCG), free beta-HCG, or unconjugated estriol (for patients with a lower risk of NTDs and those who will be under age 34½ at the time of delivery) to estimate a fetus's risk of NTD as well as possible increased risk of perinatal complications, such as premature rupture of the membranes, abruptio placentae, or fetal death.
- Ultrasound is performed when increased risk of open NTD exists, based on family history or abnormal serum screening results (not conclusive for open NTDs or ventral wall defects).

If the NTD isn't diagnosed before birth, other tests are used to make the diagnosis, including:

- palpation and spinal X-ray for spina bifida occulta
- myelography to differentiate spina bifida occulta from other spinal abnormalities, especially spinal cord tumors
- transillumination of the protruding sac to distinguish between myelomeningocele (typically doesn't transilluminate) and meningocele (typically transilluminates)
- pinprick examination of the legs and trunk to show the level of sensory and motor involvement in myelomeningocele
- skull X-rays, cephalic measurements, and computed tomography scan to demonstrate associated hydrocephalus.

Treatment

- *Spina bifida occulta:* usually no treatment
- *Meningocele:* surgical closure of protruding sac
- *Myelomeningocele:* repair of the sac (doesn't reverse neurologic defects); shunt to relieve hydrocephalus if needed; supportive measures to promote independence and prevent further complications

Spina bifida occulta

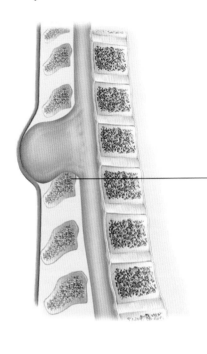

Vertebrae are incompletely fused; no external sac is present.

Meningocele

External sac contains meninges and cerebrospinal fluid (CSF).

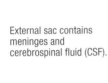

Myelomeningocele

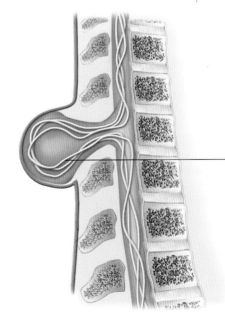

External sac contains meninges, CSF, peripheral nerves, and spinal cord tissue.

SPINAL CORD INJURY

Spinal injuries include fractures, contusions, and compressions of the vertebral column, usually as the result of trauma to the head or neck. The real danger lies in spinal cord damage — cutting, pulling, twisting, or compression. Damage may involve the entire spinal cord or be restricted to one-half, and it can occur at any level. Fractures of the C5, C6, C7, T12, and L1 vertebrae are most common.

Causes

Traumatic

- Motor vehicle accidents
- Falls
- Sports injuries or diving into shallow water
- Gunshot or stab wounds
- Lifting heavy objects

Nontraumatic

- Hyperparathyroidism
- Neoplastic lesions

Pathophysiology

Like head trauma, spinal cord trauma results from acceleration, deceleration, or other deforming forces usually applied from a distance.

Mechanisms triggered by spinal cord trauma include:

- *hyperextension* — acceleration-deceleration forces and sudden reduction in the anteroposterior diameter of the spinal cord
- *hyperflexion* — sudden and excessive force, propelling the neck forward or causing an exaggerated movement to one side
- *vertical compression* — upward or downward force along the vertical axis
- *rotation and shearing* — twisting.

Injury causes microscopic hemorrhages in the gray matter and pia-arachnoid. The hemorrhages gradually increase in size until all of the gray matter is filled with blood, which causes necrosis. From the gray matter, the blood enters the white matter, where it impedes the circulation within the spinal cord. Ensuing edema causes compression and decreases the blood supply. The edema and hemorrhage are greatest at the injury site and approximately two segments above and below it. The edema temporarily adds to the patient's dysfunction by increasing pressure and compressing the nerves. Edema near the C3 to C5 vertebrae may interfere with phrenic nerve-impulse transmission to the diaphragm and inhibit respiratory function.

In the white matter, circulation usually returns to normal in about 24 hours. However, in the gray matter, an inflammatory reaction prevents restoration of circulation. Phagocytes appear at the site within 36 to 48 hours after the injury, macrophages engulf degenerating axons, and collagen replaces the normal tissue. Scarring and meningeal thickening leave the nerves in the area blocked or tangled.

COMPLICATIONS
- Pressure ulcers
- Pulmonary embolism
- Autonomic dysreflexia
- Spinal shock
- Neurogenic shock
- Sexual dysfunction
- Deep vein thrombosis

Signs and Symptoms

- Muscle spasm and back pain that worsens with movement:
  - In cervical fractures, pain may cause point tenderness.
  - In dorsal and lumbar fractures, pain may radiate to other body areas such as the legs.
- Mild paresthesia to quadriplegia and shock, if the injury damages the spinal cord (in milder injury, such symptoms may be delayed several days or weeks)

Specific to Injury Type or Degree

- Loss of motor function; muscle flaccidity
- Loss of reflexes and sensory function below the level of injury
- Bladder and bowel atony
- Loss of perspiration below the level of injury
- Respiratory impairment

Diagnostic Test Results

- Spinal X-rays, the most important diagnostic measure, detect the fracture.
- Thorough neurologic evaluation locates the level of injury and detects cord damage.
- Lumbar puncture shows increased CSF pressure from a lesion or trauma in spinal compression.
- Computed tomography scan or magnetic resonance imaging reveals spinal cord edema and compression and may reveal a spinal mass.

Treatment

- Immediate immobilization to stabilize the spine and prevent cord damage (primary treatment), including the use of sandbags on both sides of the patient's head, a hard cervical collar, or skeletal traction with skull tongs or a halo device for cervical spine injuries
- High doses of methylprednisolone
- Bed rest on firm support (such as a bed board), analgesics, and muscle relaxants
- Plaster cast or a turning frame
- Laminectomy and spinal fusion
- Neurosurgery
- Rehabilitation
- Medications, including analgesics, anticoagulants, antiulcer agents, antidepressants, anticholinergics, antispasmodics, and laxatives

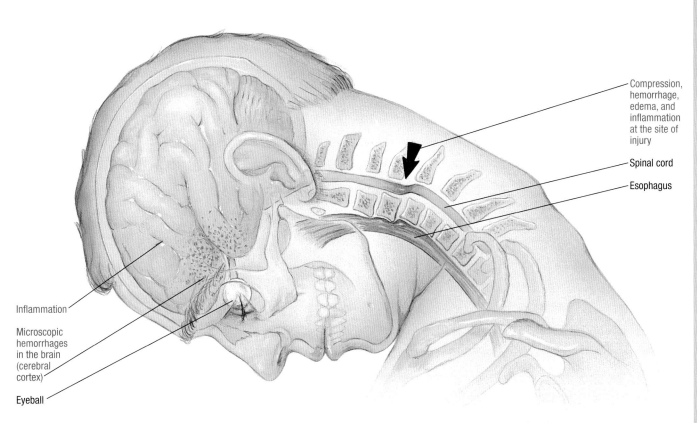

Compression, hemorrhage, edema, and inflammation at the site of injury

Spinal cord

Esophagus

Inflammation

Microscopic hemorrhages in the brain (cerebral cortex)

Eyeball

STROKE

A stroke is a sudden impairment of cerebral circulation in one or more blood vessels. Stroke interrupts or diminishes oxygen supply and commonly causes serious damage or necrosis in the brain tissues.

Causes

- Thrombosis of the cerebral arteries supplying the brain or of the intracranial vessels, occluding blood flow
- Embolism from thrombus outside the brain, such as in the heart, aorta, or common carotid artery
- Hemorrhage from an intracranial artery or vein, such as from hypertension, ruptured aneurysm, AVM trauma, hemorrhagic disorder, or septic embolism (80% to 85% of stokes are due to thrombotic events while 15% to 20% of strokes are due to hemorrhage)

Pathophysiology

Regardless of the cause, the underlying event is deprivation of oxygen and nutrients. Normally, if the arteries become blocked, autoregulatory mechanisms help maintain cerebral circulation until collateral circulation develops to deliver blood to the affected area. If the compensatory mechanisms become overworked, or if cerebral blood flow remains impaired for more than a few minutes, oxygen deprivation leads to infarction of brain tissue.

A thrombotic or embolic stroke causes ischemia. Some of the neurons served by the occluded vessel die from lack of oxygen and nutrients, resulting in cerebral infarction. Injury to surrounding cells disrupts metabolism and leads to changes in ionic transport, localized acidosis, and free radical formation. Calcium, sodium, and water accumulate in injured cells, and excitatory neurotransmitters are released. Consequent continued cellular injury and swelling may cause further damage.

When hemorrhage is the cause of stroke, impaired cerebral perfusion causes infarction, and the blood itself acts as a space-occupying mass. The brain's regulatory mechanisms attempt to maintain equilibrium by increasing blood pressure to maintain cerebral perfusion pressure. The increased ICP forces CSF out, thus restoring balance. If the hemorrhage is small, this may be enough to keep the patient alive with only minimal neurologic deficits. However, if bleeding is heavy, ICP increases rapidly and perfusion stops. Even if the pressure returns to normal, many brain cells die.

COMPLICATIONS

- Paralysis or loss of muscle movement
- Difficulty swallowing or talking
- Memory loss or trouble understanding
- Pain
- Pressure ulcers
- Infection

Signs and Symptoms

The clinical features of stroke vary according to the affected artery and the region of the brain it supplies, the severity of damage, and the extent of collateral circulation developed. A stroke in one hemisphere causes signs and symptoms on the opposite side of the body. A stroke that damages cranial nerves affects structures on the same side. Symptoms include:

- hemiparesis
- hemisensory loss
- altered level of consciousness
- headache, dizziness, and anxiety
- visual field defects
- ataxia, vertigo, and incoordination
- dysphasia (expressive and receptive)
- dysarthria
- amaurosis fugax
- dysphagia.

Diagnostic Test Results

- Computed tomography scan identifies an ischemic stroke within the first 72 hours of symptom onset and evidence of a hemorrhagic stroke (lesions larger than 1 cm) immediately.
- Magnetic resonance imaging assists in identifying areas of ischemia or infarction and cerebral swelling.
- Arteriography reveals disruption of the cerebral circulation by occlusion, such as stenosis or acute thrombus, or by hemorrhage.
- Carotid duplex scan and transcranial Doppler identify the degree of stenosis.
- Echocardiography reveals thrombi within the atrium or ventricle.

Treatment

Ischemic Stroke

- Thrombolytic therapy with tissue plasminogen activator within 3 hours after onset of symptoms
- Aspirin, warfarin, heparin
- Carotid endarterectomy
- Angioplasty and stents

Hemorrhagic Stroke

- Aneurysm clipping
- Coiling (aneurysm embolization)

ISCHEMIC STROKE

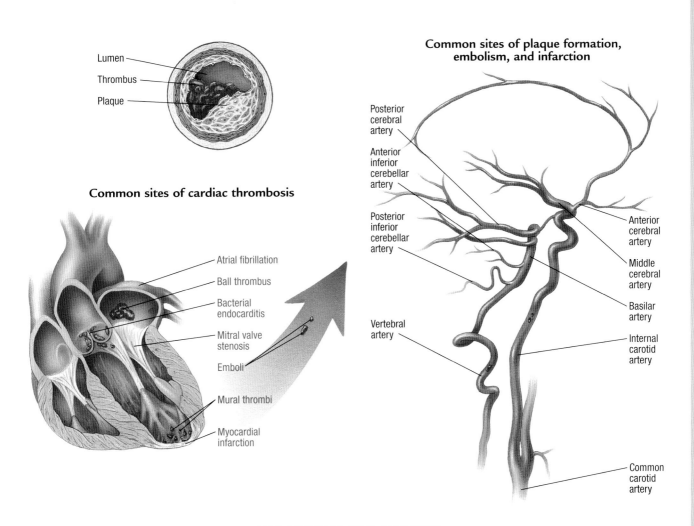

Lumen
Thrombus
Plaque

Common sites of plaque formation, embolism, and infarction

Posterior cerebral artery
Anterior inferior cerebellar artery
Posterior inferior cerebellar artery
Vertebral artery

Anterior cerebral artery
Middle cerebral artery
Basilar artery
Internal carotid artery
Common carotid artery

Common sites of cardiac thrombosis

Atrial fibrillation
Ball thrombus
Bacterial endocarditis
Mitral valve stenosis
Emboli
Mural thrombi
Myocardial infarction

HEMORRHAGIC STROKE

Common sites of cerebral hemorrhage

Intracerebral hemorrhage
Lacunar infarcts

Microaneurysm
Arterioles
Subarachnoid hemorrhage

WEST NILE VIRUS

West Nile is a virus transmitted by mosquitoes that causes an illness that can range from mild to severe. Mild, flu-like illness is commonly called *West Nile fever*. In its most severe form, West Nile virus can infect the central nervous system and cause meningitis, encephalitis, and death.

Causes

Spreads when a mosquito bites an infected bird and then bites a person

Risk Factors for Developing a Severe Form of the Disease

- Conditions that suppress the immune system, such as recent chemotherapy, recent organ transplantation, or human immunodeficiency virus
- Pregnancy
- Older age

The disease may also be spread through blood transfusions and organ transplantation. It's also possible for an infected mother to transmit the virus to her infant through breast milk.

Pathophysiology

West Nile virus is a type of organism called a flavivirus and is similar to many other mosquito-borne viruses. After infection, if encephalitis ensues, severe inflammation of the brain occurs. Intense lymphocytic infiltration of brain tissues and the leptomeninges causes cerebral edema, degeneration of the brain's ganglion cells, and diffuse nerve cell destruction.

COMPLICATIONS
- Coma
- Tremors
- Seizures
- Paralysis
- Death (rare)

Signs and Symptoms

West Nile Fever

- Fever
- Headache
- Back pain
- Muscle aches
- Lack of appetite
- Sore throat
- Nausea and vomiting
- Maculopapular or morbilliform rash on the neck
- Abdominal pain
- Diarrhea

Severe Infection

- Fever
- Weakness
- Stiff neck
- Change in mental status
- Loss of consciousness

In addition, a patient with encephalitis may have paresis or paralysis, cranial nerve deficits, sensory deficits, abnormal reflexes, seizures, and involuntary jerks.

Diagnostic Test Results

- Serology reveals the presence of antibodies against West Nile virus in CSF or serum.
- Complete blood count shows a normal or elevated white blood cell count (WBC).
- Lumbar puncture and CSF testing show elevated WBC count (especially lymphocytes) and elevated protein level.
- Magnetic resonance imaging of the head shows evidence of inflammation.

Treatment

No specific treatment

Supportive Treatment

- I.V. fluids
- Airway management
- Respiratory support
- Prevention of secondary infections
- Analgesics

Normal brain

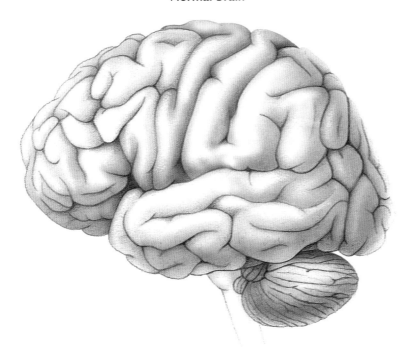

Edematous brain

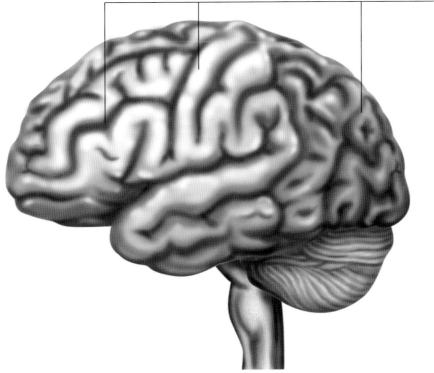

Intense lymphocytic infiltration causes cerebral edema.

GASTROINTESTINAL DISORDERS

ACHALASIA

Achalasia is a disease of the muscle of the esophagus. In achalasia, the lower esophageal sphincter (LES) "fails to relax" and open to allow food to pass into the stomach. As a result, patients with achalasia have difficulty swallowing food.

Causes

The exact cause is unknown, but theories include:

- heredity
- infection
- autoimmune disease.

Pathophysiology

In achalasia, the LES doesn't open properly to allow food to pass into the stomach and, in at least half of the patients with achalasia, the lower sphincter resting pressure also is abnormally high. The muscle of the lower half of the esophagus doesn't contract normally, and peristaltic waves don't occur. This results in food and saliva not being propelled down the esophagus and into the stomach.

Some patients with achalasia have high-pressure waves in the lower esophageal body following swallowing, but the waves aren't effective in pushing food into the stomach. This type of achalasia is called *vigorous achalasia*. These abnormalities of the lower sphincter and esophageal body are responsible for food sticking in the esophagus.

Early in achalasia, inflammation occurs in the muscle of the lower esophagus, especially around the nerves. As the disease progresses, the nerves (particularly the nerves that cause the LES to relax) begin to degenerate and ultimately disappear. This damage to the nerves may cause muscle cells to begin to degenerate as well. These changes result in a lower sphincter that can't relax and muscle in the lower esophageal body that can't support peristaltic waves. With time, the body of the esophagus stretches and becomes dilated.

COMPLICATIONS
- Aspiration
- Pneumonia
- Esophagitis
- Esophageal cancer

Signs and Symptoms

- Consistent (occurring with every meal) dysphagia (with solids and liquids)
- Heavy sensation in the chest after eating
- Chest pain
- Regurgitation
- Weight loss

Diagnostic Test Results

- Video esophagram shows esophageal dilation with a characteristic tapered narrowing of the lower end, sometimes likened to a "bird's beak." The barium also stays in the esophagus longer than normal before passing into the stomach.
- Esophageal manometry demonstrates the failure of the muscle of the esophageal body to contract with swallowing and the failure of the LES to relax.
- Endoscopy reveals high pressure in the LES, a dilated esophagus, and a lack of peristaltic waves. Endoscopy also excludes esophageal cancer.

Treatment

- Nitrates, such as isosorbide dinitrate, and calcium channel blockers, such as nifedipine and verapamil, to relax the LES
- Dilation of the LES
- Esophagomyotomy
- Endoscopic injection of botulinum toxin

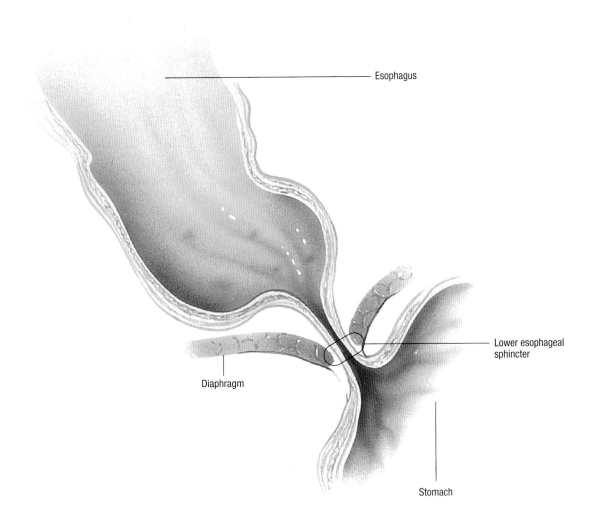

Esophagus

Lower esophageal
sphincter

Diaphragm

Stomach

APPENDICITIS

The most common major surgical disease, appendicitis, is inflammation and obstruction of the vermiform appendix. Since the advent of antibiotics, the incidence and the death rate of appendicitis have declined; if untreated, this disease is invariably fatal.

AGE ALERT
Appendicitis may occur at any age, but the majority of cases occur between ages 11 and 20. It affects both sexes equally; however, between puberty and age 25, it's more prevalent in men.

Causes

- Mucosal ulceration
- Fecal mass (fecalith)
- Stricture
- Barium ingestion
- Viral infection
- Neoplasm
- Foreign body

Pathophysiology

Mucosal ulceration triggers inflammation, which temporarily obstructs the appendix. The obstruction blocks mucus outflow. Pressure in the now distended appendix increases, and the appendix contracts. Bacteria multiply, and inflammation and pressure continue to increase, restricting blood flow to the organ and causing severe abdominal pain.

Inflammation may lead to infection, clotting, and tissue decay.

COMPLICATIONS
- Rupture or perforation of the appendix
- Peritonitis
- Appendiceal abscess
- Pyelophlebitis

Signs and Symptoms

Appendicitis

- Abdominal pain, which may become localized to the lower right quadrant (McBurney's point)

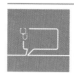

CLINICAL TIP
If a line is drawn from the umbilicus to the right superior iliac crest and divided into thirds, McBurney's point is two-thirds of the line from the umbilicus.
- Rebound tenderness
- Anorexia after the onset of pain
- Nausea or vomiting
- Low-grade fever

Rupture

- Pain
- Tenderness
- Spasm, followed by a brief cessation of abdominal pain

Diagnostic Test Results

- White blood cell count is moderately elevated with increased immature cells.
- Abdominal or transvaginal ultrasound shows inflammation of the appendix.
- Barium enema reveals a nonfilling appendix.
- Abdominal computed tomography scan shows perforation or abscess.

Treatment

- Nothing by mouth; parenteral fluids and electrolytes
- High Fowler's position
- Nasogastric intubation
- Appendectomy
- Antibiotics

Small and large intestines

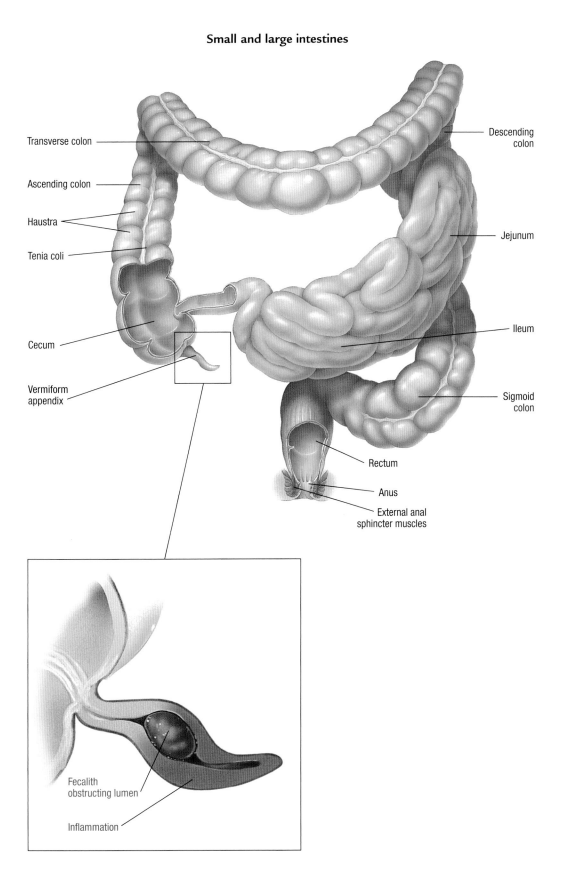

Transverse colon

Ascending colon

Haustra

Tenia coli

Cecum

Vermiform appendix

Descending colon

Jejunum

Ileum

Sigmoid colon

Rectum

Anus

External anal sphincter muscles

Fecalith obstructing lumen

Inflammation

CHOLECYSTITIS

Cholecystitis — acute or chronic inflammation causing painful distention of the gallbladder — is usually associated with a gallstone impacted in the cystic duct. Cholecystitis accounts for 10% to 25% of all gallbladder surgery. The acute form is most common among middle-aged women; the chronic form, among elderly people. The prognosis is good with treatment.

Causes

- Gallstones (the most common cause)
- Poor or absent blood flow to the gallbladder
- Abnormal metabolism of cholesterol and bile salts

Pathophysiology

In acute cholecystitis, inflammation of the gallbladder wall usually develops after a gallstone lodges in the cystic duct. Gallstones typically develop when metabolism of cholesterol and bile salts is abnormal. The liver usually makes bile continuously, and the gallbladder stores it until it's needed to help digest fat. Changes in the composition of bile may cause gallstones to form.

When gallstones block bile flow, the gallbladder becomes inflamed and distended. Growth of bacteria, usually *Escherichia coli*, may contribute to the inflammation and abscess formation or empyema.

Edema of the gallbladder (and sometimes the cystic duct) obstructs flow of bile, which chemically irritates the gallbladder. Cells in the gallbladder wall may become oxygen starved and die as the distended organ presses on vessels and impairs blood flow. The dead cells slough off, and an exudate covers ulcerated areas, causing the gallbladder to adhere to surrounding structures.

COMPLICATIONS
- Gangrene
- Perforation
- Peritonitis
- Fistula formation
- Pancreatitis

Signs and Symptoms

- Acute abdominal pain in the right upper quadrant that may radiate to the back, between the shoulders, or to the front of the chest; typically occurs after a fatty meal
- Colic
- Nausea and vomiting
- Chills and low-grade fever
- Jaundice

Diagnostic Test Results

- X-ray reveals gallstones if they contain enough calcium to be radiopaque; it also helps disclose porcelain gallbladder (hard, brittle gallbladder due to calcium deposited in wall), limy bile, and gallstone ileus.
- Computed tomography scan or magnetic resonance imaging shows calcified gallbladder and the presence of stones.
- Ultrasonography detects gallstones as small as 2 mm and distinguishes between obstructive and nonobstructive jaundice.
- Technetium scan reveals cystic duct obstruction and acute or chronic cholecystitis if ultrasound doesn't visualize the gallbladder.
- Percutaneous transhepatic cholangiography supports the diagnosis of obstructive jaundice and reveals calculi in the ducts.
- Blood chemistry reveals elevated levels of serum alkaline phosphate, lactate dehydrogenase, aspartate aminotransferase, and total bilirubin; serum amylase level slightly elevated; and icteric index elevated.
- Blood studies reveal slightly elevated white blood cell counts during cholecystitis attack.

Treatment

- Cholecystectomy
- Choledochostomy
- Percutaneous transhepatic cholecystostomy
- Endoscopic retrograde cholangiopancreatography
- Lithotripsy
- Oral chenodeoxycholic acid or ursodeoxycholic acid
- Low-fat diet
- Vitamin K
- Antibiotics
- Nasogastric intubation

Liver and gallbladder

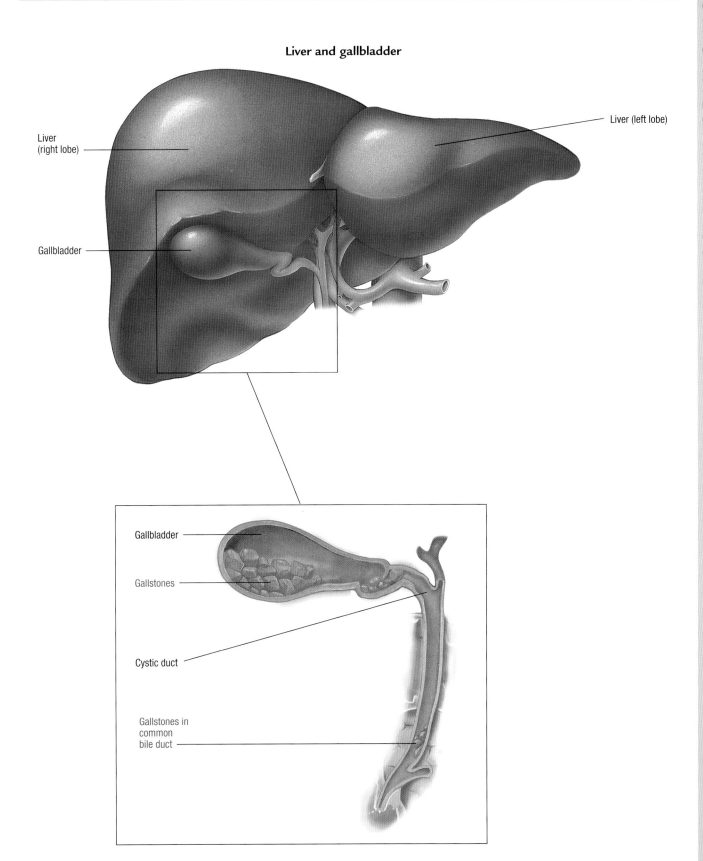

Liver
(right lobe)

Liver (left lobe)

Gallbladder

Gallbladder

Gallstones

Cystic duct

Gallstones in
common
bile duct

CIRRHOSIS

Cirrhosis is a chronic disease characterized by diffuse destruction and fibrotic regeneration of hepatic cells. Mortality is high; many patients die within 5 years of onset. As cirrhosis progresses, complications may occur; these include ascites, portal hypertension, jaundice, coagulopathy, hepatic encephalopathy, bleeding, esophageal varices, acute GI bleeding, liver failure, and renal failure.

AGE ALERT
Cirrhosis is especially prevalent among malnourished persons over age 50 with chronic alcoholism; it's also twice as common in men as in women.

Causes

- Hepatitis
- Alcoholism
- Malnutrition
- Autoimmune disease, such as sarcoidosis or chronic inflammatory bowel disease
- Diseases of the biliary tree
- Sclerosing cholangitis
- Wilson's disease
- Alpha$_1$ antitrypsin deficiency
- Hemochromatosis
- Hepatic vein obstruction
- Right-sided heart failure

Pathophysiology

The initial event in cirrhosis is hepatic scarring or fibrosis. The scar begins as an increase in extracellular matrix components — fibrin-forming collagens, proteoglycans, fibronectin, and hyaluronic acid. Hepatocyte function is eventually impaired as the matrix changes. Fat-storing cells are believed to be the source of the extracellular changes. Contraction of these cells may also contribute to disruption of the lobular architecture and obstruction of the flow of blood or bile. Cellular changes producing bands of scar tissue also disrupt the lobular structure.

COMPLICATIONS
- Portal hypertension
- Esophageal varices
- Ascites
- Hepatic encephalopathy
- Liver failure
- Death

Signs and Symptoms

Early Stage

- Anorexia, nausea and vomiting, diarrhea
- Dull abdominal ache

Late Stage

- Respiratory — pleural effusion, limited thoracic expansion, and impaired gas exchange
- Central nervous system — progressive signs or symptoms of hepatic encephalopathy, including lethargy, extreme obtundation, and coma
- Hematologic — bleeding tendency, anemia, splenomegaly, and portal hypertension
- Endocrine — testicular atrophy, menstrual irregularities, gynecomastia, and loss of chest and axillary hair
- Skin — severe pruritus, extreme dryness and poor tissue turgor, spider angiomas, and palmar erythema
- Hepatic — jaundice, hepatomegaly, ascites and edema of the legs, and hepatorenal syndrome
- Miscellaneous — musty breath, enlarged superficial abdominal veins, pain in the right upper abdominal quadrant that worsens when patient sits up or leans forward, and temperature of 101°F to 103°F (38°C to 39°C)
- Hemorrhage from esophageal varices

Diagnostic Test Results

- Liver biopsy reveals tissue destruction and fibrosis.
- Abdominal X-ray shows enlarged liver, cysts, or gas within the biliary tract or liver, liver calcification, and massive fluid accumulation (ascites).
- Computed tomography and liver scans show liver size, abnormal masses, and hepatic blood flow and obstruction.
- Esophagogastroduodenoscopy reveals bleeding esophageal varices, stomach irritation or ulceration, or duodenal bleeding and irritation.
- Blood studies reveal elevated levels of liver enzymes, total serum bilirubin, and indirect bilirubin; decreased levels of total serum albumin and protein; prolonged prothrombin time; decreased hemoglobin level, hematocrit, and serum electrolytes; and deficiency of vitamins A, C, and K.
- Urine studies show increased bilirubin and urobilinogen level.
- Fecal studies show decreased fecal urobilinogen level.

Treatment

- Vitamins and nutritional supplements
- Lactulose
- Beta-adrenergic blockers to treat portal hypertension
- Octreotide and other vasoconstrictors
- Endoscopic variceal ligation
- Surgical shunt placement
- Sclerosing agents
- Insertion of portosystemic shunts
- Liver transplantation
- Esophageal balloon tamponade

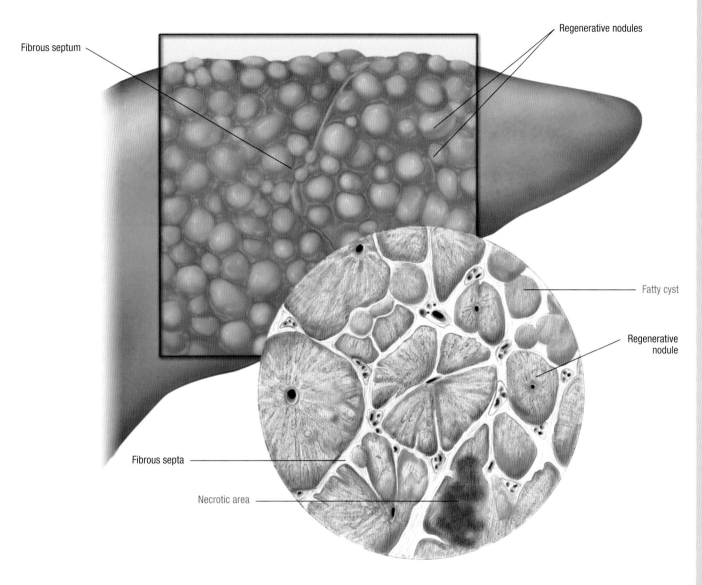

Fibrous septum

Regenerative nodules

Fatty cyst

Regenerative nodule

Fibrous septa

Necrotic area

COLONIC POLYPS

A polyp is a small tumorlike growth that projects from a mucous membrane surface. Types of polyps include common polypoid adenomas, villous adenomas, hereditary polyposis, focal polypoid hyperplasia, and juvenile polyps (hamartomas). Most rectal polyps are benign; however, villous and hereditary polyps tend to become malignant. Indeed, a striking feature of familial polyposis is its strong association with rectosigmoid adenocarcinoma.

AGE ALERT
Juvenile polyps, usually occurring among children under age 10, are characterized by rectal bleeding. Villous adenomas are most prevalent in men over age 55; common polypoid adenomas, in white women between ages 45 and 60. Incidence of non-juvenile polyps rises after age 70 in both sexes.

Causes

Unknown

Predisposing Factors

- Heredity
- Age
- Infection
- High-fat diet
- Sedentary lifestyle

Pathophysiology

Colonic polyps are masses of tissue resulting from unrestrained cell growth in the upper epithelium that rise above the mucosal membrane and protrude into the GI tract.

Polyps may be described by their appearance: pedunculated (attached by a stalk to the intestinal wall) or sessile (attached to the wall with a broad base and no stalk).

COMPLICATIONS
- Slow bleeding (can cause anemia)
- Bowel obstruction
- Gross rectal bleeding
- Intussusception
- Colorectal cancer

Signs and Symptoms

- Usually asymptomatic; discovered incidentally during a digital examination or rectosigmoidoscopy
- Rectal bleeding (high rectal polyps leave a streak of blood on the stool, whereas low rectal polyps bleed freely)
- Painful defecation
- Diarrhea

CLINICAL TIP
Although most are asymptomatic, polyps may cause symptoms by virtue of their protrusion into the bowel lumen. They may bleed, cause abdominal pain, or actually obstruct the intestine.

Diagnostic Test Results

- Barium enema identifies polyps high in the colon.
- Fecal occult blood test is positive.
- Blood studies reveal decreased hemoglobin level and hematocrit.
- Proctosigmoidoscopy or colonoscopy and rectal biopsy confirm the presence of the polyps.
- Serum analysis reveals electrolyte imbalances (villous adenomas).

Treatment

Common Polypoid Adenomas

- Less than 1 cm in size — polypectomy, commonly by fulguration during endoscopy
- Over 4 cm — abdominoperineal resection or low anterior resection

Invasive Villous Adenomas

- Abdominoperineal resection
- Low anterior resection

Focal Polypoid Hyperplasia

- Obliterated by biopsy

Hereditary Polyps

- Total abdominoperineal resection with permanent ileostomy
- Subtotal colectomy with ileoproctostomy
- Ileoanal anastomosis

Juvenile Polyps

- Often autoamputate
- Snare removal during colonoscopy

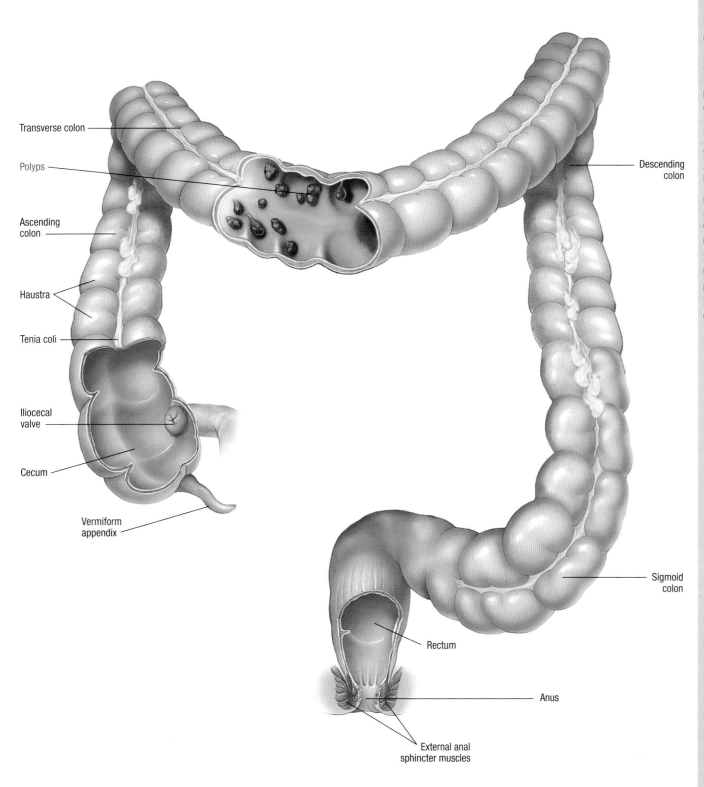

Transverse colon

Polyps

Ascending colon

Haustra

Tenia coli

Iliocecal valve

Cecum

Vermiform appendix

Descending colon

Sigmoid colon

Rectum

Anus

External anal sphincter muscles

COLORECTAL CANCER

Colorectal cancer is the second most common visceral malignant neoplasm in the United States and Europe. It tends to progress slowly and remains localized for a long time. Incidence is equally distributed between men and women. It's potentially curable in about 90% of patients if early diagnosis allows resection before nodal involvement.

Causes

Unknown

Risk Factors

- Low-fiber, high-fat, high-calorie diet
- Other diseases of the digestive tract
- History of ulcerative colitis (average interval before onset of cancer 11 to 17 years) and Crohn's disease
- Familial polyposis (cancer usually develops by age 50)
- Sedentary lifestyle and obesity
- Smoking
- Alcohol abuse
- Diabetes
- Growth hormone disorder
- Radiation therapy or history of colorectal cancer or polyps
- Family history of colorectal cancer

AGE ALERT
Age over 40 is a risk factor for colorectal cancer.

Pathophysiology

Most lesions of the large bowel are moderately differentiated adenocarcinomas. These tumors tend to grow slowly and remain asymptomatic for long periods. Tumors in the sigmoid and descending colon grow circumferentially and constrict the intestinal lumen. At diagnosis, tumors in the ascending colon are usually large and are palpable on physical examination.

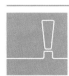

COMPLICATIONS
- Abdominal distention and intestinal obstruction
- Anemia
- Complications resulting from chemotherapy or radiation therapy

Signs and Symptoms

- Changes in bowel habits, such as bleeding, pain, anemia, and anorexia
- Symptoms of local obstruction
- Symptoms of direct extension to adjacent organs (bladder, prostate, ureters, vagina, sacrum)
- Symptoms from distant metastasis (usually liver)

Signs Specific to Site of Obstruction

- Right colon:
  - Black, tarry stools; anemia
  - Abdominal aching or pressure; dull cramps
  - Weakness, fatigue, and exertional dyspnea
  - Vomiting
- Left colon:
  - Rectal bleeding; dark or bright red blood or mucus in stools
  - Abdominal fullness or cramping
  - Rectal pressure
  - Constipation
  - Diarrhea
  - Ribbon- or pencil-shaped stools
  - Pain relieved by flatus or bowel movement

Diagnostic Test Results

- Digital rectal examination detects almost 15% of colorectal cancers; specifically, it detects suspicious rectal and perianal lesions.
- Fecal occult blood test possibly shows blood in stool.
- Barium enema studies can determine the location of lesions that aren't normally detected manually or visually.

CLINICAL TIP
Barium examination shouldn't precede colonoscopy or excretory urography because barium sulfate interferes with these tests.

- Computed tomography scan allows better visualization if a barium enema yields inconclusive results or if metastasis to the pelvic lymph nodes is suspected.
- Proctoscopy or sigmoidoscopy permits visualization of the lower GI tract, which can detect up to 66% of colorectal cancers. Colonoscopy permits visual inspection and photography of the colon up to the ileocecal valve and provides access for polypectomies and biopsies of suspected lesions.
- Carcinoembryonic antigen permits patient monitoring before and after treatment to detect metastasis or recurrence.
- Excretory urography verifies bilateral renal function and allows inspection for displacement of the kidneys, ureters, or bladder from a tumor pressing against these structures.

Treatment

- Surgery to remove tumor plus adjacent tissues and any lymph nodes that may contain cancer cells
- Chemotherapy for patients with metastasis, residual disease, or a recurrent inoperable tumor
- Radiation therapy for tumor mass reduction, done before or after surgery or combined with chemotherapy
- High-fiber diet

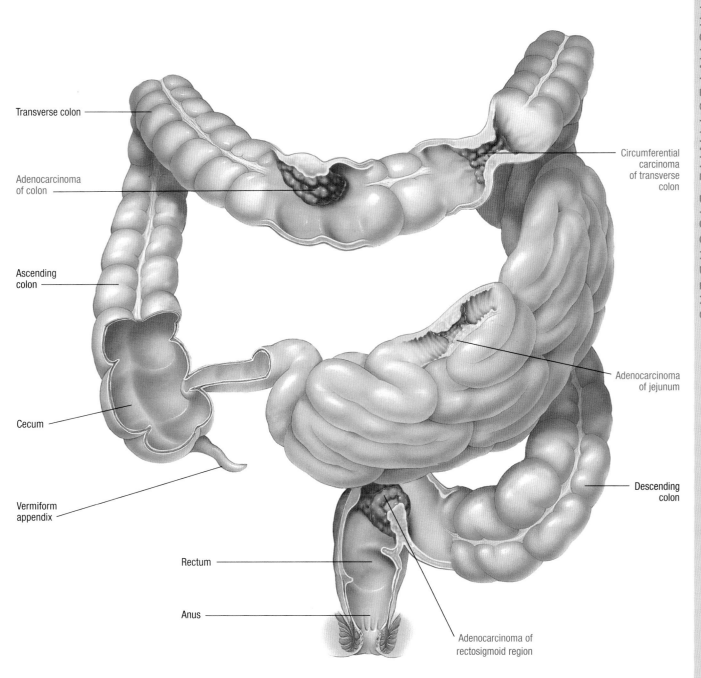

Transverse colon

Adenocarcinoma of colon

Ascending colon

Cecum

Vermiform appendix

Rectum

Anus

Circumferential carcinoma of transverse colon

Adenocarcinoma of jejunum

Descending colon

Adenocarcinoma of rectosigmoid region

CROHN'S DISEASE

Crohn's disease, also known as *regional enteritis* or *granulomatous colitis*, is inflammation of any part of the GI tract (usually the terminal ileum), extending through all layers of the intestinal wall. It may also involve regional lymph nodes and the mesentery.

AGE ALERT
Crohn's disease is most prevalent in adults ages 20 to 40.

Causes

Unknown

Possible Contributing Conditions

- Lymphatic obstruction
- Allergies and immune disorders
- Infection
- Genetic predisposition

Pathophysiology

Whatever the cause of Crohn's disease, inflammation spreads slowly and progressively. Enlarged lymph nodes block lymph flow in the submucosa. Lymphatic obstruction leads to edema, mucosal ulceration and fissures, abscesses, and sometimes granulomas. Mucosal ulcerations are called *skipping lesions* because they aren't continuous, as in ulcerative colitis.

Oval, elevated patches of closely packed lymph follicles — called Peyer's patches — develop in the lining of the small intestine. Subsequent fibrosis thickens the bowel wall and causes stenosis, or narrowing of the lumen. The serous membrane becomes inflamed (serositis), inflamed bowel loops adhere to other diseased or normal loops, and diseased bowel segments become interspersed with healthy ones. Finally, diseased parts of the bowel become thicker, narrower, and shorter.

COMPLICATIONS
- Anal fistula
- Perineal abscess
- Fistulas to the bladder, vagina, or skin
- Intestinal obstruction
- Nutritional deficiencies
- Peritonitis

Signs and Symptoms

- Steady, colicky pain in right lower quadrant
- Cramping, tenderness
- Weight loss
- Diarrhea, steatorrhea, bloody stools
- Low-grade fever
- Anal fistula
- Perineal abscess

Diagnostic Test Results

- Fecal occult blood test reveals minute amounts of blood in stools.
- Small-bowel X-ray shows irregular mucosa, ulceration, and stiffening.
- Barium enema reveals the string sign (segments of stricture separated by normal bowel) and possibly fissures and narrowing of the bowel.
- Sigmoidoscopy and colonoscopy reveal patchy areas of inflammation (helps to rule out ulcerative colitis), with cobblestonelike mucosal surface. With colon involvement, ulcers may be seen.
- Biopsy reveals granulomas in up to one-half of all specimens.
- Blood tests reveal increased white blood cell count and erythrocyte sedimentation rate and decreased potassium, calcium, magnesium, and hemoglobin levels.

Treatment

- Corticosteroids, immunosuppressants
- Aminosalicylates such as sulfasalazine
- Antidiarrheals (not in patients with significant bowel obstruction)
- Antibiotics, such as metronidazole and ampicillin
- Biologic therapies such as infliximab
- Stress reduction and reduced physical activity
- Vitamin supplements (iron supplements)
- Avoidance of fruits and vegetables; high-fiber, spicy, or fatty foods; dairy products; carbonated or caffeine-containing beverages; foods or liquids that stimulate intestinal activity
- Surgery, if necessary

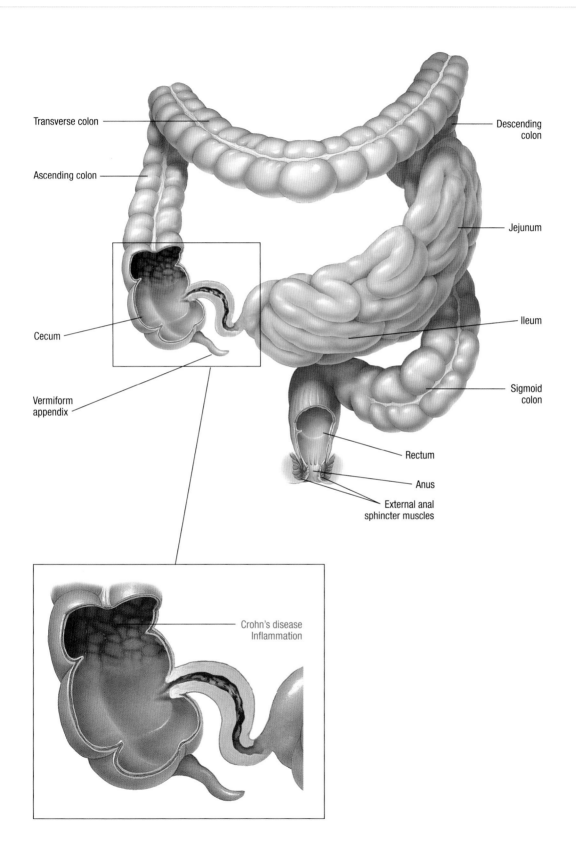

Transverse colon

Ascending colon

Cecum

Vermiform appendix

Descending colon

Jejunum

Ileum

Sigmoid colon

Rectum

Anus

External anal sphincter muscles

Crohn's disease Inflammation

DIVERTICULAR DISEASE

In diverticular disease, bulging pouches (diverticula) in the GI wall push the mucosal lining through the surrounding muscle. Although the most common site for diverticula is in the sigmoid colon, they may develop anywhere, from the proximal end of the pharynx to the anus. Common sites include the duodenum, near the pancreatic border or the ampulla of Vater, and the jejunum.

Diverticular disease of the stomach is rare and is usually a precursor of peptic or neoplastic disease. Diverticular disease of the ileum (Meckel's diverticulum) is the most common congenital anomaly of the GI tract.

Diverticular disease has two clinical forms:

- diverticulosis — diverticula present but asymptomatic
- diverticulitis — inflamed diverticula; may cause potentially fatal obstruction, infection, or hemorrhage.

AGE ALERT
Diverticular disease is most prevalent in men over age 40 and persons who eat a low-fiber diet. More than half of patients older than age 60 have colonic diverticula.

Causes

- Exact cause unknown
- Diminished colonic motility and increased intraluminal pressure
- Low-fiber diet
- Defects in colon wall strength

Pathophysiology

Diverticula probably result from high intraluminal pressure on an area of weakness in the GI wall where blood vessels enter. Diet may be a contributing factor, because insufficient fiber reduces fecal residue, narrows the bowel lumen, and leads to high intra-abdominal pressure during defecation.

In *diverticulitis*, undigested food and bacteria accumulate in the diverticular sac. This hard mass cuts off the blood supply to the thin walls of the sac, making them more susceptible to attack by colonic bacteria.

COMPLICATIONS
- Rectal hemorrhage
- Portal pyemia from artery or vein erosion
- Fistula
- Obstruction
- Perforation
- Abscess
- Peritonitis

Signs and Symptoms

Diverticulosis

- Asymptomatic

Mild Diverticulitis

- Moderate left lower abdominal pain
- Low-grade fever
- Leukocytosis
- Nausea and vomiting

Severe Diverticulitis

- Nausea and vomiting
- Left lower quadrant pain; abdominal rigidity
- High fever, chills, hypotension, and shock
- Microscopic to massive hemorrhage

Chronic Diverticulitis

- Constipation, ribbonlike stools, intermittent diarrhea, and abdominal distention
- Abdominal rigidity and pain, diminished or absent bowel sounds, nausea, and vomiting

Diagnostic Test Results

- Upper GI series reveals diverticulosis of the esophagus and upper bowel.
- Barium enema reveals filling of diverticula, which confirms diagnosis.
- Biopsy reveals evidence of benign disease, ruling out cancer.
- Blood studies show an elevated white blood cell count and elevated erythrocyte sedimentation rate in diverticulitis.

Treatment

- Liquid or bland diet, stool softeners, and occasional doses of mineral oil
- Analgesics, such as meperidine or morphine
- Antispasmodics
- Antibiotics
- Exercise
- Colon resection with removal of involved segment
- Temporary colostomy if necessary
- Blood transfusions if necessary
- High-residue diet after pain has subsided

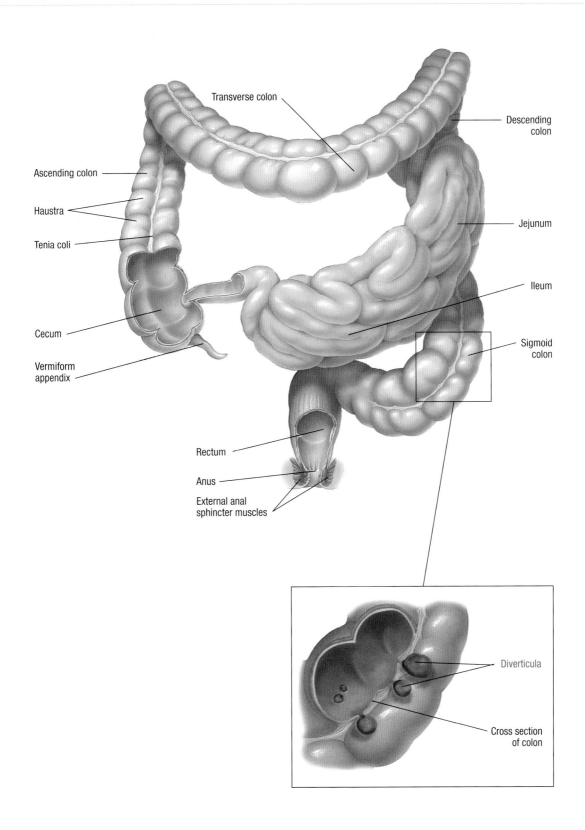

Transverse colon

Descending colon

Ascending colon

Haustra

Tenia coli

Jejunum

Cecum

Ileum

Vermiform appendix

Sigmoid colon

Rectum

Anus

External anal sphincter muscles

Diverticula

Cross section of colon

ESOPHAGEAL CANCER

Esophageal cancer is usually fatal. This disease occurs worldwide, but incidence varies geographically. It's most common in Japan, China, the Middle East, and parts of South Africa. Common sites of distant metastasis include the liver and lungs.

AGE ALERT
Esophageal cancer most commonly develops in men over age 60.

Causes

Unknown

Predisposing Factors

- Chronic irritation by heavy smoking and excessive use of alcohol
- Stasis-induced inflammation as in achalasia or stricture
- Nutritional deficiency
- Diets high in nitrosamines
- Previous head and neck tumors

Pathophysiology

Esophageal cancer includes two types of malignant tumors: squamous cell carcinoma and adenocarcinoma. Most esophageal cancers are poorly differentiated squamous cell carcinomas. Adenocarcinomas are less frequent and are contained to the lower third of the esophagus. Esophageal tumors are usually fungating and infiltrating, and they partially constrict the lumen of the esophagus.

Regional metastasis occurs early by way of submucosal lymphatics, often fatally invading adjacent vital primary organs.

COMPLICATIONS
- Inability to control secretions
- Obstruction of the esophagus
- Loss of lower esophageal sphincter control
- Aspiration pneumonia
- Mediastinitis
- Tracheoesophageal or bronchoesophageal fistula
- Aortic perforation

Signs and Symptoms

- Anorexia
- Vomiting
- Dehydration
- Regurgitation of food
- Dysphagia and weight loss (most common)
- Esophageal obstruction
- Pain
- Hoarseness and coughing
- Cachexia

Complications of Metastasis

- Tracheoesophageal fistulas
- Mediastinitis
- Aortic perforation
- Aspiration pneumonia
- Inability to control secretions

Diagnostic Test Results

- X-rays of the esophagus, with barium swallow and motility studies, delineate structural and filling defects and reduced peristalsis.
- Computed tomography shows size and location of esophageal lesions.
- Magnetic resonance imaging permits evaluation of the esophagus and adjacent structures.
- Esophagoscopy, punch and brush biopsies, and exfoliative cytologic tests confirm esophageal tumors.
- Bronchoscopy, usually performed after an esophagoscopy, reveals tumor growth in the tracheobronchial tree.
- Endoscopic ultrasonography of the esophagus combines endoscopy and ultrasound technology and reveals the depth of penetration of the tumor.

Treatment

- Usually multimodal
- Resection to maintain a passageway for food
- Palliative treatments
  - Feeding gastrostomy and chemotherapy
  - Insertion of a prosthetic tube and chemotherapy
  - Dilation of the esophagus
- Analgesics

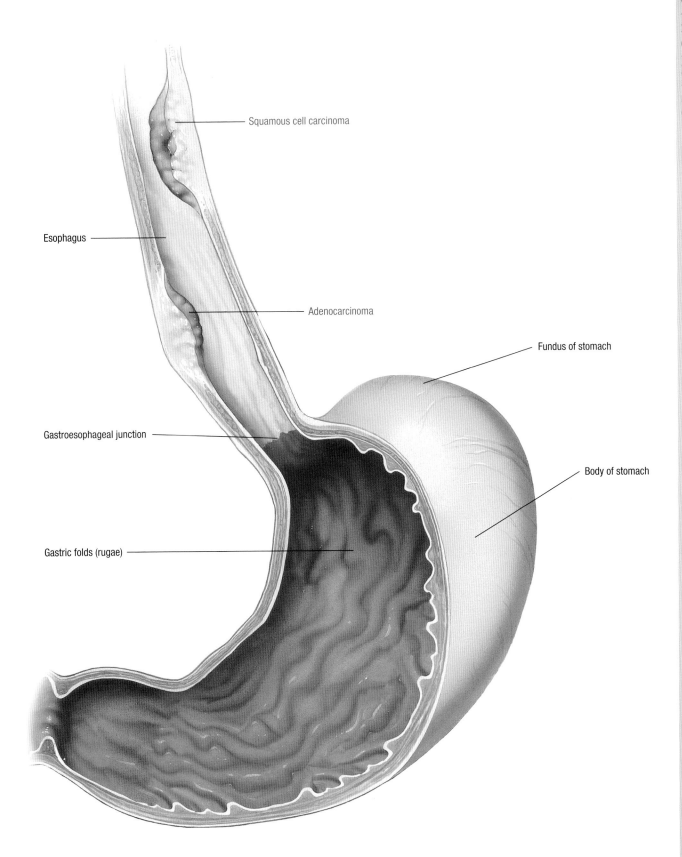

Squamous cell carcinoma

Esophagus

Adenocarcinoma

Fundus of stomach

Gastroesophageal junction

Body of stomach

Gastric folds (rugae)

GASTRIC CANCER

Gastric carcinoma is common throughout the world and affects all races; however, mortality is highest in Japan, Iceland, Chile, and Austria. In the United States, the incidence has decreased by 50% during the past 25 years and the resulting death rate is one-third of what it was 30 years ago.

AGE ALERT
Incidence of gastric cancer is highest in men over age 40.

Causes

Unknown; commonly associated with atrophic gastritis

Predisposing Factors

- Tobacco smoke
- Asbestos exposure
- High alcohol intake
- Intake of smoked, pickled, or salt-preserved foods, nitrates, and red meat
- Type A blood
- *Helicobacter pylori* infection (distal gastric cancer)
- Family history of gastric cancer
- Pernicious anemia

Pathophysiology

According to gross appearance, gastric carcinoma can be classified as polypoid, ulcerating, ulcerating and infiltrating, or diffuse. The parts of the stomach affected by gastric carcinoma, listed in order of decreasing frequency, are the pylorus and antrum, the lesser curvature, the cardia, the body of the stomach, and the greater curvature. Gastric carcinoma infiltrates rapidly to regional lymph nodes, omentum, liver, lungs, and bone.

COMPLICATIONS
- Malnutrition
- GI obstruction
- Iron deficiency anemia

Signs and Symptoms

Early Clues

- Chronic dyspepsia, epigastric discomfort

Later Clues

- Weight loss, anorexia
- Dysphagia, feeling of fullness after eating
- Anemia, fatigue
- Coffee-ground emesis
- Bloody stools

Diagnostic Test Results

- Barium X-rays of the GI tract with fluoroscopy show changes that suggest gastric cancer, including a tumor or filling defect in the outline of the stomach and loss of flexibility and distensibility, and abnormal gastric mucosa with or without ulceration.
- Gastroscopy with fiberoptic endoscope visualizes gastric mucosa including presence of gastric lesions for biopsy.
- Gastroscopic biopsy permits evaluation of gastric mucosal lesions.
- Gastric acid stimulation test discloses whether the stomach secretes acid properly.
- Complete blood count reveals anemia.
- Liver function studies possibly elevated with metastatic spread of tumor to liver.
- Radioimmunoassay reveals possibly elevated carcinoembryonic antigen.

Treatment

- Excision of lesion with appropriate margins (possible in more than one-third of patients) by subtotal or total gastrectomy or gastrojejunostomy
- Palliative surgery
- Radiation therapy with chemotherapy for patients with unresectable or partially resectable disease
- Antispasmodics, antacids for GI distress
- Antiemetics
- Opioid analgesics
- Proton pump inhibitors or histamine-2 blockers

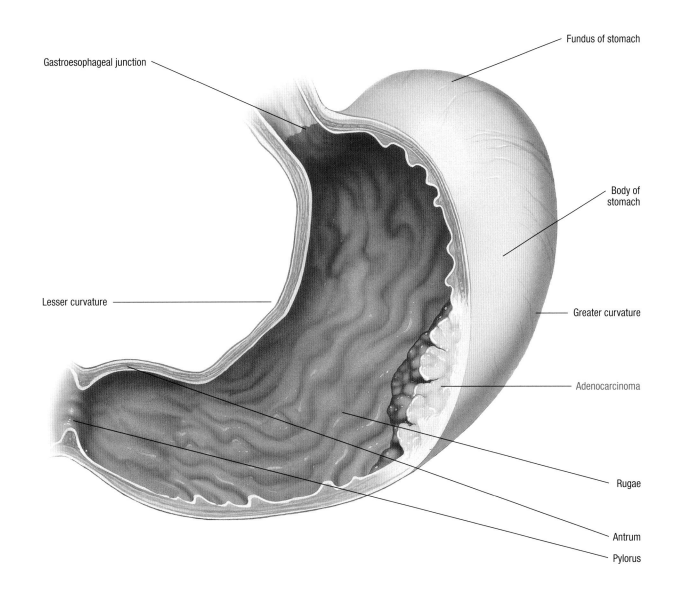

Fundus of stomach

Gastroesophageal junction

Body of stomach

Lesser curvature

Greater curvature

Adenocarcinoma

Rugae

Antrum

Pylorus

GASTRITIS

Gastritis, an inflammation of the gastric mucosa, may be acute or chronic. *Acute gastritis* produces mucosal reddening, edema, hemorrhage, and erosion; this benign, self-limiting disease is usually a response to local irritants. *Chronic gastritis* is common among elderly persons and those with pernicious anemia. It's characterized by progressive cell atrophy and commonly occurs as chronic atrophic gastritis (inflammation of all stomach mucosal layers and reduced numbers of chief and parietal cells). Acute or chronic gastritis can occur at any age.

Causes

Acute Gastritis

- Habitually ingested irritants, such as hot peppers, alcohol
- Drugs, such as aspirin, other nonsteroidal anti-inflammatory agents, cytotoxic agents, caffeine, corticosteroids, antimetabolites, phenylbutazone
- Poisons, such as DDT, ammonia, mercury, carbon tetrachloride, corrosive substances
- Bacterial endotoxins, such as staphylococci, *E. coli*, *Salmonella*
- Physiological stress, such as surgery, head trauma, renal failure, hepatic failure, or respiratory failure

Chronic Gastritis

- *H. pylori* infection
- Pernicious anemia
- Peptic ulcer disease
- Renal disease
- Diabetes mellitus

Pathophysiology

Gastritis is an inflammation of the lining of the stomach. In *acute gastritis*, the protective mucosal layer is altered. Acid secretion produces mucosal reddening, edema, and superficial surface erosion. *In chronic gastritis*, progressive thinning and degeneration of gastric mucosa occur. In either form, as mucus membranes become more eroded, gastric juices, containing pepsin and acid, come into contact with the erosion and an ulcer forms.

Pernicious anemia is often associated with atrophic gastritis, a chronic inflammation of the stomach resulting from degeneration of the gastric mucosa. In pernicious anemia, the stomach can no longer secrete intrinsic factor, which is needed for vitamin B_{12} absorption.

COMPLICATIONS
- Hemorrhage
- Shock
- Obstruction
- Perforation
- Peritonitis
- Gastric cancer

Signs and Symptoms

- Epigastric discomfort
- Indigestion, cramping
- Anorexia
- Nausea, hematemesis, vomiting
- Coffee-ground emesis or melena if GI bleeding present
- Grimacing
- Restlessness
- Pallor
- Tachycardia
- Hypotension
- Abdominal distention, tenderness, and guarding
- Normoactive to hyperactive bowel sounds

Diagnostic Test Results

- Occult blood tests reveal blood in vomitus or stools (or both) if the patient has gastric bleeding.
- Complete blood count shows decreased hemoglobin level and hematocrit.
- Urea breath test is positive for *H. pylori*.
- Upper GI endoscopy reveals gastritis when endoscopy is performed within 24 hours of bleeding.
- Biopsy reveals inflammatory process.

Treatment

- Elimination of the cause
- Bland diet
- Antacids, histamine antagonists, proton pump inhibitors
- Prostaglandins
- Vitamin B_{12}
- Antibiotics
- Blood replacement
- Iced saline lavage, possibly with norepinephrine
- Angiography with vasopressin
- Surgery — vagotomy, pyloroplasty, partial or total gastrectomy

CLINICAL TIP
Simply avoiding aspirin and spicy foods may relieve gastritis.

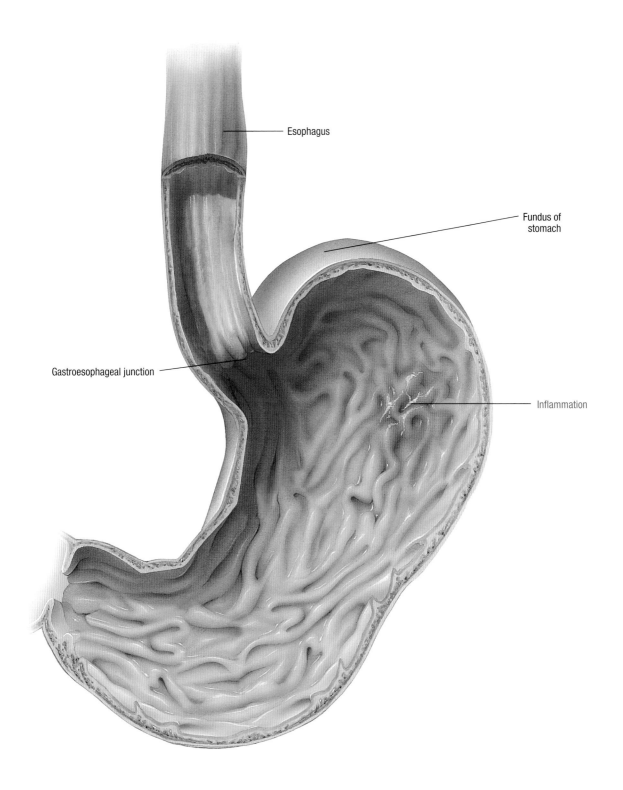

Esophagus

Fundus of stomach

Gastroesophageal junction

Inflammation

GASTROESOPHAGEAL REFLUX DISEASE

Popularly known as *heartburn*, gastroesophageal reflux disease (GERD) refers to backflow of gastric or duodenal contents or both into the esophagus and past the LES, without associated belching or vomiting. The reflux of gastric contents causes acute epigastric pain, usually after a meal. The pain may radiate to the chest or arms. It commonly occurs in pregnant or obese persons. Lying down after a meal may also contribute to reflux.

Causes

- Weak esophageal sphincter
- Increased abdominal pressure, as in obesity or pregnancy
- Hiatal hernia
- Medications, such as morphine, meperidine, diazepam, calcium channel blockers, anticholinergic agents
- Alcohol, cigarette smoke
- Nasogastric intubation for longer than 4 days
- Pyloric surgery

Pathophysiology

Normally, the LES maintains enough pressure around the lower end of the esophagus to close it and prevent reflux. Typically, the sphincter relaxes after each swallow to allow food into the stomach. In GERD, the sphincter doesn't remain closed (usually due to deficient LES pressure or pressure within the stomach exceeding LES pressure) and stomach contents flow into the esophagus. The high acidity of the stomach contents causes pain and irritation in the esophagus, and stricture or ulceration may occur.

COMPLICATIONS
- Reflux esophagitis
- Esophageal stricture
- Esophageal ulcer
- Replacement of normal squamous epithelium with columnar epithelium (Barrett's syndrome)
- Anemia
- Pulmonary complications and reflux aspiration

Signs and Symptoms

- Burning epigastric pain, possibly radiating to arms and chest, usually after a meal or when lying down

- Feeling of fluid accumulation in the throat without a sour or bitter taste
- Dyspepsia
- Chronic cough
- Laryngitis and morning hoarseness
- Wheezing
- Nausea and vomiting

Diagnostic Test Results

- Esophageal acidity test evaluates the competence of the LES and provides objective measure of reflux.
- Acid perfusion test confirms esophagitis and distinguishes it from cardiac disorders.
- Esophagoscopy allows visual examination of the lining of the esophagus to reveal the extent of the disease and confirm pathologic changes in mucosa.
- Barium swallow identifies hiatal hernia as the cause.
- Upper GI series detects hiatal hernia or motility problems.
- Esophageal manometry evaluates resting pressure of the LES and determines sphincter competence.

Treatment

- Frequent, small meals; avoidance of eating just before going to bed
- Sitting up during and after meals; sleeping with head of bed elevated
- Increased fluid intake
- Antacids, histamine-2 receptor antagonists
- Proton pump inhibitors
- Smoking cessation; reduction or cessation of alcohol intake
- Hiatal hernia repair
- Vagotomy or pyloroplasty

CLINICAL TIP
Advise patients with GERD to avoid foods that irritate the LES, such as caffeine, mint, and chocolate.

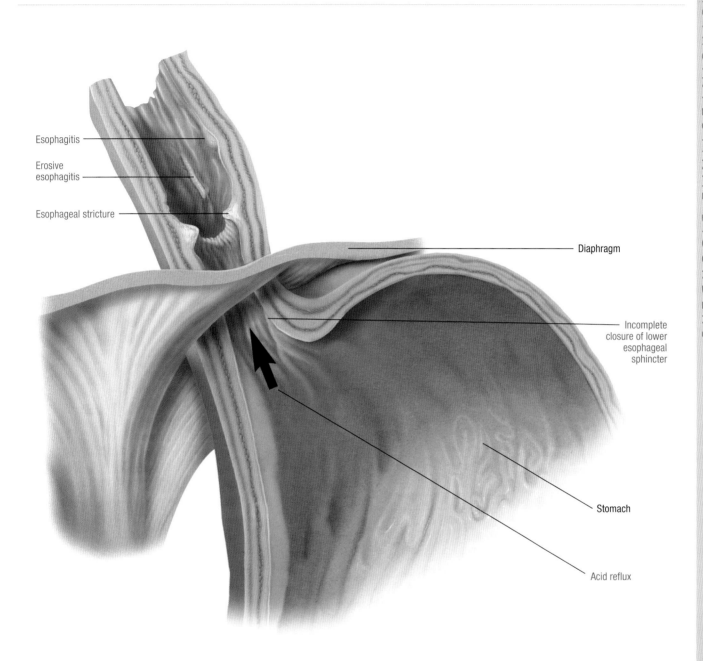

Esophagitis

Erosive esophagitis

Esophageal stricture

Diaphragm

Incomplete closure of lower esophageal sphincter

Stomach

Acid reflux

HEMORRHOIDS

Hemorrhoids are painful, swollen veins in the lower portion of the rectum or anus. They're very common, especially during pregnancy and after childbirth. They result from increased pressure in the veins of the anus, which causes the veins to bulge and expand, making them painful, especially while sitting.

AGE ALERT
Incidence of hemorrhoids is generally highest between ages 20 and 50.

Causes

- Straining at defecation, constipation, low-fiber diet
- Pregnancy
- Obesity
- Prolonged sitting

Predisposing Factors

- Hepatic disease, such as amebic abscesses or hepatitis
- Alcoholism
- Anorectal infections

Pathophysiology

Hemorrhoids are varicosities in the superior or inferior hemorrhoidal venous plexus. Dilation and enlargement of the plexus of superior hemorrhoidal veins above the dentate line cause internal hemorrhoids. Enlargement of the plexus of inferior hemorrhoidal veins below the dentate line causes external hemorrhoids, which may protrude from the rectum.

Hemorrhoids result from activities that increase intravenous pressure, causing distention and engorgement. Hemorrhoids are classified according to severity.

- *First-degree* — confined to the anal canal
- *Second-degree* — prolapse during straining but reduce spontaneously
- *Third-degree* — prolapse and require manual reduction after each bowel movement
- *Fourth-degree* — irreducible

COMPLICATIONS
- Local infection
- Bleeding
- Anemia

Signs and Symptoms

- Bright red blood on outside of the stool or on toilet tissue
- Painless, intermittent bleeding during defecation (internal hemorrhoids)
- Anal itching, vague anal discomfort
- Prolapse of rectal mucosa
- Pain
- Hard, tender lumps near anus

Diagnostic Test Results

- Physical examination confirms external hemorrhoids.
- Anoscopy shows internal hemorrhoids.
- Flexible sigmoidoscopy reveals internal hemorrhoids.
- Complete blood count shows decreased hemoglobin level and hematocrit.
- Fecal occult blood testing is positive for blood in stool.

Treatment

- High-fiber diet, increased fluid intake, bulking agents
- Avoidance of prolonged sitting on the toilet; avoidance of straining
- Local anesthetic agents, hydrocortisone cream, suppositories
- Warm sitz baths
- Injection sclerotherapy or rubber band ligation
- Hemorrhoidectomy

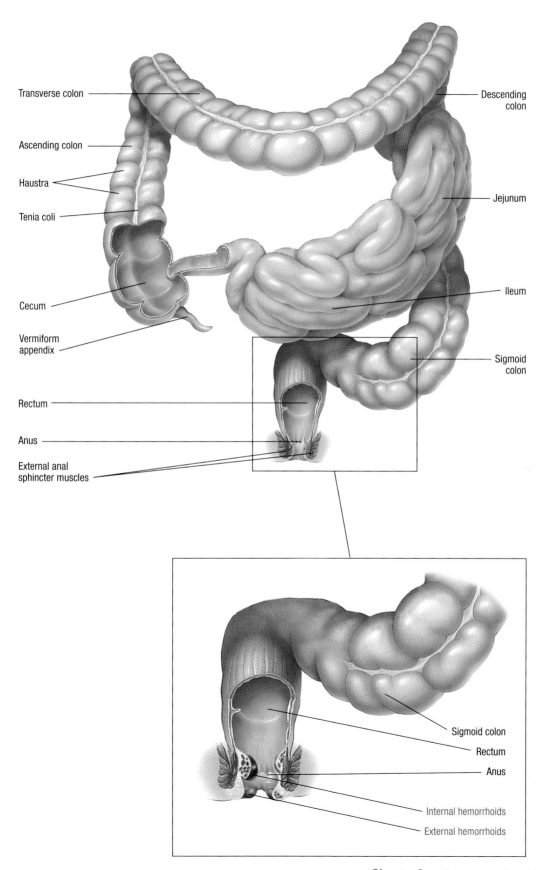

Transverse colon

Descending colon

Ascending colon

Haustra

Jejunum

Tenia coli

Cecum

Ileum

Vermiform appendix

Rectum

Sigmoid colon

Anus

External anal sphincter muscles

Sigmoid colon

Rectum

Anus

Internal hemorrhoids

External hemorrhoids

HEPATITIS

Nonviral hepatitis is an inflammation of the liver that usually results from exposure to certain chemicals or drugs. Most patients recover from this illness, although a few develop fulminating hepatitis, hepatic failure, or cirrhosis.

Viral hepatitis is a common infection, resulting in hepatic cell destruction, necrosis, and autolysis. In most patients, hepatic cells eventually regenerate with little or no residual damage. However, old age and serious underlying disorders make complications more likely. The prognosis is poor if edema and hepatic encephalopathy develop.

Causes

Nonviral

- Hepatotoxic chemicals, such as carbon tetrachloride, trichloroethylene, vinyl chloride
- Hepatotoxic drugs, such as acetaminophen
- Poisonous mushrooms
- Vinyl chloride

Viral

- Infection by hepatitis virus A, B, C, D, E, and G or transfusion transmissible virus

Pathophysiology

Nonviral

After exposure to a hepatotoxin, hepatic cellular necrosis, scarring, Kupffer cell hyperplasia, and infiltration by mononuclear phagocytes occur with varying severity. Alcohol, anoxia, and pre-existing liver disease exacerbate the effects of some toxins.

Drug-induced hepatitis may begin with a hypersensitivity reaction unique to the individual, unlike toxic hepatitis, which appears to affect all exposed people indiscriminately. Symptoms usually manifest after 2 to 5 weeks of therapy.

Viral

Hepatic damage is usually similar in all types of viral hepatitis, but extent of cell injury or necrosis varies.

The virus causes hepatocyte injury and death, either by directly killing the cells or by activating inflammatory and immune reactions. The inflammatory and immune reactions, in turn, injure or destroy hepatocytes by lysing the infected or neighboring cells. Later, direct antibody attack against the viral antigens causes further destruction of the infected cells. Edema and swelling of the interstitium lead to collapse of capillaries, decreased blood flow, tissue hypoxia, scarring, and fibrosis.

COMPLICATIONS
- Chronic persistent hepatitis
- Chronic active hepatitis
- Cirrhosis
- Hepatic failure and death
- Primary hepatocellular carcinoma

Signs and Symptoms

Nonviral

- Anorexia, nausea, vomiting
- Jaundice, dark urine, clay-colored stool
- Hepatomegaly
- Possible abdominal pain
- Pruritus

Viral, Prodromal Phase

- Easy fatigue, generalized malaise, anorexia, mild weight loss
- Arthralgia, myalgia
- Nausea, vomiting, changes in senses of taste and smell
- Fever
- Right upper quadrant tenderness
- Dark-colored urine, clay-colored stools

Viral, Icteric Phase

- Jaundice
- Worsening of prodromal symptoms
- Pruritus
- Abdominal pain or tenderness

Viral, Recovery Phase

- Symptoms subside and appetite returns.

Diagnostic Test Results

- Hepatitis profile study identifies antibodies specific to the causative virus, establishing the type of hepatitis.
- Blood chemistry reveals elevated serum aspartate aminotransferase and serum alanine aminotransferase levels in the prodromal stage.
- Serum alkaline phosphatase level is slightly increased.
- Serum bilirubin level may remain high into late disease, especially in severe cases.
- Prothrombin time is prolonged (greater than 3 seconds longer than normal indicates severe liver damage).
- White blood cell counts reveal transient neutropenia and lymphopenia followed by lymphocytosis.
- Liver biopsy identifies underlying disease.

Treatment

Nonviral

- Lavage, catharsis, or hyperventilation, depending on the route of exposure — as soon as possible after exposure
- Acetylcysteine as antidote for acetaminophen poisoning
- Corticosteroids

Viral

- Rest to minimize energy demands
- Avoidance of alcohol or other hepatotoxic drugs
- Small, high-calorie meals
- Parenteral nutrition if patient can't eat
- Standard immunoglobulin

- Antiemetics
- Alfa-2B interferon
- Cholestyramine
- Liver transplantation

CLINICAL TIP
Vaccination against hepatitis A and B provides immunity to these viruses before transmission occurs.

NONVIRAL AND VIRAL HEPATITIS

Nonviral hepatitis

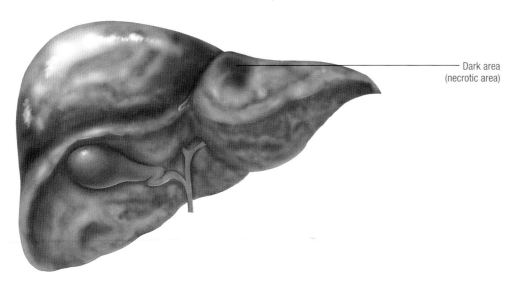

Dark area
(necrotic area)

Viral hepatitis

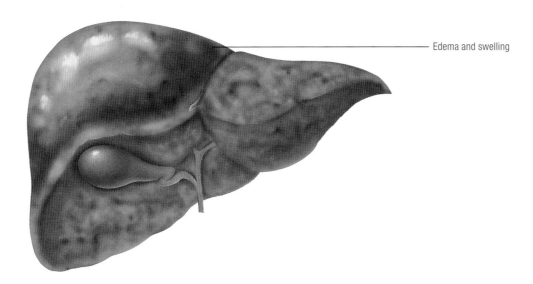

Edema and swelling

HIATAL HERNIA

Hiatal hernia is a defect in the diaphragm that permits a portion of the stomach to pass through the diaphragmatic opening into the chest. Hiatal hernia is the most common problem of the diaphragm affecting the alimentary canal. Treatment can prevent complications such as strangulation of the herniated intrathoracic portion of the stomach.

AGE ALERT
Hiatal hernias are common, especially in people over age 50.

Causes

- Esophageal carcinoma
- Kyphoscoliosis
- Trauma
- Congenital diaphragm malformations

Contributing Factors

- Aging, obesity, trauma

Pathophysiology

Hernias typically result when an organ protrudes through an abnormal opening in the muscle wall of the cavity that surrounds it. In hiatal hernias, a portion of the stomach protrudes through the diaphragm.

Three types of hiatal hernia can occur: sliding, paraesophageal (rolling), or mixed, which include features of both. In a sliding hernia, both the stomach and the gastroesophageal junction slip up into the chest, so the gastroesophageal junction is above the diaphragmatic hiatus. In paraesophageal hernia, a part of the greater curvature of the stomach rolls through the diaphragmatic defect.

COMPLICATIONS
- Gastroesophageal reflux
- Esophagitis and esophageal ulcers
- Hemorrhage
- Respiratory distress
- Aspiration pneumonia
- Esophageal stricture
- Esophageal incarceration
- Gastric ulcer
- Peritonitis

Signs and Symptoms

- Heartburn 1 to 4 hours after eating; aggravated by reclining, belching, or conditions that increase intra-abdominal pressure
- Regurgitation or vomiting
- Retrosternal or substernal chest pain (typically after meals or at bedtime)
- Feeling of fullness after eating
- Feeling of breathlessness or suffocation
- Chest pain resembling angina pectoris
- Dysphagia

Diagnostic Test Results

- Chest X-ray reveals an air shadow behind the heart in a large hernia; lower lobe infiltrates with aspiration.
- Barium swallow with fluoroscopy detects a hiatal hernia and diaphragmatic abnormalities.
- Endoscopy and biopsy results identify the mucosal junction and the edge of the diaphragm indenting the esophagus; differentiate hiatal hernia, varices, and other small gastroesophageal lesions; and rule out malignant tumors.
- Esophageal motility studies reveal esophageal motor or lower esophageal pressure abnormalities before surgical repair of the hernia.
- pH studies identify reflux of gastric contents.
- Acid perfusion (Bernstein) test identifies esophageal reflux.
- Blood chemistry reveals decreased serum hemoglobin level and hematocrit in patients with paraesophageal hernia, if bleeding from esophageal ulceration is present.
- Fecal occult blood test reveals presence of blood.
- Analysis of gastric contents possibly shows the presence of blood.

Treatment

- Restrict activities that raise intra-abdominal pressure (coughing, straining, bending)
- Pharmacologic agents: antiemetics, stool softeners, cough suppressants, antacids, and cholinergics
- Proton pump inhibitors
- Diet modifications: small, frequent, bland meals; not eating 2 hours prior to lying down; weight-loss programs
- Avoidance of foods that relax the lower esophageal sphincter, such as caffeine, mint, and chocolate
- Smoking cessation
- Surgical repair

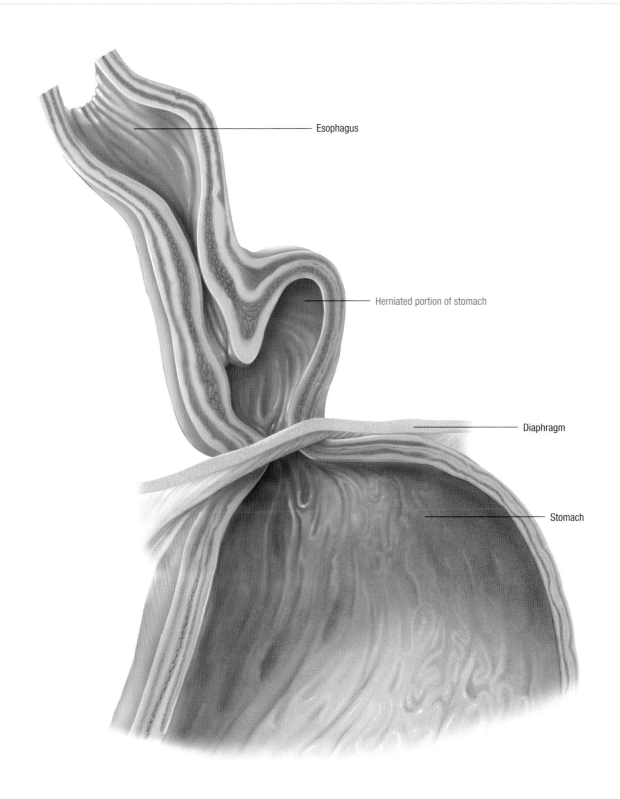

Esophagus

Herniated portion of stomach

Diaphragm

Stomach

HIRSCHSPRUNG'S DISEASE

Hirschsprung's disease, also called *congenital megacolon* or *congenital aganglionic megacolon,* is a congenital disorder of the large intestine, characterized by absence or marked reduction of parasympathetic ganglion cells in the colorectal wall. Hirschsprung's disease appears to be a familial, congenital defect, occurring in 1 in 5,000 to 1 in 8,000 live births. It's up to seven times more common in males than in females (although the aganglionic segment is usually shorter in males) and is most prevalent in whites. Total aganglionosis affects both sexes equally. Females with Hirschsprung's disease are at higher risk for having affected children. This disease usually coexists with other congenital anomalies, particularly trisomy 21 and anomalies of the urinary tract such as megaloureter.

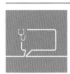

CLINICAL TIP

Without prompt treatment, an infant with colonic obstruction may die within 24 hours from enterocolitis that leads to severe diarrhea and hypovolemic shock. With prompt treatment, prognosis is good.

Causes

Familial congenital defect

Pathophysiology

In Hirschsprung's disease, parasympathetic ganglion cells in the colorectal wall are absent or markedly reduced in number. The aganglionic bowel segment contracts without the reciprocal relaxation needed to propel feces forward. Impaired intestinal motility causes severe, intractable constipation. Colonic obstruction can ensue, dilating the bowel and occluding surrounding blood and lymphatic vessels. The ensuing mucosal edema, ischemia, and infarction draw large amounts of fluid into the bowel, causing copious amounts of liquid stool. Continued infarction and destruction of the mucosa lead to infection and sepsis.

COMPLICATIONS
- Nutritional deficiencies
- Enterocolitis
- Hypovolemic shock

Signs and Symptoms

In Neonates

- Failure to pass meconium within 24 to 48 hours
- Bile-stained or fecal vomitus
- Constipation, overflow diarrhea
- Abdominal distention
- Dehydration, feeding difficulties, failure to thrive

In Children

- Intractable constipation
- Large protuberant abdomen, easily palpated fecal masses
- Wasted extremities (in severe cases)
- Loss of subcutaneous tissue (in severe cases)

In Adults (Rare)

- Abdominal distention
- Chronic intermittent constipation

Complications of Hirschsprung's disease include bowel perforation, electrolyte imbalances, nutritional deficiencies, enterocolitis, hypovolemic shock, and sepsis.

Diagnostic Test Results

- Rectal biopsy confirms diagnosis by showing the absence of ganglion cells.
- Barium enema, used in older infants, reveals a narrowed segment of distal colon with a saw-toothed appearance and a funnel-shaped segment above it. This confirms the diagnosis and assesses the extent of intestinal involvement.
- Rectal manometry detects failure of the internal anal sphincter to relax and contract.
- Upright plain abdominal X-rays show marked colonic distention.

Treatment

- Daily colonic lavage prior to surgery
- Temporary colostomy or ileostomy
- Corrective surgery
- Antibiotics
- Genetic counseling

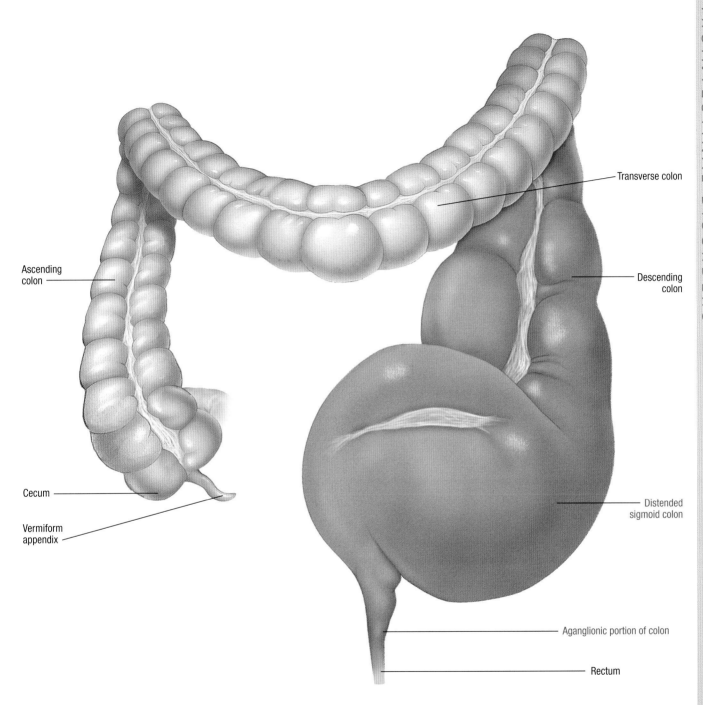

Ascending colon

Transverse colon

Descending colon

Cecum

Vermiform appendix

Distended sigmoid colon

Aganglionic portion of colon

Rectum

HYPERLIPIDEMIA

Hyperlipidemia, also called *hyperlipoproteinemia* or *lipid disorder*, occurs when excess cholesterol, triglycerides, and lipoproteins are present in the blood. The primary form includes at least five distinct and inherited metabolic disorders. Hyperlipidemia may also occur secondary to other conditions such as diabetes mellitus. It's an important risk factor in developing atherosclerosis and heart disease.

Causes

Primary Hyperlipoproteinemia

- Types I and III transmitted as autosomal recessive traits
- Types II, IV, and V transmitted as autosomal dominant traits

Secondary Hyperlipoproteinemia

- Diabetes mellitus
- Pancreatitis
- Hypothyroidism
- Renal disease
- Dietary fat intake greater than 40% of total calories; saturated fat intake greater than 10% of total calories; cholesterol intake greater than 300 mg/d
- Habitual excessive alcohol use
- Obesity

Pathophysiology

Lipids help in the production of energy, maintenance of body temperature, synthesis and repair of cell membranes, and production of steroid hormones. When lipid levels exceed what the body requires, the excess lipids form occlusive atherosclerotic plaques in blood vessels. These plaques obstruct normal blood flow, contribute to hypertension, and slow or decrease the transport of oxygen to the heart and other body organs.

COMPLICATIONS
- Coronary artery disease
- Pancreatitis
- Stroke
- Myocardial infarction
- Atherosclerosis

Signs and Symptoms

Type I

- Recurrent attacks of severe abdominal pain, usually preceded by fat intake
- Malaise and anorexia
- Papular or eruptive xanthomas over pressure points and extensor surfaces
- Ophthalmoscopic examination revealing lipemia retinalis (reddish white retinal vessels)
- Abdominal spasm, rigidity, or rebound tenderness

- Hepatosplenomegaly, with liver or spleen tenderness
- Fever may be present

Type II

- History of premature and accelerated coronary atherosclerosis
- Tendinous xanthomas on the Achilles' tendon and tendons of the hands and feet
- Tuberous xanthomas, xanthelasma
- Juvenile corneal arcus

AGE ALERT
Symptoms of hyperlipidemia typically develop in people ages 20 to 30.

Type III

- Tuberoeruptive xanthomas over elbows and knees
- Palmar xanthomas on the hands, particularly the fingertips

Type IV

- Obesity
- Xanthomas may be noted during exacerbations

Type V

- Abdominal pain associated with pancreatitis
- Complaints related to peripheral neuropathy
- Eruptive xanthomas on extensor surface of arms and legs
- Ophthalmoscopic examination revealing lipemia retinalis
- Hepatosplenomegaly

Diagnostic Test Results

- Serum lipid profiles show elevated levels of total cholesterol, triglycerides, very low–density lipoproteins, low-density lipoproteins, or high-density lipoproteins.

Treatment

- Weight reduction
- Smoking cessation
- Treatment of hypertension, diabetes mellitus, and other secondary conditions
- Avoidance of hormonal contraceptives containing estrogen
- Restriction of cholesterol and saturated animal fat intake
- Avoidance of alcohol
- Diet high in polyunsaturated fats
- Exercise and physical fitness program
- Statins, bile acid resins, cholesterol absorption inhibitors, fibrates, or nicotinic acid
- Surgical creation of an ileal bypass
- Portacaval shunt

Cholesterol transport in the blood
Lipoproteins act as "fat shuttles," transporting cholesterol through the bloodstream.

Liver cell (sectioned)
Cholesterol storage in the liver

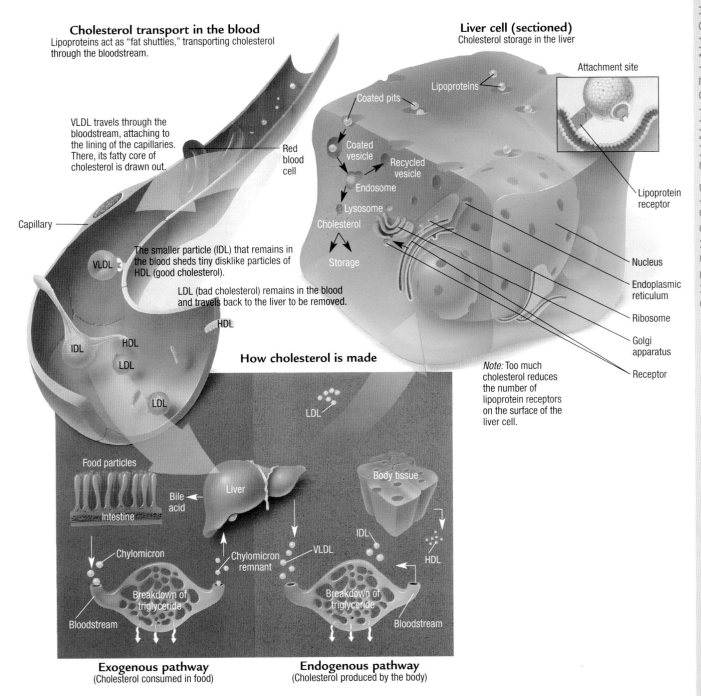

VLDL travels through the bloodstream, attaching to the lining of the capillaries. There, its fatty core of cholesterol is drawn out.

Red blood cell

Capillary

The smaller particle (IDL) that remains in the blood sheds tiny disklike particles of HDL (good cholesterol).

LDL (bad cholesterol) remains in the blood and travels back to the liver to be removed.

VLDL

IDL

HDL

HDL

LDL

LDL

Attachment site

Lipoproteins

Coated pits

Coated vesicle

Recycled vesicle

Endosome

Lysosome

Cholesterol

Storage

Lipoprotein receptor

Nucleus

Endoplasmic reticulum

Ribosome

Golgi apparatus

Receptor

Note: Too much cholesterol reduces the number of lipoprotein receptors on the surface of the liver cell.

How cholesterol is made

LDL

Food particles

Intestine

Chylomicron

Breakdown of triglyceride

Bloodstream

Bile acid

Liver

Chylomicron remnant

VLDL

IDL

Body tissue

HDL

Breakdown of triglyceride

Bloodstream

Exogenous pathway
(Cholesterol consumed in food)

Endogenous pathway
(Cholesterol produced by the body)

INGUINAL HERNIA

A hernia occurs when part of an internal organ protrudes through an abnormal opening in the wall of the cavity that surrounds it. Most hernias occur in the abdominal cavity. Although many kinds of abdominal hernias are possible, inguinal hernias (also called *ruptures*) are most common. Inguinal hernias may be direct or indirect. Indirect are more common; they may develop at any age, are three times more common in males, and are especially prevalent in infants.

Causes

- Weak fascial margin of internal inguinal ring
- Weak fascial floor of inguinal canal
- Weak abdominal muscles (caused by congenital malformation, trauma, or aging)
- Increased intra-abdominal pressure (due to heavy lifting, pregnancy, obesity, or straining)

Pathophysiology

In an inguinal hernia, the large or small intestine, omentum, or bladder protrudes into the inguinal canal. In an *indirect hernia*, abdominal viscera leave the abdomen through the inguinal ring and follow the spermatic cord (in males) or round ligament (in females); they emerge at the external ring and extend down into the inguinal canal, often into the scrotum or labia.

In a *direct inguinal hernia*, instead of entering the canal through the internal ring, the hernia passes through the posterior inguinal wall, protrudes directly through the transverse fascia of the canal (in an area known as Hesselbach's triangle), and comes out at the external ring.

In an infant, an inguinal hernia commonly coexists with an undescended testicle or hydrocele. In males, during the 7th month of gestation, the testicle normally descends into the scrotum, preceded by the peritoneal sac. If the sac closes improperly, it leaves an opening through which the intestine can slip.

Hernias can be reduced (if the hernia can be manipulated back into place with relative ease), incarcerated (if the hernia can't be reduced because adhesions have formed, obstructing the intestinal flow), or strangulated (part of the herniated intestine becomes twisted or edematous, seriously interfering with normal blood flow and peristalsis).

COMPLICATIONS
- Hernial strangulation
- Intestinal obstruction
- Necrosis

Signs and Symptoms

Reduced or Incarcerated Hernia

- Lump over the herniated area; present when the patient stands or strains; absent when the patient is in a supine position
- Sharp, steady groin pain when tension is applied to herniated contents; fades when the hernia is reduced

Strangulated Hernia

- Severe pain

Partial Bowel Obstruction

- Anorexia
- Vomiting
- Pain and tenderness in groin
- Irreducible mass
- Diminished bowel sounds

Complete Bowel Obstruction

- Shock
- High fever
- Absent bowel sounds
- Bloody stools

Diagnostic Test Results

- X-ray confirms suspected bowel obstruction.
- Complete blood count reveals elevated white blood cell count when bowel obstruction is present.

CLINICAL TIP
To detect a hernia in a male patient:

- ask the patient to stand with his ipsilateral leg slightly flexed and his weight resting on the other leg
- insert an index finger into the lower part of the scrotum and invaginate the scrotal skin so the finger can advance through the external inguinal ring to the internal ring
- tell the patient to cough. If you feel pressure against the fingertip, an indirect hernia exists; pressure felt against the side of the finger indicates that a direct hernia exists.

Treatment

Temporary Measures

- Reduction and a truss

In infants and Otherwise Healthy Adults

- Herniorrhaphy or hernioplasty

For Incarcerated or Necrotic Hernia

- Possibly bowel resection
- Antibiotics
- Parenteral fluids
- Electrolyte replacement
- Analgesics

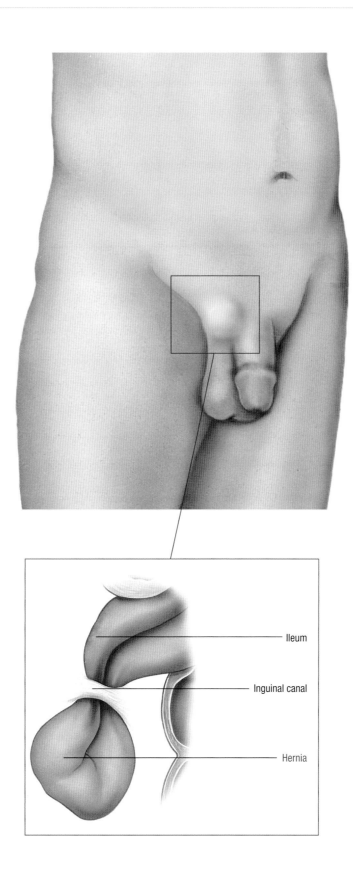

Ileum

Inguinal canal

Hernia

INTESTINAL OBSTRUCTION

Intestinal obstruction is the partial or complete blockage of the small- or large-bowel lumen. Small-bowel obstruction is far more common (90% of patients) and usually more serious. Complete obstruction in any part of the small or large bowel, if untreated, can cause death within hours due to shock and vascular collapse. Intestinal obstruction is most likely to occur after abdominal surgery or in persons with congenital bowel deformities.

Causes

- Adhesions and strangulated hernias usually causing small-bowel obstruction; large-bowel obstruction typically due to carcinoma
- Mechanical intestinal obstruction resulting from foreign bodies (fruit pits, gallstones, or worms) or compression of the bowel from intussusception, volvulus of the sigmoid or cecum, tumors, or atresia
- Nonmechanical obstruction resulting from physiologic disturbances, such as paralytic ileus, electrolyte imbalances, toxicity (uremia or generalized infection), neurogenic abnormalities (spinal cord lesions), and thrombosis or embolism of mesenteric vessels

Pathophysiology

Intestinal obstruction occurs in three forms:

- *Simple* — Blockage prevents intestinal contents from passing, with no other complications.
- *Strangulated* — *Blood* supply to part or all of the obstructed section is cut off, in addition to blockage of the lumen.
- *Close-looped* — *Both* ends of a bowel section are occluded, isolating it from the rest of the intestine.

The physiological effects are similar in all three forms of obstruction. When intestinal obstruction occurs, fluid, gas, and air collect near the obstruction. Peristalsis increases temporarily as the bowel tries to force the contents through the obstruction, injuring intestinal mucosa and causing distention at and above the site of the obstruction. Distention blocks the flow of venous blood and halts normal absorptive processes; as a result, the bowel wall becomes edematous and begins to secrete water, sodium, and potassium into fluid pooled in the ileum.

Obstruction in the small intestine results in metabolic alkalosis from dehydration and loss of gastric hydrochloric acid; lower bowel obstruction causes slower dehydration and loss of intestinal alkaline fluids, resulting in metabolic acidosis. Ultimately, intestinal obstruction may lead to ischemia, necrosis, and death.

AGE ALERT
Watch for air-fluid lock syndrome in older adults who remain recumbent for extended periods. In this syndrome, fluid collects in the dependent bowel loops. Then, peristalsis is too weak to push fluid "uphill." The resulting obstruction primarily occurs in the large bowel.

COMPLICATIONS
- Perforation
- Peritonitis
- Septicemia
- Secondary infection
- Metabolic acidosis or alkalosis
- Hypovolemia or septic shock

Signs and Symptoms

Partial Small-Bowel Obstruction

- Colicky pain
- Nausea
- Vomiting
- Constipation
- Abdominal distention
- Drowsiness
- Intense thirst
- Malaise
- Abdominal tenderness
- Borborygmi
- Rebound tenderness (strangulation with ischemia)

Complete Small-Bowel Obstruction

- Spasms every 3 to 5 minutes and lasting for about 1 hour
- Epigastric or periumbilical pain
- Passage of small amounts of mucus and blood from the site of the obstruction
- Vomitus (may first contain gastric juices, bile, and then finally bowel contents)

Large-Bowel Obstruction

- Constipation
- Colicky abdominal pain
- Continuous hypogastric pain
- Nausea
- Dramatic abdominal distention with visible bowel loops on the abdomen
- Fecal vomitus

Diagnostic Test Results

- X-ray confirms the diagnosis and reveals the presence and location of intestinal gas or fluid. Small-bowel obstruction shows a characteristic "stepladder" pattern.
- Barium enema reveals a distended, air-filled colon or a closed loop of sigmoid with extreme distention (in sigmoid volvulus) in large-bowel obstruction.
- Sodium, chloride, and potassium levels are decreased due to vomitus.
- White blood cell count is slightly elevated with necrosis, peritonitis, or strangulation.
- Serum amylase level is increased, possibly from irritation of the pancreas by a bowel loop.

Treatment

- Correction of fluid and electrolyte imbalances
- Decompression of the bowel to prevent vomiting
- Treatment of shock and peritonitis

- Passage of a nasogastric tube, followed by a weighted Miller-Abbott or Cantor tube for bowel decompression, especially in small-bowel obstruction
- Surgical resection with anastomosis, colostomy, or ileostomy in large-bowel obstruction
- Total parenteral nutrition

THREE CAUSES OF INTESTINAL OBSTRUCTION

Intussusception with invagination

The bowel is shortened by the involution of one segment of the bowel into another.

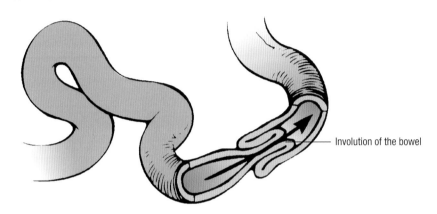

Involution of the bowel

Volvulus

In most cases, the bowel twists counterclockwise.

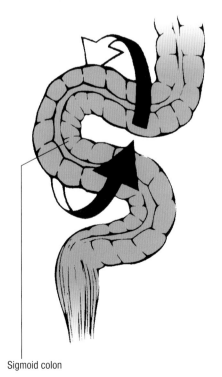

Sigmoid colon

Inguinal hernia

Intestine, omentum, and other abdominal contents pass through the hernia opening.

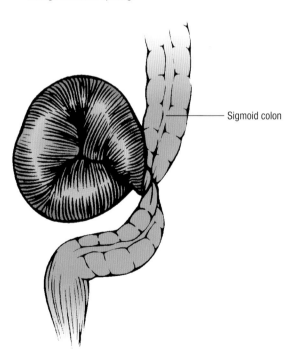

Sigmoid colon

IRRITABLE BOWEL SYNDROME

Also referred to as *spastic colon* or *spastic colitis*, irritable bowel syndrome (IBS) is marked by a group of GI symptoms often related to stress. About 20% of patients never seek medical attention for this benign condition that has no anatomical abnormality or inflammatory component. It's twice as common in women as in men.

AGE ALERT
IBS usually begins between ages 20 and 30.

Causes

- Psychological stress (most common)
- Ingested irritants (coffee, raw fruit, or vegetables)
- Lactose intolerance
- Abuse of laxatives
- Hormonal changes (menstruation)
- Allergy to certain foods or drugs

Pathophysiology

IBS appears to reflect motor disturbances of the entire colon in response to stimuli. Some muscles of the small bowel are particularly sensitive to motor abnormalities and distention; others are particularly sensitive to certain foods and drugs. The patient may be hypersensitive to the hormones gastrin and cholecystokinin. The pain of IBS seems to be caused by abnormally strong contractions of the intestinal smooth muscle as it reacts to distention, irritants, or stress.

COMPLICATIONS
- Diverticulitis
- Colon cancer
- Malnutrition

Signs and Symptoms

- Nausea and vomiting
- Crampy lower abdominal pain, occurring during the day and relieved by defecation or passage of flatus
- Pain that intensifies 1 to 2 hours after a meal
- Constipation alternating with diarrhea, with one dominant
- Passage of mucus through the rectum
- Abdominal distention and bloating

Diagnostic Test Results

- Barium enema reveals colon spasm and tubular appearance of descending colon without evidence of cancer and diverticulosis.
- Sigmoidoscopy or colonoscopy reveals spastic contractions without evidence of colon cancer or inflammatory bowel disease.

Treatment

- Stress management measures, including counseling or mild antianxiety agents
- Identification and avoidance of food irritants
- Application of heat to abdomen
- Bulking agents such as fiber supplements
- Antispasmodics
- Possibly, loperamide or alosetron
- Bowel training (if cause is chronic laxative abuse) to regain muscle control
- Antidepressant medications, such as selective serotonin reuptake inhibitors and tricyclic antidepressants

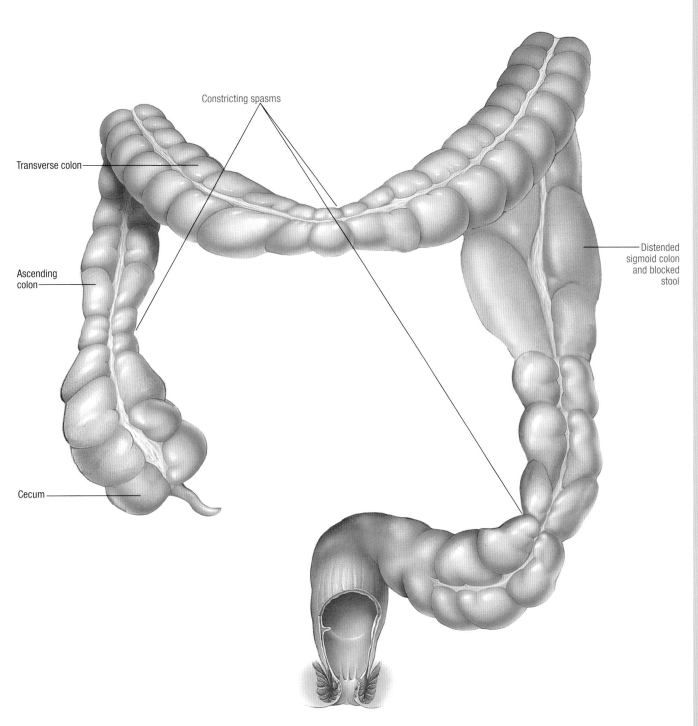

Constricting spasms

Transverse colon

Ascending colon

Cecum

Distended sigmoid colon and blocked stool

LIVER CANCER

Liver cancer, also known as *primary* or *metastatic hepatic car-cinoma*, is a rare form of cancer in the United States. It's rapidly fatal, usually within 6 months, from GI hemorrhage, progressive cachexia, liver failure, or metastasis.

AGE ALERT
Liver cancer is most prevalent in men (particularly over age 60), and incidence increases with age.

It's common for patients with hepatomas to also have cirrhosis. (Hepatomas are 40 times more likely to develop in a cirrhotic liver than in a normal one.) Whether cirrhosis is a premalignant state or alcohol and malnutrition predispose the liver to develop hepatomas is still unclear. Other risk factors are exposure to the hepatitis C or hepatitis B virus.

CLINICAL TIP
The liver is one of the most common sites of metastasis from other primary cancers, particularly those of the colon, rectum, stomach, pancreas, esophagus, lung, breast, or melanoma. In the United States, metastatic carcinoma is more than 20 times more common than primary carcinoma and, after cirrhosis, is the leading cause of death related to liver disease. Liver metastasis may appear as a solitary lesion, the first sign of recurrence after a remission.

Causes

- Immediate cause unknown
- Possibly congenital in children
- Environmental exposure to carcinogens
- Androgens
- Oral estrogens
- Cirrhosis

Pathophysiology

Most primary liver tumors (90%) originate in the parenchymal cells and are *hepatomas* (hepatocellular carcinoma, primary lower-cell carcinoma). Primary tumors that originate in the intrahepatic bile ducts are known as *cholangiomas* (cholangiocarcinoma, cholangiocellular carcinoma). Rarer tumors include a mixed-cell type, Kupffer cell sarcoma, and hepatoblastomas (which occur almost exclusively in children and are usually resectable and curable).

COMPLICATIONS
- GI hemorrhage
- Cachexia
- Liver failure

Signs and Symptoms

- Mass or enlargement in right upper quadrant
- Tender, nodular liver on palpation
- Severe epigastric or right upper quadrant pain
- Bruit, hum, or rubbing sound if tumor is large
- Weight loss, weakness, anorexia, fever
- Dependent edema
- Ascites
- Jaundice

Diagnostic Test Results

- Needle or open biopsy of the liver confirms cell type.
- Blood chemistry reveals elevated serum glutamic-oxaloacetic transaminase, serum glutamic-pyruvic transaminase, alkaline phosphatase, lactic dehydrogenase, and bilirubin, indicating abnormal liver function.
- Alpha-fetoprotein levels are elevated.
- Chest X-ray reveals possible metastasis.
- Liver scan shows filling defects.
- Serum electrolyte studies reveal hypernatremia and hypercalcemia; serum laboratory studies reveal hypoglycemia, leukocytosis, or hypocholesterolemia.

Treatment

- Resection if cancer is in early stage; few hepatic tumors are resectable.
- Liver transplantation for a small subset of patients
- Palliative measures
  - Radiation therapy, chemotherapy
  - Controlling signs and symptoms of encephalopathy
  - Caring for transhepatic catheters
  - Hospice

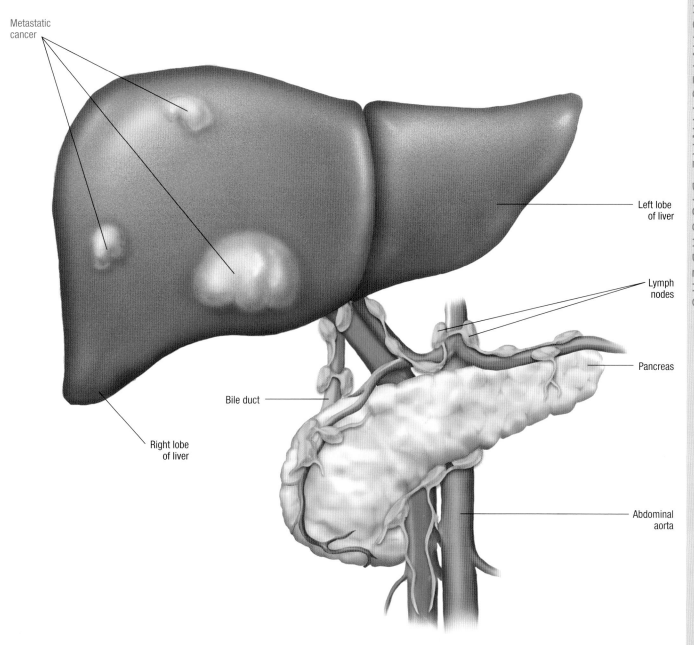

Metastatic
cancer

Left lobe
of liver

Lymph
nodes

Bile duct

Pancreas

Right lobe
of liver

Abdominal
aorta

LIVER FAILURE

Any liver disease can end in organ failure. The liver performs more than 100 separate functions in the body. When it fails, a complex syndrome involving the impairment of many different organs and body functions ensues. The only cure for liver failure is liver transplantation.

Causes

- Viral or nonviral hepatitis
- Cirrhosis
- Liver cancer

Pathophysiology

Manifestations of liver failure include hepatic encephalopathy and hepatorenal syndrome.

Hepatic encephalopathy, a set of central nervous system disorders, results when the liver can no longer detoxify the blood. Liver dysfunction and collateral vessels that shunt blood around the liver to the systemic circulation permit toxins absorbed from the GI tract to circulate freely to the brain. Ammonia, a by-product of protein metabolism, is one of the main toxins causing hepatic encephalopathy. The normal liver transforms ammonia to urea, which the kidneys excrete. When the liver fails, ammonia is delivered to the brain. Short-chain fatty acids, serotonin, tryptophan, and false neurotransmitters may also accumulate in the blood and contribute to hepatic encephalopathy.

Hepatorenal syndrome is renal failure concurrent with liver disease. The kidneys appear to be normal but abruptly cease functioning. Blood volume expands, hydrogen ions accumulate, and electrolyte disturbances ensue. It's most common in patients with alcoholic cirrhosis or fulminating hepatitis. The cause may be the accumulation of vasoactive substances that cause inappropriate constriction of renal arterioles, leading to decreased glomerular filtration and oliguria. The vasoconstriction may also be a compensatory response to portal hypertension and the pooling of blood in the splenic circulation.

COMPLICATIONS
- Coma
- Death

Signs and Symptoms

- Jaundice
- Abdominal pain or tenderness
- Nausea, anorexia, weight loss
- Fetor hepaticus
- Fatigue
- Pruritus
- Oliguria
- Splenomegaly
- Ascites, peripheral edema
- Varices of esophagus, rectum, abdominal wall
- Bleeding tendencies from thrombocytopenia (secondary to blood accumulation in the spleen), prolonged prothrombin time (from the impaired production of coagulation factors), petechiae
- Amenorrhea, gynecomastia

Complications of liver failure include variceal bleeding, GI hemorrhage, coma, and death.

Diagnostic Test Results

- Liver function tests reveal elevated levels of aspartate aminotransferase, alanine aminotransferase, alkaline phosphatase, and bilirubin.
- Blood studies reveal anemia, impaired red blood cell production, elevated bleeding and clotting times, low blood glucose levels, and increased serum ammonia levels.
- Urine analysis reveals increased urine osmolarity.

Treatment

- Liver transplantation
- Low-protein, high-carbohydrate diet
- Lactulose

For Ascites

- Salt restriction, potassium-sparing diuretics, potassium supplements
- Eliminating alcohol intake
- Paracentesis, shunt placement

For Portal Hypertension

- Shunt placement between the portal vein and another systemic vein

For Variceal Bleeding

- Vasoconstrictor drugs
- Balloon tamponade
- Surgery
- Vitamin K

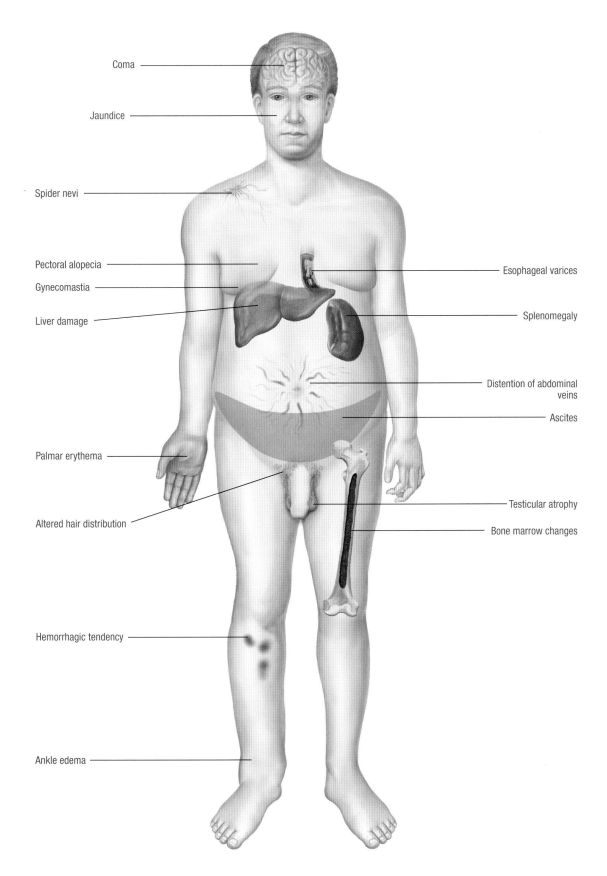

Coma

Jaundice

Spider nevi

Pectoral alopecia

Gynecomastia

Liver damage

Esophageal varices

Splenomegaly

Distention of abdominal veins

Ascites

Palmar erythema

Testicular atrophy

Altered hair distribution

Bone marrow changes

Hemorrhagic tendency

Ankle edema

ORAL CANCER

Oral cancer can occur anywhere in the mouth or throat but more than likely begins in the floor of the mouth. This includes the front two-thirds of the tongue, the upper and lower gums, the lining inside the cheeks and lips, the bottom of the mouth under the tongue, the bony top of the mouth, and the small area behind the wisdom teeth.

More than 34,000 Americans are diagnosed with oral or pharyngeal cancer each year. The death rate for oral cancer is higher than that of other cancers because it's hard to discover or diagnose. Commonly, it's only discovered when the cancer has metastasized to another location, most likely the lymph nodes of the neck. Men are affected twice as often as women, particularly men older than age 40.

Causes

- Tobacco use (smoking and smokeless)
- Alcohol use
- Poor dental and oral hygiene
- Chronic irritation from rough teeth or fillings and dentures
- Infection with human papillomavirus

Pathophysiology

Most oral cancers are caused by squamous cell carcinoma. Squamous cells normally form the lining of the mouth and throat. Squamous cell carcinoma begins as a collection of abnormal squamous cells.

Tobacco and other causative agents damage the lining of the oral cavity. The cells in this layer must grow more rapidly to repair the damage caused by tobacco and other causative agents. The more often cells need to divide, the more chances there are for them to make mistakes when copying their deoxyribonucleic acid (DNA), which may increase their chances of becoming cancerous.

Many of the chemicals found in tobacco can directly damage DNA. This direct damage to DNA can cause certain genes, such as those responsible for (starting or stopping cell growth), to malfunction. As the abnormal cells begin to build up, a tumor is formed.

COMPLICATIONS
- Disfigurement
- Metastasis

Signs and Symptoms

- Painless, usually small and pale-colored skin lesion, lump, or ulcer on the tongue, lip, or mouth area (but may be dark or discolored)
- Possible deep, hard-edged crack in the tissue
- Burning sensation or pain when the tumor is advanced
- Difficulty swallowing
- Abnormal taste

Diagnostic Test Results

- Tongue or gum biopsy confirms the presence of cancerous tissue.

Treatment

- Surgical excision of the tumor
- Radiation therapy
- Chemotherapy

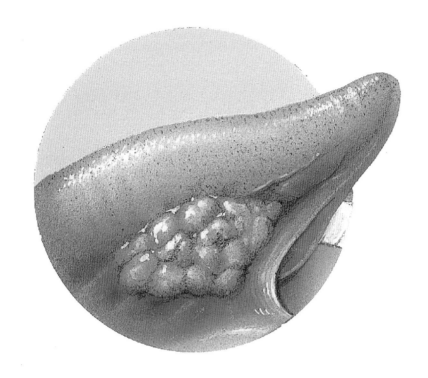

PANCREATIC CANCER

Pancreatic cancer is the fourth leading cause of cancer deaths in the United States. It occurs more frequently in blacks than whites. It occurs primarily in the head of the organ and progresses to death within 1 year of diagnosis. Rarer tumors are those of the body and tail of the pancreas and islet cell tumors.

AGE ALERT
The incidence of pancreatic cancer increases with age, peaking between ages 60 and 70.

Causes

- Inhalation or absorption of carcinogens, which are excreted by the pancreas
  - Cigarette smoke
  - Food additives
  - Industrial chemicals, such as beta-naphthalene, benzidine, and urea

Predisposing Factors

- Family or personal history of chronic pancreatitis (may be early manifestation of disease)
- Diabetes mellitus (may be early manifestation of disease)
- Chronic alcohol abuse
- Family history of pancreatic cancer
- Obesity
- Diet rich in fat and protein

Pathophysiology

Most pancreatic tumors are adenocarcinomas that arise in the head of the pancreas. The two main tissue types are cylinder cell and large, fatty, granular cell tumors. Cancers of the pancreas progress insidiously and most have metastasized before diagnosis. Cancer cells may invade the stomach, duodenum, major blood vessels, bile duct, colon, spleen, and kidney, as well as the lymph nodes.

COMPLICATIONS
- Malabsorption of nutrients
- Type 1 diabetes mellitus
- Liver and GI problems
- Mental status changes
- Metastasis

Signs and Symptoms

- Weight loss, anorexia, fatigue
- Pruritus, skin lesions (usually on the legs)
- Abdominal or low back pain
- Jaundice
- Diarrhea
- Fever
- Hyperglycemia, glucose intolerance
- Recurrent thrombophlebitis
- Clay-colored stools

Diagnostic Test Results

- Laparotomy with biopsy confirms cell type.
- Ultrasound identifies location of mass.
- Angiography reveals vascular supply of the tumor.
- Endoscopic retrograde cholangiopancreatography visualizes tumor area.
- Computed tomography scan and magnetic resonance imaging identify tumor location and size.
- Serum laboratory tests reveal increased serum bilirubin, serum amylase, and serum lipase.
- Prothrombin time is prolonged.
- Elevations of aspartate aminotransferase and alanine aminotransferase indicate necrosis of liver cells.
- Marked elevation of alkaline phosphatase indicates biliary obstruction.
- Plasma insulin immunoassay shows measurable serum insulin in the presence of islet cell tumors.
- Hemoglobin and hematocrit levels may show mild anemia.
- Fasting blood glucose reveals hypoglycemia or hyperglycemia.

Treatment

- Seldom successful because disease is usually metastatic at diagnosis
- Surgery including total pancreatectomy, cholecystojejunostomy, choledochoduodenostomy, choledochojejunostomy, pancreatoduodenectomy or Whipple's procedure, gastrojejunostomy
- Placement of a biliary stent
- Possibly, radiation therapy and chemotherapy
- Analgesics
- Antibiotics
- Anticholinergics
- Antacids
- Diuretics
- Insulin
- Pancreatic enzymes

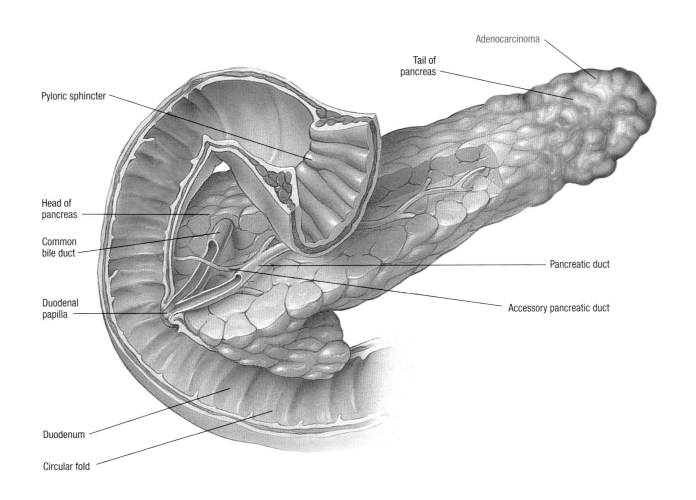

Pyloric sphincter

Head of
pancreas

Common
bile duct

Duodenal
papilla

Duodenum

Circular fold

Adenocarcinoma

Tail of
pancreas

Pancreatic duct

Accessory pancreatic duct

PANCREATITIS

Pancreatitis, inflammation of the pancreas, occurs in acute and chronic forms and may be due to edema, necrosis, or hemorrhage. In men, this disease is commonly associated with alcoholism, trauma, or peptic ulcer and carries a poor prognosis. In women, it's associated with biliary tract disease and has a good prognosis. Mortality in pancreatitis with necrosis and hemorrhage is as high as 60%.

Causes

- Biliary tract disease
- Alcoholism
- Abnormal organ structure
- Metabolic or endocrine disorders, such as high cholesterol levels or overactive thyroid
- Pancreatic cysts or tumors
- Penetrating peptic ulcers
- Blunt trauma, surgical trauma
- Drugs, such as glucocorticoids, sulfonamides, thiazides, hormonal contraceptives, nonsteroidal anti-inflammatory drugs
- Kidney failure or transplantation
- Endoscopic examination of bile ducts and pancreas
- Infection

Pathophysiology

Acute pancreatitis occurs in two forms: edematous (interstitial) and necrotizing. *Edematous* pancreatitis causes fluid accumulation and swelling. *Necrotizing* pancreatitis causes cell death and tissue damage. In both types, inappropriate activation of enzymes causes tissue damage.

Normally, the acini in the pancreas secrete enzymes in an inactive form. Two theories suggest why enzymes become prematurely activated:

- A toxic agent such as alcohol may alter the way the pancreas secretes enzymes. Alcohol probably increases pancreatic secretion, alters the metabolism of the acinar cells, and encourages duct obstruction by causing pancreatic secretory proteins to precipitate.
- *Autodigestion* may occur when duodenal contents containing activated enzymes reflux into the pancreatic duct, activating other enzymes and setting up a cycle of more pancreatic damage.

In chronic pancreatitis, persistent inflammation produces irreversible changes in the structure and function of the pancreas. It sometimes follows an episode of acute pancreatitis. Protein precipitates block the pancreatic duct and eventually harden or calcify. Structural changes lead to fibrosis and atrophy of the glands. Growths called pseudocysts contain pancreatic enzymes and tissue debris. An abscess results if pseudocysts become infected.

If pancreatitis damages the islets of Langerhans, diabetes mellitus may result. Sudden severe pancreatitis causes massive hemorrhage and total destruction of the pancreas, manifested as diabetic acidosis, shock, or coma.

COMPLICATIONS
- Diabetes mellitus
- Respiratory failure
- Pleural effusion
- GI bleeding
- Pancreatic abscess
- Pancreatic cancer

Signs and Symptoms

- Epigastric pain
- Mottled skin
- Hypotension
- Tachycardia
- Left pleural effusion
- Basilar crackles
- Abdominal distention
- Nausea and vomiting
- Cullen's sign
- Turner's sign
- Steatorrhea
- In a severe attack: persistent vomiting, abdominal distention, diminished bowel activity, crackles at lung bases, left pleural effusion

Diagnostic Test Results

- Serum amylase and lipase levels are elevated.
- Blood and urine glucose tests reveal transient glucose in urine and hyperglycemia. In chronic pancreatitis, serum glucose levels may be transiently elevated.
- White blood cell count is elevated.
- Serum bilirubin levels are elevated in both acute and chronic pancreatitis.
- Blood calcium levels may be decreased.
- Stool analysis shows elevated lipid and trypsin levels in chronic pancreatitis.
- Abdominal and chest X-rays detect pleural effusions and differentiate pancreatitis from diseases that cause similar symptoms; may detect pancreatic calculi.
- Computed tomography scan and ultrasonography show enlarged pancreas with cysts and pseudocysts.
- Endoscopic retrograde cholangiopancreatography identifies ductal system abnormalities, such as calcification or strictures, and helps differentiate pancreatitis from other disorders such as pancreatic cancer.

Treatment

- Nothing by mouth; I.V. fluids, protein, and electrolytes
- Blood transfusions
- Nasogastric suctioning
- Pain medication such as I.V. morphine
- Antacids, histamine antagonists
- Antibiotics
- Anticholinergics
- Insulin
- Surgical drainage
- Supplemental oxygen, mechanical ventilation
- Laparotomy if biliary tract obstruction causes acute pancreatitis

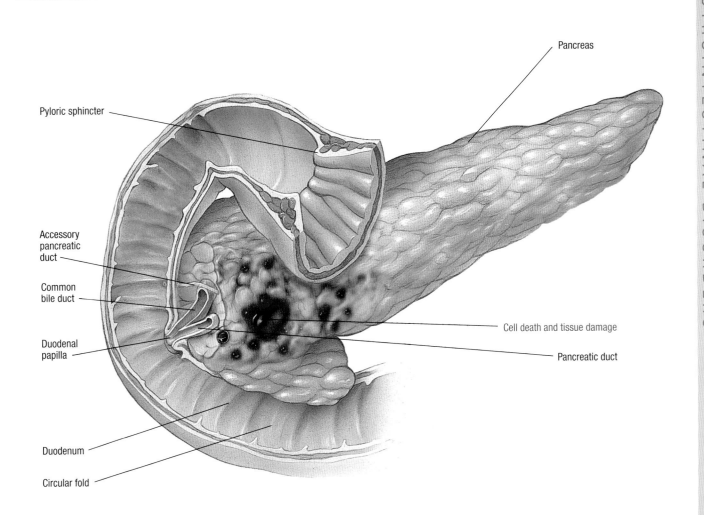

Pancreas

Pyloric sphincter

Accessory
pancreatic
duct

Common
bile duct

Duodenal
papilla

Cell death and tissue damage

Pancreatic duct

Duodenum

Circular fold

PERITONITIS

Peritonitis is an acute or chronic inflammation of the peritoneum, the membrane that lines the abdominal cavity and covers the visceral organs. Inflammation may extend throughout the peritoneum or be localized as an abscess. Peritonitis commonly decreases intestinal motility and causes intestinal distention with gas. With antibiotics, mortality is now 10%, and it's usually due to bowel obstruction.

Causes

- Chronic liver disease
- Renal failure
- Appendicitis, diverticulitis
- Chronic liver disease
- Renal failure
- Peptic ulcer, ulcerative colitis
- Volvulus, strangulated obstruction
- Abdominal neoplasm
- Penetrating trauma, such as a stab wound
- Rupture of a fallopian tube or the bladder
- Perforation of a gastric ulcer
- Released pancreatic enzymes

Pathophysiology

Although the GI tract normally contains bacteria, the peritoneum is sterile. When bacteria or chemical irritants invade the peritoneum due to inflammation and perforation of the GI tract, peritonitis is the result. Accumulated fluids containing protein and electrolytes make the transparent peritoneum opaque, red, inflamed, and edematous. Because the peritoneal cavity is so resistant to contamination, infection is commonly localized as an abscess.

COMPLICATIONS
- Abscess
- Septicemia
- Respiratory compromise
- Bowel obstruction
- Shock

Signs and Symptoms

- Sudden, severe, and diffuse abdominal pain that tends to intensify and localize in the area of the underlying disorder, such as right lower quadrant in appendicitis

- Acutely tender, distended, rigid abdomen; rebound tenderness
- Pallor, excessive sweating, cold skin
- Absent or diminished bowel sounds
- Nausea, vomiting, abdominal rigidity
- Signs and symptoms of dehydration (oliguria, thirst, dry swollen tongue, and pinched skin)
- Temperature of 103°F (39.4°C) or higher
- Shoulder pain
- Hypotension
- Tachycardia
- Cloudy peritoneal dialysis fluid

CLINICAL TIP
Abdominal distention and resulting upward displacement of the diaphragm may decrease respiratory capacity. Typically, the patient with peritonitis tends to breathe shallowly and move as little as possible to minimize pain. He may lie on his back, with knees flexed, to relax abdominal muscles.

Diagnostic Test Results

- Abdominal X-ray shows edematous and gaseous distention of the small and large bowel or in the case of visceral organ perforation, air lying under the diaphragm.
- Chest X-ray shows elevation of the diaphragm.
- Blood studies show leukocytosis.
- Paracentesis reveals bacteria, exudate, blood, pus, or urine.
- Laparotomy identifies the underlying cause.

Treatment

Emergency Treatment

- Nothing by mouth — to slow peristalsis and prevent perforation
- Nasogastric intubation
- Antibiotics, based on infecting organism
- Analgesics
- Parenteral fluids and electrolytes

When peritonitis results from perforation, surgery should be performed as soon as possible to eliminate the source of infection by evacuating the spilled contents and inserting drains.

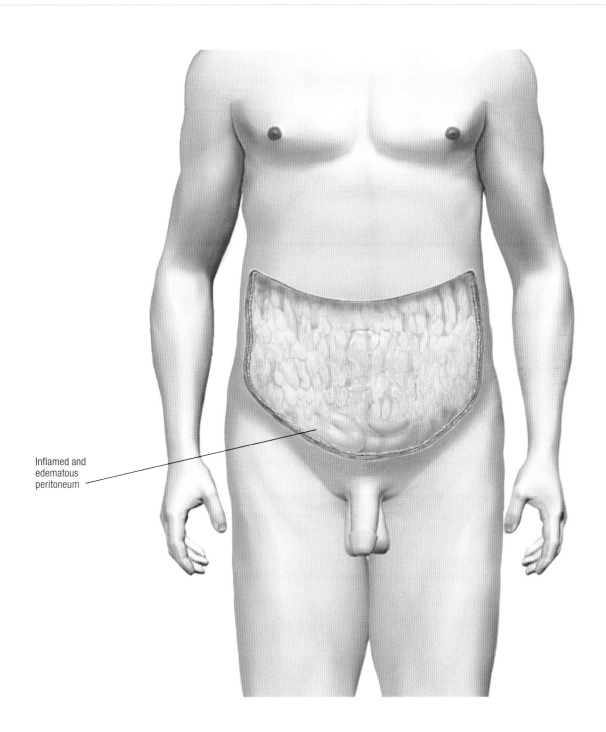

Inflamed and
edematous
peritoneum

PYLORIC STENOSIS

Pyloric stenosis is a narrowing of the pylorus — the outlet from the stomach to the small intestine. The incidence of pyloric stenosis is approximately 2 to 3 of every 1,000 infants. It occurs more frequently in whites.

AGE ALERT
Pyloric stenosis primarily occurs in infants. It occurs more commonly in boys than in girls and is rare in patients older than age 6 months.

Causes

Unknown, possibly related to genetic factors

Pathophysiology

Pyloric stenosis is caused by hypertrophy and hyperplasia of the circular and longitudinal muscles of the pylorus. When the sphincter muscles thicken, they become inelastic and this leads to a narrowing of the opening. The pyloric canal becomes lengthened and the whole pylorus becomes thickened. The mucosa usually is edematous and thickened. The extra peristaltic effort needed to empty stomach contents into the small intestine leads to hypertrophied muscle layers of the stomach.

COMPLICATIONS
- Dehydration
- Electrolyte imbalance
- Jaundice

Signs and Symptoms

- Vomiting, mild initially and then becoming projectile
- In infants: appearing hungry most of the time
- Diarrhea
- Dehydration (poor skin turgor, depressed fontanels, dry mucous membranes, decreased tearing)
- Failure to gain weight or weight loss
- Dyspepsia
- Abdominal pain
- Abdominal distention
- Visible gastric peristalsis
- Firm, nontender, and mobile 1 to 2 cm hard mass, known as an *olive*, present in the midepigastrium to the right of midline; best palpated after the infant has vomited and when calm
- Diminished stools
- Lethargy

Diagnostic Test Results

- Barium X-ray reveals a distended stomach and narrowed and elongated pylorus.
- Ultrasound shows thickened muscles of the pylorus.
- Chemistry panel often reveals hypochloremia, hypokalemia, and metabolic alkalosis. Hypernatremia or hyponatremia may also be present.

Treatment

- I.V. fluids
- Correction of electrolyte abnormalities
- Surgery
- Nothing by mouth before surgery; small frequent feedings after surgery

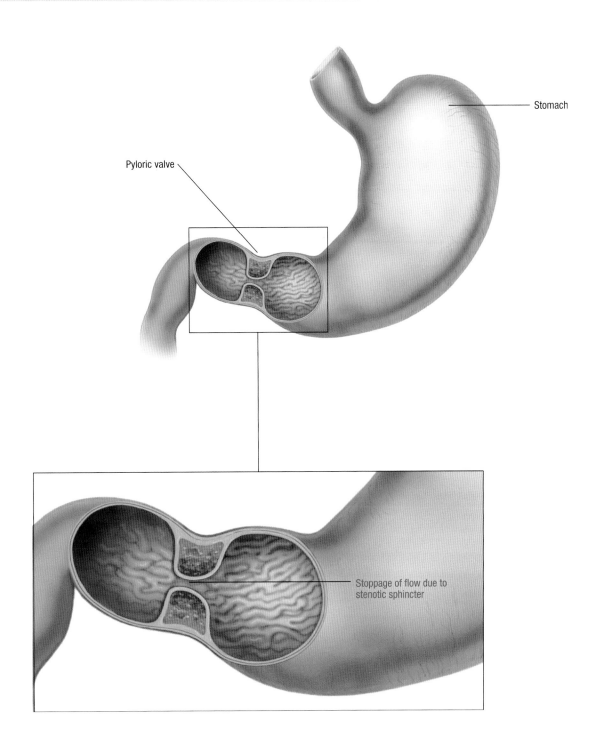

Stomach

Pyloric valve

Stoppage of flow due to stenotic sphincter

ULCERATIVE COLITIS

Ulcerative colitis is a continuous inflammatory disease that affects the mucosa of the colon and rectum. It invariably begins in the rectum and sigmoid colon and commonly extends upward into the entire colon, rarely affecting the small intestine, except for the terminal ileum. Ulcerative colitis produces edema (leading to mucosal friability) and ulcerations. Severity ranges from a mild, localized disorder to a fulminant disease that may cause a perforated colon, progressing to potentially fatal peritonitis and toxemia. The disease cycles between exacerbation and remission.

AGE ALERT
Ulcerative colitis occurs primarily in young adults, especially women. Onset of symptoms seems to peak between ages 15 and 30 and between ages 55 and 65.

Causes

- Unknown
- May be related to abnormal immune response to food or bacteria such as *E. coli*
- Heredity

Pathophysiology

Ulcerative colitis usually begins as inflammation in the base of the mucosal layer of the large intestine. The colon's mucosal surface becomes dark, red, and velvety. Inflammation leads to erosions that coalesce and form ulcers. The mucosa becomes diffusely ulcerated, with hemorrhage, congestion, edema, and exudative inflammation. Abscesses in the mucosa drain purulent pus, become necrotic, and ulcerate. Sloughing causes bloody, mucus-filled stools. As abscesses heal, scarring and thickening may appear in the bowel's inner muscle layer. As granulation tissue replaces the muscle layer, the colon narrows, shortens, and loses its characteristic pouches (hiatal folds).

COMPLICATIONS
- Nutritional deficiencies
- Anal fistula, abscess, and fissure
- Perforated colon
- Colon cancer
- Hemorrhage and toxic megacolon
- Liver disease
- Arthritis
- Coagulation defects
- Erythema nodosum of the face and arms
- Uveitis
- Pericholangitis, sclerosing cholangitis
- Cirrhosis
- Cholangiocarcinoma
- Ankylosing spondylitis
- Loss of muscle mass

Signs and Symptoms

- Weight loss
- Foul-smelling stools
- Recurrent bloody diarrhea, often containing pus and mucus (hallmark sign)
- Abdominal cramping, fecal urgency
- Weakness

Diagnostic Test Results

- Sigmoidoscopy confirms rectal involvement, specifically mucosal friability and flattening and thick, inflammatory exudate.
- Colonoscopy reveals extent of the disease, stricture areas, and pseudopolyps (not performed when the patient has active signs and symptoms).
- Biopsy with colonoscopy shows areas of inflammation.
- Barium enema reveals extent of the disease, detects complications, and identifies cancer (not performed when the patient has active signs and symptoms).
- Stool specimen analysis reveals blood, pus, and mucus but no disease-causing organisms.
- Serum potassium, magnesium, and albumin levels are decreased.
- White blood cell count is decreased.
- Hemoglobin level is decreased.
- Prothrombin time is prolonged.
- Elevated erythrocyte sedimentation rate correlates with severity of the attack.
- Abdominal X-ray may reveal loss of haustration, mucosal edema, and absence of formed stool in the diseased bowel.

Treatment

- Corticotropin and adrenal corticosteroids
- Sulfasalazine
- Antidiarrheals
- Iron supplements
- Liquid nutritional supplements

For Severe Disease

- Total parenteral nutrition and nothing by mouth
- I.V. fluids
- Proctocolectomy with ileostomy

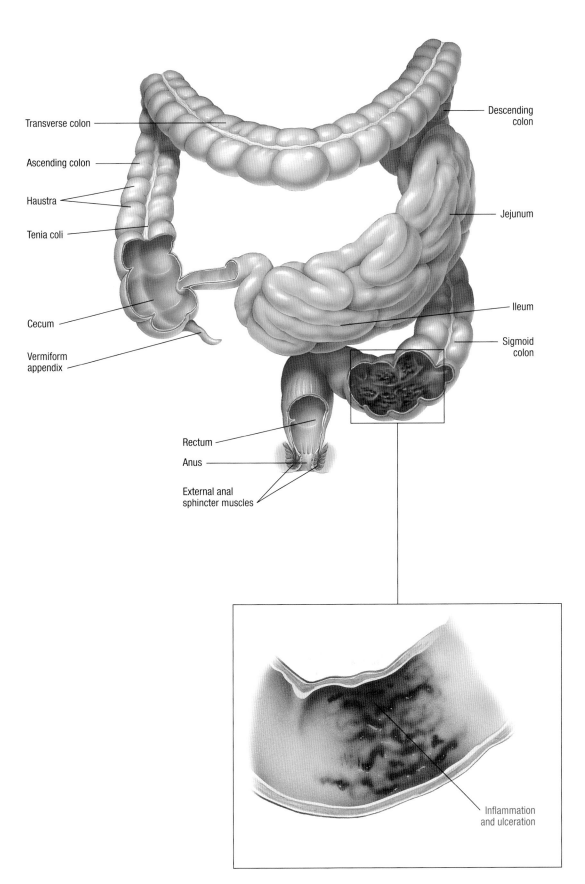

Transverse colon

Ascending colon

Haustra

Tenia coli

Cecum

Vermiform
appendix

Descending
colon

Jejunum

Ileum

Sigmoid
colon

Rectum

Anus

External anal
sphincter muscles

Inflammation
and ulceration

ULCERS

Ulcers, circumscribed lesions in the mucosal membrane extending below the epithelium, can develop in the lower esophagus, stomach, pylorus, duodenum, or jejunum. Although erosions are often referred to as ulcers, erosions are breaks in the mucosal membranes that don't extend below the epithelium. Ulcers may be acute or chronic in nature. Acute ulcers are usually multiple and superficial. Chronic ulcers are identified by scar tissue at their base.

AGE ALERT
Gastric ulcers are most common in middle-age and elderly men, especially in chronic users of nonsteroidal anti-inflammatory drugs (NSAIDs), alcohol, or tobacco.

Causes

- *H. pylori* infection
- NSAIDs
- Inadequate protection of mucous membrane
- Pathologic hypersecretory disorders

Predisposing Factors

- Blood type (gastric ulcers and type A; duodenal ulcers and type O)
- Other genetic factors
- Exposure to irritants, such as alcohol, coffee, tobacco
- Emotional stress
- Physical trauma and normal aging

Pathophysiology

Ulceration stems from inhibition of prostaglandin synthesis, increased gastric acid and pepsin secretion, reduced gastric mucosal blood flow, or decreased cytoprotective mucus production.

Although the stomach contains acidic secretions that can digest substances, intrinsic defenses protect the gastric mucosal membrane from injury. A thick, tenacious layer of gastric mucus protects the stomach from autodigestion, mechanical trauma, and chemical trauma. Prostaglandins provide another line of defense. Gastric ulcers may be a result of destruction of the mucosal barrier.

The duodenum is protected from ulceration by the function of Brunner's glands. These glands produce a viscid, mucoid, alkaline secretion that neutralizes the acid chyme. Duodenal ulcers appear to result from excessive acid production in the duodenum.

H. pylori release a toxin that destroys the gastric and duodenal mucosa, reducing the epithelium's resistance to acid digestion and causing gastritis and ulcer disease.

COMPLICATIONS
- GI hemorrhage
- Hypovolemic shock
- Perforation
- Penetration to attached structures

Signs and Symptoms

Gastric Ulcer

- Recent weight loss or loss of appetite
- Pain that worsens with eating
- Nausea and anorexia
- Pallor
- Epigastric tenderness
- Hyperactive bowel sounds

Duodenal Ulcer

- Epigastric pain that's gnawing, sharp and burning, or dull; similar to hunger
- Pain relieved by food or antacids, but usually recurring 2 to 4 hours after ingestion
- Weight gain
- Pallor
- Epigastric tenderness
- Hyperactive bowel sounds

CLINICAL TIP
Complications may occur and include hemorrhage, shock, gastric perforation, and gastric outlet obstruction.

Diagnostic Test Results

- Barium swallow or upper GI and small-bowel series reveal the presence of the ulcer.
- Esophagogastroduodenoscopy confirms the presence of an ulcer and permits cytologic studies and biopsy to rule out *H. pylori* or cancer.
- Upper GI tract X-rays reveal mucosal abnormalities.
- Stool analysis detects occult blood.
- White blood cell count is elevated.
- Gastric secretory studies show hyperchlorhydria.
- Urea breath test results reflect activity of *H. pylori*.

Treatment

- Physical and emotional rest
- For *H. pylori* infection: tetracycline, metronidazole, or clarithromycin; ranitidine, bismuth citrate, bismuth salicylate, or a proton pump inhibitor
- Misoprostol (a prostaglandin analog)
- Antacids
- Avoidance of caffeine, tobacco, and alcohol
- Anticholinergic drugs
- Histamine-2 antagonists
- Sucralfate
- Prostaglandin analogs
- Dietary therapy: small frequent meals and avoidance of eating before bedtime

Erosion — Penetration of only the superficial layer

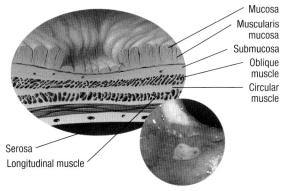

Mucosa
Muscularis mucosa
Submucosa
Oblique muscle
Circular muscle
Serosa
Longitudinal muscle

Acute ulcer — Penetration into muscle layer

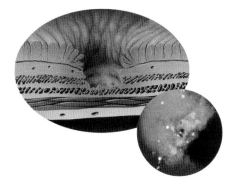

Perforating ulcer — Penetration of wall

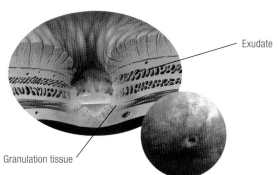

Exudate
Granulation tissue

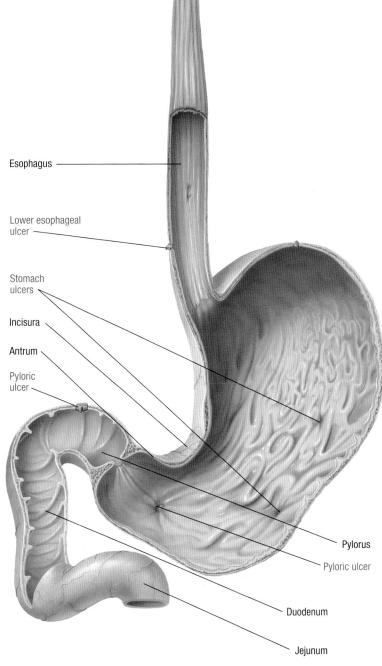

Esophagus

Lower esophageal ulcer

Stomach ulcers

Incisura

Antrum

Pyloric ulcer

Pylorus

Pyloric ulcer

Duodenum

Jejunum

MUSCULOSKELETAL DISORDERS

DEVELOPMENTAL DYSPLASIA OF THE HIP

Developmental dysplasia of the hip (DDH) is an abnormal development or dislocation of the hip joint present from birth.

DDH can be unilateral or bilateral. It affects the left hip more often (67%) than the right. This abnormality occurs in three degrees of severity:

- dislocatable — hip positioned normally but manipulation can cause dislocation
- subluxatable — femoral head rides on edge of acetabulum
- dislocated — femoral head totally outside the acetabulum.

Causes

Unknown, but genetic factors may play a role.

Risk Factors

- Breech delivery (malposition in utero; DDH is 10 times more common with breech delivery than after cephalic delivery)
- Elevated maternal relaxin
- Large neonates and twins (more common)

Pathophysiology

DDH may be related to trauma during birth, malposition in utero, or maternal hormonal factors. For example, the hormone relaxin, secreted by the corpus luteum during pregnancy, causes relaxation of pubic symphysis and cervical dilation; excessive levels may promote relaxation of the joint ligaments, predisposing the infant to DDH. Also, excessive or abnormal movement of the joint during a traumatic birth may cause dislocation. Displacement of the bones within the joint may damage joint structures, including articulating surfaces, blood vessels, tendons, ligaments, and nerves. This may lead to ischemic necrosis because of the disruption of blood flow to the joint.

COMPLICATIONS
- DDH is the most common cause of secondary osteoarthritis (Uchida et al., 2016)
  - Degenerative hip changes
  - Hip instability
- Lordosis
- Joint malformation
- Soft tissue damage and labral tears
- Progressive limp

Signs and Symptoms

- In neonates: no gross deformity or pain
  - Young patients typically complain of groin pain associated with intra-articular pathological abnormalities (Uchida et al., 2016).
  - Many young patients also have lateral hip pain due to fatigue of structures such as the iliotibial band (Poultsides et al., 2012).

- Complete dysplasia: Hip rides above the acetabulum, causing the level of the knees to be uneven.
- Limited abduction on the dislocated side as the growing child begins to walk
- Swaying from side to side ("duck waddle")
- Limp
- Asymmetry of the thigh fat folds
- Positive Ortolani's sign
- Positive Trendelenburg's sign

Eliciting Ortolani's Sign

- Place infant on his back, with hip flexed and in abduction. Adduct the hip while pressing the femur downward. This will dislocate the hip.
- Then, abduct the hip while moving the femur upward. A click or a jerk (produced by the femoral head moving over the acetabular rim) indicates subluxation in a neonate younger than 1 month. In the older infant, the sign indicates subluxation or complete dislocation.

Eliciting Trendelenburg's Sign

- When the child stands on the involved limb and lifts his other knee, the pelvis drops on the uninvolved side because the abductor muscles in the affected hip are weak.
- However, when the child stands with his weight on the uninvolved side and lifts the other knee, the pelvis remains horizontal.

Diagnostic Test Results

- X-rays show the location of the femoral head and a shallow acetabulum (also used to monitor disease or treatment progress).
- Sonography and magnetic resonance imaging (MRI) assess reduction.

Treatment

Infants Younger Than Age 3 Months

- Reduce dislocation — gentle manipulation
- Maintain reduction — splint brace or harness worn for 2 to 3 months to hold the hips in flexed and abducted position
- Tighten and stabilize joint capsule in correct alignment — night splint for another month

Beginning at Ages 3 Months to 2 Years

- Try to reduce dislocation — gradual abduction of the hips with bilateral skin traction (in infant) or skeletal traction (in child who is walking)
- Maintain immobilization — Bryant's traction or divarication traction for 2 to 3 weeks (with both extremities in traction, even if only one is affected), for children weighing less than 35 lb (16 kg)

- If traction fails — gentle closed reduction under general anesthesia to further abduct the hips, followed by spica cast for 4 to 6 months
- If closed treatment fails or in hips showing poor acetabular remodeling after closed reduction, surgery is indicated including open reduction and immobilization in spica cast for an average of 6 months or surgical division and realignment of bone (osteotomy) (Shin et al., 2016).

Beginning at Ages 2 to 5

- Skeletal traction and subcutaneous adductor tenotomy (surgical cutting of the tendon)
- Osteotomy

Delayed Until After Age 5

- Restoration of satisfactory hip function is rare.

HIP DISPLACEMENT

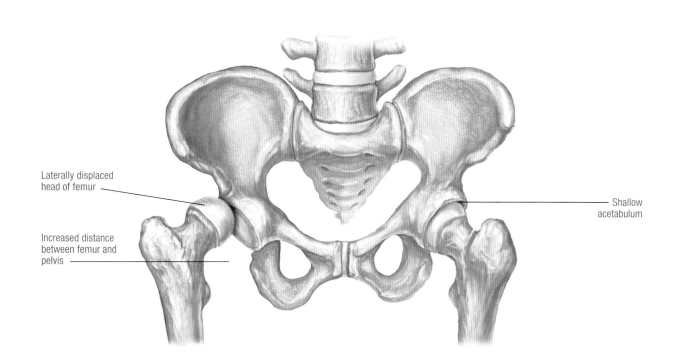

Laterally displaced head of femur

Increased distance between femur and pelvis

Shallow acetabulum

SIGNS OF DEVELOPMENTAL DYSPLASIA OF THE HIP

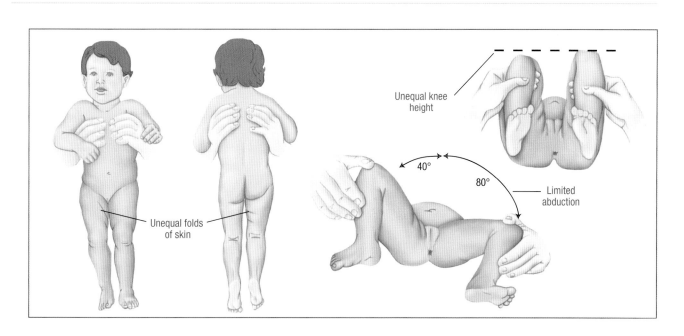

Unequal knee height

Unequal folds of skin

40°

80°

Limited abduction

MUSCULAR DYSTROPHY

Muscular dystrophy is a group of congenital disorders characterized by progressive symmetric wasting of skeletal muscles without neural or sensory defects. Paradoxically, some wasted muscles tend to enlarge (pseudohypertrophy) because connective tissue and fat replace muscle tissue, giving a false impression of increased muscle mass. The prognosis varies with the form of disease. The four main types of muscular dystrophy include:

- *Duchenne's* or *pseudohypertrophic* (50% of all cases) — strikes during early childhood, is usually fatal during the second decade of life, and affects 13 to 33 per 100,000 persons, mostly males
- *Becker's* or *benign pseudohypertrophic* (milder form of Duchenne's) — becomes apparent between ages 5 and 15, is usually fatal by age 50, and affects 1 to 3 per 100,000 persons, mostly males
- *Facioscapulohumeral (Landouzy-Dejerine)* and *limb-girdle* — usually manifests in second to fourth decades of life, doesn't shorten life expectancy, and affects both sexes equally.

Causes

Genetic Mechanisms, Typically Causing an Enzymatic or Metabolic Defect

- Duchenne's or Becker's muscular dystrophy — X-linked recessive disorders; mapped to the Xp21 locus for the muscle protein dystrophin, which is essential for maintaining muscle cell membrane; muscle cells deteriorate or die without it
- Limb-girdle muscular dystrophy — autosomal recessive disorder
- Facioscapulohumeral muscular dystrophy — autosomal dominant disorder

Pathophysiology

Abnormally permeable cell membranes allow leakage of a variety of muscle enzymes, particularly creatine kinase. The metabolic defect that causes the muscle cells to die is present from fetal life onward. The absence of progressive muscle wasting at birth suggests that other factors compound the effect of dystrophin deficiency. The specific trigger is unknown, but phagocytosis of the muscle cells by inflammatory cells causes scarring and loss of muscle function.

As the disease progresses, skeletal muscle becomes almost totally replaced by fat and connective tissue. The skeleton eventually becomes deformed, causing progressive immobility. Cardiac muscle and smooth muscle of the GI tract typically become fibrotic. The brain exhibits no consistent structural abnormalities.

COMPLICATIONS
- Scoliosis
- Joint contractures
- Decreased mobility
- Cardiomyopathy
- Respiratory failure

Signs and Symptoms

Duchenne's (Pseudohypertrophic)

- Insidious onset between ages 3 and 5
- Initial effects on legs, pelvis, shoulders
  - Enlarged, firm calf muscles
  - Delay in motor development and skeletal muscle weakness
  - Waddling gait, toe walking, and lumbar lordosis
  - Difficulty climbing stairs
  - Frequent falls
  - Positive Gower's sign — patient stands from a sitting position by "walking" hands up legs to compensate for pelvic and trunk weakness

Becker's (Benign Pseudohypertrophic)

- Similar to those of Duchenne's type but with slower progression

Facioscapulohumeral (Landouzy-Dejerine)

- Weak face, shoulder, and upper arm muscles (initial sign)
  - Pendulous lip and absent nasolabial fold
  - Abnormal facial movements; absence of facial movements when laughing or crying
  - Masklike expression
- Inability to raise arms above head

Limb-Girdle

- Weakness in upper arms and pelvis (initial sign)
- Lumbar lordosis, protruding abdomen
- Winging of scapulae
- Waddling gait, poor balance
- Inability to raise arms

Diagnostic Test Results

- Electromyography shows short, weak bursts of electrical activity in affected muscles.
- Muscle biopsy shows a combination of muscle cell degeneration and regeneration (in later stages, showing fat and connective tissue deposits).
- Immunologic and molecular biological techniques facilitate accurate prenatal and postnatal diagnosis of Duchenne's and Becker's muscular dystrophies.

Treatment

Supportive Only

- Coughing and deep-breathing exercises
- Diaphragmatic breathing
- Teaching parents to recognize early signs of respiratory complications
- Orthopedic appliances, physical therapy, possible wheelchair prescription
- Surgery to correct contractures
- Adequate fluid intake, increased dietary bulk, stool softener
- Low-calorie, high-protein, high-fiber diet
- Genetic counseling

Duchenne's

Limb-girdle

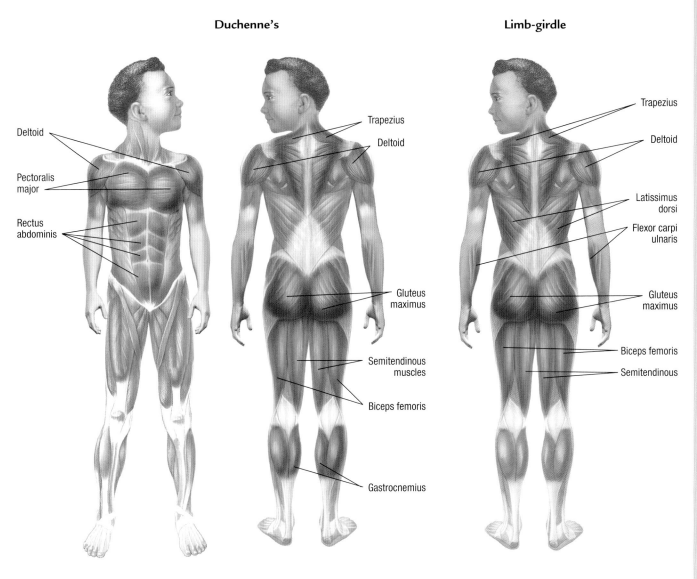

Deltoid

Pectoralis major

Rectus abdominis

Trapezius

Deltoid

Gluteus maximus

Semitendinous muscles

Biceps femoris

Gastrocnemius

Trapezius

Deltoid

Latissimus dorsi

Flexor carpi ulnaris

Gluteus maximus

Biceps femoris

Semitendinous

Facioscapulohumeral

Trapezius

Latissimus dorsi

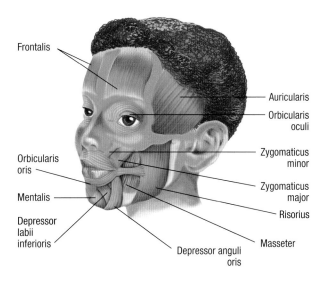

Frontalis

Auricularis

Orbicularis oculi

Zygomaticus minor

Zygomaticus major

Risorius

Masseter

Orbicularis oris

Mentalis

Depressor labii inferioris

Depressor anguli oris

OSTEOMYELITIS

Osteomyelitis is a bone infection characterized by progressive inflammatory destruction after the formation of new bone. It commonly results from a combination of local trauma — usually trivial but causing a hematoma — and an acute infection originating elsewhere in the body. Although osteomyelitis usually remains localized, it can spread through the bone to the marrow, cortex, and periosteum.

Osteomyelitis is usually classified as acute if symptoms have been present for less than 2 weeks, subacute between 2 weeks and 3 months, or chronic if greater than 3 months (Chiappini et al., 2016).

Acute osteomyelitis is usually a blood-borne disease and most commonly affects rapidly growing children, with an estimated incidence of 8 cases per 100,000 children/year and a male:female ratio of 2:1. The long bones, such as the femur, are the most frequently involved and the lower extremities are more affected than the upper extremities (Yeo & Ramachandran, 2014). Although rare, with chronic osteomyelitis, drainage of the sinus tracts may be necessary and widespread lesions may be present. Possible consequences may include amputation of an arm or leg when resistant chronic osteomyelitis causes severe, unrelenting pain and decreased function due to weakened bone cortex.

AGE ALERT

Osteomyelitis occurs more often in children (especially boys) than in adults — usually as a complication of an acute localized infection. The most common sites in children are the distal femur and the proximal tibia, humerus, and radius. The most common sites in adults are the pelvis and spinal vertebrae, usually after surgery or trauma.

The incidence of osteomyelitis is declining, except in drug abusers. With prompt treatment, prognosis is good for acute osteomyelitis but remains poor for chronic osteomyelitis.

Causes

- Minor traumatic injury
- Acute infection originating elsewhere in the body
- *Staphylococcus aureus* (most common)
- *Streptococcus pyogenes*
- *Pneumococcus* species
- *Pseudomonas aeruginosa*
- *Escherichia coli*
- *Proteus vulgaris*
- *Pasteurella multocida* (part of normal mouth flora in cats and dogs)

Pathophysiology

Typically, a pathogen finds a culture site in a hematoma after recent trauma or in a weakened area, such as the site of a local infection (for example, furunculosis). It then travels through the bloodstream to the metaphysis, the section of a long bone that is continuous with the epiphysis plates, where the blood flows into sinusoids. Pus is produced and pressure builds in the rigid medullary cavity. An abscess forms and the bone is deprived of its blood supply. Necrosis results and new bone formation is stimulated. The dead bone detaches and exits through an abscess of the sinuses resulting in chronic osteomyelitis.

COMPLICATIONS

- Septic arthritis
  - Subperiosteal abscess
  - Deep vein thrombosis (DVT)
  - Sepsis and multiorgan failure (Chiappini et al., 2016)
  - Chronic infection
- Skeletal and joint deformity
- Disturbed bone growth
- Leg length discrepancy
- Impaired mobility

Signs and Symptoms

- Sudden pain and tenderness in the affected bone is present approximately 81% of the time (Dartnell et al., 2012).
- Swelling and erythema are present approximately 70% of the time (Dartnell et al., 2012).
  - Decreased ability to bear weight through the affected bone
  - Restricted movement of the surrounding soft tissues
- Chronic infection may present intermittently for years, flaring after minor traumas or persisting as drainage of pus from a pocket in a sinus tract.
- Tachycardia
- Fever is present approximately 61% of the time in children (Dartnell et al., 2012).
- Chills, nausea, and malaise
- Drainage of pus

Diagnostic Test Results

- White blood cell (WBC) count and erythrocyte sedimentation rate (ESR) are elevated.
- Blood cultures show causative organism.
- X-ray may not show bone involvement until disease has been active for 2 to 3 weeks.
- MRI delineates bone marrow from soft tissue.
- Bone scans detect early infection.

Treatment

- Immobilization of the affected body part by cast, traction, or bed rest
- Supportive measures, such as analgesics for pain and I.V. fluids to maintain hydration
- Incision, drainage, and culture of an abscess or sinus tract

Acute Infection

- Systemic antibiotics
- Intracavitary instillation through closed system continuous irrigation with low intermittent suction
- Limited irrigation; blood drainage system with suction (Hemovac)
- Packed, wet, antibiotic-soaked dressings

Chronic Osteomyelitis

- Surgery to remove dead bone and promote drainage (prognosis remains poor even after surgery)

- Hyperbaric oxygen
- Skin, bone, and muscle grafts

STAGES OF OSTEOMYELITIS

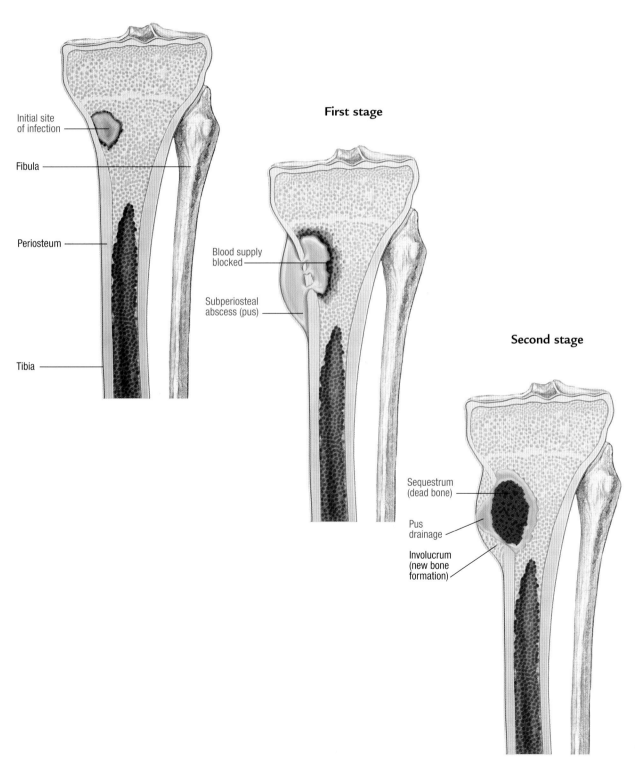

Initial infection

Initial site of infection

Fibula

Periosteum

Tibia

First stage

Blood supply blocked

Subperiosteal abscess (pus)

Second stage

Sequestrum (dead bone)

Pus drainage

Involucrum (new bone formation)

BONE TUMORS

Primary malignant bone tumors (also called *sarcomas of the bone* and *bone cancer*) are rare, and while constituting only 1% of new cancer diagnoses, it accounts for 2% of cancer deaths (Zhang et al., 2016). The incidence is approximately 8 cases per million/year (Aggerholm-Pedersen et al., 2014). Most bone tumors are secondary, caused by seeding from a primary site.

AGE ALERT
Although occurring in all ages, it has a characteristic bimodal distribution with peak incidences for both adolescents and elderly (Maretty-Nielsen et al., 2014).

Causes

Unknown

Suggested Mechanisms

- Rapid bone growth — Children and young adults with primary bone tumors are much taller than average.
- Heredity
- Trauma
- Excessive radiotherapy

Pathophysiology

Bone tumors are growths of abnormal cells in bones. These abnormal cells divide uncontrollably and healthy tissue is replaced with unhealthy tissue. Bone tumors may originate in osseous or nonosseous tissue. *Osseous* bone tumors arise from the bony structure itself and include osteogenic sarcoma (the most common), parosteal osteogenic sarcoma, chondrosarcoma, and malignant giant cell tumor. *Nonosseous* tumors arise from hematopoietic, vascular, or neural tissues and include Ewing's sarcoma, fibrosarcoma, and chordoma.

COMPLICATIONS
- Hypercalcemia
- Reduced function of limb

Signs and Symptoms

- Bone pain (most common indication of primary malignant bone tumors). Characteristics include the following:
  - greater intensity at night
  - usually associated with movement
  - dull and usually localized
  - may be referred from hip or spine and result in weakness or a limp.
- Tender, swollen, possibly palpable mass
- Pathologic fractures
- Cachexia, fever, and impaired mobility in later stages

Diagnostic Test Results

- Incisional or aspiration biopsy confirms cell type.
- Bone X-rays, radioisotope bone scan, and computed tomography (CT) scan reveal tumor size.
  - Flourine-18-fluorodeoxyglucose positron emission tomography (F-FDG PET) and PET/CT can be applied to differentiate primary bone sarcomas from benign lesions (Liu et al., 2015).
  - PET/CT is useful for the diagnosis, staging, restaging, and recurrence surveillance of bone sarcomas (Liu et al., 2015).
- Blood studies reveal hypercalcemia and elevated alkaline phosphatase.

Prognosis

- Independent adverse prognostic factors for survival include increasing age, tumor size, metastasis, soft tissue involvement, high grade, and intralesional/marginal excision or not having surgery (Aggerholm-Pedersen et al., 2014).

Treatment

- Excision of tumor with a 3-inch (7.6-cm) margin
- Radiation therapy before or after surgery
- Preoperative chemotherapy
- Postoperative chemotherapy
- Radical surgery, such as hemipelvectomy or interscapulothoracic amputation, if necessary (seldom)
- Intensive chemotherapy

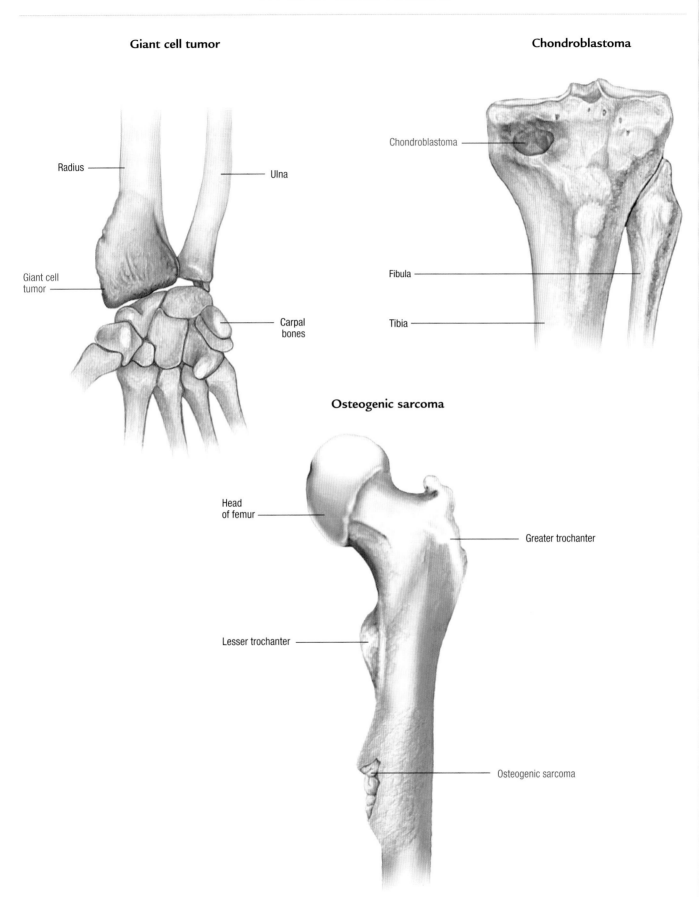

Giant cell tumor

Radius

Ulna

Giant cell tumor

Carpal bones

Chondroblastoma

Chondroblastoma

Fibula

Tibia

Osteogenic sarcoma

Head of femur

Greater trochanter

Lesser trochanter

Osteogenic sarcoma

SCOLIOSIS

Scoliosis is a lateral curvature of the thoracic, lumbar, or thoracolumbar spine. The curve may be convex to the right (more common in thoracic curves) or to the left (more common in lumbar curves). Rotation of the vertebral column around its axis may cause rib cage deformity. Scoliosis may be associated with kyphosis (humpback) and lordosis (swayback).

AGE ALERT

About 2% to 3% of adolescents have scoliosis. In general, the greater the magnitude of the curve and the younger the child at the time of diagnosis, the greater the risk for progression of the spinal abnormality. Optimal treatment usually achieves favorable outcomes.

Scoliosis may be functional (a reversible deformity) or structural (fixed deformity of spinal column). The most common curve in functional or structural scoliosis arises in the thoracic segment, with convexity to the right. As the spine curves laterally, compensatory curves (S curves) with convexity to the left develop in the cervical and lumbar segments to maintain body balance. Idiopathic scoliosis, the most common type of structural scoliosis, varies according to age at onset, as follows:

- infantile — affecting mostly male infants between birth and age 3, infantile scoliosis comprises less than 1% of all cases of idiopathic scoliosis in the Unites States. The majority of curves tend to be left sided and may be associated with other congenital anomalies (Riseborough & Wynne-Davies, 1973)
- juvenile — affects both sexes between ages 4 and 10; no typical curvature
- adolescent — generally affects girls between age 10 and skeletal maturity; no typical curvature.

Causes

Functional

- Poor posture
- Uneven leg length

Structural

- Congenital — wedge vertebrae, fused ribs or vertebrae, and hemivertebrae
- Paralytic or musculoskeletal — asymmetric paralysis of trunk muscles due to polio, cerebral palsy, or muscular dystrophy
- Idiopathic — most common; appears in a previously straight spine during the growing years; may be transmitted as an autosomal dominant or multifactorial trait

Pathophysiology

Differential stress on vertebral bone causes an imbalance of osteoblastic activity. The vertebrae rotate, forming the convex part of the curve. The rotation causes rib prominence along the thoracic spine and waistline asymmetry in the lumbar spine.

COMPLICATIONS

- Severe deformity (if untreated)
- Major thoracic deformity before the age of 5 is associated with twice the mortality rate due to compromised cardiopulmonary system (Alsiddiky, 2015).
- Cor pulmonale (curvature greater than 80 degrees)

Signs and Symptoms

- Backache
- Lower back pain
- Fatigue
- Dyspnea
- Uneven hemlines or pant legs that appear unequal in length
- Apparent discrepancy in hip height
- Unequal shoulder heights, elbow levels, and heights of iliac crests
- Asymmetric thoracic cage and misalignment of the spinal vertebrae when patient bends forward — commonly known as a rib hump
- Asymmetric paraspinal muscles, rounded on the convex side of the curve and flattened on the concave side
- Asymmetric gait

Diagnostic Test Results

- Anterior, posterior, and lateral spinal X-rays, taken with the patient standing upright and bending, confirm scoliosis and determine the degree of curvature and flexibility of the spine.
- CT provides three-dimensional information that can allow evaluation of the curvature, thoracic cage, and lung volumes (Gollogly et al., 2004).
- An MRI may be performed to further investigate underlying spinal anomalies (Pahys 2009).
- Scoliosiometry measures the angle of trunk rotation.

Treatment

Mild Scoliosis (Less Than 25 Degrees)

- Observation — X-rays to monitor curve and re-examination every 3 months
- Physical therapy and exercise to strengthen torso muscles and prevent curve progression

Moderate Scoliosis (30 to 50 Degrees)

- Spinal exercises and a brace (may halt progression but doesn't correct established curvature); braces can be adjusted as the patient grows and worn until bone growth is complete
- Alternative therapy using transcutaneous electrical nerve stimulation (TENS) for pain
- Physical therapy

Severe Scoliosis (50 Degrees or More)

- Surgery — supportive instrumentation; spinal fusion in severe cases
- Physical therapy is often indicated after surgery to regain motion and improve trunk strength

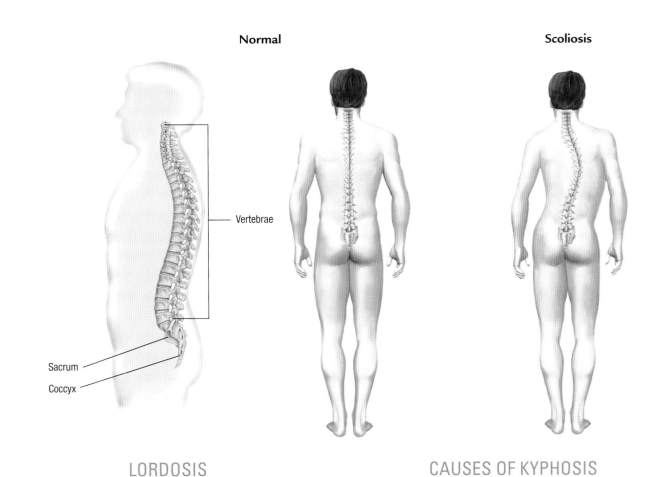

Normal

Scoliosis

Vertebrae

Sacrum

Coccyx

LORDOSIS

CAUSES OF KYPHOSIS

Absence of a corner or flattening by compression

Incomplete vertebral segmentation

Absence of a vertebra (T12)

T10

T11

L1

L2

L3

L4

FRACTURES

When a force exceeds the compressive or tensile strength of the bone, a fracture will occur. An estimated 25% of the population has a traumatic musculoskeletal injury each year, and a significant number of these involve fractures. The prognosis varies depending on the extent of disability or deformity, amount of tissue and vascular damage, adequacy of reduction and immobilization, and the patient's age, health, and nutritional status.

AGE ALERT

Children's bones usually heal rapidly and without deformity. However, epiphyseal plate fractures in children are likely to cause deformity because they interfere with normal bone growth. In elderly people, underlying systemic illness, impaired circulation, or poor nutrition may cause slow or poor healing.

Causes

- Falls, motor vehicle accidents (MVA), and sports
- Drugs that impair judgment or mobility
- Young age (immaturity of bone)
- Bone tumors
- Metabolic illnesses (such as hypoparathyroidism or hyperparathyroidism)
- Medications that cause iatrogenic osteoporosis such as corticosteroids

AGE ALERT

The highest incidence of fractures occurs in young males between the ages of 15 and 24 (tibia, clavicle, and distal humerus); these fractures are usually the result of trauma. In older and aging adults, fractures of the proximal femur, proximal humerus, vertebrae, distal radius, or pelvis are often associated with osteoporosis.

Pathophysiology

A fracture disrupts the periosteum and blood vessels in the cortex, marrow, and surrounding soft tissue. A hematoma forms between the broken ends of the bone and beneath the periosteum, and granulation tissue eventually replaces the hematoma.

Damage to bone tissue triggers an intense inflammatory response in which cells from surrounding soft tissue and the marrow cavity invade the fracture area, and blood flow to the entire bone increases. Osteoblasts in the periosteum, endosteum, and marrow produce osteoid (collagenous, young bone that hasn't yet calcified, also called callus). The osteoid hardens along the outer surface of the shaft and over the broken ends of the bone. Osteoclasts reabsorb material from previously formed bones and osteoblasts rebuild bone. Osteoblasts then transform into osteocytes (mature bone cells).

COMPLICATIONS

- Arterial damage
- Nonunion
- Fat embolism
- Infection
- Shock
- Avascular necrosis
- Peripheral nerve damage
- Heterotopic ossification (HO) is an abnormal formation of mature bone at extraskeletal sites, which can lead to pain, stiffness, decreased motion, and functional impairments (Robinson et al., 2010). HO may develop in any bone after a fracture but is especially common in those with major elbow fractures (with up to 1/3 of patients affected — Hong et al., 2015), hip arthroplasty (up to 24% affected — Pavlou et al., 2012), and femoral head fractures (up to 16.8% affected — Giannoudis et al., 2009).

Signs and Symptoms

- Pain
- Broken skin with bone protruding (open fracture)
- Deformity
- Swelling, muscle spasm, and tenderness
- Ecchymosis
- Impaired sensation distal to fracture site
- Limited range of motion
- Crepitus or clicking sounds on movement
- Functional impairment

Diagnostic Test Results

- X-rays confirm the diagnosis and, after treatment, confirm alignment.

Treatment

Emergency Treatment for Arm or Leg Fractures

- Splinting the limb above and below the suspected fracture
- Applying a cold pack and elevating the limb

For Severe Fractures That Cause Blood Loss

- Direct pressure to control bleeding
- Fluid replacement as soon as possible

Closed Reduction

- Local anesthetic, analgesic, muscle relaxants, or a sedative
- Manual manipulation

Open Reduction (If Closed Reduction Is Impossible or Unsuccessful)

- Prophylactic tetanus immunization and antibiotics
- Surgery
  - Thorough wound debridement
  - Immobilization by rods, plates, screws, or external fixation devices

FRACTURES OF THE ELBOW

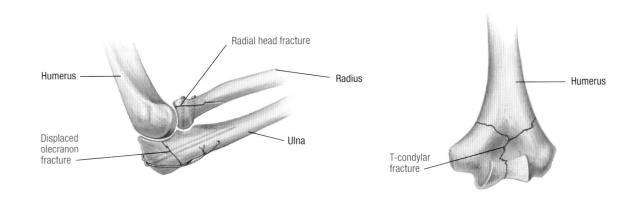

Humerus

Radial head fracture

Radius

Ulna

Displaced olecranon fracture

Humerus

T-condylar fracture

FRACTURES OF THE HAND AND WRIST

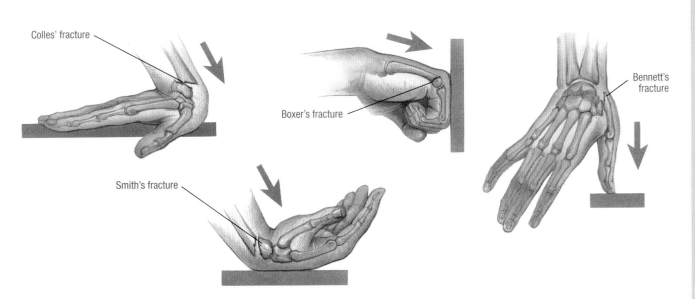

Colles' fracture

Boxer's fracture

Bennett's fracture

Smith's fracture

FRACTURES OF THE HIP

FRACTURES OF THE FOOT AND ANKLE

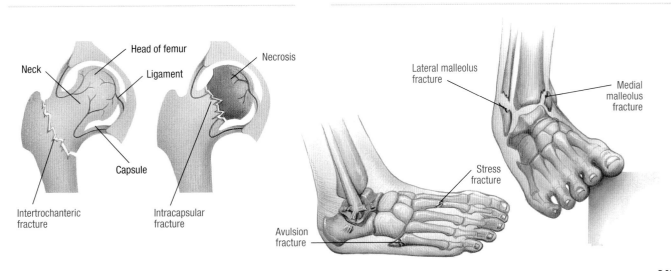

Neck

Head of femur

Ligament

Capsule

Intertrochanteric fracture

Necrosis

Intracapsular fracture

Lateral malleolus fracture

Medial malleolus fracture

Stress fracture

Avulsion fracture

OSTEOPOROSIS

Osteoporosis is a metabolic bone disorder in which the rate of bone resorption accelerates while the rate of bone formation slows, causing a net loss of bone mass. Bones affected by this disease lose calcium and phosphate salts and become porous, brittle, and abnormally vulnerable to fractures. It is defined by the World Health Organization (WHO) as a bone mineral density (BMD) T score of less than or equal to –2.5 standard deviations (SD) below the average value for premenopausal women using dual-energy X-ray absorptiometry (Kanis, 2002). The term osteopenia refers to bone density that is lower than normal but does not reach the –2.5 SD threshold to be classified as osteoporosis. As estimated, 200 million people have osteoporosis worldwide, with 44 million in the United States (Reginster & Burlet, 2006).

Osteoporosis may be primary or secondary to an underlying disease, such as Cushing's syndrome or hyperthyroidism. It primarily affects the weight-bearing bones such as spinal vertebrae, femoral heads, and pelvic acetabula. Only when the condition is advanced or severe, as in secondary disease, do similar changes occur in the skull, ribs, and long bones.

AGE ALERT
Osteoporosis is most apparent with the aging population, and although historically afflicting women more than men, it is now a serious health problem affecting both genders (Kanis, 2002).

Causes

Primary Osteoporosis

* Unknown
* Contributing factors:
  * Mild but prolonged negative calcium balance
  * Declining gonadal and adrenal function
  * Relative or progressive estrogen deficiency
  * Sedentary lifestyle
* Smoking

Secondary Osteoporosis

* Prolonged therapy with corticosteroids, heparin, and anticonvulsants
* Total immobilization or disuse of a bone (as in hemiplegia)
* Alcoholism, malnutrition, malabsorption, and scurvy
* Lactose intolerance
* Endocrine disorders such as hyperthyroidism, hyperparathyroidism, Cushing's syndrome, and diabetes mellitus (DM)
* Osteogenesis imperfecta
* Sudeck's atrophy (localized to hands and feet)

Pathophysiology

In normal bone, the rates of bone formation and resorption are constant; replacement follows resorption immediately, and the amount of bone replaced equals the amount of bone resorbed. The endocrine system maintains plasma and bone calcium and phosphate balance. Estrogen also supports normal bone metabolism by stimulating osteoblastic activity and limiting the osteoclastic-stimulating effects of parathyroid hormones. Osteoporosis develops when new bone formation falls behind resorption. For example, heparin promotes bone resorption by inhibiting collagen synthesis or enhancing collagen breakdown. Elevated levels of cortisone, either endogenous or exogenous, inhibit GI absorption of calcium.

COMPLICATIONS
* The major complication of osteoporosis is fragility fracture. Common fracture sites include the spine, hip, and wrist.
* Loss of mobility

CLINICAL TIP
When the rate of bone resorption exceeds that of bone formation, the bone becomes less dense. Men have approximately 30% greater bone mass than women, which may explain why osteoporosis develops later in men.

Signs and Symptoms

* Typically, asymptomatic until a fracture occurs
* Spontaneous fractures or those involving minimal trauma to spinal vertebrae, the distal radius, or the femoral neck
* Progressive deformity — kyphosis and loss of height
* Decreased exercise tolerance
* Low back pain
* Neck pain

Diagnostic Test Results

* Dual-energy X-ray absorptiometry test measures bone mass of the extremities, hips, and spine.
* X-rays show typical degeneration in the lower thoracic and lumbar vertebrae (vertebral bodies may appear flattened and may look more dense than normal; bone mineral loss is evident only in later stages); X-rays also reveal fractures.
* Computed tomography scan (CT scan) detects spinal bone loss.
* Laboratory studies reveal elevated parathyroid hormone.
* Bone biopsy shows thin, porous, but otherwise normal-looking bone.

Treatment

Early prevention to control bone loss, prevent fractures, control pain. The US Preventive Services Task Force recommends osteoporosis screening for all women aged 65 years and older and for those who have a fracture risk (Nelson et al., 2010). The National Osteoporosis Foundation guidelines recommend BMD testing in women aged 65 years and older and men aged 70 and older (Cosman et al., 2014).

* Limited alcohol and tobacco use
* High-calcium diet
* Prevention of falls
* Early mobilization after surgery, trauma, or illness
* Identification and treatment of risk factors
* Physical therapy emphasizing regular, moderate weight-bearing exercise including walking and stair-climbing
* Supportive devices, such as a back brace
* Prompt, effective treatment of underlying disorders to prevent secondary osteoporosis

Pharmacotherapy

- Estrogen; selective estrogen receptor modulators such as raloxifene; bisphosphonates, such as alendronate and risedronate

- Analgesics and local heat to relieve pain
- Calcium and vitamin D supplements
- Calcitonin

MUSCULOSKELETAL DISORDERS

CALCIUM METABOLISM IN OSTEOPOROSIS

Normally, blood absorbs calcium from the digestive system and deposits it in the bones. In osteoporosis, blood levels of calcium are reduced. To maintain blood calcium levels as normal as possible, reabsorption from the bones increases.

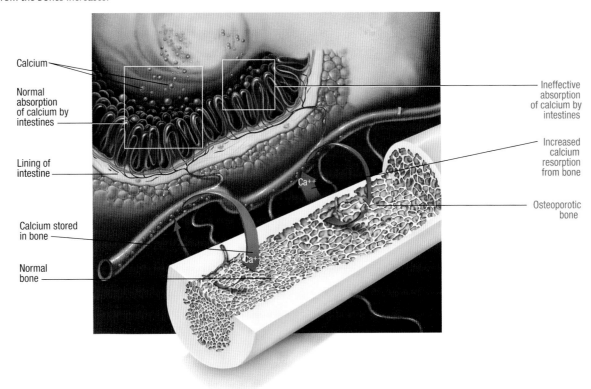

Bone formation and resorption
The organic portion of bone, called *osteoid,* acts as the matrix or framework for the mineral portion.

Bone cells called *osteoblasts* produce the osteoid matrix. The mineral portion, which consists of calcium and other minerals, hardens the osteoid matrix.

Large bone cells called *osteoclasts* reshape mature bone by resorbing the mineral and organic components. However, in osteoporosis, osteoblasts continue to produce bone, but resorption by osteoclasts exceeds bone formation.

Chapter 10 • Musculoskeletal Disorders **245**

OSTEOARTHRITIS

Osteoarthritis (OA) is the most common form of arthritis and the fastest growing cause of worldwide disability (Kalunian, 2016). Accounting for approximately 25% of primary care visits annually, it is a chronic condition caused by deterioration of joint cartilage (Leahy, 2012). Usually affecting weight-bearing joints, osteoarthritis is widespread (affecting more than 20 million persons in the United States) and is more common in women. Typically, its earliest symptoms manifest in middle age and is most common in the older adult with the knee being the most frequently affected joint (Smith et al., 2014). Osteoarthritis may be secondary to the wear and tear of aging (idiopathic) or to some abnormal initiating event. The rate of progression varies, and joints may remain stable for years in an early stage of deterioration.

Causes

Idiopathic (Contributing Factors)

- Metabolic — endocrine disorders such as hyperparathyroidism
- Genetic — decreased collagen synthesis
- Chemical — drugs that stimulate collagen-digesting enzymes in synovial membranes, such as corticosteroids
- Mechanical factors — repeated stress

Secondary (Identifiable Predisposing Event)

- Trauma (most common)
- Congenital deformity
- Obesity and poor posture
- Occupational stress

Pathophysiology

Osteoarthritis occurs in synovial joints. The joint cartilage deteriorates as a result of damage to chondrocytes, and reactive new bone forms at the margins and subchondral areas of the joints. Cartilage softens with age, narrowing the joint space. Mechanical injury erodes articular cartilage, leaving the underlying bone unprotected. This causes sclerosis or thickening and hardening of the bone underneath the cartilage.

Cartilage particles irritate the synovial lining, which becomes fibrotic and limits joint movement. Synovial fluid may be forced into defects in the bone, causing cysts. New bone, called *osteophyte* (bone spur), forms at joint margins as the articular cartilage erodes, causing gross alteration of the bony contours and enlargement of the joint.

COMPLICATIONS

- Flexion contractures and loss of motion
- Subluxation and deformity
- Ankylosis
- Bony cysts
- Gross bony overgrowth
- Central cord syndrome (with cervical spine osteoarthritis)
- Nerve root compression
- Cauda equina syndrome

Signs and Symptoms

- Deep, aching joint pain
- Stiffness in the morning and after exercise (relieved by rest)
- Crepitus or grating of the joint during motion
- Heberden's nodes (bony enlargements of distal interphalangeal joints)
- Altered gait from contractures
- Decreased range of motion
- Joint enlargement
- Localized headaches (may be direct result of cervical spine arthritis)
- Bouchard's nodes (bony enlargement of proximal interphalangeal joint)

Diagnostic Test Results

- Erythrocyte sedimentation rate (ESR) is elevated.
- X-rays show:
    - narrowing of joint space or margins
    - cystlike bony deposits in joint space and margins and sclerosis of the subchondral space
    - joint deformity
    - bony growths
    - joint fusion.
- Arthroscopy reveals bone spurs and narrowing of the joint space.

Treatment

- Weight loss to reduce stress on the joint
- Physical therapy
- Balanced rest and exercise
- Medications, including aspirin and other nonsteroidal anti-inflammatory drugs (NSAIDs); propoxyphene, acetaminophen, glucosamine, and celecoxib. There is also emerging evidence that methotrexate may be beneficial (Kalunian, 2016).
- Support, unloading, and stabilization of the involved joint with crutches, braces, cane, walker, cervical collar, or traction
- Intra-articular injections of corticosteroids (every 4 to 6 months) to try to delay node formation in the fingers

Surgical Treatment (For Severe Disability or Uncontrollable Pain)

- Arthroplasty — partial or total replacement of joint with prosthetic appliance
- Arthrodesis or laminectomy — fusion of bones, primarily in spine
- Osteoplasty — scraping and lavage of deteriorated bone
- Osteotomy — changing alignment of bone to relieve stress on joint

Hand

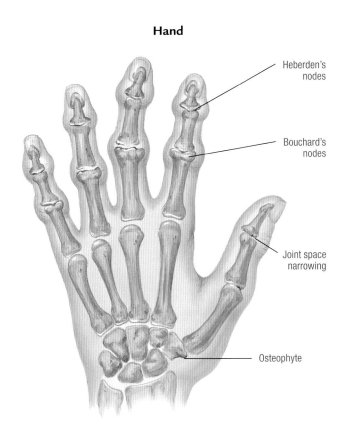

Heberden's nodes

Bouchard's nodes

Joint space narrowing

Osteophyte

Right knee

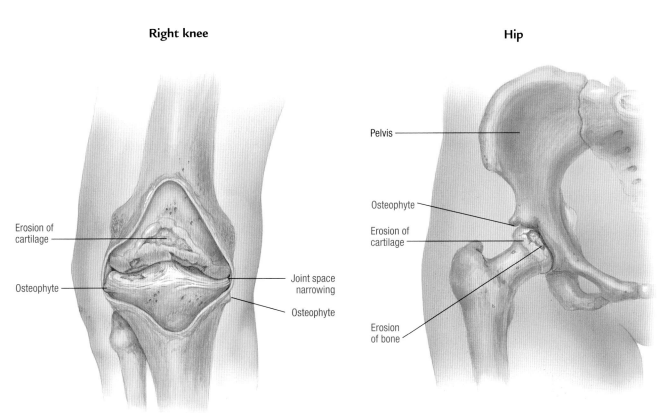

Erosion of cartilage

Osteophyte

Joint space narrowing

Osteophyte

Hip

Pelvis

Osteophyte

Erosion of cartilage

Erosion of bone

GOUT

Gout is the most common inflammatory arthropathy affecting more than 8 million Americans (Zhu et al., 2011). Primary gout is a metabolic disease marked by urate crystals deposited in a joint space. This triggers an immune and inflammatory response, which over time can damage the joint leading to chronic pain and disability (Hainer et al., 2014). Secondary gout develops during the course of another disease. Gout most commonly affects the foot, especially the great toe, ankle, or midfoot, knees, fingers, wrists, and elbows, but it may affect any joint. Gout follows an intermittent course, and patients may be completely free of symptoms for years between attacks. The prognosis is good with treatment. However, renal tubular damage by aggregates of urate crystals may result in progressively poorer excretion of uric acid and chronic renal dysfunction.

AGE ALERT

Primary gout usually occurs in men after age 30 (95% of cases) and in postmenopausal women; secondary gout occurs in older and aging adults.

Causes

Primary Gout

- Possibly genetic defect in purine metabolism, causing overproduction of uric acid (hyperuricemia), retention of uric acid, or both

Secondary Gout

- Obesity, diabetes mellitus (DM), hypertension (HTN), sickle cell anemia, and renal disease
- Drug therapy, especially hydrochlorothiazide or pyrazinamide, which decreases excretion of urate (ionic form of uric acid)

Pathophysiology

When uric acid becomes supersaturated in blood and other body fluids, it crystallizes and forms tophi — accumulations of urate salts in connective tissue throughout the body. The presence of these crystals triggers an acute inflammatory response in which neutrophils begin to ingest the crystals. With the release of lysosomes from the neutrophils, tissue damage occurs and inflammation is perpetuated. The prevalence of gout increases with age and peaks at more than 12% of those older than 80 years (Zhu et al., 2011).

COMPLICATIONS

- Renal calculi
- Atherosclerotic disease
- Cardiovascular lesions
- Stroke
- Coronary thrombosis
- Hypertension (HTN)
- Infection with tophi rupture and nerve entrapment

Signs and Symptoms

- Joint pain, redness, and swelling
- Tophi in great toe, ankle, and pinna of ear
- Elevated skin temperature
- Hypertension
- Chills
- Fever
- When occurring in the lower limb, difficulty bearing weight and ambulating may occur.

Diagnostic Test Results

- Needle aspiration of synovial fluid shows needlelike intracellular crystals.
- X-rays of the articular cartilage and subchondral bone shows evidence of chronic gout.
- Serum analysis reveals elevated uric acid levels and elevated white blood cell counts.
- Urine analysis shows elevated uric acid levels.

Treatment

Acute Gout

- Immobilization and protection of the inflamed, painful joints; local application of heat or cold
- Increased fluid intake to prevent kidney stone formation
- Oral corticosteroids, intravenous corticosteroids, and/or NSAIDs are optimally started within 24 hours of onset (Hainer et al., 2014).
- Colchicine (oral or I.V.) is used to inhibit phagocytosis of uric acid crystals by neutrophils (doesn't affect uric acid level) (Hainer et al., 2014).

Chronic Gout

- Allopurinol is a first-line agent, which acts to suppress uric acid formation or control uric acid levels, preventing further attacks (use cautiously in renal failure).
- Colchicine to prevent recurrent acute attacks until uric acid level subsides (doesn't affect uric acid level)
- Uricosuric agents (probenecid or sulfinpyrazone) to promote uric acid excretion and inhibit uric acid accumulation (of limited value in patients with renal impairment)
- Pegloticase, xanthine, and Febuxostat are also commonly prescribed (Hainer et al., 2014).
- Weight gain is a significant risk factor for gout in men and weight loss reduces this risk (Choi et al., 2005).
- Dietary modifications including restricted high-fructose corn syrup, purine-rich animal protein (shellfish, liver, sardines, anchovies), and alcohol. Vegetables and low-fat or nonfat dairy products should be encouraged (Khanna et al., 2012).

GOUT OF THE KNEE

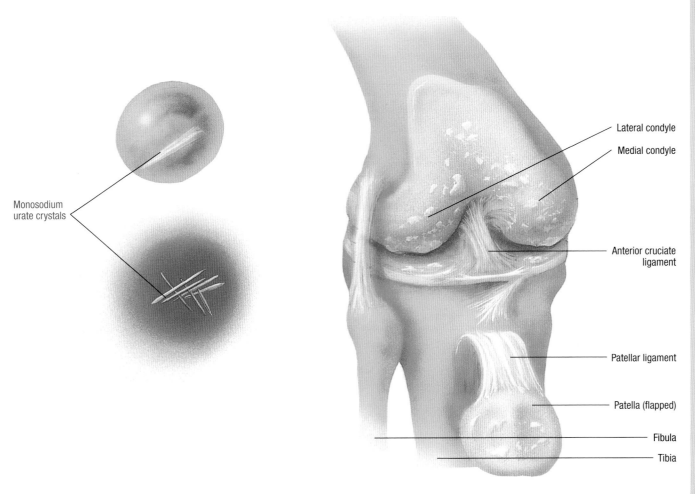

Monosodium urate crystals

Lateral condyle

Medial condyle

Anterior cruciate ligament

Patellar ligament

Patella (flapped)

Fibula

Tibia

GOUT OF THE FOOT

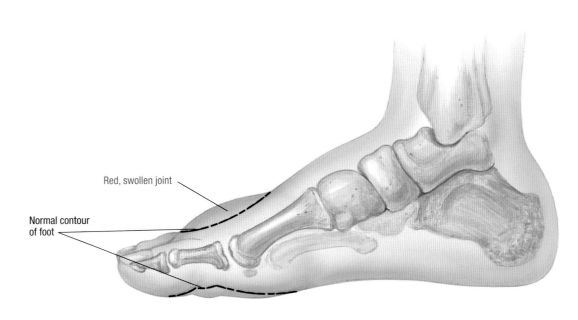

Red, swollen joint

Normal contour of foot

CARPAL TUNNEL SYNDROME

The carpal tunnel is a channel for the median nerve and nine flexor tendons, which travel into the hand. Carpal tunnel syndrome (CTS), a form of repetitive stress injury involving the median nerve, is the most common of the nerve entrapment syndromes. The incidence of CTS is reported to be between 2.7% and 5.8% (Bardak et al., 2009).

AGE ALERT
Carpal tunnel injury usually occurs in women between ages 30 and 60 and poses a serious occupational health problem.

At-risk groups include those who repetitively use their hands and upper extremities, especially assembly line workers and those who repeatedly use poorly designed tools. Computer keyboard and mouse users are also frequently affected. Any strenuous use of the hands — sustained grasping, twisting, or flexing — aggravates this condition.

Causes

Mostly idiopathic or may result from:

- repetitive stress injury
- rheumatoid arthritis
- flexor tenosynovitis (commonly associated with rheumatic disease)
- nerve compression
- pregnancy
- multiple myeloma
- diabetes mellitus
- acromegaly
- hypothyroidism
- amyloidosis
- obesity
- benign tumor
- other conditions that increase fluid pressure in the wrist, including alterations in the endocrine or immune systems
- wrist dislocation or sprain, including Colles' fracture followed by edema.

Pathophysiology

The carpal bones and the transverse carpal ligament form the carpal tunnel. Inflammation or fibrosis of the tendon sheaths that pass through the carpal tunnel often cause edema and compression of the median nerve. This compression neuropathy causes pain as well as sensory and motor changes in the median distribution of the hand. There is often initial impairment of the sensory transmission to the thumb, index finger, second finger, and inner aspect of the third finger.

COMPLICATIONS
- Decrease in wrist and hand function
- In more chronic cases, atrophy of the thenar eminence may be present.
- Permanent nerve damage with loss of movement and sensation
- CTS can have a negative effect on quality of life (Horng et al., 2011).

Signs and Symptoms

- Weakness, pain, burning, numbness, or tingling in one or both hands
- Paresthesia in thumb, forefinger, middle finger, and half of the fourth finger
- Inability to clench fist
- Pain extending to forearm and, in severe cases, to shoulder
- Pain usually relieved by shaking or rubbing hands vigorously or dangling arms
- Symptoms typically worse at night and in the morning (vasodilation, stasis, and prolonged wrist flexion during sleep may contribute to compression of the carpal tunnel)
- Possibly atrophic nails
- Dry, shiny skin

Diagnostic Test Results

- Electromyography shows a median nerve motor conduction delay of more than 5 ms.
- Digital electrical stimulation shows median nerve compression by measuring the length and intensity of stimulation from the fingers to the median nerve in the wrist.

CLINICAL TIP
These tests provide rapid diagnosis of carpal tunnel syndrome:

- Tinel's sign — tingling over the median nerve on light percussion of the carpal tunnel
- Phalen's wrist flexion test — holding the forearms vertically and allowing both hands to drop into complete flexion at the wrists for 1 minute reproduces symptoms of carpal tunnel syndrome
- Compression test — blood pressure cuff inflated above systolic pressure on the forearm for 1 to 2 minutes provokes pain and paresthesia along the distribution of the median nerve.

Treatment

- Conservative treatment — resting the hands by splinting the wrists in neutral extension especially at night for 1 to 2 weeks, along with gentle daily range-of-motion exercises
- Physical therapy including the use of nerve gliding exercises (Kim, 2015)
- Nonsteroidal anti-inflammatory drugs for symptomatic relief
- Injection of the carpal tunnel with hydrocortisone and lidocaine
- Treatment of any underlying disorder
- Surgical decompression of the nerve by resecting the entire transverse carpal tunnel ligament or by using endoscopic surgical techniques
- Possibly, neurolysis (freeing of the nerve fibers)
- Modification of the work area

Cross section of normal wrist

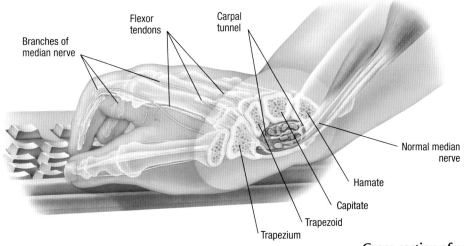

Branches of median nerve

Flexor tendons

Carpal tunnel

Normal median nerve

Hamate

Capitate

Trapezoid

Trapezium

Cross section of wrist with carpal tunnel syndrome

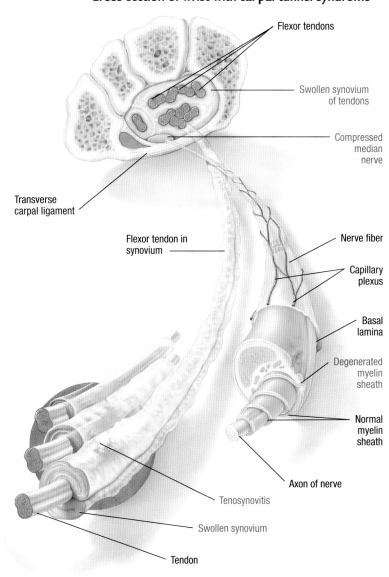

Flexor tendons

Swollen synovium of tendons

Compressed median nerve

Transverse carpal ligament

Flexor tendon in synovium

Nerve fiber

Capillary plexus

Basal lamina

Degenerated myelin sheath

Normal myelin sheath

Axon of nerve

Tenosynovitis

Swollen synovium

Tendon

HOW CARPAL TUNNEL SYNDROME OCCURS

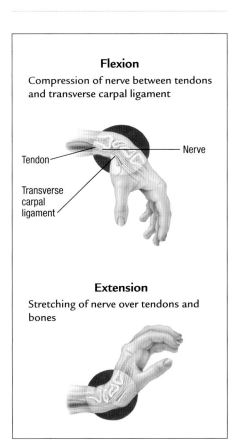

Flexion

Compression of nerve between tendons and transverse carpal ligament

Tendon

Nerve

Transverse carpal ligament

Extension

Stretching of nerve over tendons and bones

SPRAINS

A ligament is a band of connective tissue that connects two bones, spanning and offering support to joints. A sprain occurs when a joint is forced beyond its normal range of motion, resulting in an incomplete or complete tear to the supporting ligaments. Joint dislocations and fractures may accompany a severe sprain. The ankle is the most commonly sprained joint. Finger, wrist, knee, and shoulder sprains are also common.

Causes

- Trauma including falls
- Motor vehicle accidents (MVA)
- Sports injuries

Pathophysiology

A ligament may tear at any point along its length or at its attachment to bone (with or without avulsion of bone). Bleeding and formation of a hematoma are followed by formation of an inflammatory exudate and development of granulation tissue. Collagen formation begins 4 to 5 days after the injury, eventually organizing fibers parallel to the lines of stress. However, swelling, stretching, or impingement on nerves or vessels around the joint may cause neurovascular compromise. Further reorganization results in eventual strengthening of the damaged ligament, although persistent laxity may result in chronic joint instability.

COMPLICATIONS
- Avulsion fracture
- Chronic instability

Signs and Symptoms

- Localized pain (especially during joint movement) and tenderness
- Swelling and warmth
- Progressive loss of motion
- Ecchymosis
- Function will be impacted to varying degrees depending on the location and extent of the injury.

CLINICAL TIP
Sprains are graded according to the degree of swelling and instability:
Grade I — stable and minimal swelling
Grade II — moderate instability and swelling
Grade III — gross instability, extensive swelling, and ecchymosis.

Diagnostic Test Results

- Stress radiography visualizes the injury in motion.
- X-ray confirms damage to ligaments.
- Although not standard for most sprains, an MRI can be used if further tissue damage is suspected or if surgery may be indicated as in the case of anterior cruciate ligament (ACL) tears.

Treatment

- PRICE: Protection, Rest, Ice, Compression, Elevation
- Elevate the joint above the level of the heart for 48 to 72 hours (immediately after the injury)
- Intermittent ice packs for 12 to 48 hours
- Immobilizer or splint during the acute phase (up to 1 week)
- Nonsteroidal anti-inflammatory drugs (NSAIDs) and analgesics
- Early range-of-motion (ROM) exercises as tolerated
- Physical therapy may be indicated depending on the severity of the injury
- Acute surgical repair if indicated — notably, for the ulnar collateral ligament (UCL) of thumb and multiple ligamentous injuries of the knee or elbow due to dislocation
- Late surgical reconstruction may be indicated for chronic instability of the shoulder, knee, and ankle.

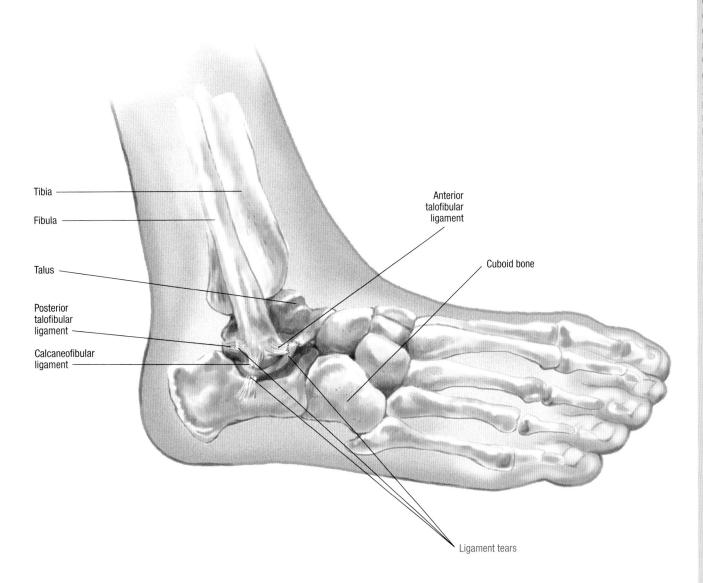

Tibia

Fibula

Talus

Posterior
talofibular
ligament

Calcaneofibular
ligament

Anterior
talofibular
ligament

Cuboid bone

Ligament tears

STRAINS

A strain is an injury to a muscle-tendon unit. The mechanism is described as a sudden forceful contraction of a muscle under stretch that overloads its tensile strength, resulting in failure at the muscle-tendon junction. Muscles that cross two joints are the most susceptible to strain. These include the hamstrings, rectus femoris of the thigh, gastrocnemius of the calf, and biceps brachialis of the upper arm.

Causes

- Sudden or unanticipated muscle contraction due to falling, sprinting, throwing, or other forceful activity
- Inadequate warm-ups and conditioning
- Degenerative changes in muscle-tendon units secondary to aging or anabolic steroid use

Pathophysiology

When a tendon or muscle is torn, bleeding occurs into the muscle and surrounding tissues and an inflammatory exudate develops between the torn ends. Granulation tissue grows inward from the surrounding soft tissue and cartilage. Collagen formation begins 4 to 5 days after the injury, eventually organizing fibers parallel to the lines of stress. With the aid of vascular fibrous tissue, the new tissue eventually fuses with the surrounding tissues. As further reorganization takes place, the new tendon or muscle separates from the surrounding tissue and eventually becomes strong enough to withstand normal muscle strain.

COMPLICATIONS
- Calcium deposits in muscle (with repeated injury)
- Limited movement and stiffness
- Muscle fatigue

Signs and Symptoms

- Pain
- Inflammation
- Erythema
- Ecchymosis
- Elevated skin temperature
- Function is impacted to varying degrees depending on the severity and location of injury.

CLINICAL TIP
Strains are usually graded on a scale of I to III.

- Grade I strains are characterized by small tears with mild pain and minimal to no swelling. Treatment is often not necessary.
- A grade II strain is a moderate strain and although partially torn, the muscle and tendon are intact. There is marked pain and swelling.
- Grade III strains are the most severe and occur when a majority of fibers are torn or there is a complete tear.
- Health care professionals should be consulted for grade II and III strains.

Diagnostic Test Results

- Stress radiography visualizes the injury in motion.
- X-ray detects the presence of fracture.
- Muscle biopsy, which is rarely done, shows muscle regeneration and connective tissue repair.
- MRI may be used depending on the severity of the injury and patient presentation.

Treatment

- PRICE: Protection, Rest, Ice, Compression, Elevation
- Physical therapy depending on the severity of injury and functional impairment
- Analgesics
- Application of ice for up to 48 hours. Heat may be applied after inflammation has subsided
- Surgery to suture tendon or muscle ends in close approximation.

Chronic Strains

- Treatment is usually unnecessary, but physical therapy may assist in recovery
- Heat, nonsteroidal anti-inflammatory drugs, and analgesic muscle relaxants to relieve discomfort

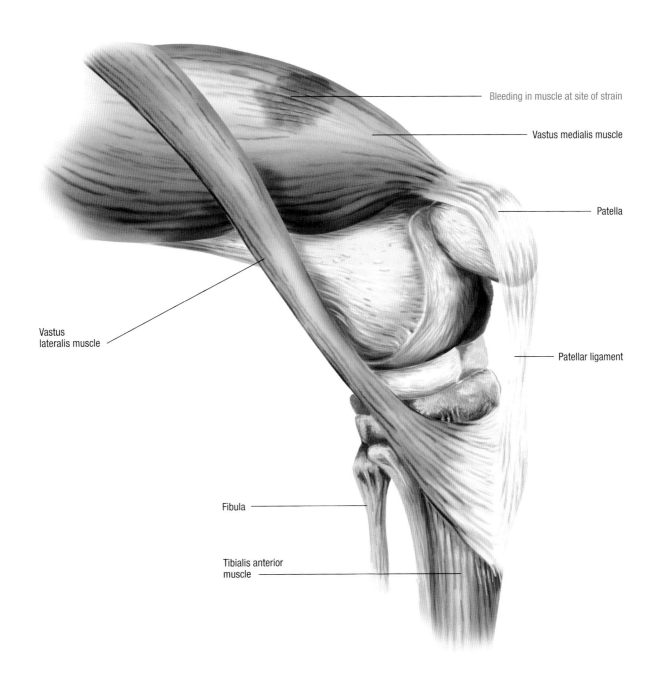

Bleeding in muscle at site of strain

Vastus medialis muscle

Patella

Vastus
lateralis muscle

Patellar ligament

Fibula

Tibialis anterior
muscle

TENDINOPATHY

A tendon is a type of connective tissue that transfers muscle forces to the skeleton (Ryan et al., 2015). Tendinopathy refers to a condition characterized by localized pain over an injured tendon that is associated with loading of the tendon (Vicenzino, 2015). When injured, the tendon shows a disorganization of collagen fibers, an increase in the number of blood vessels and nerves, and a breakdown of tissue (Scott et al., 2015).

Tendinopathy progresses in stages. Reactive tendinopathy is the mildest form and is reversible and characterized by minimal changes to collagen integrity. If not treated correctly, this may progress to tendon disrepair where more significant structural changes are observed. The final stage is degenerative tendinopathy, which is characterized by fibroblast degeneration and greater disarray of collagen fibers.

Tendon injuries are estimated to be as high as 50% of all sports-related and running injuries (Couppe et al., 2015; Lopes et al., 2012).

Causes

- Overuse or a rapid increase in load to the tendon
- Other musculoskeletal disorders, such as rheumatic diseases and congenital defects
- Postural misalignment
- Abnormal body development
- Hypermobility

Pathophysiology

A tendon is a band of dense fibrous connective tissue that attaches muscle to bone. Tendons are extremely strong, flexible, and inelastic. Tendinopathy describes an injury to the tendon characterized by pain and dysfunction with increased load.

AGE ALERT
Common forms of tendinopathy in adolescents (both males and females) include patellar (quadriceps tendon) and Achilles tendinopathy.

COMPLICATIONS
- Scar tissue
- Disability and loss of function

Signs and Symptoms

- Restricted range of motion
- Localized pain especially when the tendon is loaded
- Swelling
- Crepitus
- Calcific tendinitis
- Proximal weakness (due to calcium deposits in the tendon)
- Calcium erosion into adjacent bursae (acute calcific bursitis)

Diagnostic Test Results

- X-rays may be normal at first but later show bony fragments, osteophyte sclerosis, or calcium deposits.
- Arthrography shows irregularities on the undersurface of the tendon.
- CT scan and MRI identify tears, partial tears, and inflammation.

Treatment

Treatment varies with the stage of tendinopathy but may include:

- Physical therapy with an emphasis on tendon loading and remodeling
- Immobilization with a sling, splint, or cast
- Systemic analgesics
- Application of cold or heat
- Injection of a corticosteroid and an anesthetic such as lidocaine into the tendon sheath
- Oral nonsteroidal anti-inflammatory drugs (NSAIDs) until the patient is free of pain and able to perform range-of-motion exercises without difficulty
- Surgical debridement of degenerative tendon or excision of calcific deposits may be needed.

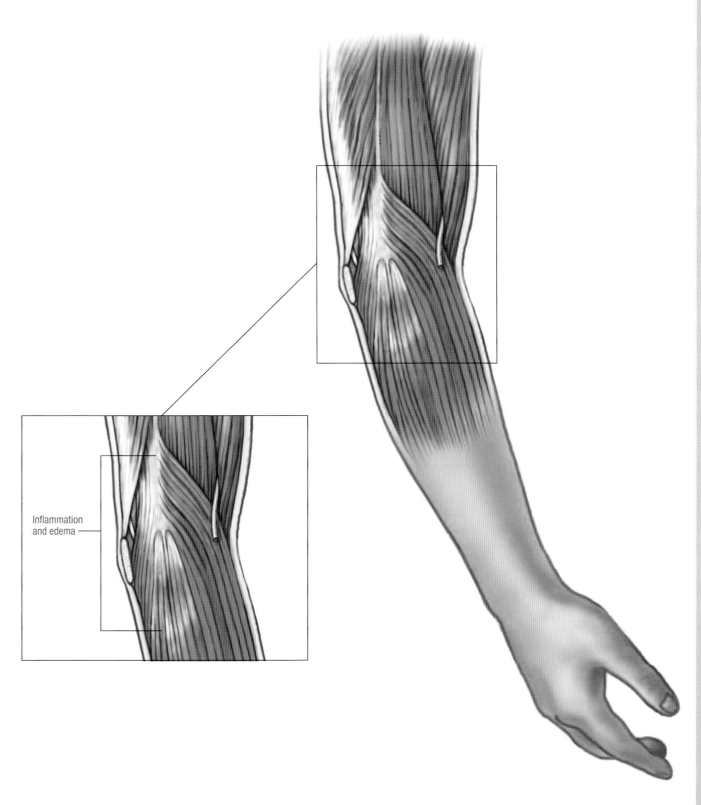

Inflammation and edema

BURSITIS

Bursitis is a painful inflammation of one or more of the bursae — closed sacs lubricated with small amounts of synovial fluid that facilitate the motion of muscles and tendons over bony prominences. Bursitis can occur wherever bursae are located; however, they are commonly seen in the subdeltoid, olecranon, trochanteric, calcaneal, prepatellar, or Achilles tendon regions.

Causes

- Recurrent or direct trauma to a joint or the soft tissues surrounding the joint
- Inflammatory joint disease, such as rheumatoid arthritis or gout
- Chronic bursitis — repeated attacks of acute bursitis, trauma, or infection
- Septic bursitis — wound infection; bacterial invasion of overlying skin

Pathophysiology

The role of the bursa is to act as a cushion and to suppress friction allowing the tendon to move over bone as the muscle contracts and relaxes. It's a fibrous sac lined with synovial fluid. Bursitis is an inflammation of the bursa. The inflammation leads to excessive production of fluid in the sac, which becomes distended and presses on sensory nerve endings, causing pain.

COMPLICATIONS
- Extreme pain
- Restricted joint movement

Signs and Symptoms

- Tenderness and irritation
- Inflammation
- Swelling
- Warmth over the affected joint
- Sudden or gradual onset of pain and limited movement

Site-Specific

- Subdeltoid bursa — limited arm abduction
- Prepatellar bursa — so-called *housemaid's knee;* pain when climbing stairs and kneeling
- Trochanteric bursa (hip bursa) — pain when climbing, squatting, and crossing legs

Diagnostic Test Results

Bursitis frequently occurs concurrently with tendinitis, and the two may be difficult to distinguish as distinct problems. X-rays are usually normal in the early stages. In calcific bursitis, calcium deposits may be present. MRI and ultrasonography can be used to view deep bursae or to differentiate other causes of pain in recalcitrant cases.

Treatment

- Rest, which may include immobilization with a sling, splint, or cast
- Physical therapy
- Application of cold or heat
- Therapeutic ultrasonography
- Mixture of a corticosteroid and an anesthetic such as lidocaine injected into bursal sac for immediate pain relief. Diagnostic ultrasound may be used to guide the injections to assure proper placement of the medication (Hsieh et al., 2013)
- Nonsteroidal anti-inflammatory drugs until the patient is free of pain and able to perform range-of-motion exercises easily
- Short-term analgesics, such as propoxyphene, codeine, acetaminophen with codeine, and, occasionally, oxycodone
- For chronic bursitis, lifestyle changes to prevent recurring joint irritation
- Antibiotics
- Surgical drainage of the bursa

Hip

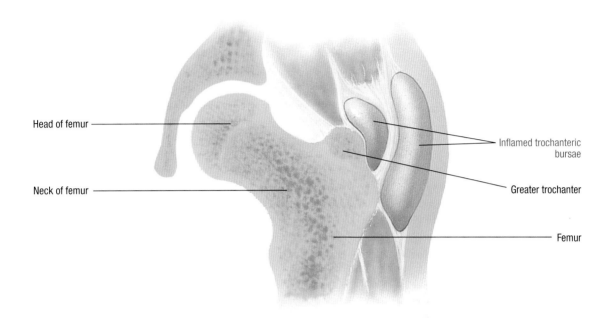

Head of femur

Neck of femur

Inflamed trochanteric bursae

Greater trochanter

Femur

Knee

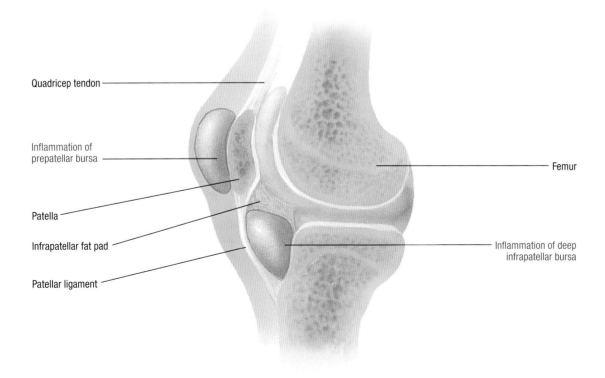

Quadricep tendon

Inflammation of prepatellar bursa

Patella

Infrapatellar fat pad

Patellar ligament

Femur

Inflammation of deep infrapatellar bursa

Suggested References

Aggerholm-Pedersen, N., Maretty-Nielsen, K., Keller, J., Baerentzen, S., & Safwat, A. (2014). Comorbidity in adult bone sarcoma patients: A population-based cohort study. *Sarcoma, 2014*, 690316. doi:10.1155/2014/690316

Alsiddiky, A. M. (2015). An insight into early onset of scoliosis: New update information—a review. *European Review for Medical and Pharmacological Sciences, 19*(15), 2750–2765.

Bardak, A. N., Alp, M., Erhan, B., Paker, N., Kaya, B., & Onal, A. E. (2009). Evaluation of the clinical efficacy of conservative treatment in the management of carpal tunnel syndrome. *Advances in Therapy, 26*(1), 107–116. doi:10.1007/s12325-008-0134-7

Chiappini, E., Mastrangelo, G., & Lazzeri, S. (2016). A case of acute osteomyelitis: An update on diagnosis and treatment. *International Journal of Environmental Research and Public Health, 13*(6). doi:10.3390/ijerph13060539

Choi, H. K., Atkinson, K., Karlson, E. W., & Curhan, G. (2005). Obesity, weight change, hypertension, diuretic use, and risk of gout in men: The health professionals follow-up study. *Archives of Internal Medicine, 165*(7), 742–748. doi:10.1001/archinte.165.7.742

Cosman, F., de Beur, S. J., LeBoff, M. S., Lewiecki, E. M., Tanner, B., Randall, S., …, National Osteoporosis. (2014). Clinician's guide to prevention and treatment of osteoporosis. *Osteoporosis International, 25*(10), 2359–2381. doi:10.1007/s00198-014-2794-2

Couppe, C., Svensson, R. B., Silbernagel, K. G., Langberg, H., & Magnusson, S. P. (2015). Eccentric or concentric exercises for the treatment of tendinopathies? *Journal of Orthopaedic and Sports Physical Therapy, 45*(11), 853–863. doi:10.2519/jospt.2015.5910

Dartnell, J., Ramachandran, M., & Katchburian, M. (2012). Haematogenous acute and subacute paediatric osteomyelitis: A systematic review of the literature. *Journal of Bone and Joint Surgery. British Volume, 94*(5), 584–595. doi:10.1302/0301-620X.94B5.28523

Giannoudis, P. V., Kontakis, G., Christoforakis, Z., Akula, M., Tosounidis, T., & Koutras, C. (2009). Management, complications and clinical results of femoral head fractures. *Injury, 40*(12), 1245–1251. doi:10.1016/j.injury.2009.10.024

Gollogly, S., Smith, J. T., & Campbell, R. M. (2004). Determining lung volume with three-dimensional reconstructions of CT scan data: A pilot study to evaluate the effects of expansion thoracoplasty on children with severe spinal deformities. *Journal of Pediatric Orthopedics, 24*(3), 323–328.

Hainer, B. L., Matheson, E., & Wilkes, R. T. (2014). Diagnosis, treatment, and prevention of gout. *American Family Physician, 90*(12), 831–836.

Hong, C. C., Nashi, N., Hey, H. W., Chee, Y. H., & Murphy, D. (2015). Clinically relevant heterotopic ossification after elbow fracture surgery: A risk factors study. *Orthopaedics and Traumatology: Surgery and Research, 101*(2), 209–213. doi:10.1016/j.otsr.2014.10.021

Horng, Y. S., Hsieh, S. F., Tu, Y. K., Lin, M. C., Horng, Y. S., & Wang, J. D. (2011). The comparative effectiveness of tendon and nerve gliding exercises in patients with carpal tunnel syndrome: A randomized trial. *American Journal of Physical Medicine and Rehabilitation, 90*(6), 435–442. doi:10.1097/PHM.0b013e318214eaaf

Hsieh, L. F., Hsu, W. C., Lin, Y. J., Wu, S. H., Chang, K. C., & Chang, H. L. (2013). Is ultrasound-guided injection more effective in chronic subacromial bursitis? *Medicine and Science in Sports and Exercise, 45*(12), 2205–2213. doi:10.1249/MSS.0b013e31829b183c

Kalunian, K. C. (2016). Current advances in therapies for osteoarthritis. *Current Opinion in Rheumatology, 28*(3), 246–250. doi:10.1097/BOR.0000000000000273

Kanis, J. A. (2002). Diagnosis of osteoporosis and assessment of fracture risk. *Lancet, 359*(9321), 1929–1936. doi:10.1016/S0140-6736(02)08761-5

Khanna, D., Fitzgerald, J. D., Khanna, P. P., Bae, S., Singh, M. K., Neogi, T., …, Terkeltaub, R. (2012). 2012 American College of Rheumatology guidelines for management of gout. Part 1: Systematic nonpharmacologic and pharmacologic therapeutic approaches to hyperuricemia. *Arthritis Care and Research, 64*(10), 1431–1446. doi:10.1002/acr.21772

Kim, S. D. (2015). Efficacy of tendon and nerve gliding exercises for carpal tunnel syndrome: A systematic review of randomized controlled trials. *Journal of Physical Therapy Science, 27*(8), 2645–2648. doi:10.1589/jpts.27.2645

Liu, F., Zhang, Q., Zhu, D., Li, Z., Li, J., Wang, B., …, Dong, J. (2015). Performance of positron emission tomography and positron emission tomography/computed tomography using fluorine-18-fluorodeoxyglucose for the diagnosis, staging, and recurrence assessment of bone sarcoma: A systematic review and meta-analysis. *Medicine (Baltimore), 94*(36), e1462. doi:10.1097/MD.0000000000001462

Lopes, A. D., Hespanhol Junior, L. C., Yeung, S. S., & Costa, L. O. (2012). What are the main running-related musculoskeletal injuries? A systematic review. *Sports Medicine, 42*(10), 891–905. doi:10.2165/11631170-000000000-00000

Maretty-Nielsen, K., Aggerholm-Pedersen, N., Keller, J., Safwat, A., Baerentzen, S., & Pedersen, A. B. (2013). Population-based Aarhus Sarcoma Registry: Validity, completeness of registration, and incidence of bone and soft tissue sarcomas in western Denmark. *Clinical Epidemiology, 5*, 45–56. doi:10.2147/CLEP.S41835

Nelson, H. D., Haney, E. M., Dana, T., Bougatsos, C., & Chou, R. (2010). Screening for osteoporosis: An update for the U.S. Preventive Services Task Force. *Annals of Internal Medicine, 153*(2), 99–111. doi:10.7326/0003-4819-153-2-201007200-00262

Pahys, J. M., Samdani, A. F., & Betz, R. R. (2009). Intraspinal anomalies in infantile idiopathic scoliosis: Prevalence and role of magnetic resonance imaging. *Spine (Phila Pa 1976), 34*(12), E434–E438. doi:10.1097/BRS.0b013e3181a2b49f

Pavlou, G., Salhab, M., Murugesan, L., Jallad, S., Petsatodis, G., West, R., & Tsiridis, E. (2012). Risk factors for heterotopic ossification in primary total hip arthroplasty. *Hip International, 22*(1), 50–55. doi:10.5301/HIP.2012.9057

Poultsides, L. A., Bedi, A., & Kelly, B. T. (2012). An algorithmic approach to mechanical hip pain. *HSS Journal, 8*(3), 213–224. doi:10.1007/s11420-012-9304-x

Reginster, J. Y., & Burlet, N. (2006). Osteoporosis: A still increasing prevalence. *Bone, 38*(2 Suppl 1), S4–S9. doi:10.1016/j.bone.2005.11.024

Riseborough, E. J., & Wynne-Davies, R. (1973). A genetic survey of idiopathic scoliosis in Boston, Massachusetts. *Journal of Bone and Joint Surgery (American Volume), 55*(5), 974–982.

Robinson, C. G., Polster, J. M., Reddy, C. A., Lyons, J. A., Evans, P. J., Lawton, J. N., ..., Suh, J. H. (2010). Postoperative single-fraction radiation for prevention of heterotopic ossification of the elbow. *International Journal of Radiation Oncology, Biology, Physics, 77*(5), 1493–1499. doi:10.1016/j.ijrobp.2009.06.072

Ryan, M., Bisset, L., & Newsham-West, R. (2015). Should we care about tendon structure? The disconnect between structure and symptoms in tendinopathy. *Journal of Orthopaedic and Sports Physical Therapy, 45*(11), 823–825. doi:10.2519/jospt.2015.0112

Scott, A., Backman, L. J., & Speed, C. (2015). Tendinopathy: Update on pathophysiology. *Journal of Orthopaedic and Sports Physical Therapy, 45*(11), 833–841. doi:10.2519/jospt.2015.5884

Shin, C. H., Yoo, W. J., Park, M. S., Kim, J. H., Choi, I. H., & Cho, T. J. (2016). Acetabular remodeling and role of osteotomy after closed reduction of developmental dysplasia of the hip. *Journal of Bone and Joint Surgery (American Volume), 98*(11), 952–957. doi:10.2106/JBJS.15.00992

Smith, T., Kirby, E., & Davies, L. (2014). A systematic review to determine the optimal type and dosage of land-based exercises for treating knee osteoarthritis. *Physical Therapy Reviews, 19*(2), 105–113.

The Pediatric Orthopedic Society of North America (POSNA). (2013). *Acute Osteomyelitis.* Retrieved from www.posna.org/education/StudyGuide/acuteOsteomyelitis.asp

Uchida, S., Utsunomiya, H., Mori, T., Taketa, T., Nishikino, S., Nakamura, T., & Sakai, A. (2016). Clinical and radiographic predictors for worsened clinical outcomes after hip arthroscopic labral preservation and capsular closure in developmental dysplasia of the hip. *American Journal of Sports Medicine, 44*(1), 28–38. doi:10.1177/0363546515604667

Vicenzino, B. (2015). Tendinopathy: Evidence-informed physical therapy clinical reasoning. *Journal of Orthopaedic and Sports Physical Therapy, 45*(11), 816–818. doi:10.2519/jospt.2015.0110

Yeo, A., & Ramachandran, M. (2014). Acute haematogenous osteomyelitis in children. *British Medical Journal, 348*, g66. doi:10.1136/bmj.g66

Zhang, X., Du, G., Xu, Y., Li, X., Fan, W., Chen, J., ..., Liu, P. (2016). Inhibition of notch signaling pathway prevents cholestatic liver fibrosis by decreasing the differentiation of hepatic progenitor cells into cholangiocytes. *Laboratory Investigation, 96*(3), 350–360. doi:10.1038/labinvest.2015.149

Zhu, Y., Pandya, B. J., & Choi, H. K. (2011). Prevalence of gout and hyperuricemia in the US general population: The National Health and Nutrition Examination Survey 2007–2008. *Arthritis and Rheumatism, 63*(10), 3136–3141. doi:10.1002/art.30520

HEMATOLOGIC DISORDERS

ANEMIA

Anemia is a condition associated with lower than normal levels of erythrocytes in the blood. There are several types of anemia, including aplastic, iron deficiency, and pernicious.

Causes

Aplastic Anemia

- Congenital or acquired
- Autoimmune reactions or other severe disease (hepatitis)
- Drugs, radiation, and toxic agents

Iron Deficiency Anemia

- Inadequate iron intake or iron malabsorption
- Blood loss
- Pregnancy, which diverts maternal iron to fetus
- Intravascular hemolysis-induced hemoglobinuria or paroxysmal nocturnal hemoglobinuria
- Trauma by prosthetic heart valve or vena cava filters

Pernicious Anemia

- Vitamin B_{12} deficiency due to lack of intrinsic factor in stomach lining
- Genetic predisposition and age over 60
- Immunologically related disorder
- Partial gastrectomy

Pathophysiology

Aplastic anemia usually develops when damaged or destroyed stem cells inhibit blood cell production. Less commonly, damage to bone marrow microvasculature creates an unfavorable environment for cell growth and maturation.

Iron deficiency anemia occurs when the supply of iron is inadequate for optimal formation of red blood cells (RBCs); the result is microcytic (smaller-sized) cells with pale color (hypochromic) on staining. Body stores of iron, including plasma iron, become depleted, and the concentration of serum transferrin, which binds with and transports iron, decreases. Insufficient iron stores lead to a depleted RBC mass with low hemoglobin (Hb) concentration and impaired oxygen-carrying capacity.

Decreased production of hydrochloric acid in the stomach and a deficiency of intrinsic factor characterize pernicious anemia. The resulting vitamin B_{12} deficiency inhibits cell growth, leading to the production of scant, deformed, macrocytic (larger-sized) RBCs having poor oxygen-carrying capacity.

COMPLICATIONS
Aplastic Anemia
- Life-threatening hemorrhage
- Major infection

Iron Deficiency Anemia
- Infection and pneumonia
- Pica and lead poisoning in children
- Bleeding
- Hemochromatosis (from overreplacement of iron)

Pernicious Anemia
- Psychotic behavior
- Neurologic disability

Signs and Symptoms

Although fatigue, weakness, pallor, and tachycardia, chest pain, and shortness of breath may occur in individuals with all types of anemia, the following signs and symptoms have been more closely associated with one of the types of anemia.

Aplastic Anemia

- Progressive weakness, fatigue, and altered level of consciousness
- Ecchymosis, pallor, petechiae, and hemorrhage from the mucous membranes or into the retina (may result in visual disturbances)
- Fever, oral and rectal ulcers, and sore throat
- Bibasilar crackles and tachycardia

Iron Deficiency Anemia

- Spoon-shaped, brittle nails
- Unusual craving for nonnutritious items (for example, dirt, ice, or chalk)
- Uncomfortable tingling or crawling feeling in the legs
- Burning or smooth tongue, with sores at the corners of the mouth

Pernicious Anemia

- Weakness, numbness, and tingling of extremities in areas that would be covered by socks or gloves
- Gingival bleeding and tongue inflammation
- Disturbed position sense, lack of coordination, impaired fine finger movement, and altered vision, taste, and hearing
- Irritability, poor memory, headache, depression, delirium, and ataxia; changes may have occurred before treatment

Diagnostic Test Results

Aplastic Anemia

- Laboratory studies show 1 million/mm³ or fewer RBCs of normal color and size with a very low absolute reticulocyte count, elevated serum iron level, normal or slightly reduced total iron-binding capacity, and decreased platelet, neutrophil, and lymphocyte counts.
- Bone marrow biopsy may show severely hypocellular or aplastic marrow and depression of RBCs and precursors.

PERIPHERAL BLOOD SMEAR IN APLASTIC ANEMIA

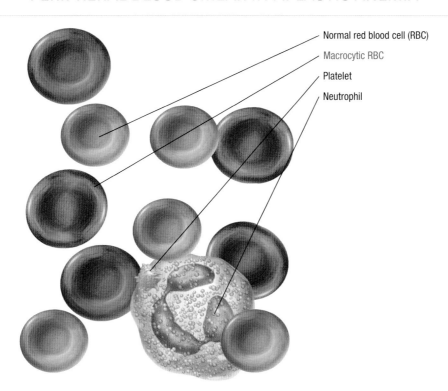

Normal red blood cell (RBC)

Macrocytic RBC

Platelet

Neutrophil

PERIPHERAL BLOOD SMEAR IN IRON DEFICIENCY ANEMIA

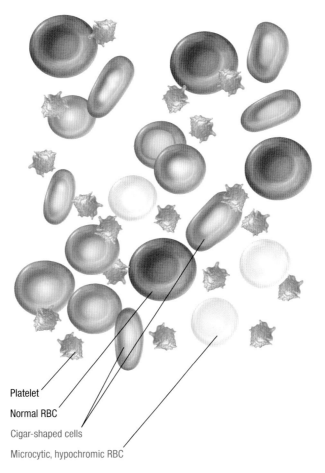

Platelet

Normal RBC

Cigar-shaped cells

Microcytic, hypochromic RBC

Iron Deficiency Anemia

- Laboratory analysis reveals low hematocrit, low Hb, low serum ferritin and serum iron with high iron-binding capacity (TIBC), low RBC count with microcytic (low MCV) and hypochromic cells (low MCHC) due to decreased mean corpuscular Hb., and depleted or absent iron stores.
- Bone marrow studies show hyperplasia of precursor cells.

Pernicious Anemia

- Laboratory analysis shows low hematocrit (Hct), low Hb, low RBC count, mean corpuscular volume (MCV) greater than 120 mm^3, and serum vitamin B_{12} less than 0.1 $\mu g/mL$.
- Schilling test evaluates excretion of radiolabeled vitamin B_{12}.
- Gastric analysis shows the absence of free hydrochloric acid after histamine or pentagastrin injection.
- Bone marrow aspiration shows erythroid hyperplasia with increased megaloblasts but few normally developing RBCs.
- Antibody testing reveals intrinsic factor antibodies and anti-parietal cell antibodies.

Treatment

Aplastic Anemia

- Blood or platelet transfusion
- Bone marrow transplantation
- Measures to prevent infection and antibiotics
- Respiratory support with oxygen
- Corticosteroids, marrow-stimulating agents, immunosuppressive agents, and colony-stimulating factors

Iron Deficiency Anemia

- Oral or parenteral iron
- Blood transfusions in cases of severe anemia

Pernicious Anemia

- Early parenteral vitamin B_{12} replacement
- After initial response, lifelong monthly dose of vitamin B_{12}
- Blood transfusions in cases of severe anemia

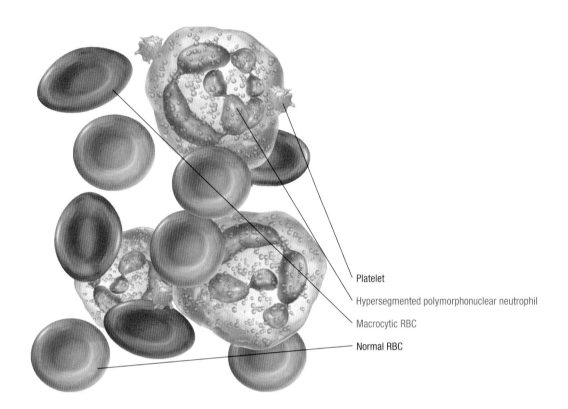

Platelet

Hypersegmented polymorphonuclear neutrophil

Macrocytic RBC

Normal RBC

SICKLE CELL ANEMIA

A congenital hemolytic anemia that occurs primarily, but not exclusively, in blacks, sickle cell anemia results from a defective hemoglobin molecule (Hb S) that causes RBCs to become sickle-shaped. Such cells clog capillaries and impair circulation, resulting in chronic ill health (fatigue, dyspnea on exertion, swollen joints), periodic crises, long-term complications, and early death.

If both parents are carriers of sickle cell trait (or another hemoglobinopathy), each child has a 25% chance of developing sickle cell anemia. Approximately 1 out of every 500 blacks has sickle cell anemia. The defective Hb S–producing gene may have persisted because, in areas where malaria is endemic, the heterozygous sickle cell trait provides resistance to malaria and is actually beneficial.

AGE ALERT
Half of patients with sickle cell anemia once died by their early 20s; few lived to middle age. Earlier diagnosis and more effective treatment have improved the prognosis of sickle cell anemia. Most patients now survive well into adulthood.

Causes

- Homozygous inheritance of the gene that produces Hb S
- Heterozygous inheritance of this gene results in sickle cell trait, which is usually asymptomatic

Pathophysiology

Hb S becomes insoluble whenever hypoxia occurs. As a result, these RBCs become rigid and elongated, forming a crescent or sickle shape. Such sickling can produce hemolysis (cell destruction). In addition, these altered cells make blood more viscous and tend to accumulate in smaller blood vessels and capillaries. The result is loss of normal circulation, swelling, tissue infarctions, and pain. Furthermore, the blockage causes anoxic changes that lead to further sickling and obstruction. Each patient with sickle cell anemia has a different hypoxic threshold and particular factors that trigger a sickle cell crisis. Illness, exposure to cold, stress, acidotic states, or a pathophysiologic process that pulls water out of the sickle cells precipitates a crisis in most patients. The blockages then cause anoxic changes that lead to further sickling and obstruction.

COMPLICATIONS
- Chronic obstructive pulmonary disease
- Heart failure and heart murmurs
- Splenic infarction and splenomegaly (splenic sequestration)
- Retinopathy
- Nephropathy
- Major organ infarction
- Stroke
- Acute chest syndrome
- Pulmonary infarctions, which may result in cor pulmonale
- Ischemic leg ulcers (especially around the ankles)
- Increased susceptibility to infection
- Iron overload from recurrent blood transfusions

Signs and Symptoms

- Tachycardia, cardiomegaly, and systolic and diastolic murmurs
- Chronic fatigue and unexplained dyspnea or dyspnea on exertion
- Joint pain
- Delayed growth
- Irritability in children

Occlusive or Infarctive Crises

- Severe abdominal, thoracic, muscular, or bone pain
- Worsening jaundice, dark urine

Aplastic Crisis

- Pallor
- Lethargy, sleepiness, and coma
- Dyspnea
- Markedly decreased bone marrow activity and RBC hemolysis

Diagnostic Test Results

- Electrophoresis shows Hb S.
- Stained peripheral blood smear shows the presence of sickled cells.
- Laboratory studies show low RBC count, elevated white blood cell (WBC) and platelet counts, decreased erythrocyte sedimentation rate, increased serum iron levels, decreased RBC survival, and reticulocytosis.
- Lateral chest X-ray shows "Lincoln log" deformity in the vertebrae of many adults and some adolescents.

Treatment

- Prophylactic penicillin before age 4 months
- Oral hydroxyurea to reduce the number of painful crises
- Packed RBC transfusions for severe anemia
- Sedation
- Analgesics
- Oxygen
- Oral or I.V. fluids
- Folic acid supplements
- Antibiotics
- Infectious disease prevention, through immunizations, proper food preparation, and frequent handwashing
- Bone marrow-stem cell transplant

PERIPHERAL BLOOD SMEAR IN SICKLE CELL ANEMIA

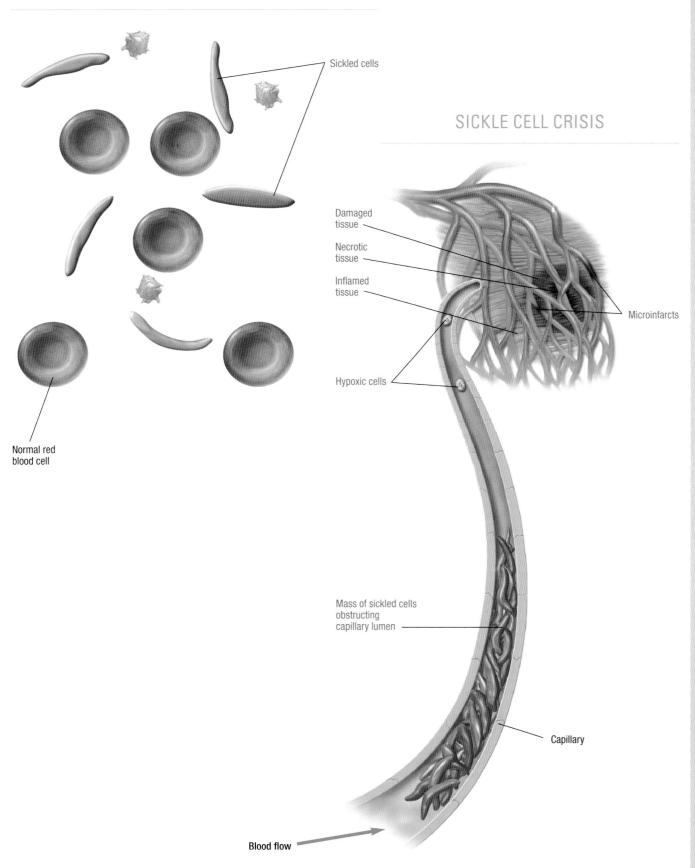

Sickled cells

Normal red blood cell

SICKLE CELL CRISIS

Damaged tissue

Necrotic tissue

Inflamed tissue

Microinfarcts

Hypoxic cells

Mass of sickled cells obstructing capillary lumen

Capillary

Blood flow

THALASSEMIA

Thalassemia, a group of hereditary hemolytic anemias, is characterized by defective synthesis in the polypeptide chains of the protein component of Hb. RBC synthesis is also impaired.

Thalassemias are most common in people of Mediterranean ancestry (especially Italian and Greek, who develop the form called *beta-thalassemia*). People whose ancestors originated in Africa, southern China, southeast Asia, and India develop the form called *alpha-thalassemia*, which reflects deletion of one or more of four Hb genes. Prognosis varies with the number of deleted genes.

In beta-thalassemia, the most common form of this disorder, synthesis of the beta-polypeptide chain is defective. It occurs in three clinical forms: *major*, *intermedia*, and *minor*. The severity of the resulting anemia depends on whether the patient is homozygous or heterozygous for the thalassemic trait. The prognosis varies:

- thalassemia major — patients seldom survive to adulthood
- thalassemia intermedia — children develop normally into adulthood; puberty usually delayed
- thalassemia minor — normal life span.

Causes

Beta-Thalassemia

- Thalassemia major or intermedia — homozygous inheritance of a partially dominant autosomal gene
- Thalassemia minor — heterozygous inheritance of the same gene

Alpha-Thalassemia

- Deletion of one or more of four genes

Pathophysiology

In beta-thalassemia, total or partial deficiency of beta-polypeptide chain production impairs Hb synthesis and results in continual production of fetal Hb beyond the neonatal period. Normally, immunoglobulin synthesis switches from gamma- to beta-polypeptides at the time of birth. This conversion doesn't happen in thalassemic infants. Their RBCs are hypochromic and microcytic. In alpha-thalassemia, a much reduced quantity of alpha-globin chains is produced.

COMPLICATIONS
- Pathologic fractures and bone deformities
- Cardiac arrhythmias and heart failure
- Iron overload from multiple blood transfusion
- Growth and developmental delays in children
- Infections
- Splenomegaly

Signs and Symptoms

Thalassemia Major

- At birth — no symptoms
- Infants ages 3 to 6 months — pallor; yellow skin and sclera
- Infants ages 6 to 12 months — severe anemia, bone abnormalities, failure to thrive, and life-threatening complications
- Splenomegaly or hepatomegaly, with abdominal enlargement; frequent infections; bleeding tendencies (especially nosebleeds); anorexia
- Small body, large head (characteristic features); possible mental retardation
- Facial features similar to Down syndrome in infants, due to thickened bone at the base of the nose from bone marrow hyperactivity

Thalassemia Intermedia

- Some degree of anemia, jaundice, and splenomegaly
- Signs of hemosiderosis, such as hemoptysis, iron deficiency anemia, or paroxysmal nocturnal hemoglobinemia — due to increased intestinal absorption of iron

Thalassemia Minor

- Usually produces no symptoms
- Mild anemia, often overlooked

Alpha-Thalassemia Syndromes

- Reflect the number of gene deletions present
- Range from asymptomatic to incompatible with life

Diagnostic Test Results

- Laboratory analysis reveals low RBC and Hb level, microcytosis, and high reticulocyte count; elevated bilirubin and urinary and fecal urobilinogen levels; and low serum folate level.
- Peripheral blood smear shows target cells; microcytes; pale, nucleated RBCs; and marked anisocytosis.
- Skull and long bone X-rays show thinning and widening of the marrow space due to overactive bone marrow, granular appearance of bones of skull and vertebrae, areas of osteoporosis in long bones, and deformed (rectangular or biconvex) phalanges.
- Quantitative Hb studies (hemoglobin electrophoresis) reveal significantly increased fetal Hb level and slightly increased Hb A_2 level.
- Family studies of DNA analysis may be conducted to evaluate carrier status and confirm mutations in the alpha- or beta-globin–producing genes.

Thalassemia Intermedia

- Peripheral blood smear shows hypochromic, microcytic RBCs (less severe than in thalassemia major).

Thalassemia Minor

- Peripheral blood smear shows hypochromic, microcytic RBCs.
- Quantitative Hb studies (hemoglobin electrophoresis) reveal significantly increased Hb A_2 level and moderately increased fetal Hb level.

Treatment

- Iron supplements contraindicated in all forms of thalassemia

Beta-Thalassemia Major: Essentially Supportive

- Prompt treatment with appropriate antibiotics for infections
- Folic acid supplements

- Transfusions of packed RBCs to increase Hb levels (used judiciously to minimize iron overload)
- Splenectomy and bone marrow transplantation (effectiveness hasn't been confirmed)

Beta-Thalassemia Intermedia and Thalassemia Minor

- No treatment

Alpha-Thalassemia

- Blood transfusions
- In utero transfusion for hydrops fetalis

PERIPHERAL BLOOD SMEAR IN THALASSEMIA MAJOR

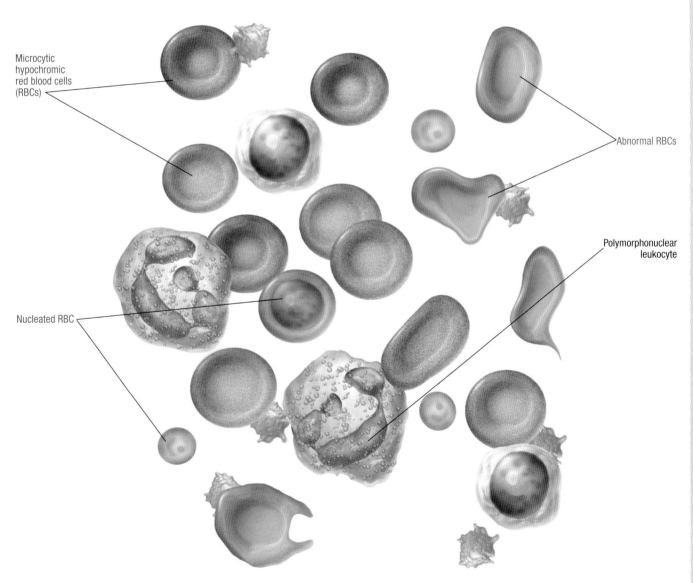

Microcytic hypochromic red blood cells (RBCs)

Abnormal RBCs

Polymorphonuclear leukocyte

Nucleated RBC

POLYCYTHEMIA VERA

Polycythemia vera is a chronic disorder characterized by increased RBC mass, erythrocytosis, leukocytosis, thrombocytosis, elevated Hb level, and low or normal plasma volume. This disease is also known as *primary polycythemia, erythremia,* or *polycythemia rubra vera.* It occurs most commonly among Jewish males of European descent.

AGE ALERT
Polycythemia vera usually occurs between ages 40 and 60; it seldom affects children.

Prognosis depends on age at diagnosis, treatment, and complications. In untreated polycythemia, mortality is high and associated with thrombosis, hyperviscosity, or expanded blood volume. Additionally, myeloid metaplasia (ectopic hematopoiesis in the liver and spleen) with myelofibrosis (fibrous tissue in bone marrow) and acute leukemia may develop.

Causes

Unknown, but probably related to a clonal stem cell defect. Nearly all patients have a mutation on the JAK2 gene, which results in altered signal within the Janus kinase pathway.

Pathophysiology

In polycythemia vera, uncontrolled and rapid cellular reproduction and maturation cause proliferation or hyperplasia of all bone marrow cells (panmyelosis). Increased RBC mass makes the blood abnormally viscous and inhibits blood flow through the microcirculation. Diminished blood flow and thrombocytosis set the stage for intravascular thrombosis.

CLINICAL TIP
Secondary polycythemia is excessive production of circulating RBCs due to hypoxia, tumor, or disease. It occurs in approximately 2 of every 100,000 people living at or near sea level; the incidence increases among those living at high altitudes.

Spurious polycythemia is characterized by an increased hematocrit but decreased plasma volume. It usually affects the middle-aged population and is more common in men than in women. Causes include dehydration, hypertension, thromboembolic disease, or elevated serum cholesterol or uric acid.

COMPLICATIONS
- Renal calculi
- Abdominal thrombosis
- Hemorrhage
- Stroke or myocardial infarction
- Peptic ulcer disease
- Acute myelogenous leukemia
- Myelofibrosis (bone marrow scarring, hepato- and splenomegaly, and severe anemia)

Signs and Symptoms

- Feeling of fullness in the head, dizziness, and headache
- Ruddy cyanosis (plethora) of nose
- Clubbing of digits
- Painful pruritus
- Ecchymosis
- Hepatosplenomegaly
- Alterations in vision
- Abdominal fullness
- Cramping in legs while walking (intermittent claudication)
- Chest pain (angina pectoris)

Diagnostic Test Results

- Laboratory studies reveal:
  - increased RBC mass
  - increased hemoglobin (greater than 18.5 g/dL in men or greater than 16.5 g/dL in women)
  - normal arterial oxygen saturation
  - increased uric acid level
  - increased blood histamine levels
  - decreased serum iron concentration
  - decreased or absent urinary erythropoietin.
- Bone marrow biopsy shows excess production of myeloid stem cells.

Treatment

- Phlebotomy to reduce RBC mass and keep hematocrit below 45% in men and 42% in women
- Low-dose aspirin
- Myelosuppressive therapy with hydroxyurea or a Janus kinase inhibitor. Interferon alpha has been used off-label

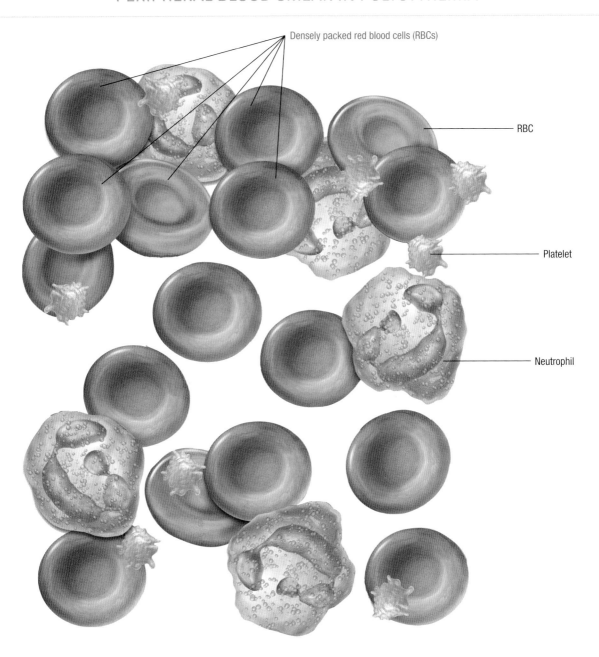

Densely packed red blood cells (RBCs)

RBC

Platelet

Neutrophil

DISSEMINATED INTRAVASCULAR COAGULATION

Disseminated intravascular coagulation (DIC) occurs as a complication of diseases and conditions that accelerate clotting. DIC causes small blood vessel occlusion, organ necrosis, depletion of circulating clotting factors and platelets, activation of the fibrinolytic system, and consequent severe hemorrhage. Clotting in the microcirculation usually affects the kidneys and extremities but may occur in the brain, lungs, pituitary and adrenal glands, and GI mucosa. DIC, also called *consumption coagulopathy* or *defibrination syndrome*, is generally an acute condition but may be chronic in cancer patients (Trousseau's syndrome). Prognosis depends on early detection and treatment, the severity of the hemorrhage, and treatment of the underlying disease.

Causes

Etiology unclear (however, in many patients, the triggering mechanisms may be the entrance of foreign protein into the circulation and vascular endothelial injury). Several underlying etiologies may lead to the development of DIC, but the coagulation disorder is generally initiated through (a) a systemic inflammatory response, which leads to activation of inflammatory mediators (for example, cytokines) and subsequent activation of coagulation pathways or (b) a release or exposure to materials that promote coagulation in the circulatory system.

DIC may result from:

- infections — gram-negative or gram-positive septicemia; viral, fungal, rickettsial, and protozoal infection (malaria)
- obstetric complications — abruptio placenta, amniotic fluid embolism, retained dead fetus, septic abortion, and eclampsia
- neoplasia — acute leukemia, metastatic carcinoma, and especially adenocarcinoma
- necrosis — extensive burns or trauma, brain tissue destruction, transplant rejection, and hepatic necrosis
- other causes — heatstroke, shock, poisonous snakebite, cirrhosis, fat embolism, incompatible blood transfusion, cardiac arrest, surgery necessitating cardiopulmonary bypass, giant hemangioma, severe venous thrombosis, and purpura fulminans.

Pathophysiology

Regardless of how DIC begins, the typical accelerated clotting results in generalized activation of prothrombin and a consequent excess of thrombin. The thrombin converts fibrinogen to fibrin, producing fibrin clots in the microcirculation. This process uses huge amounts of coagulation factors (especially fibrinogen, prothrombin, platelets, and factors V and VIII), causing hypofibrinogenemia, hypoprothrombinemia, thrombocytopenia, and deficiencies in factors V and VIII. Circulating thrombin also activates the fibrinolytic system, which dissolves fibrin clots into fibrin degradation products. Hemorrhage may be mostly the result of the anticoagulant activity of fibrin degradation products as well as depletion of plasma coagulation factors.

COMPLICATIONS

- Renal failure
- Hepatic damage
- Stroke or intracerebral hemorrhage
- Ischemic bowel
- Respiratory dysfunction or failure
- Gangrene and loss of digits
- Shock and coma
- Death

Signs and Symptoms

- Abnormal bleeding:
  - Cutaneous oozing of serum, bleeding from surgical or I.V. sites, and bleeding from the GI tract
  - Petechiae or blood blisters (purpura), epistaxis, and hemoptysis
- Cyanosis; cold, mottled fingers and toes
- Severe muscle, back, abdominal, and chest pain
- Nausea and vomiting (may be a manifestation of GI bleeding)
- Vital sign changes consistent with shock
- Confusion
- Dyspnea
- Oliguria
- Hematuria

Diagnostic Test Results

Laboratory analysis reveals:

- complete blood count showing decreased hemoglobin levels (less than 10 g/dL) and decreased serum platelet count (less than 100,000/mm³)
- prolonged prothrombin time [PT] (more than 15 seconds)
- prolonged activated partial thromboplastin time [aPTT] (more than 80 seconds)
- decreased serum fibrinogen level (less than 150 mg/dL)
- positive D-dimer test (specific fibrinogen test for DIC) at less than 1:8 dilution
- increased fibrin degradation products (commonly greater than 45 µg/mL, or positive at less than 1:100 dilution)
- diminished blood clotting factors V and VIII (and factor VII in some studies)
- elevated blood urea nitrogen (greater than 25 mg/dL) and elevated serum creatinine levels (greater than 1.3 mg/dL).

Treatment

- Prompt recognition and treatment of underlying disorder
- Blood transfusions: fresh frozen plasma, platelet, packed red blood cell transfusions, or cryoprecipitate to support hemostasis in active bleeding
- I.V. fluids
- Vasopressors, such as dopamine
- Inhibitors of fibrinolysis, such as epsilon-aminocaproic acid
- Unfractionated or low molecular weight heparin in early stages to prevent microclotting and as a last resort in hemorrhage (controversial in acute DIC after sepsis)

NORMAL CLOTTING PROCESS

Blood vessel walls

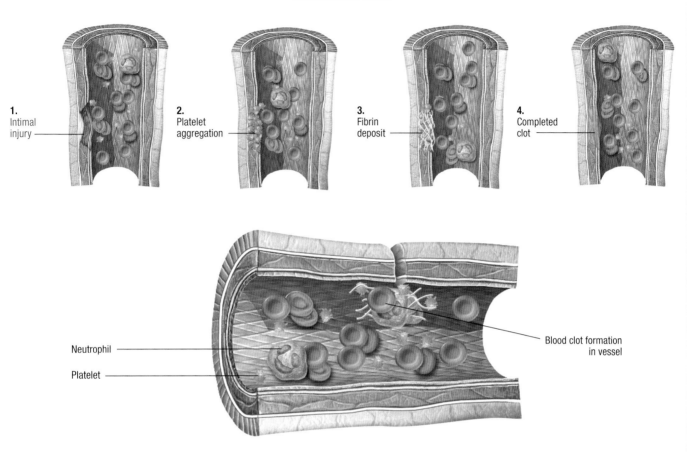

1. Intimal injury

2. Platelet aggregation

3. Fibrin deposit

4. Completed clot

Neutrophil

Platelet

Blood clot formation in vessel

UNDERSTANDING DISSEMINATED INTRAVASCULAR COAGULATION

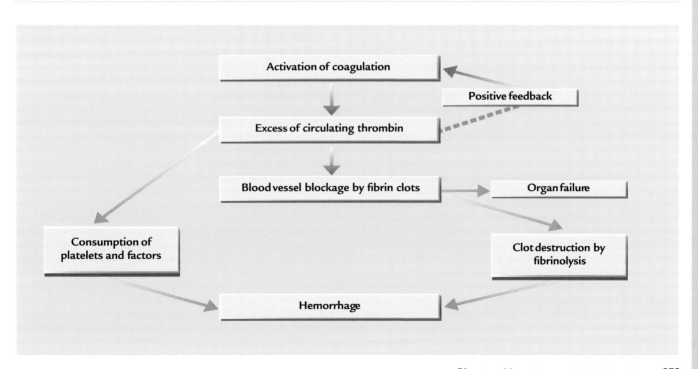

Activation of coagulation

Positive feedback

Excess of circulating thrombin

Blood vessel blockage by fibrin clots

Organ failure

Consumption of platelets and factors

Clot destruction by fibrinolysis

Hemorrhage

HEMOPHILIA

Hemophilia, a hereditary bleeding disorder, results from a deficiency of specific clotting factors. The severity of bleeding and the prognosis vary with the degree of deficiency, or nonfunction, and the site of bleeding. Hemophilia occurs in 20 of 100,000 male births.

There are several types of haemophilia, but two most common types are hemophilia A and hemophilia B. Hemophilia A (classic hemophilia) results from a deficiency of factor VIII. More common than type B, it affects more than 80% of all hemophiliacs and is the most common X-linked genetic disease. Hemophilia B (Christmas disease) affects approximately 15% of all hemophiliacs and results from a deficiency of factor IX. Hemophilia C results from a deficiency of factor X.

Advances in treatment have greatly improved the prognosis for hemophiliacs, many of whom live normal life spans. Surgical procedures can be done safely at special treatment centers under the guidance of a hematologist.

Causes

Hemophilia types A and B: X-linked recessive genetic traits. Hemophilia A and B almost always occurs in boys and is passed from women who are hemophilia carriers to their male children. Hemophilia C can be passed to offspring from either parent, and although it is much less prevalent, it may occur in both boys and girls.

Pathophysiology

Hemophilia is an X-linked recessive genetic disease causing abnormal bleeding because of a specific clotting factor malfunction. Factors VIII and IX are components of the intrinsic clotting pathway; factor IX is an essential factor and factor VIII is a critical cofactor that accelerates the activation of factor X by several thousandfold. Excessive bleeding occurs when these clotting factors are reduced by more than 75%. A deficiency or nonfunction of factor VIII causes hemophilia A, and a deficiency or nonfunction of factor IX causes hemophilia B.

Hemophilia may be severe, moderate, or mild, depending on the degree of activation of clotting factors. Patients with severe disease have no detectable factor VIII or factor IX activity. Moderately afflicted patients have 1% to 4% of normal clotting activity, and mildly afflicted patients have 5% to 25% of normal clotting activity.

A patient with hemophilia forms a platelet plug at a bleeding site, but clotting factor deficiency impairs the ability to form a stable fibrin clot. Bleeding occurs primarily into large joints, especially after trauma or surgery. Delayed bleeding is more common than immediate hemorrhage.

COMPLICATIONS
- Intracranial bleeding, shock, and death
- Neuropathies
- Paresthesia
- Muscle atrophy
- Ischemia and gangrene of the major vessels
- Adverse reactions to clotting factor therapies
- Hepatitis or other infectious disease related to blood product infusion

Signs and Symptoms

- Spontaneous bleeding in severe hemophilia (prolonged or excessive bleeding after circumcision is often the first sign)
- Excessive or continued bleeding or bruising after minor trauma or surgery
- Large subcutaneous and deep I.M. hematomas due to mild trauma
- Prolonged bleeding in mild hemophilia after major trauma or surgery, but no spontaneous bleeding after minor trauma
- Pain, swelling, and tenderness due to bleeding into joints (especially weight-bearing joints)
- Internal bleeding, often manifested as abdominal, chest, or flank pain
- Hematuria
- Hematemesis or tarry stools
- Epistaxis without a known cause

Diagnostic Test Results

- Specific coagulation factor assays show the type and severity of hemophilia; most children are diagnosed by age 2.
- Laboratory analysis reveals low serum factor VIII activity of normal and prolonged aPTT (hemophilia A).
- Laboratory analysis reveals deficient factor IX and normal factor VIII levels (hemophilia B).

Treatment

- Regular infusions or intranasal administration of desmopressin (DDAVP) or lyophilized factor VIII or IX to increase clotting factor levels and to permit normal hemostasis levels
- Factor IX concentrate during bleeding episodes (hemophilia B)
- Aminocaproic acid (Amicar) for oral bleeding (inhibits plasminogen activator substances)
- Prophylactic DDAVP before dental procedures or minor surgery to release stored von Willebrand's factor and factor VIII (to reduce bleeding)
- Fresh frozen plasma
- Immunization with hepatitis A and B vaccine
- Prompt first aid for minor cuts; fibrin sealants may be applied to promote healing (fibrin sealants are helpful for patients undergoing dental procedures)

Normal **Hemophilia**

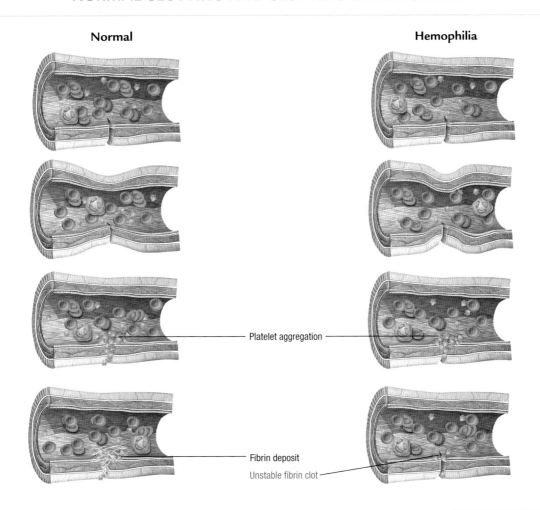

Platelet aggregation

Fibrin deposit

Unstable fibrin clot

CLINICAL TIP

X-LINKED RECESSIVE INHERITANCE

The diagram shows the children of a normal parent and those of a parent with a recessive gene on the X chromosome (shown by an open dot). All daughters of an affected male will be carriers. The son of a female carrier may inherit a recessive gene on the X chromosome and be affected by the disease. Unaffected sons can't transmit the disorder.

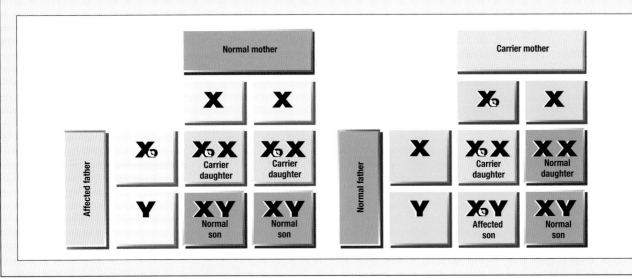

HODGKIN'S DISEASE

Hodgkin's disease is a neoplastic disease characterized by painless, progressive enlargement of lymph nodes, spleen, and other lymphoid tissue resulting from proliferation of lymphocytes, histiocytes, eosinophils, and Reed-Sternberg giant cells. Untreated, Hodgkin's disease follows a variable but relentlessly progressive and, ultimately, fatal course. With appropriate treatment, the 5-year survival rate for stage I and II is approximately 90% and for stage III is 80%.

Causes

Unknown; however, viral etiology is suspected (Epstein-Barr virus is a leading candidate)

AGE ALERT
Hodgkin's disease is most common in young adults, and more common in males than in females. Incidence peaks in two age-groups: ages 15 to 38 and after age 50 (in Japan, where it occurs exclusively among people over age 50).

Pathophysiology

Hodgkin's disease is characterized by proliferation of a tumor in which only a small proportion of the cells are malignant and most are normal lymphocytes. The characteristic malignant cells — called Reed-Sternberg cells — are most likely multinucleated, giant-cell mutations of the T lymphocyte. Infiltration of the nodes with eosinophils and plasma cells is associated with lymph node necrosis and fibrosis.

COMPLICATIONS
- Secondary cancers
- Cardiac disease
- Liver failure
- Pulmonary disease
- Infertility
- Thyroid disorders

These long-term complications are most commonly associated with the treatment for the disease (radiation and chemotherapy), rather than the disease itself.

Signs and Symptoms

- Painless swelling in one of lymph nodes in the neck, axilla, or groin
- Persistent fever
- Night sweats
- Fatigue
- Weight loss
- Malaise
- Pruritus
- Extremity pain
- Nerve irritation
- Absence of pulse due to rapid enlargement of lymph nodes
- Pericardial friction rub
- Pericardial effusion
- Neck vein engorgement
- Enlargement of retroperitoneal nodes, spleen, and liver resulting in a feeling of abdominal fullness

Diagnostic Test Results

- Lymph node biopsy confirms presence of Reed-Sternberg cells (abnormal B lymphocytes), nodular fibrosis, and necrosis.
- Bone marrow, liver, mediastinal, lymph node, and spleen biopsies reveal histologic presence of Reed-Sternberg cells.
- Chest X-ray, abdominal computed tomography (CT) scan, lung scan, bone scan, and lymphangiography detect lymph and organ involvement.
- PET scan (has replaced some of the testing listed above)
- Hematologic tests show:
  - mild to severe normocytic anemia
  - normochromic anemia
  - elevated, normal, or reduced WBC count
  - differential with any combination of neutrophilia, lymphocytopenia, monocytosis, and eosinophilia.
- Elevated serum alkaline phosphatase indicates bone or liver involvement.

Tests of heart and lung function may be ordered as a baseline prior to initiating chemotherapy (MUGA [multigated acquisition] scan and pulmonary function tests)

Treatment

- Chemotherapy, radiation, or both (appropriate to stage of the disease — based on histologic interpretation and clinical staging) are considered standard therapy
- Concomitant antiemetics, sedatives, or antidiarrheals to combat adverse GI effects
- Autologous bone marrow (stem cell) transplant combined with high-dose chemotherapy
- Immunotherapy (for those who relapse or do not respond to traditional chemotherapy and radiation)
- Autologous peripheral blood sternal transfusions, as an alternative to autologous stem cell transplantation

Cotswold Modification of Ann Arbor Staging System

STAGE	AREA OF INVOLVEMENT
I	Single lymph node group
II	Multiple lymph node groups on same side of diaphragm
II	Multiple lymph node groups on both sides of diaphragm
IV	Multiple extranodal sites or lymph nodes and extranodal disease
X	Bulk > 10 cm
E	Extranodal extension or single, isolated site of extranodal disease
A/B	B symptoms: weight loss > 10%, fever, drenching night sweats

NON-HODGKIN'S LYMPHOMAS

Like Hodgkin's lymphoma, non-Hodgkin's lymphomas refer to a heterogeneous group of malignant diseases originating in lymph nodes and other lymphoid tissue. Non-Hodgkin's lymphomas are three times more common than Hodgkin's disease. The incidence is increasing, especially in patients with autoimmune disorders and those receiving immunosuppressant treatment. The 10-year survival rate for non-Hodgkin's lymphoma is 59%.

Causes

- Direct cause unknown
- Possible viral etiology
- Exposure to chemical toxins — benzene, pesticides, and herbicides
- Exposure to radiation
- Deficiencies or abnormalities of the immune system (HIV, immunosuppressant therapies, and autoimmune diseases)

AGE ALERT
Malignant lymphomas occur in all age-groups, but incidence rises with age (median age is 50). The American Cancer Society notes that 95% of all cases occur in adults and nearly one-half of all those affected are older than age 66.

Pathophysiology

Non-Hodgkin's lymphoma is pathophysiologically similar to Hodgkin's disease, but Reed-Sternberg cells aren't present, and the specific mechanism of lymph node destruction is different. Both B lymphocytes and T lymphocytes can develop into lymphoma cells and different types of lymphomas can develop from each type of lymphocyte depending on how mature the cells were when they became cancerous. Non-Hodgkin's lymphomas have been most recently classified by a system that includes microscopic features of tissue architecture and patterns of infiltration, chromosomal features of the cells, and the presence of specific proteins on the cells' surface.

COMPLICATIONS
- Hypercalcemia
- Hyperuricemia
- Lymphomatosis
- Meningitis
- Anemia
- Increased intracranial pressure
- Respiratory problems
- Liver and kidney problems
- Increased risk of infection
- Infertility related to chemotherapy and radiation
- Second cancers related to chemotherapy and radiation

Signs and Symptoms

Signs and symptoms will vary depending on the location of the cancer, but common signs and symptoms include:

- painless, rubbery enlargement of lymphatic tissue (lymphadenopathy), usually cervical or supraclavicular nodes
- abdominal fullness or swelling
- chest pain, pressure, or shortness of breath
- fever
- night sweats
- fatigue
- weight loss
- anemia.

In Children
- Cervical nodes usually affected first
- Dyspnea and coughing

In Advancing Disease
- Symptoms specific to involved structure
- Systemic complaints — fatigue, malaise, weight loss, fever, and night sweats

Diagnostic Test Results

- Lymph node biopsy (excisional or fine needle aspiration) reveals cell type.
- Biopsy of tonsils, bone marrow, liver, bowel, or skin reveals malignant cells.
- Pleural or peritoneal fluid sampling reveals malignant cells.
- Complete blood count detects anemia.
- Uric acid level is elevated or normal.
- Lactate dehydrogenase (LDH) is often increased in patient with lymphomas.
- Blood chemistry shows elevated serum calcium levels if bone lesions are present.
- Bone and chest X-rays, lymphangiography, liver and spleen scans, abdominal **or chest** CT scan, PET scans, gallium scans, and excretory urography show evidence of metastasis.
- Tests of heart and lung function may be ordered as a baseline prior to initiating chemotherapy (MUGA [multigated acquisition] scan and pulmonary function tests).

Treatment

- Radiation therapy — mainly in the early, localized stage of disease
- Total nodal irradiation
- Chemotherapy with combinations of antineoplastic agents
- Autologous or allogeneic stem cell transplantation

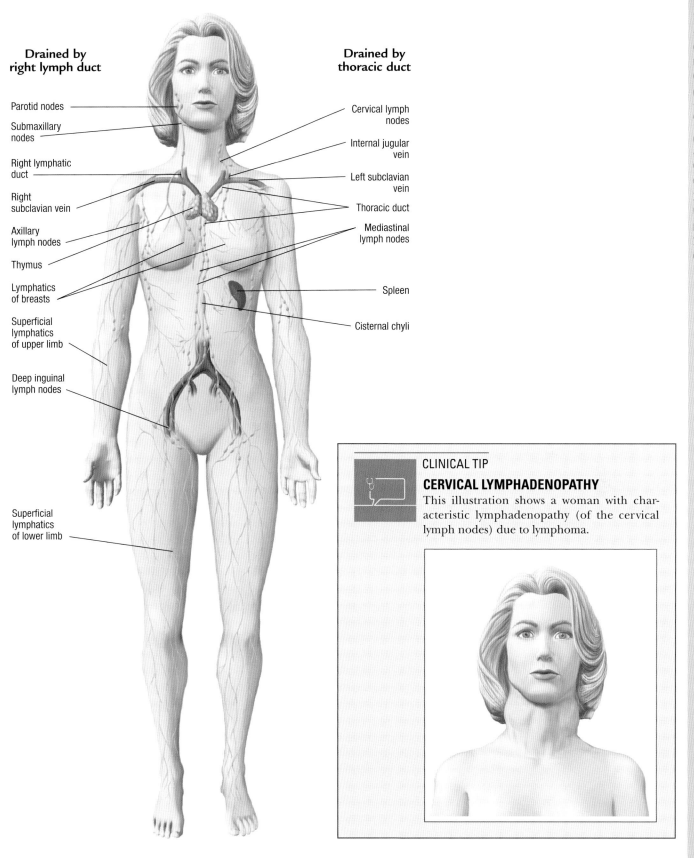

Drained by right lymph duct

Parotid nodes

Submaxillary nodes

Right lymphatic duct

Right subclavian vein

Axillary lymph nodes

Thymus

Lymphatics of breasts

Superficial lymphatics of upper limb

Deep inguinal lymph nodes

Superficial lymphatics of lower limb

Drained by thoracic duct

Cervical lymph nodes

Internal jugular vein

Left subclavian vein

Thoracic duct

Mediastinal lymph nodes

Spleen

Cisternal chyli

CLINICAL TIP

CERVICAL LYMPHADENOPATHY

This illustration shows a woman with characteristic lymphadenopathy (of the cervical lymph nodes) due to lymphoma.

LEUKEMIA

Leukemia is a group of diseases caused by malignant proliferation of WBCs; each is classified by the dominant cell type. The course of a leukemia may be acute or chronic.

- Acute — large numbers of immature leukocytes; rapid onset and progression
- Chronic — excessive mature leukocytes in the periphery and bone marrow; slower onset and progression

AGE ALERT
Leukemias are the most common malignancies in children. Each specific type has its own prognosis, but generally, the prognosis in children is better than in adults.

Causes

No definitive cause identified

Risk Factors

- Genetic predisposition
- Immunologic factors
- Environmental exposure to chemicals and radiation
- Predisposing disease

Chronic Myeloid Leukemia (CML)

- In almost 90% of patients, Philadelphia, or Ph¹ chromosome; translocated long arm of chromosome 22, usually to chromosome 9

Pathophysiology

Acute leukemia is characterized by malignant proliferation of WBC precursors (blasts) in bone marrow or lymph tissue and their accumulation in peripheral blood, bone marrow, and body tissues. Leukemic cells inhibit normal bone marrow production of erythrocytes, platelets, and immune function. Its most common forms and the characteristic cells include:

- *Acute lymphoblastic (or lymphocytic) leukemia (ALL)*: lymphocyte precursors (lymphoblasts)
- *Acute myeloid leukemia (AML)*, known collectively as *acute non-lymphocytic leukemia:*
  - acute myeloblastic (or myelogenous) leukemia: myeloid precursors (myeloblasts)
  - acute monoblastic (monocytic) leukemia: monocyte precursors (monoblasts)
  - other types: acute myelomonocytic leukemia and acute erythroleukemia.
- *Chronic myeloid leukemia (CML)* proceeds in two distinct phases:
  - insidious chronic phase: anemia and bleeding disorders
  - blastic crisis or acute phase: rapid proliferation of myeloblasts, the most primitive granulocyte precursors.
- *Chronic lymphocytic leukemia (CLL):* abnormal small lymphocytes in lymphoid tissue, blood, and bone marrow.

Chronic myelomonocytic leukemia (CMML): previously recognized as a type of myelodysplastic syndrome, individuals with CMML have significantly elevated monocytes in their blood, which will increase the total WBC count.

COMPLICATIONS
- Infection
- Organ malfunction
- Weight loss
- Anemia
- Adverse effects of treatment
- Tumor lysis syndrome

Signs and Symptoms

Signs and symptoms will vary based on the type of leukemia but commonly include:

AML and ALL

- Sudden high fever, thrombocytopenia, and abnormal bleeding
- Nonspecific signs and symptoms, including weakness, pallor, and chills
- Also, in acute monoblastic leukemia: possible dyspnea, anemia, fatigue, malaise, tachycardia, palpitations, systolic ejection murmur, and abdominal and bone pain

CML

- Anemia, thrombocytopenia, and hepatosplenomegaly
- Sternal and rib tenderness
- Low-grade fever
- Anorexia and weight loss
- Renal calculi or gouty arthritis
- Prolonged infection
- Ankle edema

CLL

- Early stages: fatigue, malaise, fever, and nodular enlargement
- Late stages: severe fatigue, weight loss, liver or spleen enlargement, and bone tenderness
- With disease progression and bone marrow involvement: anemia, pallor, weakness, dyspnea, tachycardia, palpitations, bleeding, and opportunistic fungal, viral, and bacterial infections

Diagnostic Test Results

AML and ALL

- Laboratory studies (CBC and peripheral smear) show thrombocytopenia and neutropenia. WBC differential shows cell type (increased myeloblasts in AML and lymphoblasts in ALL).
- CT scan, MRI, PET scan, or ultrasound can show affected organs.
- Bone marrow biopsy shows proliferation of immature WBCs.

Chromosomal testing of bone marrow aspirates in AML and ALL may identify translocations that can be targeted by specific therapies.

CML

- Chromosomal studies of peripheral blood or bone marrow show the Philadelphia chromosome.
- Laboratory studies reveal low leukocyte alkaline phosphate, leukocytosis, leukopenia, neutropenia, decreased Hb and hematocrit, increased circulating myeloblasts, thrombocytosis, and increased serum uric acid level.
- CT scan, MRI, PET scan, or ultrasound can show affected organs.
- Bone marrow biopsy reveals hypercellular showing bone marrow infiltration by increased number of myeloid elements.

CLL

- Laboratory studies show increased WBC, granulocytopenia, decreased Hb, neutropenia, lymphocytosis, and thrombocytopenia.
- CT scan shows affected organs.
- Bone marrow biopsy shows lymphocytic invasion.
- Serum protein electrophoresis shows hypogammaglobulinemia.

Treatment

Treatment of leukemia is highly variable and dependent on cell type, stage of disease, and age and general health of the patient. Some adults with CLL benefit from watchful waiting. General treatment principles for individuals with leukemia include:

- systemic chemotherapy (for ALL, this includes induction therapy, consolidation therapy, and maintenance therapy)
- biological therapy to help the immune system recognize and attack leukemia cells
- targeted therapy (specific drugs that kill leukemia cells contain the Philadelphia chromosome or other chromosomal translocation abnormalities)
- radiation therapy
- interferon
- supportive care to offset side effects of treatment: granulocyte injections and transfusion of blood and blood products
- stem cell transplantation.

HISTOLOGIC FINDINGS OF LEUKEMIAS

Acute lymphocytic leukemia

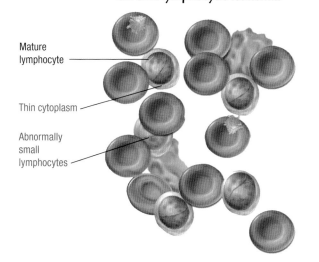

Lymphoblast

Minimal cytoplasm

Nucleolus (usually 1 or 2)

Acute myelogenous leukemia

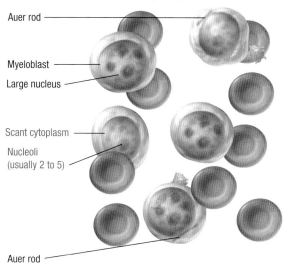

Auer rod

Myeloblast

Large nucleus

Scant cytoplasm

Nucleoli (usually 2 to 5)

Auer rod

Chronic lymphocytic leukemia

Mature lymphocyte

Thin cytoplasm

Abnormally small lymphocytes

Chronic myeloid leukemia

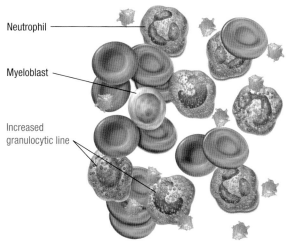

Neutrophil

Myeloblast

Increased granulocytic line

MULTIPLE MYELOMA

Multiple myeloma, also known as *malignant plasmacytoma* or *plasma cell myeloma*, is a disseminated malignant neoplasia of marrow plasma cells that infiltrates bone to produce osteolytic lesions throughout the skeleton (flat bones, vertebrae, skull, pelvis, and ribs). It's a rare disease with only three new cases occurring per 100,000 people a year.

AGE ALERT
Men are slightly more likely to be diagnosed with multiple myeloma than women. Most people diagnosed are at least 65 years of age. Less than 1% of all cases are diagnosed in individuals younger than 35 years of age. Prognosis is usually poor because diagnosis is typically made after the disease has already infiltrated the vertebrae, pelvis, skull, ribs, clavicles, and sternum. By then, skeletal destruction is widespread and vertebral collapse is imminent. Without treatment, about half of all patients die within 6 months of diagnosis. Early diagnosis and treatment prolong the lives of many patients by 3 to 5 years. Death usually follows complications, such as infection, renal failure, hematologic imbalance, fractures, hypercalcemia, hyperuricemia, or dehydration.

Causes

Primary cause unknown, but linked to DNA mutations that turn on oncogenes or turn off suppressor genes.

Possible Links

- Genetic factors (African Americans are more than twice as likely to get multiple myeloma than Whites; individuals with a sibling or parent with multiple myeloma are four times more likely to develop multiple myeloma.)
- Autoimmune diseases or allergies
- Radiation exposure
- Environmental toxins
- Chemicals in agricultural products or added during food processing

Pathophysiology

Plasma cells are normal leukocytes that secrete immunoglobulins. When plasma cells become malignant, they reproduce uncontrollably and create many abnormal immunoglobulins. During this process, they invade the bone marrow, and then the bone matrix, causing osteolytic lesions of the bone. Myeloma cells then proliferate outside of the bone marrow in all lymphatic tissues where plasma cells are normally present. Because plasma cells exist in virtually all body organs, all body systems may be affected by this proliferation and abnormal immunoglobulin production. The severity of renal failure correlates with the amount of immunoglobulin protein found in the urine. Infiltration and precipitation of immunoglobulin light chains (Bence Jones protein) in the distal tubules cause myeloma nephrosis.

COMPLICATIONS
- Infections
- Pyelonephritis
- Hematologic imbalance
- Fractures
- Hypercalcemia
- Hyperuricemia
- Dehydration
- Renal calculi
- Renal failure
- Spinal cord compression

Signs and Symptoms

- Severe, constant back and rib pain that increases with exercise and may be worse at night
- Arthritic symptoms — achy pain; swollen, tender joints
- Fever and malaise
- Evidence of peripheral neuropathy (such as paresthesia)
- Evidence of diffuse osteoporosis and pathologic fractures

In Advanced Disease

- Acute symptoms of vertebral compression; loss of body height — 5 inches (12.5 cm) or more
- Thoracic deformities (ballooning)
- Anemia
- Bleeding
- Weight loss
- Severe, recurrent infection, such as pneumonia, may follow damage to nerves associated with respiratory function.

Diagnostic Test Results

- Complete blood count shows moderate to severe anemia; differential may show 40% to 50% lymphocytes but seldom more than 3% plasma cells.
- Differential smear reveals *rouleaux* formation from elevated erythrocyte sedimentation rate.
- Urine studies reveal Bence Jones protein and hypercalciuria.
- Bone marrow aspiration detects myelomatous cells (abnormal number of immature plasma cells; 60% or more plasma cells in the bone marrow is a diagnostic criteria).
- Serum electrophoresis shows elevated globulin spike that's electrophoretically and immunologically abnormal.
- Serum quantitative antibodies may detect altered immunoglobulin levels.
- Bone X-rays in early stages may reveal diffuse osteoporosis; in later stages, they show multiple sharply circumscribed osteolytic lesions, particularly in the skull, pelvis, and spine.
- MRI or PET scans are helpful in identifying disease within the bone marrow when simple X-rays are negative.

Treatment

- Chemotherapy to suppress plasma cell growth and control pain
- Corticosteroids

- Immunotherapy/biologics to stimulate the immune system to destroy myeloma cells
- Targeted therapy to promote myeloma cell death
- Autologous hematopoietic blood cell transfusion
- Autologous stem cell transplantation
- Adjuvant local radiation to decrease bone pain
- Plasmapheresis to remove myeloma proteins and reduce viscosity
- Management of complications with bisphosphonates, dialysis, and analgesics

BONE MARROW ASPIRATE IN MULTIPLE MYELOMA

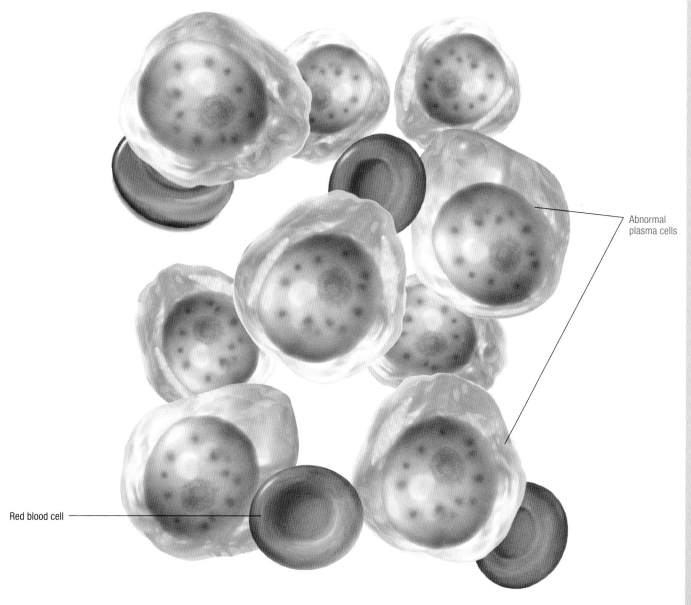

Abnormal plasma cells

Red blood cell

Suggested References

Bartlett, N. (2016). Fine-tuning the treatment of Hodgkin's lymphoma. *New England Journal of Medicine*, 374(25), 2490–2492.

Geyer, H., Scherber, R., Kosiorek, H., Dueck, A. C., Kiladjian, J.-J., Xiao, Z.,... Mesa, R. A. (2016). Symptomatic profiles of patients with polycythemia vera: Implications of inadequately controlled disease. *Journal of Clinical Oncology*, 34(2), 151–159.

Koch, J. A., & Munden, L. (2016). Hematology. In J. G. Stewart, & N. L. Dennert (Eds.), *Family nurse practitioner certification review*. Burlington, MA: Jones & Bartlett Learning.

Minard-Colin, V., Brugières, L., Reiter, A., Cairo, M. S., Gross, T. G., Woessmann, W.,... Patte, C. (2015). Non-Hodgkin lymphoma in children and adolescents: Progress through effective collaboration, current knowledge, and challenges ahead. *Journal of Clinical Oncology*, 33(27), 2963–2974.

Muncie, H., & Campbell, J. (2009). Alpha and beta thalassemia. *American Family Physician*, 80(4), 339–344.

National Heart Lung and Blood Institute. (2013). *What is hemophilia?* Available at http://www.nhlbi.nih.gov/health/health-topics/topics/hemophilia

National Hemophilia Foundation. (n.d.). *Types of bleeding disorders*. Available at www.hemophilia.org/Bleeding-Disorders/Types-of-Bleeding-Disorders

Patnaik, M. M., & Tefferi, A. (2016). Chronic myelomonocytic leukemia: Focus on clinical practice. *Mayo Clinic Proceedings*, 91(2), 259–272.

Peyvandi, R., Garagiola, I., & Young, G. (2016). The past and future of haemophilia: Diagnosis, treatments, and its complications. *Lancet*, 388(10040), 187–197.

Rajkumar, S. V., & Kumar, S. (2016). Multiple myeloma: Diagnosis and treatment. *Mayo Clinic Proceedings*, 91(1), 101–119.

Rees, D. C., Williams, T. N., & Gladwin, M. T. (2010). Sickle-cell disease. *The Lancet*, 376, 2018–2031.

Solheim, J. (2009). DIC: When the coagulation cascade goes horribly wrong. *Nursing Spectrum*, 21(10), 20–25.

Tefferi, A., & Barbuie, T. (2015). Essential thrombocythemia and polycythemia vera: Focus on clinical practice. *Mayo Clinic Proceedings*, 90(9), 1283–1293.

Vieth, J. T., & Lane, D. R. (2014). Anemia. *Emergency Medicine Clinics of North America*, 32, 613–628.

ACQUIRED IMMUNODEFICIENCY SYNDROME

Human immunodeficiency virus (HIV) infection is the virus that causes acquired immunodeficiency syndrome (AIDS). Although characterized by gradual destruction of cell-mediated (T-cell) immunity, AIDS also affects humoral immunity and even autoimmunity through the central role of the $CD4^+$ (helper) T lymphocyte in all immune reactions. The resulting immunodeficiency makes the patient susceptible to opportunistic infections, cancers, and other abnormalities that define AIDS.

Causes

- There are two species of HIV: HIV-1 and HIV-2. HIV-1 is the most common of the two. HIV-1 and HIV-2 retrovirus are transmitted by contact with infected blood or body fluids (semen, breast milk, rectal, or vaginal fluids), although HIV-2 has a slightly lower risk of transmission and typically progresses slower.

High-Risk Populations

- Homosexual or bisexual men
- I.V. drug users
- Neonates of infected women
- Recipients of contaminated blood or blood products
- Heterosexual partners of persons in high-risk groups

Pathophysiology

The natural history of AIDS begins with infection by the HIV retrovirus, which is detectable only by laboratory tests, and ends with death. The HIV virus may enter the body by any of several routes involving the transmission of blood or body fluids, for example:

- direct inoculation during intimate unprotected sexual contact
- transfusion of contaminated blood or blood products
- use of contaminated needles
- transplacental or postpartum transmission.

HIV strikes helper T cells bearing the $CD4^+$ antigen. Normally a receptor for major histocompatibility complex molecules, the antigen serves as a receptor for the retrovirus and allows it to enter the cell. Viral binding also requires the presence of a coreceptor on the cell surface (CCR5, CXCR4, or both).

Like other retroviruses, HIV copies its genetic material in a reverse manner compared with other viruses and cells. Through the action of reverse transcriptase, HIV produces deoxyribonucleic acid (DNA) from its viral ribonucleic acid (RNA). Transcription is often poor, leading to mutations, some of which make HIV resistant to antiviral drugs. The viral DNA enters the nucleus of the cell and is incorporated into the host cell's DNA, where it's transcribed into more viral RNA. If the host cell reproduces, it duplicates the HIV DNA along with its own and passes it on to the daughter cells. Thus, the host cell carries this information and, if activated, replicates the virus. Viral enzymes and proteases arrange the structural components and RNA into viral particles that move to the periphery of the host cell, where the virus buds and emerges from the host cell — free to infect other cells. Reservoirs of HIV include gut-associated lymphoid tissue (GALT) and peripheral lymphoid tissues. The reproductive tract, bone marrow, reticuloendothelial system, peripheral blood dendritic cells, and microglial cells of the central nervous system are sites that are believed to be reservoirs of HIV.

HIV replication may lead to cell death or the virus may become latent. HIV infection leads to profound pathology, either directly through destruction of $CD4^+$ cells, other immune cells, and neuroglial cells or indirectly through the secondary effects of $CD4^+$ T-cell dysfunction and resulting immunosuppression.

COMPLICATIONS

- Opportunistic infections
- Wasting syndrome
- Kaposi's sarcoma and non-Hodgkin's lymphoma
- Lymphoid interstitial pneumonia
- Arthritis
- Hypergammaglobulinemia
- AIDS dementia complex
- HIV encephalopathy
- Peripheral neuropathy
- HIV associated nephropathy

Clinical Manifestations

Acute Retroviral Syndrome

- Over 50% of those infected with HIV develop a mononucleosislike syndrome, which may be attributed to flu or another virus and which occurs 1 to 6 weeks post exposure; may remain asymptomatic for years

Latency

During this time period, which can last for a decade or more, the virus is replicating at low levels, but people are often asymptomatic. People who are taking antiretroviral therapy can remain in this phase for decades.

Symptomatic Phase

- Persistent generalized lymphadenopathy
- Nonspecific symptoms, including weight loss, fatigue, and night sweats
- Fevers related to altered function of $CD4^+$ cells, immunodeficiency, and infection of other $CD4^+$ antigen-bearing cells
- Neurologic symptoms

Diagnostic Test Results

- Laboratory studies reveal $CD4^+$ T-cell count less than 200 cells/μL and the presence of HIV antibodies.

Treatment

Antiretroviral Agents

- Protease inhibitors
- Nucleoside reverse transcriptase inhibitors
- Nonnucleoside reverse transcriptase inhibitors

- Entry inhibitors
- Fusion inhibitors
- Integrase inhibitors

Additional Treatment

- Immunomodulatory agents
- Human granulocyte colony-stimulating growth factor

- Anti-infective and antineoplastic agents
- Supportive therapy, including nutritional support, fluid and electrolyte replacement therapy, pain relief, and psychological support
- Prevention and treatment of opportunistic infections
- Preexposure prophylaxis
- Postexposure prophylaxis

MANIFESTATIONS OF HIV INFECTION AND AIDS

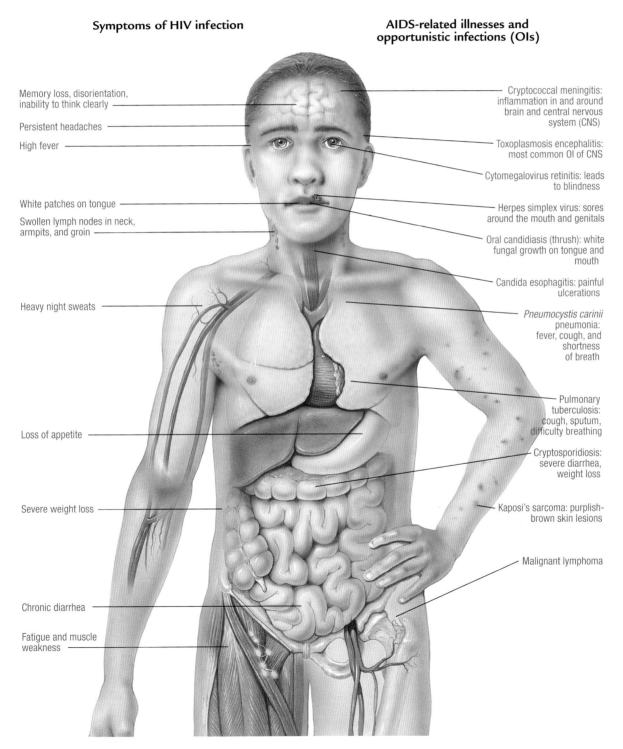

Symptoms of HIV infection

Memory loss, disorientation, inability to think clearly

Persistent headaches

High fever

White patches on tongue

Swollen lymph nodes in neck, armpits, and groin

Heavy night sweats

Loss of appetite

Severe weight loss

Chronic diarrhea

Fatigue and muscle weakness

AIDS-related illnesses and opportunistic infections (OIs)

Cryptococcal meningitis: inflammation in and around brain and central nervous system (CNS)

Toxoplasmosis encephalitis: most common OI of CNS

Cytomegalovirus retinitis: leads to blindness

Herpes simplex virus: sores around the mouth and genitals

Oral candidiasis (thrush): white fungal growth on tongue and mouth

Candida esophagitis: painful ulcerations

Pneumocystis carinii pneumonia: fever, cough, and shortness of breath

Pulmonary tuberculosis: cough, sputum, difficulty breathing

Cryptosporidiosis: severe diarrhea, weight loss

Kaposi's sarcoma: purplish-brown skin lesions

Malignant lymphoma

ALLERGIC RHINITIS

Allergic rhinitis is a reaction to airborne (inhaled) allergens. Depending on the allergen, the resulting rhinitis and conjunctivitis may occur seasonally (hay fever) or year-round (perennial allergic rhinitis). Allergic rhinitis is the most common atopic allergic reaction, affecting over 20 million US residents.

AGE ALERT
Allergic rhinitis is most prevalent in young children and adolescents but occurs in all age groups.

Causes

- Immunoglobulin (Ig) E–mediated type I hypersensitivity response to an environmental antigen (allergen) in a genetically susceptible person

Common Triggers

- Wind-borne pollens:
  - Spring — oak, elm, maple, alder, birch, and cottonwood
  - Summer — grasses, sheep sorrel, and English plantain
  - Autumn — ragweed and other weeds
- Perennial allergens and irritants:
  - Dust mite excreta, fungal spores, and molds
  - Feather pillows
  - Cigarette smoke
  - Animal dander

Pathophysiology

During primary exposure to an allergen, T cells recognize the foreign allergens and release chemicals that instruct B cells to produce specific antibodies called *IgE*. IgE antibodies attach themselves to mast cells. Mast cells with attached IgE can remain in the body for years, ready to react when they next encounter the same allergen.

The second time the allergen enters the body, it comes into direct contact with the IgE antibodies attached to the mast cells. This stimulates the mast cells to release chemicals, such as histamine, which initiate a response that causes tightening of the smooth muscles in the airways, dilation of small blood vessels, increased mucus secretion in the nasal cavity and airways, and itching.

COMPLICATIONS
- Secondary sinus and middle ear infections
- Nasal polyps

Signs and Symptoms

Seasonal Allergic Rhinitis

- Paroxysmal sneezing
- Profuse watery rhinorrhea; nasal obstruction or congestion
- Pruritus of nose and eyes
- Pale, cyanotic, edematous nasal mucosa
- Red, edematous eyelids and conjunctivae
- Excessive lacrimation
- Headache or sinus pain
- Itching of the throat
- Malaise

Perennial Allergic Rhinitis

- Chronic nasal obstruction, commonly extending to eustachian tube
- Conjunctivitis and other extranasal effects rare

CLINICAL TIP
In both types of allergic rhinitis, dark circles may appear under the patient's eyes ("allergic shiners") because of venous congestion in the maxillary sinuses.

Diagnostic Test Results

A definitive diagnosis is based on the patient's personal and family history of allergies as well as physical findings during a symptomatic phase.

- Microscopic examination of sputum and nasal secretions reveals large numbers of eosinophils.
- Blood chemistry shows normal or elevated IgE.
- Skin testing paired with tested responses to environmental stimuli pinpoints the responsible allergens given the patient's history.

Treatment

- Antihistamines such as fexofenadine
- Inhaled intranasal steroids, such as beclomethasone, flunisolide, and fluticasone
- Immunotherapy or desensitization with injections of extracted allergens
- Nasal decongestants

Primary exposure

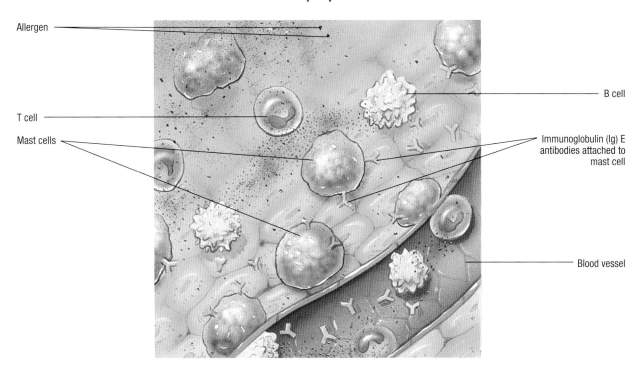

Allergen

T cell

Mast cells

B cell

Immunoglobulin (Ig) E antibodies attached to mast cell

Blood vessel

Reexposure

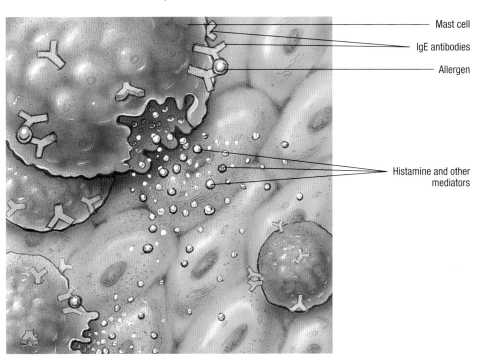

Mast cell

IgE antibodies

Allergen

Histamine and other mediators

ANAPHYLAXIS

Anaphylaxis is an acute, potentially life-threatening type I (immediate) hypersensitivity reaction marked by sudden onset of rapidly progressive urticaria (vascular swelling in skin, accompanied by itching) and respiratory distress. With prompt recognition and treatment, prognosis is good. Typically occurring within minutes, the reaction can occur up to 1 hour after reexposure to an antigen.

Causes

Ingestion of or other systemic exposure to sensitizing drugs or other substances, such as:

- serums (usually horse serum), vaccines, and allergen extracts
- diagnostic chemicals, such as sulfobromophthalein, sodium dehydrocholate, and radiographic contrast media
- enzymes such as L-asparaginase in chemotherapeutic regimens
- hormones such as insulin
- penicillin or other antibiotic and sulfonamides
- salicylates
- food proteins, as in legumes, nuts, berries, seafood, and egg albumin
- sulfite food additives, common in dried fruits and vegetables and salad bars
- insect venom
- nonimmunologic triggers such as cold air or water, heat, exercise, and ethanol

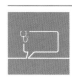

CLINICAL TIP
Latex allergy is a hypersensitivity reaction to products that contain natural latex derived from the sap of a rubber tree, not synthetic latex. Natural latex is increasingly present in products in the home and workplace. Hypersensitivity reactions can range from local dermatitis to a life-threatening anaphylactic reaction.

Pathophysiology

Anaphylaxis requires previous sensitization or exposure to the specific antigen, resulting in immunoglobulin (Ig) E production by plasma cells in the lymph nodes and enhancement by helper T cells. IgE antibodies then bind to membrane receptors on mast cells in connective tissue and basophils in the blood.

On reexposure, IgM and IgG recognize the antigen as foreign and bind to it. Destruction of the antigen by the complement cascade begins. Continued antigen presence activates IgE on basophils, which promotes the release of mediators, including histamine, serotonin, and eosinophil chemotactic factor of anaphylaxis (ECF-A) and platelet-activating factor. The sudden release of histamine causes vasodilation and increases capillary permeability.

Activated IgE also stimulates mast cells in connective tissue along the venule walls to release more histamine and ECF-A. These substances produce disruptive lesions that weaken the venules.

In the lungs, histamine causes endothelial cells to burst and endothelial tissue to tear away from surrounding tissue. Fluids leak into the alveoli, and leukotrienes prevent the alveoli from expanding, thus reducing pulmonary compliance.

At the same time, basophils and mast cells begin to release prostaglandins and bradykinin along with histamine and serotonin. These chemical mediators spread through the body in the circulation, triggering systemic responses: vasodilation, smooth muscle contraction, and increased mucus production. The mediators also induce vascular collapse by increasing vascular permeability, which leads to decreased peripheral resistance and plasma leakage from the vessels to the extravascular tissues.

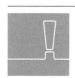

COMPLICATIONS
- Hypovolemic shock
- Cardiac dysfunction
- Death

Signs and Symptoms

- Sudden physical distress within seconds or minutes after exposure to an allergen
- Delayed or persistent reaction may occur up to 24 hours later (severity of the reaction relates inversely to the interval between exposure to the allergen and the onset of symptoms).

Usual Initial Symptoms

- Feeling of impending doom or fright
- Sweating
- Sneezing, shortness of breath, nasal pruritus, urticaria, and angioedema

Systemic Manifestations

- Hypotension, shock, and cardiac arrhythmias
- Edema of the upper respiratory tract, resulting in hypopharyngeal and laryngeal obstruction
- Hoarseness, stridor, wheezing, and accessory muscle use
- Severe stomach cramps, nausea, diarrhea, and urinary urgency and incontinence

Diagnostic Test Results

No single diagnostic test can identify anaphylaxis. The following tests provide clues to the patient's risk of anaphylaxis:

- Skin tests show hypersensitivity to a certain allergen.
- Laboratory studies reveal elevated serum IgE levels.
- Monitoring diagnostics include pulse oximetry, EKG, arterial blood gases, plasma histamine, serum tryptase level, and chest X-ray.

Treatment

- Immediate administration of epinephrine to reverse bronchoconstriction and cause vasoconstriction
- Airway patency is vital. Preparation for tracheostomy or endotracheal intubation and mechanical ventilation
- Oxygen therapy
- I.V. access and isotonic saline. Vasopressors, such as norepinephrine and dopamine may be required
- Longer-acting epinephrine, corticosteroids, antihistamines, and histamine-2 blocker
- Albuterol mini-nebulizer treatment
- Volume expanders
- Cardiopulmonary resuscitation

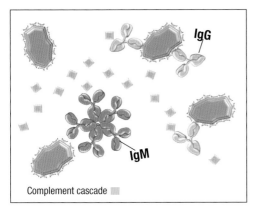

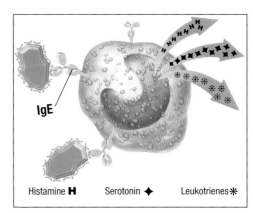

1. Response to antigen
Immunoglobulins (Ig) M and G recognize and bind the antigen. The patient has no signs or symptoms.

2. Release of chemical mediators
Activated IgE on basophils promotes the release of mediators: histamine, serotonin, and leukotrienes. The patient develops nasal congestion, itchy and watery eyes, flushing, weakness, and anxiety.

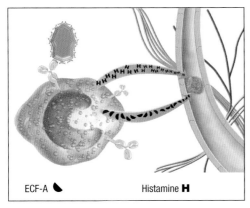

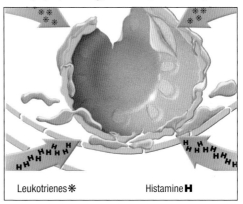

3. Intensified response
Mast cells release more histamine and eosinophil chemotactic factor of anaphylaxis (ECF-A), which create venule-weakening lesions. Signs and symptoms worsen; swelling and wheals appear.

4. Respiratory distress
In the lungs, histamine causes endothelial cell destruction and fluid leak into alveoli. The patient develops changes in level of consciousness, respiratory distress and, possibly, seizures.

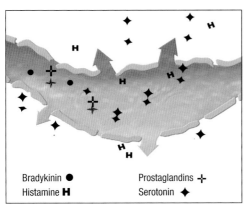

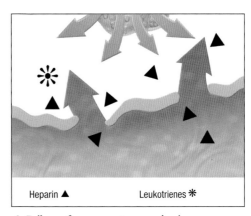

5. Deterioration
Meanwhile, mediators increase vascular permeability, causing fluid to leak from the vessels. Shock, confusion, tachycardia, and hypotension signal vascular collapse.

6. Failure of compensatory mechanisms
Endothelial cell damage causes basophils and mast cells to release heparin and mediator-neutralizing substances. However, anaphylaxis is now irreversible. Hemorrhage, disseminated intravascular coagulation, and cardiac arrest can occur.

ANKYLOSING SPONDYLITIS

A chronic, usually progressive inflammatory bone disease, ankylosing spondylitis primarily affects the sacroiliac, apophyseal, and costovertebral joints, along with adjacent soft tissue. The disease (also known as *rheumatoid spondylitis* and *Marie-Strümpell disease*) usually begins in the sacroiliac joints and gradually progresses to the lumbar, thoracic, and cervical regions of the spine. Deterioration of bone and cartilage can lead to formation of fibrous tissue and eventual fusion of the spine or peripheral joints.

Ankylosing spondylitis affects men two to three times more than it does women. Progressive disease is well recognized in men, but the diagnosis is commonly overlooked or missed in women, who tend to have more peripheral joint involvement.

Causes

- Direct cause unknown
- Familial tendency. More than 90% of patients are positive for human leukocyte antigen (HLA)-B27
- Presence of circulating immune complexes suggests immunologic activity.

Pathophysiology

Spondylitis involves inflammation of one or more vertebrae. Ankylosing spondylitis is a chronic inflammatory disease that predominantly affects the joints between the vertebrae of the spine and the joints between the spine and the pelvis. Fibrous tissue of the joint capsule is infiltrated by inflammatory cells that erode the bone and fibrocartilage. Repair of the cartilaginous structures begins with the proliferation of fibroblasts, which synthesize and secrete collagen. The collagen forms fibrous scar tissue that eventually undergoes calcification and ossification, causing the joint to fuse or lose flexibility.

Involvement of the peripheral joints or soft tissues is a rare occurrence. The disease waxes and wanes; it can go into remission, exacerbation, or arrest at any stage.

COMPLICATIONS
- Severe physical restrictions
- Inflammatory bowel disease
- Iritis
- Osteopenia

Signs and Symptoms

- Intermittent low back pain most severe in the morning or after inactivity and relieved by exercise
- Mild fatigue, fever, anorexia, and weight loss
- Pain in shoulders, hips, knees, and ankles
- Pain over the symphysis pubis
- Stiffness or limited motion of the lumbar spine
- Pain and limited chest expansion
- Kyphosis
- Iritis
- Warmth, swelling, or tenderness of affected joints
- Small joints, such as toes, may become sausage-shaped
- Aortic murmur caused by regurgitation
- Cardiomegaly
- Upper lobe pulmonary fibrosis, which mimics tuberculosis, that may reduce vital capacity to 70% or less of predicted volume

Diagnostic Test Results

Modified New York Criteria for AS (1984) defined AS if the patient has at least one clinical criterion with sacroiliitis grade greater than or equal to 2 bilaterally or greater than or equal to grade 3 unilaterally. Clinical criteria include low back pain with stiffness for greater than 3 months not relieved by resting but improves with exercise, motion of the lumbar spines in the sagittal and frontal planes limited, and chest expansion limited relative to gender and age.

The SpondyloArthritis International Society (ASAS) Classification Criteria for Axial Spondyloarthritis (SpA) in patients with back pain for 3 months or longer and age at onset younger than 45 years includes either HLA-B27 plus greater than or equal to 2 other features of SpA or sacroiliitis on imaging plus greater than or equal to 1 SpA feature.

- HLA typing test shows serum findings that include HLA-B27 in about 95% of patients with primary ankylosing spondylitis and up to 80% of patients with secondary disease.
- Laboratory tests show slightly elevated erythrocyte sedimentation rate, serum alkaline phosphate levels, and creatine kinase levels in active disease.
- Serum immunoglobulin (Ig) profile shows elevated serum IgA levels.
- X-ray studies define characteristic changes, such as bilateral sacroiliac involvement (the hallmark of the disease), blurring of the joints' bony margins in early disease, patchy sclerosis with superficial bony erosions, eventual squaring of vertebral bodies, and "bamboo spine" with complete ankylosis.

Treatment

- No treatment that reliably halts progression
- Physical therapy to delay further deformity — good posture, stretching and deep-breathing exercises, and, in some patients, braces and lightweight supports
- Heat, warm showers, baths, and ice
- Nerve stimulation
- Nonsteroidal anti-inflammatory analgesics, such as aspirin, indomethacin, and sulfasalazine
- Corticosteroids
- Anti–tumor necrosis factor agents
- Hip replacement
- Spinal wedge osteotomy

Lateral view

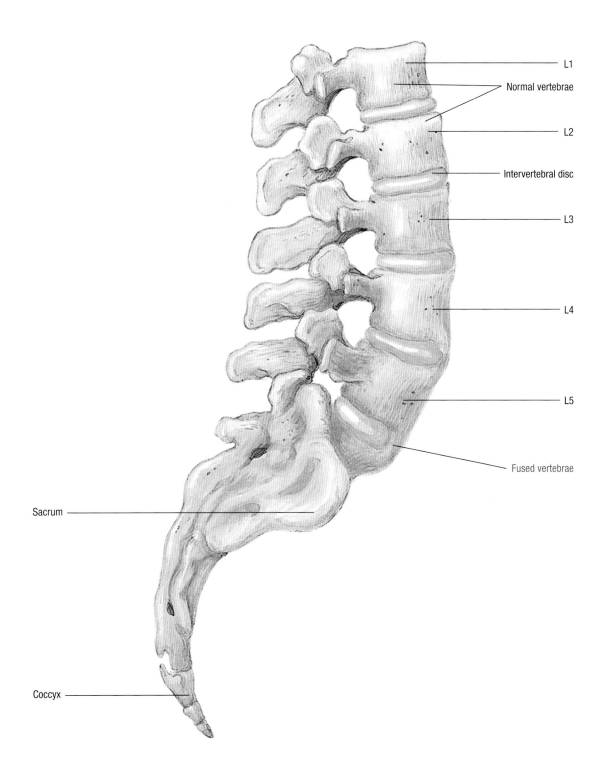

L1

Normal vertebrae

L2

Intervertebral disc

L3

L4

L5

Fused vertebrae

Sacrum

Coccyx

RHEUMATOID ARTHRITIS

Rheumatoid arthritis (RA) is a chronic, systemic inflammatory disease that primarily attacks peripheral joints and the surrounding muscles, tendons, ligaments, and blood vessels. Partial remissions and unpredictable exacerbations mark the course of this potentially crippling disease. RA strikes women three times more often than it does men.

AGE ALERT
RA can occur at any age, but it begins most often between ages 25 and 55.

Causes

Direct cause unknown

Proposed Mechanisms

- Abnormal immune activation (in a genetically susceptible person) leading to inflammation, complement activation, and cell proliferation in joints and tendon sheaths
- Infection (viral or bacterial), hormone action, or lifestyle factors

Pathophysiology

The body develops immunoglobulin (Ig) M antibody against the body's own IgG (also called *rheumatoid factor [RF]*). RF aggregates into complexes and generates inflammation, causing eventual cartilage damage and triggering other autoimmune responses.

If not arrested, the inflammatory process in the joints occurs in four stages:

- Congestion and edema of the synovial membrane and joint capsule cause synovitis. Infiltration by lymphocytes, macrophages, and neutrophils continues the local inflammatory response. These cells, as well as fibroblastlike synovial cells, produce enzymes that help to degrade bone and cartilage.
- Pannus — thickened layers of granulation tissue — covers and invades cartilage and eventually destroys the joint capsule and bone.
- Fibrous ankylosis — fibrous invasion of the pannus and scar formation — occludes the joint space. Bone atrophy and misalignment cause visible deformities and disrupt the articulation of opposing bones, causing muscle atrophy and imbalance and, possibly, partial dislocations (subluxations).
- Fibrous tissue calcifies, resulting in bony ankylosis and total immobility.

COMPLICATIONS
- Joint deformities
- Vasculitis
- Pericarditis
- Peripheral neuropathy

Signs and Symptoms

- Nonspecific symptoms (most likely related to the initial inflammatory reactions) precede inflammation of the synovium, including fever, weight loss, malaise, fatigue, and lymphadenopathy.

As the Disease Progresses

- Specific localized, bilateral, and symmetric articular symptoms, frequently in the fingers at the proximal interphalangeal, metacarpophalangeal, and metatarsophalangeal joints, possibly extending to the wrists, knees, elbows, and ankles from inflammation of the synovium
- Stiffening of affected joints after inactivity, especially on arising in the morning
- Joint pain and tenderness, at first only with movement but eventually even at rest
- Gradual appearance of rheumatoid nodules — subcutaneous, round or oval, nontender masses (20% of RF-positive patients), usually on elbows, hands, or Achilles' tendon

Diagnostic Test Results

- X-rays show bone demineralization and soft tissue swelling (early stages), cartilage loss and narrowed joint spaces, and, finally, cartilage and bone destruction and erosion, subluxations, and deformities (later stages).
- RF titer is positive in 75% to 80% of patients (titer of 1:160 or higher).
- Synovial fluid analysis shows increased volume and turbidity but decreased viscosity and elevated white blood cell (WBC) counts (usually greater than 10,000/μL).
- Serum protein electrophoresis shows elevated serum globulin levels.
- Erythrocyte sedimentation rate and C-reactive protein levels are elevated in 85% to 90% of patients (may be useful to monitor response to therapy because elevation frequently parallels disease activity).
- Complete blood count reveals moderate anemia, slight leukocytosis, and slight thrombocytosis.

Treatment

- Nonsteroidal anti-inflammatory agents
- Immunosuppressants
- Corticosteroids
- Disease-modifying antirheumatic drugs
- Anakinra
- Tumor necrosis factor inhibitors
- Abatacept
- Supportive measures, including rest, splinting to rest inflamed joints, range-of-motion exercises, physical therapy, heat applications for chronic disease, and ice application for acute episodes
- Rituximab
- Synovectomy, osteotomy, and tendon repair
- Joint reconstruction or total joint replacement

Left knee
Patella removed to visualize

Erosion of bone

Erosion of cartilage

Pannus covers
synovial membrane

Hand and wrist

Pannus

Swelling

Erosion

Joint space
narrowing

Pannus

Left hip

Pelvis

Pannus
Erosion of cartilage
Erosion of bone
Femur

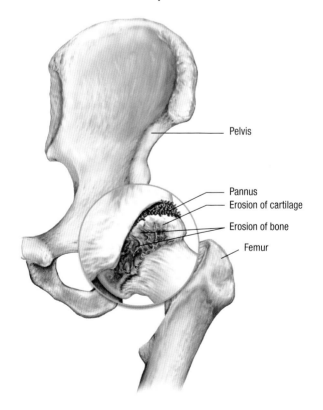

SCLERODERMA

Scleroderma (also known as *systemic sclerosis*) is an uncommon disease of diffuse connective tissue. Degenerative and fibrotic changes in the skin, blood vessels, synovial membranes, skeletal muscles, and internal organs (especially the esophagus, intestinal tract, thyroid, heart, lungs, and kidneys) follow the initial inflammation. The seven forms of scleroderma are diffuse systemic sclerosis, localized, linear, chemically induced localized, eosinophilia myalgia syndrome, toxic oil syndrome, and graft-versus-host disease.

AGE ALERT
Scleroderma affects women three to four times more often than it does men, especially between ages 30 and 50. The peak incidence is in people ages 50 to 60.

Causes

Unknown

Possible Causes

- Systemic exposure to silica dust or polyvinyl chloride
- Anticancer agents such as bleomycin; nonnarcotic analgesics such as pentazocine hydrochloride
- Abnormal immune response
- Underlying vascular cause with tissue changes initiated by persistent perfusion defect

Pathophysiology

Scleroderma usually begins in the fingers and extends proximally to the upper arms, shoulders, neck, and face. The skin atrophies, edema, and infiltrates containing CD4+ T cells surround the blood vessels, and inflamed collagen fibers become edematous and degenerative, losing strength and elasticity. The dermis becomes tightly bound to the underlying structures, resulting in atrophy of the affected appendages and destruction of the distal phalanges by osteoporosis. As the disease progresses, the fibrosis and atrophy can affect other areas, including muscles and joints.

Signs and Symptoms

- Skin thickening, commonly limited to the distal extremities and face but possibly involving internal organs
- CREST syndrome (a benign subtype of limited systemic sclerosis): calcinosis, Raynaud's phenomenon, esophageal dysfunction, sclerodactyly, and telangiectasia
- Patchy skin changes with a teardroplike appearance known as *morphea* (localized scleroderma)
- Band of thickened skin on the face or extremities that severely damages underlying tissues, causing atrophy and deformity (linear scleroderma)
- Raynaud's phenomenon (blanching, cyanosis, and erythema of the fingers and toes); progressive phalangeal resorption that may shorten the fingers (early symptoms)
- Taut, shiny skin over the entire hand and forearm due to skin thickening

- Tight and inelastic facial skin, causing a masklike appearance and "pinching" of the mouth
- Thickened skin over proximal limbs and trunk (diffuse systemic sclerosis)
- Abdominal distention
- Pain, stiffness, and swelling of fingers and joints (later symptoms)
- Frequent reflux, heartburn, dysphagia, and bloating after meals due to GI dysfunction
- Diarrhea, constipation, and malodorous floating stool

COMPLICATIONS
- Arrhythmias
- Dyspnea
- Malignant hypertension
- Renal failure
- Bowel obstruction
- Aspiration pneumonia
- Pulmonary hypertension
- Respiratory failure
- Cor pulmonale
- Heart failure
- Cardiomyopathy

Diagnostic Test Results

- Laboratory analysis reveals slightly elevated erythrocyte sedimentation rate, positive RF in 25% to 35% of patients, and positive antinuclear antibody (ANA).
- Urinalysis shows proteinuria, microscopic hematuria, and casts.
- Hand X-rays show terminal phalangeal tuft resorption, subcutaneous calcification, and joint space narrowing and erosion.
- Chest X-rays show bilateral basilar pulmonary fibrosis.
- GI X-rays show distal esophageal hypomotility and stricture, duodenal loop dilation, small bowel malabsorption pattern, and large diverticula.
- Pulmonary function studies show decreased diffusion and vital capacity.
- Electrocardiogram reveals nonspecific abnormalities related to myocardial fibrosis and possible arrhythmias.
- Skin biopsy shows changes consistent with disease progression, such as marked thickening of the dermis and occlusive vessel changes.

Treatment

No cure

To Preserve Normal Body Functions and Minimize Complications

- Immunosuppressants, vasodilators, and antihypertensives
- Digital sympathectomy and cervical sympathetic blockade
- Possible surgical debridement
- Antacids and soft, bland diet
- Angiotensin-converting enzyme inhibitors
- Physical therapy and heat therapy
- Broad-spectrum antibiotics

Thin, shiny skin on fingers

Flexed, stiff fingers

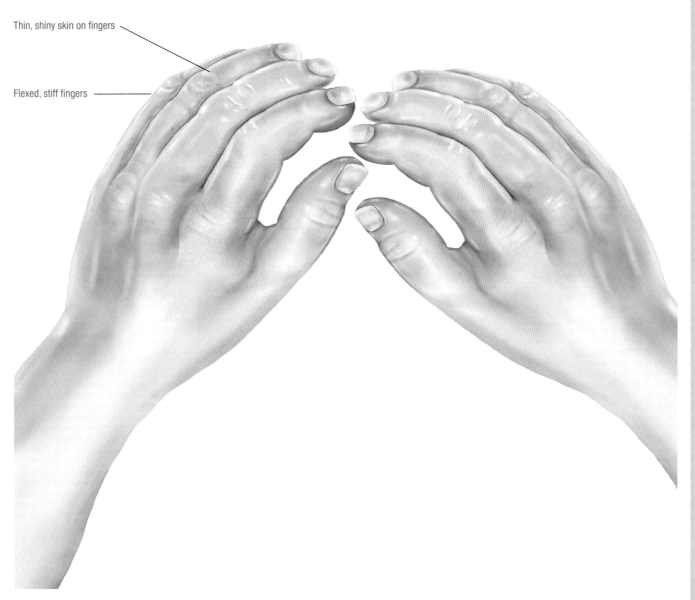

SYSTEMIC LUPUS ERYTHEMATOSUS

Systemic lupus erythematosus (SLE) is a chronic inflammatory autoimmune disorder that affects the connective tissues.

SLE is characterized by recurring remissions and exacerbations, which are especially common during the spring and summer. It strikes women 10 times as often as it does men, increasing to 15 times as often during child-bearing years. The prognosis improves with early detection and treatment but remains poor for patients who develop cardiovascular, renal, or neurologic complications or severe bacterial infections.

Causes

Direct cause unknown

Predisposing Factors

- Physical or mental stress
- Streptococcal or viral infections
- Exposure to sunlight or ultraviolet light
- Immunization
- Pregnancy
- Abnormal estrogen and androgen metabolism
- Drugs, including procainamide, hydralazine, and anticonvulsants; less commonly, penicillins, sulfa drugs, and oral contraceptives
- Associated with certain HLA haplotypes

Pathophysiology

Autoimmunity is believed to be the prime mechanism in SLE. The body produces antibodies against components of its own cells, such as the ANA, and immune complex disease follows. Patients with SLE may produce antibodies against many different tissue components, such as red blood cells (RBCs), neutrophils, platelets, lymphocytes, or almost any organ or tissue in the body. The disease presents in various clinical symptoms and is characterized by remissions and relapses.

COMPLICATIONS

- Pleurisy, pleural effusion, pneumonitis, pulmonary hypertension, and pulmonary infection
- Pericarditis, myocarditis, endocarditis, and coronary atherosclerosis
- Renal failure
- Seizures and mental dysfunction
- Infection
- Cancer
- Avascular necrosis
- Deep vein thrombosis, pulmonary embolism, and cerebral vascular accident

Signs and Symptoms

- Joint pain
- Raynaud's phenomenon
- Photosensitivity
- Tachycardia, central cyanosis, and hypotension
- Altered level of consciousness, weakness of the extremities, and speech disturbances
- Skin lesions
- Malar rash
- Ulcers in the mouth or nose
- Patchy alopecia (common)
- Vasculitis
- Lymph node enlargement (diffuse or local and nontender)
- Fever
- Pericardial friction rub
- Irregular menstruation or amenorrhea, particularly during flareups
- Chest pain and dyspnea
- Emotional instability, psychosis, organic brain syndrome, headaches, irritability, and depression
- Oliguria and urinary frequency; dysuria and bladder spasms

Diagnostic Test Results

- Complete blood count with differential reveals anemia and a reduced WBC count, decreased platelet count, elevated erythrocyte sedimentation rate, and serum electrophoresis showing hypergammaglobulinemia
- Positive ANA, DNA, and lupus erythematosus cell test findings in most patients with active SLE but only slightly useful in diagnosing the disease (the ANA test is sensitive but not specific for SLE)
- Urine studies showing RBCs, WBCs, urine casts and sediment, and significant protein loss
- Blood studies detect decreased serum complement (C3 and C4) levels, indicating active disease, increased C-reactive protein during flareups, and positive RF
- Chest X-rays reveal pleurisy or lupus pneumonitis
- Electrocardiogram reveals a conduction defect with cardiac involvement or pericarditis
- Renal biopsy shows the progression of SLE and the extent of renal involvement
- Skin biopsy shows immunoglobulin and complement deposition in the dermal-epidermal junction in 90% of patients

Treatment

- Nonsteroidal anti-inflammatory compounds
- Topical corticosteroid creams
- Intralesional corticosteroids or antimalarials
- Systemic corticosteroids
- High-dose steroids and cytotoxic therapy
- Dialysis or renal transplant
- Antihypertensives
- Dietary changes
- Sunscreen use

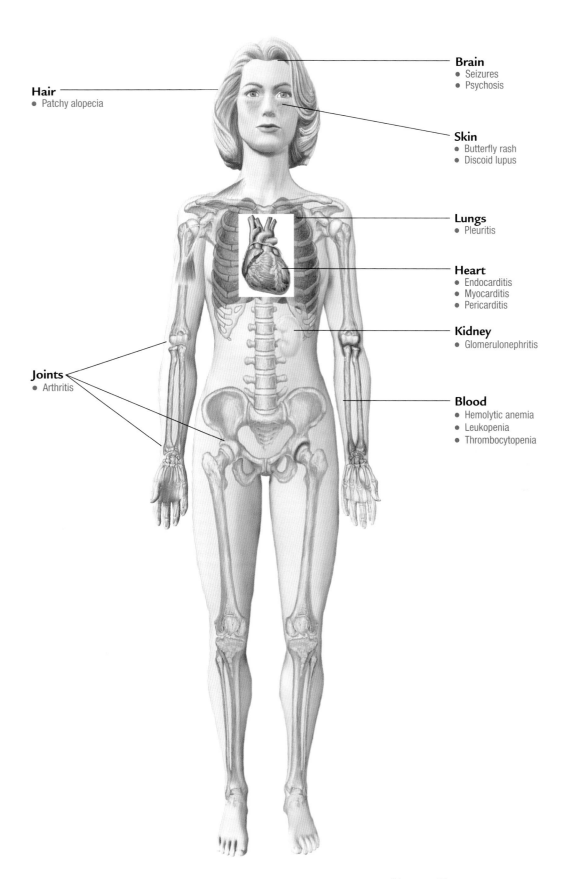

Brain
- Seizures
- Psychosis

Hair
- Patchy alopecia

Skin
- Butterfly rash
- Discoid lupus

Lungs
- Pleuritis

Heart
- Endocarditis
- Myocarditis
- Pericarditis

Kidney
- Glomerulonephritis

Joints
- Arthritis

Blood
- Hemolytic anemia
- Leukopenia
- Thrombocytopenia

Suggested References

Buttaro, T. M., Trybulski, J., Bailey, P. P., & Sandberg-Cook, J. (2017). *Primary care: A collaborative approach* (5th ed.). St. Louis, MO: Elsevier.

Centers for Disease Control (CDC).

Mandell, J., Dolin, R., & Blaser, M. (2015). *Mandell, Douglas, and Bennett's principles and practice of infectious diseases* (8th ed.). St. Louis, MO: Elsevier.

Wallace, D. (August 2015). Patient education: Systemic lupus erythematosus (beyond the basics). *UpToDate*. Retrieved from http://www.uptodate.com/contents/systemic-lupus-erythematosus-sle-beyond-the-basics

ADRENAL HYPOFUNCTION

Adrenal hypofunction is classified as primary or secondary. *Primary* adrenal hypofunction or insufficiency (Addison's disease) originates within the adrenal gland and is characterized by the decreased secretion of mineralocorticoids, glucocorticoids, and androgens. It's defined as destruction of more than 90% of both adrenal glands and is usually caused by an autoimmune process. Addison's disease is relatively uncommon and can occur at any age and in both sexes. *Secondary* adrenal hypofunction is due to impaired pituitary secretion of adrenocorticotropin (ACTH) and is characterized by decreased glucocorticoid secretion.

With early diagnosis and adequate replacement therapy, the prognosis for adrenal hypofunction is good.

CLINICAL TIP
Adrenal crisis (addisonian crisis) is a critical deficiency of mineralocorticoids and glucocorticoids that generally follows sepsis, trauma, surgery, omission of steroid therapy, or other acute physiologic stress. This medical emergency mandates immediate, vigorous treatment.

Causes

Primary Hypofunction (Addison's Disease)

- Bilateral adrenalectomy
- Hemorrhage into adrenal gland
- Neoplasms
- Tuberculosis, histoplasmosis, and cytomegalovirus
- Family history of autoimmune disease

Secondary Hypofunction (Glucocorticoid Deficiency)

- Hypopituitarism (causing decreased ACTH secretion)
- Abrupt withdrawal of long-term corticosteroid therapy
- Removal of an ACTH-secreting tumor
- Pituitary injury by tumor or infiltrative or autoimmune process

Pathophysiology

Addison's disease is a chronic condition that results from partial or complete adrenal destruction. In most cases, cellular atrophy is limited to the cortex, although medullary involvement may occur, resulting in catecholamine deficiency.

ACTH acts primarily to regulate the adrenal release of glucocorticoids (primarily cortisol); mineralocorticoids, including aldosterone; and sex steroids that supplement those produced by the gonads. ACTH secretion is controlled by corticotrophin-releasing hormone from the hypothalamus and by negative feedback control by the glucocorticoids.

Cortisol deficiency causes decreased liver gluconeogenesis. Glucose levels of patients on insulin may be dangerously low.

Aldosterone deficiency causes increased renal sodium loss and enhances potassium reabsorption. Sodium excretion causes a reduction in water volume that leads to hypotension.

Androgen deficiency may result in decreased hair growth in axillary and pubic areas, loss of erectile function, or decreased libido.

Signs and Symptoms

Primary Hypofunction

- Weakness, fatigue
- Nausea, vomiting, anorexia, weight loss
- Conspicuous bronze color of the skin, especially on hands, elbows, and knees; darkening of scars
- Cardiovascular abnormalities, including orthostatic hypotension, decreased cardiac size and output, and weak, irregular pulse
- Decreased tolerance for even minor stress
- Fasting hypoglycemia
- Craving for salty food

Secondary Hypofunction

- Similar to primary hypofunction; differences include:
  - hyperpigmentation absent because ACTH and melanocyte-stimulating hormone levels are low
  - possibly normal blood pressure and electrolyte balance because aldosterone secretion is near normal
  - usually normal androgen secretion.

COMPLICATIONS
- Adrenal crisis (profound weakness and fatigue, nausea, vomiting, dehydration, hypotension, confusion)

Diagnostic Test Results

- Blood test for plasma cortisol levels confirms adrenal insufficiency.
- Metyrapone test is used to detect secondary adrenal hypofunction.
- Rapid corticotropin stimulation test by I.V. or I.M. administration of cosyntropin, a synthetic form of corticotropin, after baseline sampling for cortisol and corticotropin (samples drawn for cortisol 30 and 60 minutes after injection), differentiates between primary and secondary adrenal hypofunction. A low corticotropin level indicates a secondary disorder. An elevated level is indicative of a primary disorder.
- Laboratory studies reveal decreased plasma cortisol level (less than 10 µg/dL in the morning; less in the evening) and decreased serum sodium and fasting blood glucose levels.
- Serum chemistry reveals increased serum potassium, calcium, and blood urea nitrogen levels.
- Complete blood count shows elevated hematocrit and increased lymphocyte and eosinophil counts.
- X-rays show adrenal calcification if the cause is infectious.

Treatment

Primary or Secondary Adrenal Hypofunction

- Lifelong corticosteroid replacement, usually with cortisone or hydrocortisone, which have a mineralocorticoid effect
- I.V. hydrocortisone

Primary Adrenal Hypofunction

- Oral fludrocortisone, a synthetic mineralocorticoid, to prevent dangerous dehydration, hypotension, hyponatremia, and hyperkalemia

ADRENAL HORMONE SECRETION

Adrenal hormones

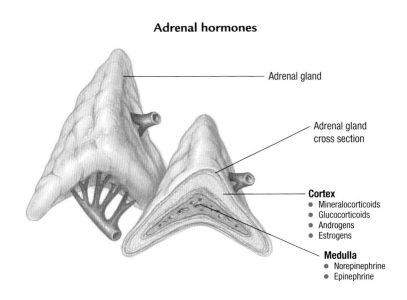

- Adrenal gland
- Adrenal gland cross section

Cortex
- Mineralocorticoids
- Glucocorticoids
- Androgens
- Estrogens

Medulla
- Norepinephrine
- Epinephrine

Blocked secretion of cortisol in primary adrenal hypofunction

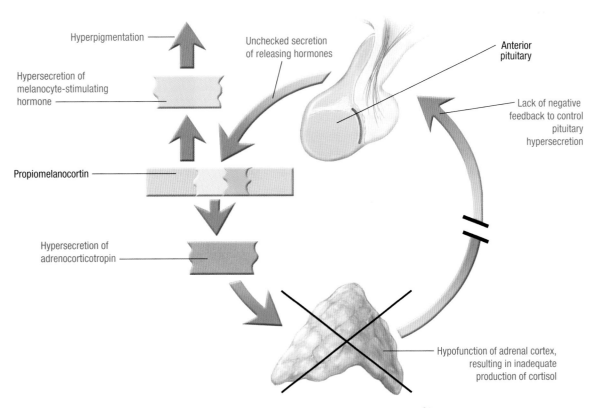

Hyperpigmentation

Hypersecretion of melanocyte-stimulating hormone

Unchecked secretion of releasing hormones

Anterior pituitary

Lack of negative feedback to control pituitary hypersecretion

Propiomelanocortin

Hypersecretion of adrenocorticotropin

Hypofunction of adrenal cortex, resulting in inadequate production of cortisol

CUSHING'S SYNDROME

ushing's syndrome is a cluster of clinical abnormalities caused by excessive adrenocortical hormones (particularly cortisol) or related corticosteroids and, to a lesser extent, androgens and aldosterone. Cushing's disease (ACTH excess) accounts for about 70% of the cases of Cushing's syndrome.

AGE ALERT
Cushing's syndrome caused by ectopic corticotropin secretion is most common in adult men, with the peak incidence between ages 40 and 60. In 30% of patients, Cushing's syndrome results from a cortisol-secreting tumor. Adrenal tumors, rather than pituitary tumors, are more common in children, especially girls.

Causes

- Pituitary hypersecretion of ACTH
- Autonomous, ectopic ACTH secretion by a tumor outside the pituitary (usually malignant, frequently a pancreatic tumor or oat cell carcinoma of the lung)
- Administration of synthetic glucocorticoids or steroids
- Adrenal adenoma or a cancerous adrenal tumor

Pathophysiology

Cortisol excess results in anti-inflammatory effects and excessive catabolism of protein and peripheral fat to support hepatic glucose production. The mechanism may be ACTH-dependent, in which elevated plasma ACTH levels stimulate the adrenal cortex to produce excess cortisol, or ACTH-independent, in which excess cortisol is produced by the adrenal cortex or exogenously administered. This suppresses the hypothalamic-pituitary-adrenal axis, also present in ectopic ACTH-secreting tumors.

COMPLICATIONS
- Osteoporosis
- Peptic ulcer
- Diabetes mellitus or impaired glucose tolerance
- Ischemic heart disease and heart failure

Signs and Symptoms

- Fat pads above the clavicles, over the upper back (buffalo hump), on the face (moon face), and throughout the trunk (truncal obesity); slender arms and legs
- Increased susceptibility to infection; decreased resistance to stress

- Hypertension, left ventricular hypertrophy, bleeding and ecchymosis, and dyslipidemia
- Increased androgen production — clitoral hypertrophy, mild virilism, hirsutism, and amenorrhea or oligomenorrhea in women; sexual dysfunction
- Sodium and secondary fluid retention, increased potassium excretion, and ureteral calculi
- Irritability and emotional lability
- Little or no scar formation; poor wound healing
- Purple striae, facial plethora, and acne
- Muscle weakness
- Pathologic fractures; skeletal growth retardation in children

Diagnostic Test Results

- Laboratory studies reveal hyperglycemia, hypernatremia, glucosuria, hypokalemia, and metabolic acidosis; elevated urinary free cortisol levels; elevated salivary free cortisol; and elevated serum cortisol.
- Dexamethasone suppression test confirms the diagnosis and determines the cause, possibly an adrenal tumor or a nonendocrine, corticotropin-releasing tumor.
- Ultrasound, computed tomography scan, and magnetic resonance imaging detect the presence of a pituitary or adrenal tumor.

Treatment

- Specific for cause of hypercortisolism — pituitary, adrenal, and ectopic
- Surgery for tumors of adrenal or pituitary glands or other tissue, such as lung
- Radiation therapy for tumor
- Cortisol replacement therapy after surgery
- Antihypertensives
- Potassium supplements
- Diuretics
- Antineoplastic and antihormone agents
- For inoperable tumor, drugs such as mitotane or aminoglutethimide to block steroid synthesis

CLINICAL TIP
Most patients with Cushing's syndrome are treated with transsphenoidal surgery, which has a high cure rate (80%). Pharmacotherapy is usually used as adjunctive rather than primary therapy.

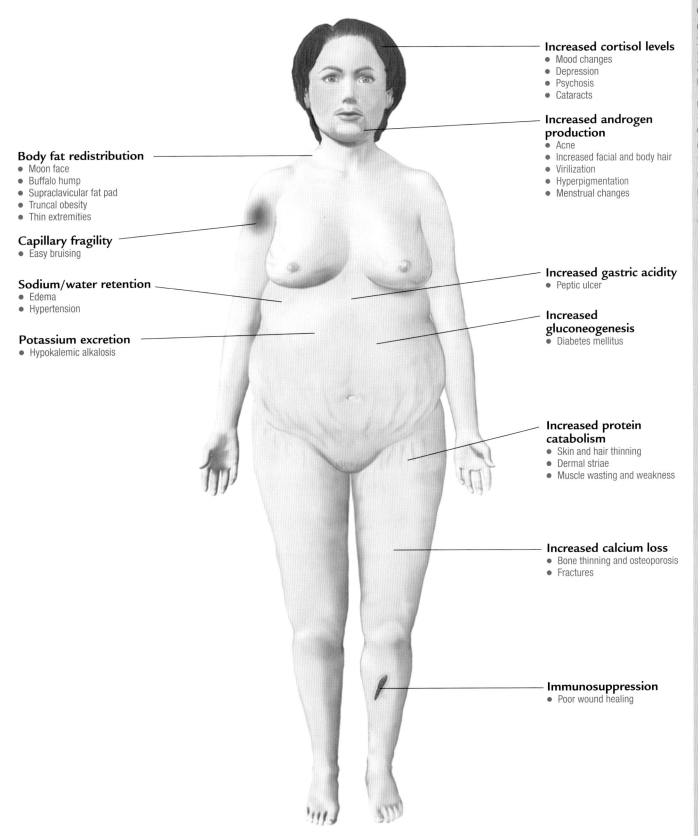

Increased cortisol levels
- Mood changes
- Depression
- Psychosis
- Cataracts

Increased androgen production
- Acne
- Increased facial and body hair
- Virilization
- Hyperpigmentation
- Menstrual changes

Body fat redistribution
- Moon face
- Buffalo hump
- Supraclavicular fat pad
- Truncal obesity
- Thin extremities

Capillary fragility
- Easy bruising

Increased gastric acidity
- Peptic ulcer

Sodium/water retention
- Edema
- Hypertension

Increased gluconeogenesis
- Diabetes mellitus

Potassium excretion
- Hypokalemic alkalosis

Increased protein catabolism
- Skin and hair thinning
- Dermal striae
- Muscle wasting and weakness

Increased calcium loss
- Bone thinning and osteoporosis
- Fractures

Immunosuppression
- Poor wound healing

DIABETES INSIPIDUS

A disorder of water metabolism, diabetes insipidus results from a deficiency of circulating vasopressin (also called *antidiuretic hormone*, or *ADH*) or from renal resistance to this hormone. The three forms of diabetes insipidus are neurogenic, nephrogenic, and psychogenic. Neurogenic diabetes insipidus is caused by a deficiency of ADH; nephrogenic diabetes insipidus, by the resistance of renal tubules to ADH. Diabetes insipidus is characterized by excessive fluid intake and hypotonic polyuria. A decrease in ADH levels leads to altered intracellular and extracellular fluid control, causing renal excretion of a large amount of urine.

AGE ALERT
Diabetes insipidus may begin at any age and is slightly more common in men than in women.

In uncomplicated diabetes insipidus, the prognosis is good with adequate water replacement, and patients usually lead normal lives.

Causes

- Neurogenic: stroke, hypothalamic or pituitary tumor, cranial trauma, or surgery
- Nephrogenic: X-linked recessive trait, end-stage renal failure
- Psychogenic: primary polydipsia or sarcoidosis
- Transient diabetes insipidus: certain drugs, such as lithium, phenytoin, or alcohol

Pathophysiology

Diabetes insipidus is related to an insufficiency of ADH, leading to polydipsia and polyuria.

Neurogenic or *central*, diabetes insipidus is an inadequate ADH response to changes in plasma osmolarity. A lesion of the hypothalamus, infundibular stem, or posterior pituitary partially or completely blocks ADH synthesis, transport, or release.

Neurogenic diabetes insipidus has an acute onset. A three-phase syndrome can occur, which involves:

- progressive loss of nerve tissue and increased diuresis
- normal diuresis
- polyuria and polydipsia, reflecting permanent loss of the ability to secrete adequate ADH.

Nephrogenic diabetes insipidus is caused by an inadequate renal response to ADH. The collecting duct's permeability to water doesn't increase in response to ADH. Nephrogenic diabetes insipidus is generally related to disorders and drugs that damage the renal tubules or inhibit the generation of cyclic adenosine monophosphate in the tubules. In addition, hypokalemia or hypercalcemia impairs the renal response to ADH. A rare genetic form of nephrogenic diabetes insipidus is an X-linked recessive trait.

Psychogenic diabetes insipidus is caused by an extremely large fluid intake. This primary polydipsia may be idiopathic or reflect psychosis or sarcoidosis. The polydipsia and resultant polyuria wash out ADH more quickly than it can be replaced. Chronic polyuria may overwhelm the renal medullary concentration gradient, rendering the kidneys partially or totally unable to concentrate urine.

Regardless of the cause, insufficient ADH causes the immediate excretion of large volumes of dilute urine and consequent plasma hyperosmolality. In conscious individuals, the thirst mechanism is stimulated, usually for cold liquids.

COMPLICATIONS
- Severe dehydration
- Shock
- Renal failure
- Central nervous system damage
- Bladder distention
- Hydronephrosis

Signs and Symptoms

- Polydipsia and polyuria up to 20 L/d (cardinal symptoms)
- Nocturia
- Sleep disturbance and fatigue
- Headache and visual disturbance
- Abdominal fullness, anorexia, and weight loss
- Fever
- Changes in level of consciousness
- Hypotension
- Tachycardia

Diagnostic Test Results

- Urinalysis shows almost colorless urine of low osmolality and low specific gravity.
- Water deprivation test identifies vasopressin deficiency, resulting in renal inability to concentrate urine.

Treatment

- Vasopressin to control fluid balance and prevent dehydration until the cause of diabetes insipidus can be identified and eliminated
- Hydrochlorothiazide with potassium supplement
- Desmopressin acetate
- Chlorpropamide
- Fluid intake to match output

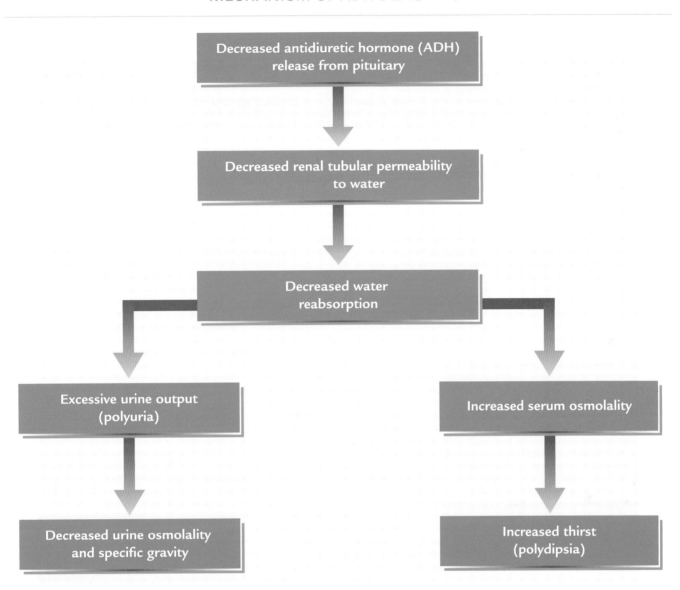

CLINICAL TIP

LABORATORY VALUES FOR PATIENTS WITH DIABETES INSIPIDUS

Value	Normal	Diabetes Insipidus (DI)
Serum ADH	<2.5 pg/mL	Decreased in central DI; may be normal with nephrogenic or psychogenic DI
Serum osmolality	285–300 mOsm/kg	>300 mOsm/kg
Serum sodium	136–145 mEq/L	>145 mEq/L
Urine osmolality	300–900 mOsm/kg	<300 mOsm/kg
Urine specific gravity	1.005–1.030	<1.005
Urine output	1–1.5 L/24 h	30–40 L/24 h
Fluid intake	1–1.5 L/24 h	>50 L/24 h

DIABETES MELLITUS

Diabetes mellitus is a metabolic disorder characterized by hyperglycemia resulting from lack of insulin, lack of insulin effect, or both. Three general classifications are recognized:

- type 1 — absolute insulin insufficiency
- type 2 — insulin resistance with varying degrees of insulin secretory defects
- gestational diabetes — manifested during pregnancy.

AGE ALERT
Although possible at any age, type 1 usually manifests before age 30. Type 2 usually occurs in obese adults after age 40.

Causes

- Heredity
- Environment (infection, toxins)
- Stress, diet, and lack of exercise in genetically susceptible persons
- Pregnancy

Pathophysiology

Type 1 and type 2 diabetes mellitus are two separate and distinct pathophysiological entities. In persons genetically susceptible to *type 1* diabetes, a triggering event, possibly a viral infection, causes production of autoantibodies, which kill the beta cells of the pancreas. This leads to a decline in and an ultimate lack of insulin secretion. Insulin deficiency, when more than 90% of the beta cells have been destroyed, leads to hyperglycemia, enhanced lipolysis, and protein catabolism.

Type 2 diabetes mellitus is a chronic disease caused by one or more of the following factors: impaired insulin production, inappropriate hepatic glucose production, or peripheral insulin receptor insensitivity.

Gestational diabetes mellitus is glucose intolerance during pregnancy in a woman not previously diagnosed with diabetes. This may occur if placental hormones counteract insulin, causing insulin resistance.

COMPLICATIONS
- Cardiovascular disease
- Nephropathy
- Retinopathy
- Neuropathy
- Ketoacidosis and hyperosmolar coma
- Infections

Signs and Symptoms

- Polyuria and polydipsia
- Nausea; anorexia (common) or polyphagia (occasional)
- Weight loss (usually 10% to 30%; persons with type 1 diabetes often have almost no body fat at diagnosis)
- Headaches, fatigue, lethargy, reduced energy levels, and impaired school or work performance
- Muscle cramps, irritability, and emotional lability
- Vision changes such as blurring
- Numbness and tingling

- Abdominal discomfort and pain; diarrhea or constipation
- Recurrent vaginal candidiasis

Diagnostic Test Results

In Men and Nonpregnant Women

- Two of the following criteria obtained more than 24 hours apart, using the same test twice or any combination, are indicators of the disease:
    - fasting plasma glucose level of 126 mg/dL or more
    - typical symptoms of uncontrolled diabetes and random blood glucose level of 200 mg/dL or more
    - blood glucose level of 200 mg/dL or more 2 hours after ingesting 75 g of oral dextrose.
- Other criteria include:
    - diabetic retinopathy on ophthalmologic examination
    - other diagnostic and monitoring tests, including urinalysis for acetone and glycosylated hemoglobin (reflects glycemic control over the past 2 to 3 months).

In Pregnant Women

- Positive glucose tolerance test reveals high peak blood sugar levels after ingestion of glucose (1 g/kg body weight) and delayed return to fasting levels.

Treatment

Type 1 Diabetes Mellitus

- Insulin replacement, meal planning, and exercise (current forms of insulin replacement include mixed-dose, split mixed-dose, inhaled, and multiple daily injection regimens and continuous subcutaneous insulin infusions)
- Islet cell transplantation (currently requires chronic immunosuppression)

Type 2 Diabetes Mellitus

- Oral antidiabetic drugs to stimulate endogenous insulin production, increase insulin sensitivity at the cellular level, suppress hepatic gluconeogenesis, and delay GI absorption of carbohydrates (drug combinations may be used)
- Exogenous insulin, alone or with oral antidiabetic drugs, to optimize glycemic control

Type 1 and Type 2 Diabetes Mellitus

- Individualized meal plan designed to meet nutritional needs, control blood glucose and lipid levels, and reach and maintain appropriate body weight
- Weight reduction (obese patient with type 2 diabetes mellitus) or high calorie allotment, depending on growth stage and activity level (type 1 diabetes mellitus)

Gestational Diabetes

- Medical nutrition therapy and exercise
- Alpha glucosidase inhibitors, injected insulin, or both (if euglycemia not achieved)
- Counseling on the high risk for gestational diabetes in subsequent pregnancies and type 2 diabetes later in life
- Exercise and weight control to help avert type 2 diabetes

Type 1 diabetes

Pancreas with no insulin production

Cell

Glucose

Closed glucose channel

Open glucose channel

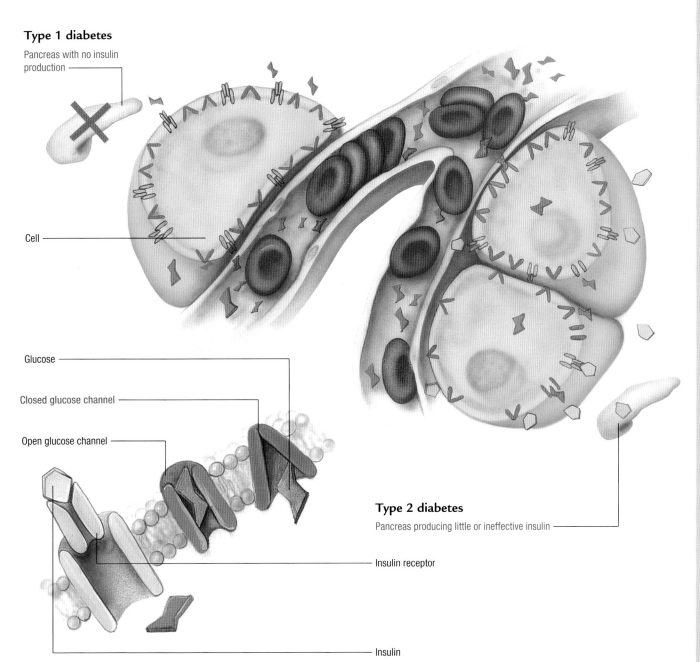

Type 2 diabetes

Pancreas producing little or ineffective insulin

Insulin receptor

Insulin

GROWTH HORMONE EXCESS

Growth hormone (GH) excess that begins in adulthood (after epiphyseal closure) is called *acromegaly*. GH excess that's present before closure of the epiphyseal growth plates of the long bones causes *pituitary gigantism*. In both cases, the result is increased growth of bone, cartilage, and other tissues, as well as increased carbohydrate catabolism and protein synthesis. In gigantism, a proportional overgrowth of all body tissues before epiphyseal closure causes remarkable height increases — as much as 6 inches (15 cm) a year. Acromegaly is rare; its prevalence is about 70 people per million in the United States, affecting men and women equally. GH excess is a slow but progressive disease that shortens life if untreated. Morbidity and mortality tend to be related to coronary artery disease and hypertension secondary to prolonged exposure to excessive GH.

AGE ALERT
Most cases of acromegaly are diagnosed in the fourth and fifth decades, but the disease is usually present for years before diagnosis. Gigantism affects infants and children, causing them to reach as much as three times the normal height for their age. Affected adults may reach a height of more than 7/2′ (7.6 m).

Causes

Eosinophilic or mixed cell adenomas of the anterior pituitary gland

Pathophysiology

A GH-secreting tumor creates an unpredictable GH secretion pattern, which replaces the usual peaks at 1 to 4 hours after the onset of sleep. Elevated GH and somatomedin levels stimulate growth of all tissues. In pituitary gigantism, the epiphyseal plates aren't closed, and so the excess GH stimulates linear growth. It also increases the bulk of bones and joints and causes enlargement of internal organs and metabolic abnormalities. In acromegaly, the excess GH increases bone density and width and the proliferation of connective and soft tissues.

COMPLICATIONS
- Arthritis
- Carpal tunnel syndrome
- Osteoporosis
- Kyphosis
- Hypertension
- Diabetes mellitus
- Arteriosclerosis
- Heart enlargement
- Heart failure

Signs and Symptoms

Acromegaly

- Soft tissue thickening that causes enlargement of hands, feet, nose, mandible, supraorbital ridge, and ears
- Severe headache, central nervous system impairment, bitemporal hemianopia (defective vision), and loss of visual acuity
- Marked prognathism and malocclusion of teeth; may interfere with chewing
- Laryngeal hypertrophy, paranasal sinus enlargement, and thickening of the tongue — causing the voice to sound deep and hollow
- Arrowhead appearance of distal phalanges on X-rays and thickened fingers
- Sweating, oily skin, hypertrichosis, and new skin tags (typical)
- Irritability, hostility, and various psychological disturbances
- Bow legs, barrel chest, arthritis, osteoporosis, and kyphosis
- Glucose intolerance
- Hypertension and arteriosclerosis (effects of prolonged excessive GH secretion)
- Hypermetabolism
- Weakness, arthralgia

Gigantism

- Backache, arthralgia, and arthritis
- Excessive height
- Headache, vomiting, seizure activity, visual disturbances, and papilledema
- Deficiencies of other hormone systems if GH-producing tumor destroys other hormone-secreting cells
- Glucose intolerance

Diagnostic Test Results

- Laboratory studies reveal elevated plasma GH level measured by radioimmunoassay, the presence of somatomedin C, and elevated blood glucose levels.
- Glucose suppression test confirms hyperpituitarism.
- Skull X-rays, computed tomography scan, or magnetic resonance imaging shows the presence and extent of pituitary lesion.
- Bone X-rays show a thickening of the cranium (especially frontal, occipital, and parietal bones) and long bones and osteoarthritis in the spine.

Treatment

- Tumor removal by cranial or transsphenoidal hypophysectomy or pituitary radiation therapy
- Mandatory surgery for a tumor causing blindness or other severe neurologic disturbances
- Postoperative replacement of thyroid, cortisone, and gonadal hormones
- Bromocriptine and octreotide to inhibit GH synthesis

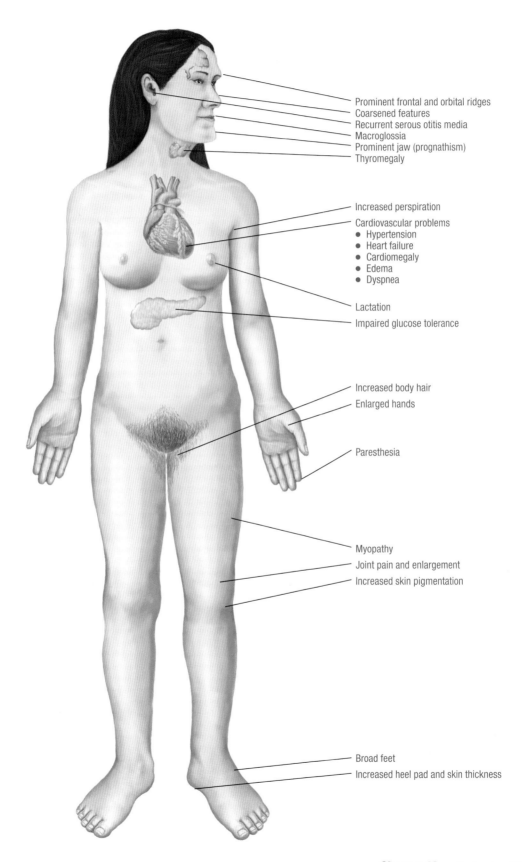

Prominent frontal and orbital ridges
Coarsened features
Recurrent serous otitis media
Macroglossia
Prominent jaw (prognathism)
Thyromegaly

Increased perspiration
Cardiovascular problems
- Hypertension
- Heart failure
- Cardiomegaly
- Edema
- Dyspnea

Lactation
Impaired glucose tolerance

Increased body hair
Enlarged hands

Paresthesia

Myopathy
Joint pain and enlargement
Increased skin pigmentation

Broad feet
Increased heel pad and skin thickness

HYPERPARATHYROIDISM

Hyperparathyroidism results from excessive secretion of parathyroid hormone (PTH) from one or more of the four parathyroid glands. PTH promotes bone resorption, and hypersecretion leads to hypercalcemia and hypophosphatemia. Renal and GI absorption of calcium increase. Primary hyperparathyroidism is commonly diagnosed when an asymptomatic patient has elevated calcium levels in routine laboratory tests.

AGE ALERT
Hyperparathyroidism affects women two to three times more frequently than it does men and is usually seen in women older than age 40.

Causes

Primary Hyperparathyroidism

- Most commonly a single adenoma
- Multiple endocrine neoplasia (all four glands usually involved)

Secondary Hyperparathyroidism

- Rickets, vitamin D deficiency, chronic renal failure, and osteomalacia due to phenytoin

Pathophysiology

Overproduction of PTH by a tumor or hyperplastic tissue increases intestinal calcium absorption, reduces renal calcium clearance, and increases bone calcium release. Response to this excess varies for each patient for unknown reasons.

Hypophosphatemia results when excessive PTH inhibits renal tubular phosphate reabsorption. It aggravates hypercalcemia by increasing the sensitivity of the bone to PTH. Pathologic fractures may be a presenting symptom.

A hypocalcemia-producing abnormality outside the parathyroids can cause excessive compensatory production of PTH or secondary hyperparathyroidism.

COMPLICATIONS
- Renal calculi and renal failure
- Peptic ulcer
- Cholelithiasis
- Cardiac arrhythmias, vascular damage, and heart failure
- Central nervous system changes

Signs and Symptoms

Primary Hyperparathyroidism

- Polyuria, nephrocalcinosis, or recurring nephrolithiasis and consequent renal insufficiency
- Chronic low back pain and easy fracturing
- Bone tenderness and chondrocalcinosis
- Osteopenia and osteoporosis, especially of vertebrae
- Erosions of juxta-articular (adjoining joint) surface
- Subchondral fractures
- Traumatic synovitis
- Pseudogout

- Pancreatitis causing constant, severe epigastric pain that radiates to the back
- Peptic ulcers, causing abdominal pain, anorexia, nausea, and vomiting
- Muscle weakness and atrophy, particularly in the legs
- Psychomotor and personality disturbances, depression, and overt psychosis
- Skin necrosis, cataracts, calcium microthrombi to lungs and pancreas, anemia, and subcutaneous calcification

Secondary Hyperparathyroidism

- Same features of calcium imbalance as in primary hyperparathyroidism
- Skeletal deformities of the long bones (such as rickets)
- Symptoms of the underlying disease

Diagnostic Test Results

Primary Hyperparathyroidism

- Hypercalcemia and high concentrations of serum PTH on radioimmunoassay confirm the diagnosis.
- X-rays show diffuse demineralization of bones, bone cysts, outer cortical bone absorption, and subperiosteal erosion of the phalanges and distal clavicles.
- Microscopic bone examination by X-ray spectrophotometry typically shows increased bone turnover.
- Laboratory studies detect elevated urine and serum calcium, chloride, and alkaline phosphatase levels; decreased serum phosphorus levels; elevated uric acid and creatinine levels; and increased serum amylase levels.

Secondary Hyperparathyroidism

- Laboratory analysis reveals normal or slightly decreased serum calcium level and variable serum phosphorus level, especially when the cause is rickets, osteomalacia, or kidney disease.

Treatment

Primary Hyperparathyroidism

- Surgery to remove the adenoma or, depending on the extent of hyperplasia, all but half of one gland, to provide normal PTH levels
- Treatments to decrease calcium levels — forcing fluids, limiting dietary intake of calcium, and promoting sodium and calcium excretion through forced diuresis
- Oral sodium or potassium phosphate; subcutaneous calcitonin; I.V. mithramycin or bisphosphonate
- I.V. magnesium and phosphate; sodium phosphate solution by mouth or retention enema; possibly supplemental calcium, vitamin D, or calcitriol

Secondary Hyperparathyroidism

- Vitamin D to correct the underlying cause of parathyroid hyperplasia; oral calcium preparation to correct hyperphosphatemia in the patient with kidney disease
- Dialysis in patient with renal failure to decrease phosphorus levels
- Calcitonin
- Pamidronate

Tumor or hyperplastic tissue secretes excess parathyroid hormone

Thyroid cartilage

Superior parathyroid glands

Thyroid gland

Inferior parathyroid glands

Renal tubule
Enhanced calcium reabsorption and phosphate excretion

Bone
Enhanced calcium and phosphate resorption

GI tract
Enhanced calcium absorption

Serum calcium level rises

CLINICAL TIP

BONE RESORPTION IN PRIMARY HYPERPARATHYROIDISM

In hyperparathyroidism, body mechanisms sacrifice bone to preserve intracellular calcium levels. X-rays may show diffuse demineralization of bones, bone cysts, outer cortical bone absorption, and subperiosteal erosion of the phalanges and distal clavicles. Microscopic examination of the bone with tests — such as X-ray spectrophotometry — typically demonstrates increased bone turnover.

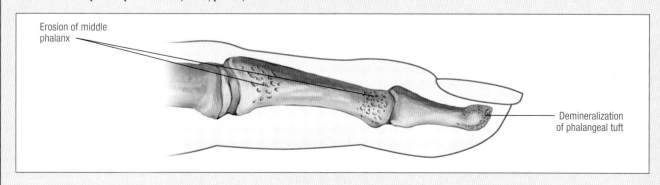

Erosion of middle phalanx

Demineralization of phalangeal tuft

HYPERTHYROIDISM

Hyperthyroidism, or thyrotoxicosis, is a metabolic imbalance that results from the overproduction of thyroid hormone. The most common form is Graves' disease, an autoimmune disorder that increases thyroxine (T_4) production, enlarges the thyroid gland (goiter), and causes multiple system changes.

AGE ALERT
Incidence of Graves' disease is greatest in women between ages 30 and 60, especially those with a family history of thyroid abnormalities; only 5% of patients are younger than age 15.

Causes

- Inherited predisposition, probably autosomal recessive gene
- Other endocrine abnormalities
- Defect in suppressor T-lymphocyte function and consequent production of autoantibodies
- Excessive dietary intake of iodine
- Stress, such as surgery, infection, toxemia of pregnancy, or diabetic ketoacidosis — can precipitate thyroid storm
- Medications, such as lithium and amiodarone
- Toxic nodules or tumors

Pathophysiology

The thyroid gland secretes the thyroid precursor T_4, the thyroid hormone triiodothyronine (T_3), and thyrocalcitonin. T_4 and T_3 stimulate protein, lipid, and carbohydrate metabolism primarily through catabolic pathways. Thyrocalcitonin removes calcium from the blood and incorporates it into bone. Biosynthesis, storage, and release of thyroid hormones are controlled by the hypothalamic-pituitary axis through a negative feedback loop.

Thyrotropin-releasing hormone (TRH) from the hypothalamus stimulates the release of thyroid-stimulating hormone (TSH) by the pituitary. Circulating T_3 levels provide negative feedback through the hypothalamus to decrease TRH levels and through the pituitary to decrease TSH levels.

In Graves' disease, autoantibodies are produced that attach to and then stimulate TSH receptors on the thyroid gland. This process leads to increased stimulation of the gland and increased hormone production.

COMPLICATIONS
- Thyroid storm (extreme irritability, hypertension, tachycardia, vomiting, temperature up to 106°F [41.1°C], delirium, and coma)

Signs and Symptoms

- Enlarged thyroid (goiter)
- Nervousness, tremor, and palpitations
- Heat intolerance and sweating
- Weight loss despite increased appetite
- Frequent bowel movements
- Exophthalmos (characteristic, but absent in many patients with thyrotoxicosis)

Other Signs and Symptoms, Common Because Thyrotoxicosis Profoundly Affects Virtually Every Body System

- Difficulty concentrating; fine tremor, shaky handwriting, and clumsiness; emotional instability and mood swings ranging from occasional outbursts to overt psychosis
- Moist, smooth, warm, flushed skin; fine, soft hair; premature patchy graying and increased hair loss in both sexes; friable nails and onycholysis; pretibial myxedema, producing thickened skin; accentuated hair follicles; sometimes itchy or painful raised red patches of skin with occasional nodule formation; microscopic examination showing increased mucin deposits
- Systolic hypertension, tachycardia, full bounding pulse, wide pulse pressure, cardiomegaly, increased cardiac output and blood volume, visible point of maximal impulse, paroxysmal supraventricular tachycardia and atrial fibrillation (especially in elderly people), and occasional systolic murmur at the left sternal border
- Increased respiratory rate, dyspnea on exertion and at rest, nausea and vomiting, soft stools or diarrhea, and liver enlargement
- Weakness, fatigue, and muscle atrophy; rare coexistence with myasthenia gravis; possibly generalized or localized paralysis associated with hypokalemia and, rarely, acropachy
- Oligomenorrhea or amenorrhea, decreased fertility, increased incidence of spontaneous abortion (females), gynecomastia (males), and diminished libido (both sexes)

Diagnostic Test Results

- Radioimmunoassay shows increased serum T_4 and T_3 levels.
- Laboratory studies reveal low TSH levels.
- Thyroid scan shows increased uptake of radioactive iodine (^{131}I) in Graves' disease and, usually, in toxic multinodular goiter and toxic adenoma; low radioactive uptake in thyroiditis and thyrotoxic factitia (test contraindicated in pregnancy).
- Ultrasonography confirms subclinical ophthalmopathy.

Treatment

- Antithyroid drugs — thyroid hormone antagonists, including propylthiouracil and methimazole, to block thyroid hormone synthesis; propranolol until antithyroid drugs reach their full effect — to manage tachycardia and other peripheral effects of excessive hypersympathetic activity
- Single oral dose of ^{131}I
- Surgery and lifelong regular medical supervision — most patients become hypothyroid, sometimes as long as several years after surgery

CLINICAL TIP
With treatment, most patients with hyperthyroidism can lead normal lives. However, thyroid storm — an acute, severe exacerbation of thyrotoxicosis — is a medical emergency that may have life-threatening cardiac, hepatic, or renal consequences.

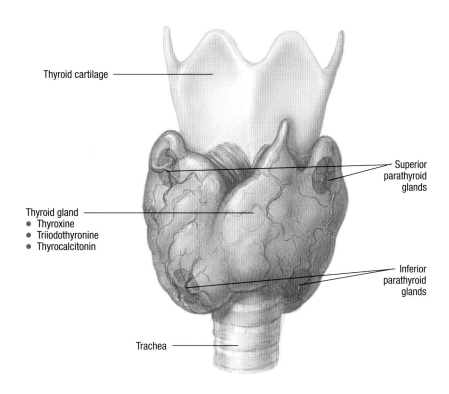

Thyroid cartilage

Superior
parathyroid
glands

Thyroid gland
- Thyroxine
- Triiodothyronine
- Thyrocalcitonin

Inferior
parathyroid
glands

Trachea

HISTOLOGIC CHANGES IN GRAVES' DISEASE

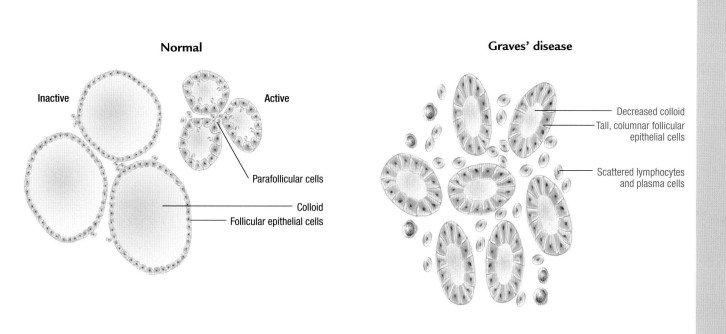

Normal

Inactive

Active

Parafollicular cells

Colloid

Follicular epithelial cells

Graves' disease

Decreased colloid

Tall, columnar follicular
epithelial cells

Scattered lymphocytes
and plasma cells

HYPOPITUITARISM

Hypopituitarism, also known as *panhypopituitarism*, is a complex syndrome marked by metabolic dysfunction, sexual immaturity, and growth retardation (when it occurs in childhood). The cause is a deficiency of the hormones secreted by the anterior pituitary gland. Panhypopituitarism is a partial or total failure of all six of this gland's vital hormones — ACTH, thyroid-stimulating hormone (TSH), luteinizing hormone (LH), follicle-stimulating hormone (FSH), GH, and prolactin.

AGE ALERT
Partial and complete forms of hypopituitarism affect adults and children; in children, these diseases may cause dwarfism and delayed puberty. The prognosis may be good with adequate replacement therapy and correction of the underlying causes.

Primary hypopituitarism usually develops in a predictable pattern. It generally begins with decreased gonadotropin (FSH and LH) levels and consequent hypogonadism, reflected by cessation of menses in women and impotence in men. GH deficiency follows, causing short stature, delayed growth, and delayed puberty in children. Subsequent decreased TSH levels cause hypothyroidism and, finally, decreased ACTH levels result in adrenal insufficiency, possibly leading to adrenal crisis. When hypopituitarism follows surgical ablation or trauma, the pattern of hormonal events may not necessarily follow that sequence. Damage to the hypothalamus or neurohypophysis may cause diabetes insipidus.

Causes

Primary Hypopituitarism

- Tumor of the pituitary gland
- Congenital defect (hypoplasia or aplasia of the pituitary gland)
- Pituitary infarction (most often from postpartum hemorrhage)
- Partial or total hypophysectomy by surgery, irradiation, or chemical agents
- Granulomatous disease such as tuberculosis
- Idiopathic or autoimmune origin (occasionally)

Secondary Hypopituitarism

- Deficiency of releasing hormones produced by the hypothalamus, either idiopathic or resulting from infection, trauma, or a tumor

Pathophysiology

The pituitary gland is highly vascular and therefore extremely vulnerable to ischemia and infarction. Any event that leads to circulatory collapse and compensatory vasospasm may result in gland ischemia, tissue necrosis, or edema. Expansion of the pituitary gland within the fixed compartment of the *sella turcica* further impedes its blood supply. An absence or decrease of one or more pituitary hormones leads to a loss of function in the gland or organ that it controls.

COMPLICATIONS
- Pituitary apoplexy
- Shock
- Coma
- Death

Signs and Symptoms

- ACTH deficiency: weakness, fatigue, weight loss, fasting hypoglycemia, and altered mental function; loss of axillary and pubic hair; orthostatic hypotension and hyponatremia
- TSH deficiency: weight gain, constipation, cold intolerance, fatigue, and coarse hair
- Gonadotropin deficiency: sexual dysfunction and infertility
- Antidiuretic hormone deficiency: diabetes insipidus
- Prolactin deficiency: lactation dysfunction or gynecomastia

Diagnostic Test Results

- Blood test reveals decreased serum thyroxin levels in diminished thyroid gland function due to lack of TSH.
- Radioimmunoassay shows decreased plasma levels of some or all of the pituitary hormones.
- Increased prolactin levels possibly indicating a lesion in the hypothalamus or pituitary stalk.
- Computed tomography scans, magnetic resonance imaging, or cerebral angiography may show the presence of intrasellar or extrasellar tumors.
- Oral administration of metyrapone shows the source of low hydroxycorticosteroid levels.
- Insulin administration shows low levels of corticotropin, indicating pituitary or hypothalamic failure.
- Dopamine antagonist administration evaluates prolactin secretory reserve.
- I.V. administration of gonadotropin-releasing hormone distinguishes pituitary and hypothalamic causes of gonadotropin deficiency.
- Provocative testing shows persistently low GH and insulin-like growth factor-1 levels confirming GH deficiency.

Treatment

- Replacement of hormones (cortisol, thyroxine, androgen or cyclic estrogen) secreted by the target glands; prolactin not replaced
- Clomiphene or cyclic gonadotropin-releasing hormone to induce ovulation in female patient of reproductive age
- Surgery for pituitary tumor

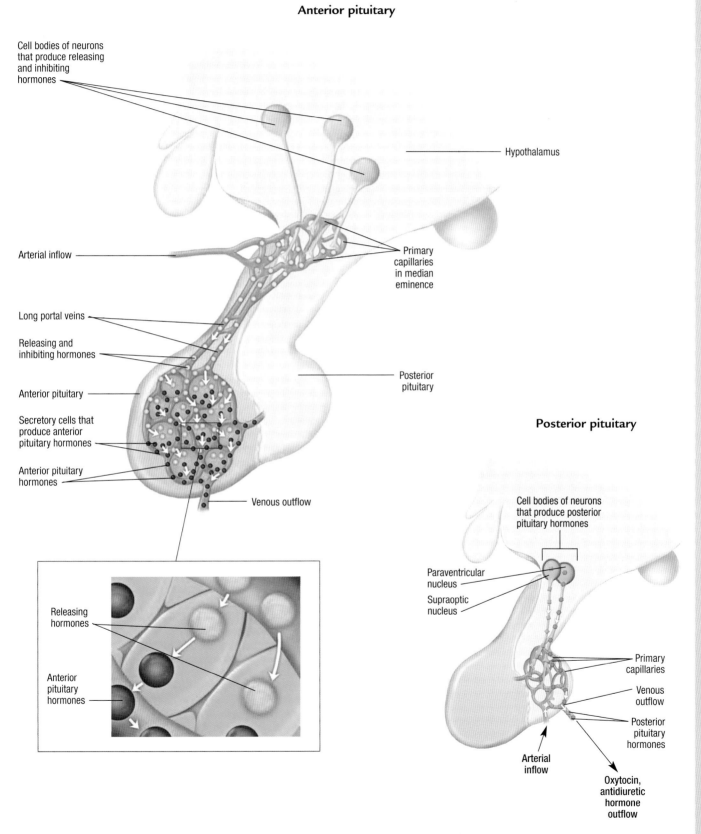

Anterior pituitary

Cell bodies of neurons that produce releasing and inhibiting hormones

Hypothalamus

Arterial inflow

Primary capillaries in median eminence

Long portal veins

Releasing and inhibiting hormones

Posterior pituitary

Anterior pituitary

Secretory cells that produce anterior pituitary hormones

Anterior pituitary hormones

Venous outflow

Releasing hormones

Anterior pituitary hormones

Posterior pituitary

Cell bodies of neurons that produce posterior pituitary hormones

Paraventricular nucleus

Supraoptic nucleus

Primary capillaries

Venous outflow

Posterior pituitary hormones

Arterial inflow

Oxytocin, antidiuretic hormone outflow

HYPOTHYROIDISM

Hypothyroidism results from hypothalamic, pituitary, or thyroid insufficiency or resistance to thyroid hormone. Hypothyroidism is more prevalent in women than men; in the United States, the incidence is increasing significantly in people ages 40 to 50.

AGE ALERT
Hypothyroidism occurs primarily after age 50 and is particularly underdiagnosed in elderly persons. After age 65, prevalence increases to as much as 10% in females and 3% in males.

A deficiency of thyroid hormone secretion during fetal development and early infancy results in infantile cretinism (congenital hypothyroidism). Subacute thyroiditis, painless thyroiditis, and postpartum thyroiditis are self-limited conditions that may follow an episode of hyperthyroidism.

Causes

Primary (Disorder of Thyroid Gland)

- Thyroidectomy or radiation therapy (particularly with radioactive iodine)
- Inflammation, chronic autoimmune thyroiditis (Hashimoto's thyroiditis), or such conditions as amyloidosis and sarcoidosis (rare)

Secondary (Failure to Stimulate Normal Thyroid Function)

- Inadequate production of thyroid hormone
- Use of such antithyroid medications as propylthiouracil
- Pituitary failure to produce TSH
- Inborn errors of thyroid hormone synthesis
- Iodine deficiency (usually dietary)
- Hypothalamic failure to produce TRH

Pathophysiology

Hypothyroidism may reflect a malfunction of the hypothalamus, pituitary, or thyroid gland, all of which are part of the same negative feedback mechanism. However, disorders of the hypothalamus and pituitary rarely cause hypothyroidism. Primary hypothyroidism is most common.

Chronic autoimmune thyroiditis, also called *chronic lymphocytic thyroiditis*, occurs when autoantibodies destroy thyroid gland tissue. Chronic autoimmune thyroiditis associated with goiter is called *Hashimoto's thyroiditis*. The cause of this autoimmune process is unknown, although heredity plays a role, and specific human leukocyte antigen subtypes are associated with greater risk.

Outside the thyroid, antibodies can reduce the effect of thyroid hormone in two ways. First, antibodies can block the TSH receptor and prevent the production of TSH. Second, cytotoxic antithyroid antibodies may trigger thyroid destruction.

COMPLICATIONS
- Myxedema coma
- Pernicious anemia
- Impaired fertility
- Achlorhydria
- Anemia
- Goiter
- Psychiatric disturbances

Signs and Symptoms

- Typical, vague, early clinical features — weakness, fatigue, forgetfulness, sensitivity to cold, unexplained weight gain, and constipation
- Myxedema — decreasing mental stability; coarse, dry, flaky, inelastic skin; puffy face, hands, and feet; hoarseness; periorbital edema; upper eyelid droop; dry, sparse hair; thick, brittle nails (as disorder progresses)
- Cardiovascular involvement — decreased cardiac output, slow pulse rate, signs of poor peripheral circulation, congestive heart failure, and cardiomegaly (occasionally)

Other Common Effects

- Anorexia, abdominal distention, menorrhagia, decreased libido, infertility, ataxia, and nystagmus; reflexes with delayed relaxation time (especially Achilles' tendon)

Diagnostic Test Results

- Radioimmunoassay shows decreased serum levels of triiodothyronine (T_3) and thyroxine (T_4).
- Serum TSH level is increased with thyroid insufficiency and decreased with hypothalamic or pituitary insufficiency.
- Serum cholesterol, alkaline phosphatase, and triglycerides levels are elevated.
- Blood chemistry shows low serum sodium levels in myxedema coma.
- Arterial blood gases show decreased pH and increased partial pressure of carbon dioxide in myxedema coma.
- Skull X-ray, computed tomography scan, and magnetic resonance imaging may show pituitary or hypothalamic lesions.
- Chest X-ray detects cardiomegaly.

Treatment

- Gradual lifelong thyroid hormone replacement with T_4 and, occasionally, T_3
- Surgery for underlying cause such as pituitary tumor

AGE ALERT
Elderly patients should be started on a very low dose of T_4, such as 25 μg every morning, to avoid cardiac problems. TSH levels guide gradual increases in the dosage.

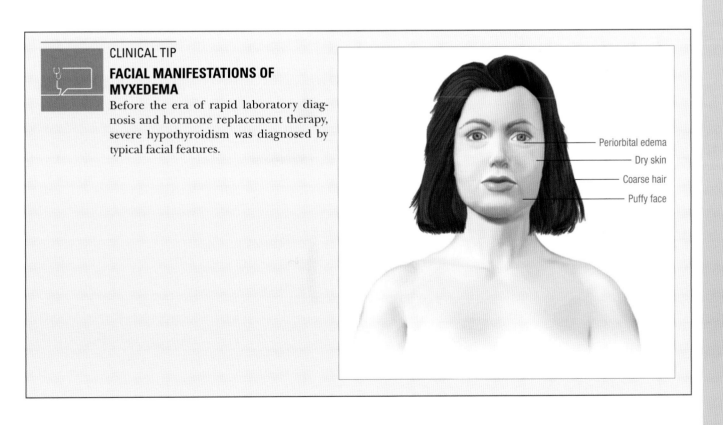

Normal

Inactive

Active

Parafollicular cells

Colloid

Follicular epithelial cells

Hashimoto's thyroiditis

Lymphocytes and plasma cells

Atrophied follicles

Metaplasia of follicular epithelial cells

Inflammation with progressive fibrosis

CLINICAL TIP

FACIAL MANIFESTATIONS OF MYXEDEMA

Before the era of rapid laboratory diagnosis and hormone replacement therapy, severe hypothyroidism was diagnosed by typical facial features.

Periorbital edema

Dry skin

Coarse hair

Puffy face

METABOLIC SYNDROME

Metabolic syndrome is a common condition in which obesity, high blood pressure, high blood glucose, and an abnormal cholesterol profile cluster together in one person. When these risk factors occur together, the chance of developing heart disease, stroke, and diabetes is much greater than when these risk factors develop independently. According to the American Heart Association, almost 25% of U.S. residents are affected by metabolic syndrome.

Causes

Some studies suggest that metabolic syndrome is closely tied to an individual's metabolism. Normally, food is absorbed into the bloodstream in the form of glucose and other basic substances. When glucose levels in the bloodstream rise, the pancreas releases insulin. Insulin attaches to the body's cells, allowing glucose to enter, where it's used for energy. In some people, the body's cells aren't able to respond to insulin. As suggested by recent studies, this insulin resistance is behind the development of metabolic syndrome.

Pathophysiology

When insulin resistance occurs, the body is unable to process glucose and the pancreas responds by creating more insulin. This cycle leads to high glucose levels and hyperinsulinemia. The increase in circulating insulin causes hypertrophy and vascular remodeling. It also leads to increased cholesterol and triglyceride levels, increased serum uric acid, increased platelet adhesion, increased response to angiotensin II, and decreased amounts of nitric oxide.

COMPLICATIONS
- Coronary artery disease
- Stroke
- Peripheral vascular disease
- Type 2 diabetes mellitus

Signs and Symptoms

- Abdominal obesity
- *Acanthosis nigricans* (darkening of the skin on the neck or under the arms)
- Irregular or absent menstrual periods
- Ovarian cysts
- Infertility
- Acne
- Hirsutism
- Alopecia

Diagnostic Test Results

- Measurement of waist circumference is greater than 35 inches in females or greater than 40 inches in males.
- Blood tests reveal triglyceride levels that are greater than or equal to 150 mg/dL.
- Blood tests reveal fasting blood glucose that's greater than or equal to 100 mg/dL.
- Blood test reveals high-density lipoprotein level that's less than 50 mg/dL in females and less than 40 mg/dL in males.
- Blood pressure 130/85 mm Hg or greater suggests disorder.

Treatment

- Weight loss through diet and exercise or, if needed, weight loss drugs, such as sibutramine or orlistat
- Exercise
- Antihypertensive medications such as diuretics, angiotensin-converting enzyme inhibitors, calcium channel blockers, or beta-adrenergic blockers
- Cholesterol-lowering medications, such as statins, fibrates, or niacin
- Thiazolidinediones or metformin to decrease insulin resistance
- Aspirin
- Smoking cessation
- Reduction of saturated fats, cholesterol, and salt intake
- Increase of high fiber foods like fruits, vegetables, and grains

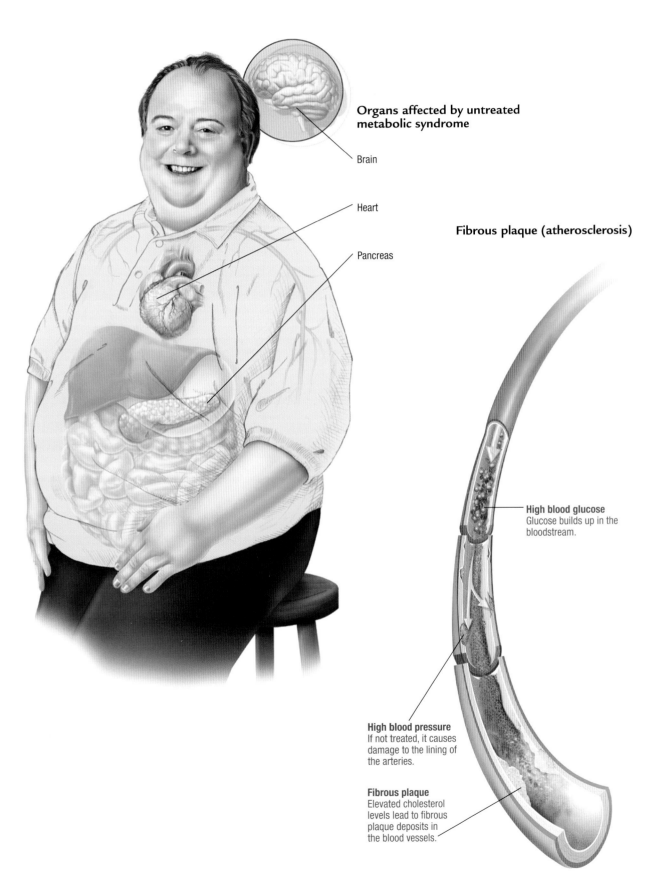

Organs affected by untreated metabolic syndrome

Brain

Heart

Pancreas

Fibrous plaque (atherosclerosis)

High blood glucose
Glucose builds up in the bloodstream.

High blood pressure
If not treated, it causes damage to the lining of the arteries.

Fibrous plaque
Elevated cholesterol levels lead to fibrous plaque deposits in the blood vessels.

SIMPLE GOITER

Simple (or nontoxic) goiter is a thyroid gland enlargement that isn't caused by inflammation or a neoplasm and is commonly classified as endemic or sporadic. Inherited defects may be responsible for insufficient thyroxine (T_4) synthesis or impaired iodine metabolism. Because families tend to congregate in a single geographic area, this familial factor may contribute to the incidence of both endemic and sporadic goiters.

Causes

Endemic Goiter

- Inadequate dietary iodine

Sporadic Goiter

- Large amounts of foods containing agents that inhibit T_4 production, such as rutabagas, cabbage, soybeans, peanuts, peaches, peas, strawberries, spinach, and radishes
- Drugs, such as propylthiouracil, iodides, phenylbutazone, para-aminosalicylic acid, cobalt, lithium; may cross placenta and affect fetus

Pathophysiology

Goiters can occur in the presence of hypothyroidism, hyperthyroidism, or normal levels of thyroid hormone. In the presence of a severe underlying disorder, compensatory responses may cause both thyroid enlargement (goiter) and hypothyroidism. Simple goiter occurs when the thyroid gland can't secrete enough thyroid hormone to meet metabolic requirements. As a result, the thyroid gland enlarges to compensate for inadequate hormone synthesis, a compensation that usually overcomes mild to moderate hormonal impairment.

COMPLICATIONS

- Respiratory distress
- Hypothyroidism
- Hyperthyroidism
- Thyroid cancer

Signs and Symptoms

- Enlarged thyroid
- Dysphagia
- Venous engorgement; development of collateral venous circulation in the chest
- Dizziness or syncope (Pemberton's sign) when the patient raises the arms above the head

Diagnostic Test Results

Laboratory tests reveal:

- normal serum thyroid levels
- high or normal TSH levels
- low-normal or normal T_4 concentrations
- normal or increased radioactive iodine uptake.

Treatment

- Exogenous thyroid hormone replacement with levothyroxine (treatment of choice) — inhibits TSH secretion and allows gland to rest
- Small doses of iodide (Lugol's iodine or potassium iodide solution) — commonly relieves goiter due to iodine deficiency
- Avoidance of known goitrogenic drugs and foods
- For large goiter that's unresponsive to treatment, subtotal thyroidectomy

Toxic goiter (Graves' disease)

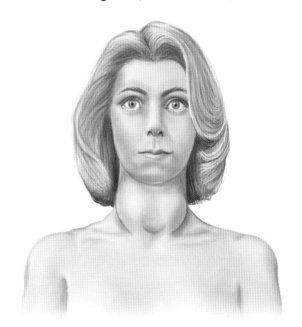

Simple (nontoxic) goiter

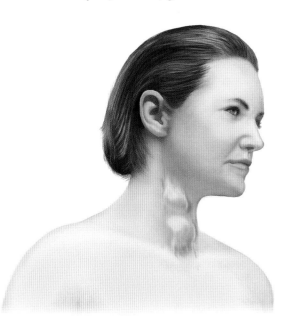

Nodular goiter

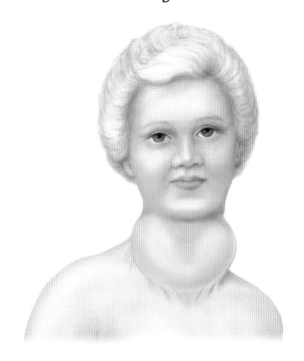

THYROID CANCER

Thyroid carcinoma is the most common endocrine malignancy. It occurs in all age groups, especially in people who have had radiation treatment of the neck area.

Causes

Direct cause unknown

Predisposing Factors

- Prolonged TSH stimulation due to radiation exposure or heredity
- Familial predisposition
- Chronic goiter

Pathophysiology

Papillary carcinoma accounts for approximately 80% of all thyroid cancers in adults. Most common in young adult females, it's the least virulent form of thyroid cancer and metastasizes slowly. *Follicular carcinoma* is less common (accounting for approximately 10% to 15% of all thyroid cancers) but more likely to recur and metastasize to the regional nodes and through blood vessels into the bones, liver, and lungs. Papillary plus follicular cancer accounts for approximately 90% of all thyroid cancers. *Medullary carcinoma* originates in the parafollicular cells derived from the last branchial pouch and contains amyloid and calcium deposits. It can produce thyrocalcitonin, histaminase, ACTH (producing Cushing's syndrome), and prostaglandin E_2 and F_3 (producing diarrhea). This rare form of thyroid cancer is familial, associated with pheochromocytoma, and completely curable when detected before it causes symptoms. Untreated, it progresses rapidly. Seldom curable by resection, anaplastic tumors resist radiation and metastasize rapidly.

COMPLICATIONS
- Metastasis
- Stridor

Signs and Symptoms

- Painless nodule; hard nodule in an enlarged thyroid gland; or palpable lymph nodes and thyroid enlargement
- Hoarseness, dysphagia, dyspnea, and pain on palpation
- Cough
- Hypothyroidism (low metabolism, mental apathy, sensitivity to cold) or hyperthyroidism (hyperactivity, restlessness, sensitivity to heat)
- Diarrhea, anorexia, irritability, and vocal cord paralysis

Diagnostic Test Results

- Calcitonin assay identifies silent medullary carcinoma; calcitonin level measuring during a resting state and during a calcium infusion (15 mg/kg over a 4-hour period) showing an elevated fasting calcitonin level and an abnormal response to calcium stimulation — a high release of calcitonin from the node in comparison with the rest of the gland — indicates medullary cancer.
- Thyroid scan differentiates functional nodes, which are rarely malignant, from hypofunctional nodes, which are commonly malignant.
- Ultrasonography shows changes in the size of thyroid nodules after thyroxine suppression therapy and is used to guide fine needle aspiration and to detect recurrent disease.
- Magnetic resonance imaging and computed tomography scans provide a basis for treatment planning because they establish the extent of the disease within the thyroid and in surrounding structures.
- Fine needle aspiration biopsy differentiates benign from malignant thyroid nodules.
- Histologic analysis stages the disease and guides treatment plans.

Treatment

- Papillary or follicular cancer — total or subtotal thyroidectomy; modified node dissection (bilateral or unilateral) on the side of the primary cancer

CLINICAL TIP
Before surgery, tell the patient to expect temporary voice loss or hoarseness lasting several days after surgery.

- Medullary, giant, or spindle cell cancer — total thyroidectomy and radical neck excision
- Inoperable cancer or postoperatively in lieu of radical neck excision — radiation (^{131}I) or external radiation
- To increase tolerance to surgery and radiation — adjunctive thyroid suppression with exogenous thyroid hormones and simultaneous administration of an adrenergic blocking agent such as propranolol
- Metastasis — ^{131}I; chemotherapy for symptomatic, widespread metastasis is rare

CLINICAL TIP
Hypocalcemia may develop if parathyroid glands are removed during surgery.

- Thyroid hormone replacement after surgeries

Anterior view

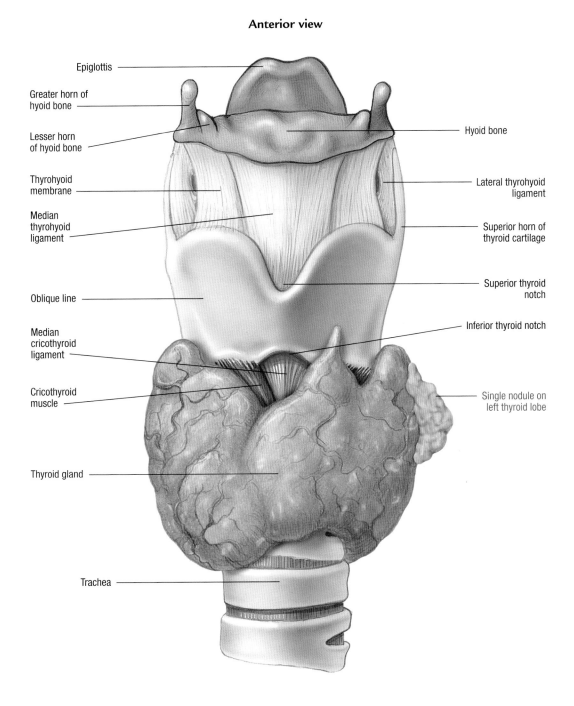

Epiglottis

Greater horn of
hyoid bone

Lesser horn
of hyoid bone

Thyrohyoid
membrane

Median
thyrohyoid
ligament

Oblique line

Median
cricothyroid
ligament

Cricothyroid
muscle

Thyroid gland

Trachea

Hyoid bone

Lateral thyrohyoid
ligament

Superior horn of
thyroid cartilage

Superior thyroid
notch

Inferior thyroid notch

Single nodule on
left thyroid lobe

REPRODUCTIVE DISORDERS

AMENORRHEA

Amenorrhea is the *abnormal* absence of menstruation. Absence of menstruation is normal before puberty, after menopause, or during pregnancy and lactation; it's pathologic at any other time. Primary amenorrhea is the absence of menarche in an adolescent by age 14 without the development of secondary sex characteristics or by age 16 with normal development of secondary sex characteristics. Secondary amenorrhea is the absence of menstruation for at least 6 months after the normal onset of menarche. Primary amenorrhea occurs in 0.3% of women; secondary amenorrhea occurs in about 4% of women. Prognosis is variable, depending on the specific cause. In the case of obstructive causes, surgical correction of outflow tract obstruction is usually curative.

Causes

- Anovulation due to deficient secretion of:
  - estrogen
  - gonadotropins
  - luteinizing hormone (LH)
  - follicle-stimulating hormone (FSH).
- Lack of ovarian response to gonadotropins
- Constant presence of progesterone or other endocrine abnormalities
- Endometrial adhesions (Asherman's syndrome)
- Ovarian, adrenal, or pituitary tumor
- Emotional disorders — common in patients with depression or anorexia nervosa:
  - Mild emotional disturbances such as stress tend to distort the ovulatory cycle.
  - Severe psychic trauma may abruptly change the bleeding pattern or completely suppress one or more full ovulatory cycles.
- Malnutrition or intense exercise — suppresses hormonal changes initiated by the hypothalamus
- Pregnancy
- Excessive weight loss
- Thyroid disorder
- Obesity or excessive weight gain
- Ovarian or adrenal tumor
- Anatomic defects

Pathophysiology

The mechanism varies depending on the cause and whether the defect is structural, hormonal, or both. Women who have adequate estrogen levels but a progesterone deficiency don't ovulate and are thus infertile. In primary amenorrhea, the hypothalamic-pituitary-ovarian axis is dysfunctional. Because of anatomic defects of the central nervous system, the ovary doesn't receive the hormonal signals that normally initiate the development of secondary sex characteristics and the beginning of menstruation.

Secondary amenorrhea can result from any of several mechanisms, including:

- central — hypogonadotropic, hypoestrogenic anovulation

- uterine — such as Asherman's syndrome, in which severe scarring has replaced functional endometrium
- premature ovarian failure.

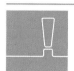

COMPLICATIONS
- Infertility

Signs and Symptoms

- Absence of menstruation
- Vasomotor flushes
- Vaginal atrophy
- Hirsutism
- Acne (secondary amenorrhea)

Diagnostic Test Results

- Physical and pelvic examination and sensitive pregnancy test rule out pregnancy as well as anatomic abnormalities (such as cervical stenosis) that may cause false amenorrhea (cryptomenorrhea), in which menstruation occurs without external bleeding.
- Onset of menstruation (spotting) within 1 week after giving pure progestational agents such as medroxyprogesterone (Provera) indicates enough estrogen to stimulate the lining of the uterus (if menstruation doesn't occur, special diagnostic studies such as gonadotropin levels are indicated).
- Blood and urine studies show hormonal imbalances, such as elevated pituitary gonadotropin levels, low pituitary gonadotropin levels, and abnormal thyroid levels (without suspicion of premature ovarian failure or central hypogonadotropism, gonadotropin levels aren't clinically meaningful because they're released in a pulsatile fashion).
- Complete medical workup, including appropriate X-rays, computed tomography scans, or magnetic resonance imaging; laparoscopy; and a biopsy, identifies ovarian, adrenal, and pituitary tumors.
- Tests to identify dominant or missing hormones include:
  - "ferning" of cervical mucus on microscopic examination (an estrogen effect)
  - LH levels
  - vaginal cytologic examination
  - endometrial biopsy
  - serum progesterone level
  - serum androgen levels
  - elevated urinary 17-ketosteroid levels with excessive androgen secretions
  - plasma FSH level more than 50 International Units/L, depending on the laboratory (suggests primary ovarian failure), or normal or low FSH level (possible hypothalamic or pituitary abnormality, depending on the clinical situation).

Treatment

- Appropriate hormone replacement to reestablish menstruation
- Treatment of the cause of amenorrhea not related to hormone deficiency — for example, surgery for amenorrhea due to a tumor
- Inducing ovulation — for example, with clomiphene citrate in women with intact pituitary gland and amenorrhea secondary to gonadotropin deficiency, polycystic ovarian disease, or excessive weight loss or gain
- FSH and human menopausal gonadotropins for women with pituitary disease
- Reassurance and emotional support (psychiatric counseling if amenorrhea results from emotional disturbances)
- Teaching the patient how to keep an accurate record of her menstrual cycles

PRIMARY AMENORRHEA

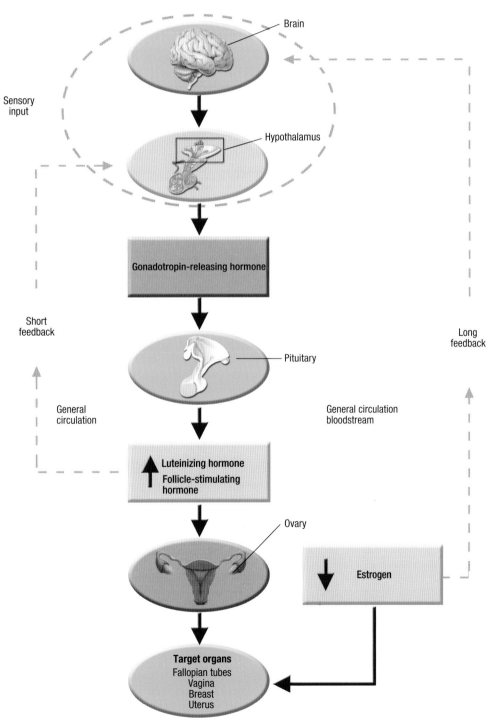

BREAST CANCER

Breast cancer is the most common cancer affecting women. It is estimated that one in eight women in the United States will develop breast cancer during her lifetime. Male breast cancer accounts for 1% of all male cancers and less than 1% of all breast cancers. The 5-year survival rate for localized breast cancer is 98% because of early diagnosis and a variety of treatments. Lymph node involvement is the most valuable prognostic predictor. With adjuvant therapy, 70% to 75% of women with negative nodes will survive 10 years or more, compared with 20% to 25% of women with positive nodes.

AGE ALERT
Breast cancer may develop any time after puberty but is most common after age 50.

Causes

High Risk Factors

- Family history of breast cancer, particularly first-degree relatives (mother, sister, and/or maternal aunt)
- Positive tests for genetic mutations (BRCA1 and BRCA2)
- Long menstrual cycles, early menarche, late menopause
- Nulliparous or first pregnancy after age 30
- History of unilateral breast cancer or ovarian cancer
- Exposure to low-level radiation

Low Risk Factors

- Pregnancy before age 20, history of multiple pregnancies
- Native American or Asian ancestry

Pathophysiology

Breast cancer occurs more commonly in the left breast than the right and more commonly in the outer upper quadrant. Slow-growing breast cancer spreads by way of the lymphatic system and the bloodstream, through the right side of the heart to the lungs, and eventually to the other breast, the chest wall, liver, bone, and brain.

Most breast cancers arise from the ductal epithelium. Tumors of the infiltrating ductal type don't grow to a large size, but metastasize early (70% of breast cancers).

Breast cancer is classified by histologic appearance and location of the lesion, as follows:

- adenocarcinoma — arising from the epithelium
- intraductal — within the ducts (includes Paget's disease)
- infiltrating — in parenchymal tissue of the breast
- inflammatory (rare) — overlying skin becomes edematous, inflamed, and indurated; reflects rapid tumor growth
- lobular carcinoma in situ — involves glandular lobes
- medullary or circumscribed — large tumor, rapid growth rate.

The descriptive terms should be coupled with a staging or nodal status classification system. The most commonly used staging system is the TNM (tumor size, nodal involvement, metastatic progress).

COMPLICATIONS
- Infection
- Decreased mobility with bone metastasis
- Central nervous system effects with brain metastasis
- Respiratory difficulty with lung involvement
- Potential death from metastatic changes

Signs and Symptoms

- Painless lump or mass in the breast, breast pain
- Change in symmetry or size of the breast
- Change in skin — thickening, scaly skin around the nipple, dimpling, edema (peau d'orange), ulceration, or temperature
- Unusual drainage or discharge
- Change in nipple (itching, burning, erosion, or retraction)
- Pathologic bone fractures, hypercalcemia
- Edema of the arm, axillary node enlargement
- Dilated blood vessels visible through the skin of the breast
- Bone pain

Diagnostic Test Results

- Alkaline phosphatase levels and liver function tests uncover distant metastases.
- Hormonal receptor assay determines whether the tumor is estrogen or progesterone dependent.
- Mammography reveals a tumor that is too small to palpate.
- Ultrasonography distinguishes between a fluid-filled cyst and solid mass.
- Chest X-rays pinpoint metastases in the chest.
- Scans of the bone, brain, liver, and other organs detect distant metastases.
- Fine-needle aspiration and excisional biopsy provide cells for histologic examination may confirm the diagnosis.

Treatment

Surgical

- Lumpectomy — in many cases, radiation therapy is combined with this surgery
- Lumpectomy and dissection of axillary lymph nodes
- Quadrant excision
- Simple mastectomy — removes breast but not lymph nodes or pectoral muscles
- Modified radical mastectomy — removes breast and axillary lymph nodes
- Radical mastectomy (now seldom used) — removes breast, axillary lymph nodes, and pectoralis major and minor muscles
- Therapy after tumor mapping

Other Treatments

- Reconstructive surgery if no advanced disease
- Chemotherapy — adjuvant or primary therapy

- Selective estrogen receptor modulators such as tamoxifen
- Aromatase inhibitors, such as anastrozole and letrozole
- Peripheral stem cell therapy for advanced disease
- Primary radiation therapy before or after tumor removal:
  - effective for small tumors in early stages
- helps make inflammatory breast tumors more surgically manageable
- also used to prevent or treat local recurrence.
- Biotherapy with such drugs as trastuzumab, bevacizumab, and lapatinib

UNDERSTANDING BREAST CANCER

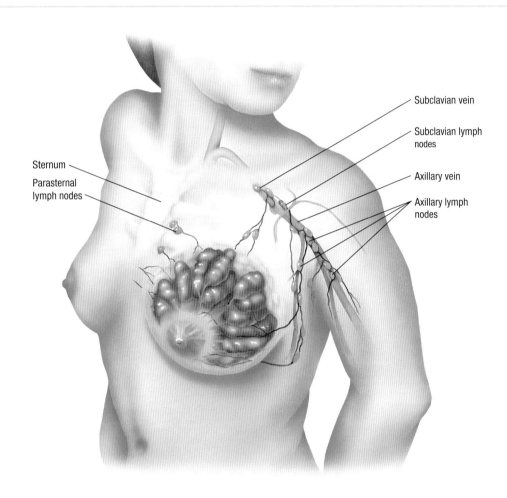

Sternum

Parasternal lymph nodes

Subclavian vein

Subclavian lymph nodes

Axillary vein

Axillary lymph nodes

Ductal carcinoma in situ

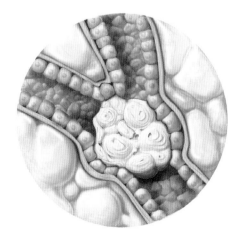

Infiltrating (invasive) ductal carcinoma

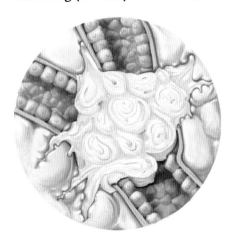

Also known as *fibrocystic disease of the breast*, this disorder of benign changes in breast tissue is usually bilateral.

AGE ALERT
Fibrocystic change is the most common benign breast disorder, affecting an estimated 10% of women ages 21 and younger, 25% of women ages 22 and older, and 50% of postmenopausal women.

Although most lesions are benign, some may proliferate and show atypical cellular growth. Fibrocystic change by itself isn't a precursor to breast cancer, but if atypical hyperplasia is present, the risk for breast carcinoma increases.

Causes

Exact cause unknown

Proposed Causes

- Estrogen excess and progesterone deficiency during luteal phase of menstrual cycle
- Environmental toxins that inhibit cyclic guanosine monophosphate enzymes:
  - methylxanthines — caffeine (coffee), theophylline (tea), theobromine (chocolate)
  - tyramine — in cheese, wine, nuts
  - tobacco.

Pathophysiology

Breast tissue appears to respond to hormonal stimulation, although the exact mechanism is unknown. Fibrocystic breast changes involve three types: cystic, fibrous, and epithelial proliferation. Cysts, fluid-filled sacs, are the most common feature and are easily treated. Fibrous tissue increases progressively until menopause and regresses thereafter. Epithelial proliferation diseases include structurally diverse lesions, such as sclerosing adenosis and the lobular and ductal hyperplasias.

COMPLICATIONS
- Possible increased risk of breast cancer

Signs and Symptoms

- Breast pain due to inflammation and nerve root stimulation (most common symptom), beginning 4 to 7 days into the luteal phase of the menstrual cycle and continuing until the onset of menstruation
- Pain in the upper outer quadrant of both breasts (common site)
- Palpable lumps that increase in size premenstrually and are freely moveable (about 50% of all menstruating women)
- Granular feeling of breasts on palpation
- Occasional greenish-brown to black nipple discharge that contains fat, proteins, ductal cells, and erythrocytes (ductal hyperplasia)

Diagnostic Test Results

- Ultrasonography distinguishes cystic (fluid-filled) from solid masses.
- Tissue biopsy distinguishes benign from malignant changes.
- Cytologic analysis of bloody aspirate rules out malignancy.

Treatment

- Symptomatic to relieve pain, including:
  - diet low in caffeine and fat and high in fruits and vegetables
  - support bra.
- Draining of painful cysts under local anesthesia
- Synthetic androgens (danazol) for severe pain (occasionally)
- Oral contraceptives

BENIGN BREAST CONDITIONS

Fibrocystic changes

- Dense fibrous tissue
- Pectoralis muscle
- Fat
- Normal lobules

Breast cyst

- Cyst
- Pectoralis muscle
- Fat
- Normal lobules

BENIGN BREAST TUMORS

Intraductal papilloma

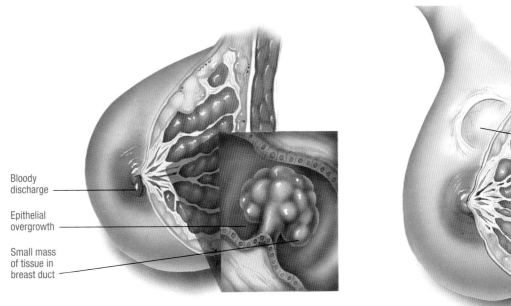

- Bloody discharge
- Epithelial overgrowth
- Small mass of tissue in breast duct

Fibroadenoma

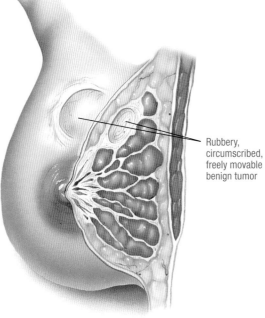

- Rubbery, circumscribed, freely movable benign tumor

Chapter 14 • Reproductive Disorders **331**

CERVICAL CANCER

The third most common cancer of the female reproductive system, cervical cancer is classified as either microinvasive or invasive. Precancerous dysplasia, also called *cervical intraepithelial carcinoma* or *cervical carcinoma in situ*, is more frequent than invasive cancer and occurs more often in younger women.

Causes

- Human papillomavirus (HPV)

Predisposing Factors

- Frequent intercourse at a young age (under age 16)
- Multiple sexual partners and/or partner with multiple partners
- Multiple pregnancies
- Sexually transmitted infections
- Smoking

Pathophysiology

Preinvasive disease ranges from mild cervical dysplasia, in which the lower third of the epithelium contains abnormal cells, to carcinoma in situ, in which the full thickness of epithelium contains abnormally proliferating cells. Other names for carcinoma in situ include *cervical intraepithelial neoplasia* and *squamous intraepithelial lesion*. Preinvasive disease detected early and properly treated is curable in 75% to 90% of cases. If preinvasive disease remains untreated (and depending on the form in which it appears), it may progress to invasive cervical cancer.

In invasive carcinoma, cancer cells penetrate the basement membrane and can spread directly to contiguous pelvic structures or disseminate to distant sites by lymphatic routes.

In almost all cases of cervical cancer (95%), the histologic type is squamous cell carcinoma, which varies from well-differentiated cells to highly anaplastic spindle cells. Only 5% are adenocarcinomas.

AGE ALERT
Usually, invasive carcinoma occurs in women between ages 30 and 50 and, rarely, in those under age 25.

COMPLICATIONS
- Hematuria
- Renal failure
- Infertility

Signs and Symptoms

Preinvasive Disease

- Often produces no symptoms or other clinically apparent changes

Early Invasive Cervical Cancer

- Abnormal vaginal bleeding
- Persistent vaginal discharge
- Postcoital pain and bleeding

Advanced Disease

- Pelvic pain
- Vaginal leakage of urine and stool through a fistula
- Anorexia, weight loss, and anemia

Diagnostic Test Results

- Papanicolaou (Pap) test screens for abnormal cells.
- Colposcopy shows the source of the abnormal cells seen on the Pap test.
- Cone biopsy is performed if endocervical curettage is positive.
- ViraPap test permits examination of the specimen's deoxyribonucleic acid structure to detect HPV.
- Lymphangiography and cystography detect metastasis.
- Organ and bone scans show metastasis.

Treatment

Preinvasive Lesions

- Loop electrosurgical excision procedure
- Cryosurgery
- Laser destruction
- Conization (with frequent Pap smear follow-up)
- Hysterectomy

Invasive Carcinoma

- Radical hysterectomy
- Radiation therapy (internal, external, or both)
- Chemotherapy
- Combination of the above procedures

Carcinoma in situ

Squamous cell carcinoma

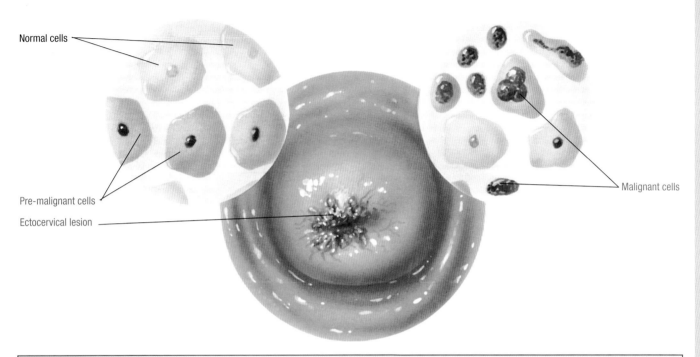

Normal cells

Pre-malignant cells

Ectocervical lesion

Malignant cells

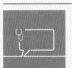

CLINICAL TIP

PAP SMEAR FINDINGS

Normal
- Large, surface-type squamous cells
- Small, pyknotic nuclei

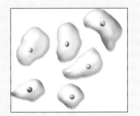

Mild Dysplasia
- Mild increase in nuclear:cytoplasmic ratio
- Hyperchromasia
- Abnormal chromatin pattern

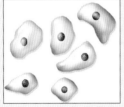

Severe Dysplasia, Carcinoma in Situ
- Basal type cells
- Very high nuclear:cytoplasmic ratio
- Marked hyperchromasia
- Abnormal chromatin

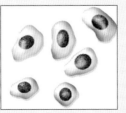

Invasive Carcinoma
- Marked pleomorphism
- Irregular nuclei
- Clumped chromatin
- Prominent nucleoli

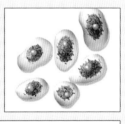

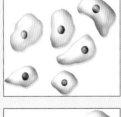

Endocervix
Columnar epithelium

External os

Squamocolumnar junction

Ectocervix
Stratified squamous epithelium

CRYPTORCHIDISM

Cryptorchidism is a congenital disorder in which one or both testes fail to descend into the scrotum, remaining in the abdomen inguinal canal or at the external ring. Although this condition may be bilateral, it more commonly affects the right testis. True undescended testes remain along the path of normal descent; ectopic testes deviate from that path.

Undescended testes are susceptible to neoplastic changes. The risk of testicular cancer is greater for men with cryptorchidism than for the general male population.

AGE ALERT
Cryptorchidism occurs in 30% of premature male neonates but in only 3% of those born at term. In about 80% of affected infants, the testes descend spontaneously during the first year; in the rest, the testes may descend later. If indicated, surgical therapy is successful in up to 95% of the cases if the infant is treated early enough.

Causes

Primary cause unknown

Possible Causes

- Testosterone deficiency resulting in a defect in the hypothalamic-pituitary-gonadal axis, causing failure of gonadal differentiation and gonadal descent
- Structural factors impeding gonadal descent, such as ectopic testis or short spermatic cord
- Genetic predisposition in a small number of cases; greater incidence of cryptorchidism in infants with neural tube defects
- In premature neonates — early gestational age; normal descent of testes into the scrotum is in seventh month of gestation

Pathophysiology

A prevalent but still unsubstantiated theory links undescended testes to the development of the gubernaculum, a fibromuscular band that connects the testes to the scrotal floor and probably helps pull the testes into the scrotum by shortening as the fetus grows. Normally in the male fetus, testosterone stimulates the formation of the gubernaculum. Thus, cryptorchidism may result from inadequate testosterone levels or a defect in the testes or the gubernaculum. Because the undescended testis is maintained at a higher temperature, spermatogenesis is impaired, leading to reduced fertility.

COMPLICATIONS
- Sterility
- Testicular cancer
- Testicular trauma

Signs and Symptoms

Unilateral Cryptorchidism

- Testis on affected side not palpable in scrotum; scrotum underdeveloped
- Enlarged scrotum on unaffected side due to compensatory hypertrophy (occasionally)

Uncorrected Bilateral Cryptorchidism

- Infertility after puberty despite normal testosterone levels

Diagnostic Test Results

Physical examination confirms cryptorchidism after sex is determined by these laboratory tests:

- Buccal smear (cells from oral mucosa) determines genetic sex (a male sex chromatin pattern).
- Blood test of serum gonadotropin level confirms the presence of testes by showing presence of circulating hormone.

Treatment

AGE ALERT
If the testes don't descend spontaneously by age 1, surgical correction is generally indicated. Surgery should be performed before age 2; by this time, about 40% of undescended testes can no longer produce viable sperm.

- Orchiopexy to secure the testes in the scrotum and prevent sterility, excessive trauma from abnormal positioning, and harmful psychological effects (usually before age 4 years; optimum age, 1 to 2 years)
- Human chorionic gonadotropin (HCG) I.M. to stimulate descent (rarely); ineffective for testes located in the abdomen

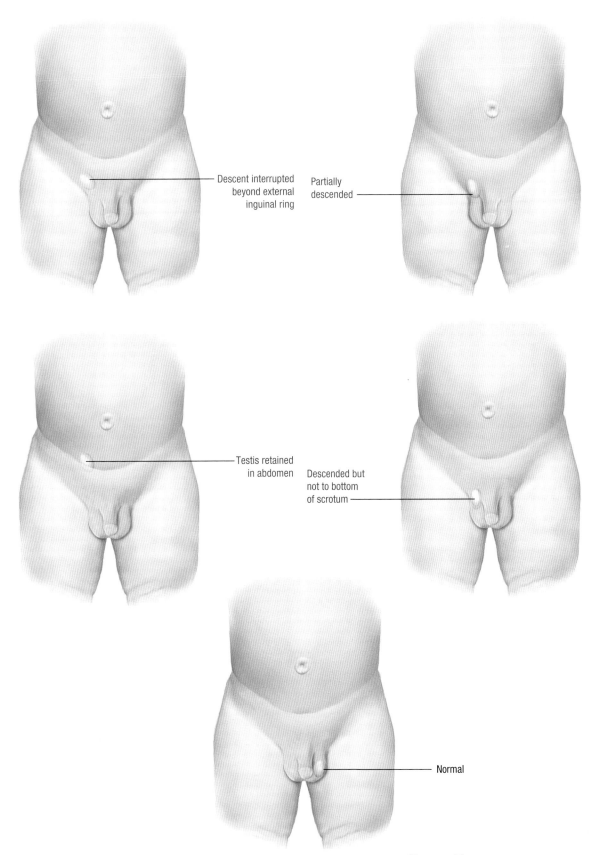

Descent interrupted beyond external inguinal ring

Partially descended

Testis retained in abdomen

Descended but not to bottom of scrotum

Normal

ECTOPIC PREGNANCY

An ectopic pregnancy occurs when a fertilized ovum implants outside the uterine cavity, most commonly in the fallopian tube. Prognosis is good with prompt diagnosis, appropriate surgical intervention, and control of bleeding. Few ectopic pregnancies are carried to term; rarely, with abdominal implantation, the fetus survives to term.

In whites, ectopic pregnancy occurs in about 1 of 200 pregnancies. In nonwhites, the incidence is about 1 of 120 pregnancies.

Causes

- Endosalpingitis
- Diverticula
- Tumors pressing against the tube
- Previous surgery, such as tubal ligation or resection
- Transmigration of the ovum
- Congenital defects in reproductive tract
- Ectopic endometrial implants in the tubal mucosa
- Sexually transmitted tubal infection or history of STIs and/or PID
- Intrauterine device

Pathophysiology

In ectopic pregnancy, transport of a blastocyst to the uterus is delayed and the blastocyst implants at another available vascularized site, usually the fallopian tube lining. Normal signs of pregnancy are initially present and uterine enlargement occurs in about 25% of cases. Human chorionic gonadotropin (HCG) hormonal levels are lower than in uterine pregnancies.

COMPLICATIONS
- Rupture of fallopian tube
- Internal hemorrhage
- Shock potentially leading to death
- Peritonitis
- Infertility

Signs and Symptoms

- Abdominal tenderness and discomfort
- Amenorrhea
- Abnormal menses (after fallopian tube implantation)
- Slight vaginal bleeding
- Unilateral pelvic pain over the mass
- If fallopian tube ruptures, sharp lower abdominal pain, possibly radiating to the shoulders and neck

CLINICAL TIP

Ectopic pregnancy sometimes produces symptoms of normal pregnancy or no symptoms other than mild abdominal pain (especially in abdominal pregnancy).

- Possible extreme pain when cervix is moved and adnexa palpated
- Boggy and tender uterus
- Adnexa may be enlarged.

Diagnostic Tests

- Blood test reveals abnormally low serum HCG; when repeated in 48 hours, level remains lower than levels found in a normal intrauterine pregnancy.
- Real-time ultrasonography shows intrauterine pregnancy, tubal pregnancy, or ovarian cyst.
- Culdocentesis shows free blood in the peritoneum.
- Laparoscopy reveals pregnancy outside the uterus.

Treatment

- Transfusion with whole blood or packed red blood cells
- Broad-spectrum I.V. antibiotics
- Supplemental iron
- Methotrexate
- Analgesics
- Rh$_O$ immune globulin if the patient is Rh negative
- Laparotomy and salpingectomy if culdocentesis shows blood in the peritoneum; possibly after laparoscopy to remove affected fallopian tube and control bleeding
- Microsurgical repair of the fallopian tube for patients who wish to have children
- Oophorectomy for ovarian pregnancy
- Hysterectomy for interstitial pregnancy
- Laparotomy to remove the fetus for abdominal pregnancy

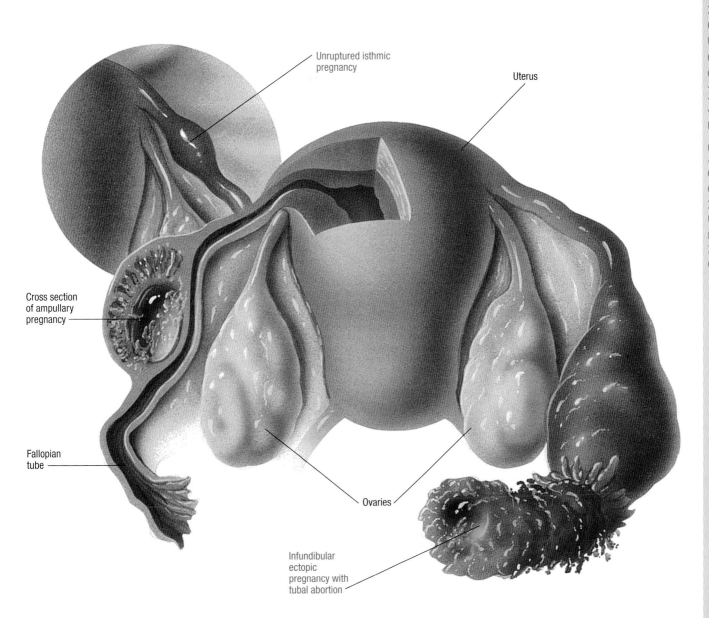

Unruptured isthmic
pregnancy

Uterus

Cross section
of ampullary
pregnancy

Fallopian
tube

Ovaries

Infundibular
ectopic
pregnancy with
tubal abortion

ENDOMETRIAL CANCER

Also known as *uterine cancer* (cancer of the endometrium), endometrial cancer is the most common gynecologic cancer.

AGE ALERT
Uterine cancer usually affects postmenopausal women between ages 50 and 60; it's uncommon between ages 30 and 40 and extremely rare before age 30. Most premenopausal women who develop uterine cancer have a history of anovulatory menstrual cycles or other hormonal imbalance.

Causes

Primary cause unknown

Predisposing Factors

- Anovulation, abnormal uterine bleeding
- History of atypical endometrial hyperplasia
- Unopposed estrogen stimulation
- Nulliparity
- Polycystic ovarian syndrome
- Familial tendency
- Obesity, hypertension, diabetes

Pathophysiology

In most cases, uterine cancer is an adenocarcinoma that metastasizes late, usually from the endometrium to the cervix, ovaries, fallopian tubes, and other peritoneal structures. It may spread to distant organs, such as the lungs and the brain, through the blood or the lymphatic system. Lymph node involvement can also occur. Less common are adenoacanthoma, endometrial stromal sarcoma, lymphosarcoma, mixed mesodermal tumors (including carcinosarcoma), and leiomyosarcoma.

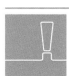

COMPLICATIONS
- Intestinal obstruction
- Ascites
- Hemorrhage

Signs and Symptoms

- Uterine enlargement
- Persistent and unusual premenopausal bleeding
- Any postmenopausal bleeding
- Other signs or symptoms, such as pain and weight loss, don't appear until the cancer is well advanced

Diagnostic Test Results

- Endometrial, cervical, or endocervical biopsy confirms the presence of cancer cells.
- Fractional dilation and curettage identifies cancer when biopsy is negative.
- Cervical biopsies and endocervical curettage pinpoint cervical involvement.

Treatment

- Surgery — generally total abdominal hysterectomy, bilateral salpingo-oophorectomy, or possibly omentectomy with or without pelvic or para-aortic lymphadenectomy
- Radiation therapy — intracavitary or external (or both):
  - if tumor is poorly differentiated or histology is unfavorable
  - if tumor has deeply invaded uterus or spread to extra-uterine sites
  - may be curative in some patients
- Hormonal therapy:
  - synthetic progesterones, such as medroxyprogesterone or megestrol, for recurrent disease
  - tamoxifen as a second-line treatment; 20% to 40% response rate
- Chemotherapy — usually tried when other treatments have failed:
  - varying combinations of cisplatin, doxorubicin, etoposide, dactinomycin
  - no evidence that they are curative.

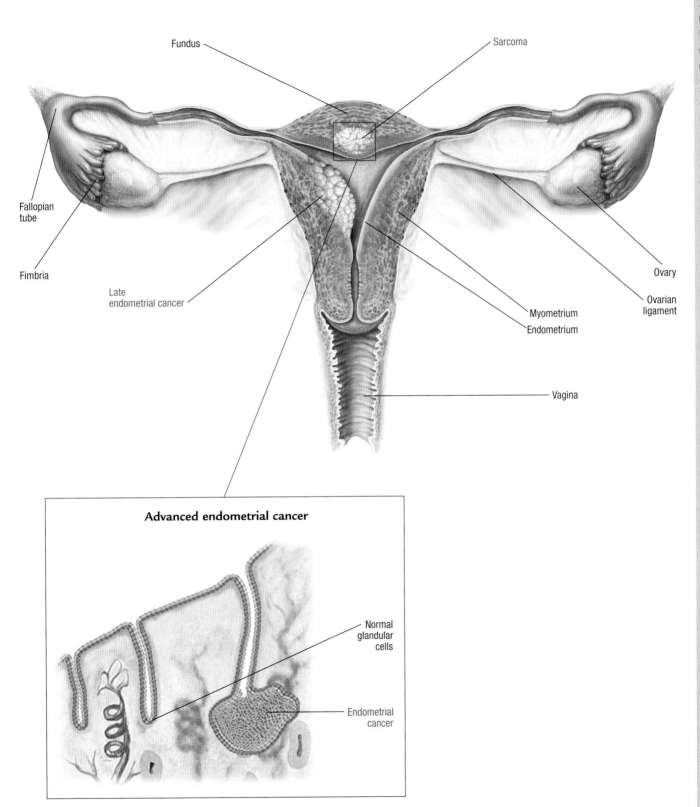

Fundus

Sarcoma

Fallopian tube

Fimbria

Late endometrial cancer

Myometrium

Endometrium

Ovary

Ovarian ligament

Vagina

Advanced endometrial cancer

Normal glandular cells

Endometrial cancer

ENDOMETRIOSIS

Endometriosis is the presence of endometrial tissue outside the lining of the uterine cavity, which occurred during fetal development of the woman. Ectopic tissue is generally confined to the pelvic area, usually around the ovaries, uterovesical peritoneum, uterosacral ligaments, and cul-de-sac, but it can appear anywhere in the body.

Active endometriosis may occur at any age, including adolescence. As many as 50% of infertile women may have endometriosis, although the true incidence in both fertile and infertile women remains unknown.

Severe symptoms of endometriosis may have an abrupt onset or may develop over many years. Of women with endometriosis, 30% to 40% become infertile. Endometriosis usually manifests during the menstrual years; after menopause, it tends to subside.

Causes

Primary cause unknown

Suggested Causes (One or More may be True in Different Women)

- Retrograde menstruation with implantation at ectopic sites; may not be causative alone; occurs in women with no clinical evidence of endometriosis
- Genetic predisposition and depressed immune system
- Coelomic metaplasia (metaplasia of mesothelial cells to the endometrial epithelium caused by repeated inflammation)
- Lymphatic or hematogenous spread to extraperitoneal sites

Pathophysiology

The ectopic endometrial tissue responds to normal stimulation in the same way as the endometrium, but less predictably. The endometrial cells respond to estrogen and progesterone with proliferation and secretion. During menstruation, the ectopic tissue bleeds as does the endometrium, which causes inflammation of the surrounding tissues. This inflammation causes fibrosis, leading to adhesions that produce pain and infertility.

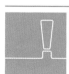

COMPLICATIONS
- Infertility
- Spontaneous abortion
- Anemia
- Emotional problems

Signs and Symptoms

- Classic symptoms — dysmenorrhea, abnormal uterine bleeding, infertility
- Pain — begins 5 to 7 days before menses, peaks, and lasts for 2 to 3 days; severity doesn't reflect extent of disease
- Depending on site of ectopic tissue:
  - ovaries and oviducts: infertility, profuse menses
  - ovaries or cul-de-sac: deep-thrust dyspareunia
  - bladder: suprapubic pain, dysuria, hematuria
  - large bowel, appendix: abdominal cramps, pain on defecation, constipation, bloody stools
  - cervix, vagina, perineum: bleeding from endometrial deposits, painful intercourse

Diagnostic Test Results

- Laparoscopy or laparotomy reveals multiple tender nodules on uterosacral ligaments or in the rectovaginal septum and ovarian enlargement in the presence of endometrial cysts on the ovaries.
- A pelvic ultrasound test detects an endometrial tissue on an ovary.
- Empiric trial of gonadotropin-releasing hormone (GnRH) agonist therapy confirms or refutes the impression of endometriosis before resorting to laparoscopy.
- Biopsy at the time of laparoscopy may be helpful to confirm the diagnosis.

Treatment

Conservative Therapy for Young Women who Want to Have Children

- Androgens such as danazol
- Progestins and continuous combined oral contraceptives (pseudopregnancy regimen) to relieve symptoms by causing regression of endometrial tissue
- GnRH agonists to induce pseudomenopause (medical oophorectomy), causing remission of the disease (commonly used)
- Analgesics
- Antigonadotropin drugs

To Rule Out Cancer, When Ovarian Masses Are Present

- Laparoscopic removal of endometrial implants

Treatment of Last Resort for Women who Don't Want to Bear Children or With Extensive Disease

- Total abdominal hysterectomy with or without bilateral salpingo-oophorectomy; success rates vary; unclear whether ovarian conservation is appropriate

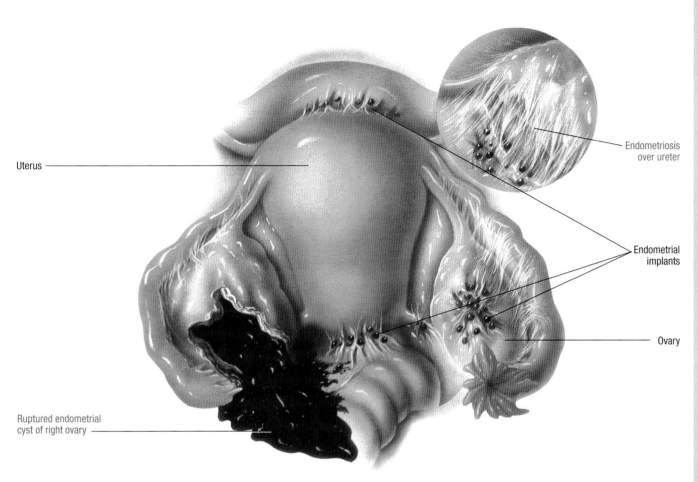

Uterus

Endometriosis over ureter

Endometrial implants

Ovary

Ruptured endometrial cyst of right ovary

CLINICAL TIP

COMMON SITES OF ENDOMETRIOSIS

Ectopic endometrial tissue can implant almost anywhere in the pelvic peritoneum. It can even invade distant sites such as the lungs.

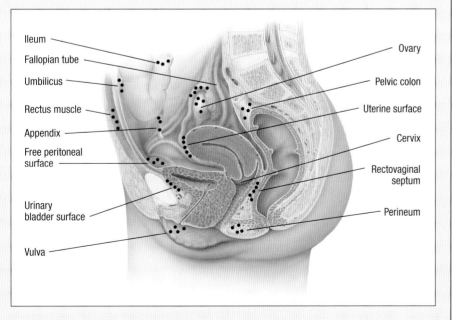

Ileum

Fallopian tube

Umbilicus

Rectus muscle

Appendix

Free peritoneal surface

Urinary bladder surface

Vulva

Ovary

Pelvic colon

Uterine surface

Cervix

Rectovaginal septum

Perineum

ERECTILE DYSFUNCTION

Erectile dysfunction, or impotence, refers to a male's inability to attain or maintain penile erection sufficient to complete intercourse. The patient with primary impotence has never achieved a sufficient erection. Secondary impotence is more common but no less disturbing than the primary form, and implies that the patient has succeeded in completing intercourse in the past.

Transient periods of impotence aren't considered dysfunction and probably occur in half of adult males. The prognosis for erectile dysfunction patients depends on the severity and duration of their impotence and the underlying causes.

AGE ALERT
Erectile dysfunction affects men of all age groups but increases in frequency with age.

Causes

Psychogenic

- Personal sexual anxieties that generally involve guilt, fear, depression, or feelings of inadequacy resulting from previous traumatic sexual experience, rejection by parents or peers, exaggerated religious orthodoxy, abnormal mother-son intimacy, or homosexual experiences
- Disturbed sexual relationship, possibly stemming from differences in sexual preferences between partners, lack of communication, insufficient knowledge of sexual function, or nonsexual personal conflicts
- Situational impotence, a temporary condition in response to stress

Organic

- Chronic diseases that cause neurologic and vascular impairment, such as cardiopulmonary disease, diabetes, multiple sclerosis, or renal failure
- Liver cirrhosis causing increased circulating estrogen due to reduced hepatic inactivation
- Spinal cord trauma
- Complications of surgery, particularly radical prostatectomy
- Drug- or alcohol-induced dysfunction
- Genital anomalies or central nervous system defects

Pathophysiology

Upon stimulation, chemicals are released in the brain that cause signals to pass down the spinal cord and outward through special nerves into the penis. These nerves release another chemical (nitric oxide) that causes the smooth muscles of the penis to relax and blood to rush into the erectile bodies, causing erection. Neurologic dysfunction results in lack of the autonomic signal and, in combination with vascular disease, interferes with arteriolar dilation. The blood is shunted around the sacs of the corpus cavernosum into medium-sized veins, which prevents the sacs from filling completely. Also, perfusion of the corpus cavernosum is initially compromised because of partial obstruction of small arteries, leading to loss of erection before ejaculation.

Anxiety or fear can prevent the brain signals from reaching the level required to induce erection. Medical conditions can block the erection arteries or cause scarring of the spongy erection tissue and prevent proper blood flow or trapping of blood and, therefore, limit the erection.

COMPLICATIONS
- Disruption of sexual relationships
- Depression

Signs and Symptoms

- Inability to achieve or sustain a full erection
- Anxiety
- Perspiration
- Palpitations
- Loss of interest in sexual activity
- Depression

Diagnostic Test Results

- A detailed sexual history helps differentiate between organic and psychogenic factors and primary and secondary impotence.
- Fulfilling the diagnostic criteria for the *Diagnostic and Statistical Manual of Mental Disorders*, Fourth edition, Text Revision by meeting either of two criteria:
  - persistent or recurrent partial or complete failure to attain or maintain erection until completion of sexual activity
  - marked distress or interpersonal difficulty occurs as a result of erectile dysfunction.

Treatment

Psychogenic Impotence

- Sex therapy including both partners (course and content of therapy depend on the specific cause of dysfunction and nature of the partner relationship)
- Teaching or helping the patient to improve verbal communication skills, eliminate unreasonable guilt, or reevaluate attitudes toward sex and sexual roles

Organic Impotence

- Reversing the cause if possible
- Psychological counseling to help the couple deal realistically with their situation and explore alternatives for sexual expression if reversing the cause isn't possible
- Sildenafil, tadalafil, or vardenafil to cause vasodilatation within the penis
- Adrenergic antagonist, yohimbine, to enhance parasympathetic neurotransmission
- Testosterone supplementation for hypogonadal men (not for men with prostate cancer)
- Prostaglandin E injected directly into the corpus cavernosum (may induce an erection for 30 to 60 minutes in some men)
- Surgically inserted inflatable or noninflatable penile implants

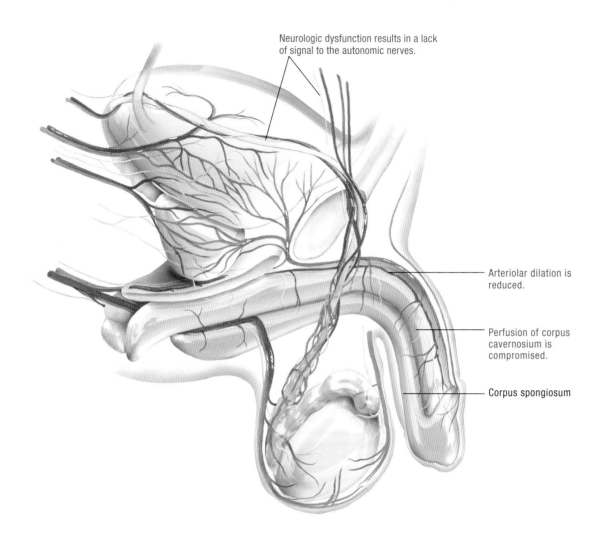

Neurologic dysfunction results in a lack of signal to the autonomic nerves.

Arteriolar dilation is reduced.

Perfusion of corpus cavernosium is compromised.

Corpus spongiosum

FIBROID DISEASE OF UTERUS

Uterine leiomyomas, also known as *myomas*, *fibromyomas*, or *fibroids*, are the most common benign tumors in women. They are most common in the uterine corpus, although they may appear on the cervix or on the round or broad ligament.

The tumors become malignant (leiomyosarcoma) in less than 0.1% of patients, which should serve to comfort women concerned with the possibility of a uterine malignancy in association with a fibroid.

AGE ALERT
Fibroids of the uterus may be present in 15% to 20% of reproductive-age women and 30% to 40% of women over age 30.

Causes

Primary cause unknown

Implicated Regulators of Leiomyoma Growth

- Several growth factors, including epidermal growth factor
- Steroid hormones, including estrogen and progesterone

Pathophysiology

Leiomyomas are masses of smooth muscle and fibrous connective tissue. They're classified according to location: in the uterine wall (intramural), protruding into the endometrial cavity (submucous), or protruding from the serosal surface of the uterus (subserous). Their size varies greatly. They're usually firm and surrounded by a pseudocapsule composed of compressed but otherwise normal uterine myometrium. The uterine cavity may become larger, increasing the endometrial surface area and causing increased uterine bleeding.

COMPLICATIONS
- Infertility
- Anemia
- Intestinal obstruction
- During pregnancy: spontaneous abortion, premature labor, dystocia

Signs and Symptoms

- Mostly asymptomatic
- Abnormal bleeding, typically menorrhagia with disrupted submucosal vessels (most common symptom)

- Pain only with:
  - torsion of a pedunculated (stemmed) subserous tumor
  - degenerating leiomyomas (fibroid outgrows its blood supply and shrinks down in size; after myolysis, a laparoscopic procedure to shrink fibroids; after uterine artery embolization)
- Pelvic pressure and impingement on adjacent viscera leads to mild hydronephrosis

Diagnostic Test Results

- Blood studies show anemia from abnormal bleeding.
- Bimanual examination reveals an enlarged, firm, nontender, and irregularly contoured uterus.
- Ultrasound and magnetic resonance imaging accurately assess the dimension, number, and location of tumors.

Treatment

Nonsurgical

- Gonadotropin-releasing hormone agonists (not a cure, as tumors increase in size after cessation of therapy)
- Nonsteroidal anti-inflammatory drugs

Surgical

- Hysteroscopic resection of fibroids
- Abdominal, laparoscopic, or hysteroscopic myomectomy (removal of tumors in the uterine muscle)
- Myolysis (a laparoscopic procedure, performed on an outpatient basis); contraindicated in women who desire fertility
- Uterine artery embolization (a promising alternative to surgery, but no existing long-term studies confirm effect on fertility or establish long-term success)
- Hysterectomy (usually isn't the only available option)
- Blood transfusions for severe anemia due to excessive bleeding

CLINICAL TIP
WARNING: After a uterine resection for fibroids, depending on their size and the area of resection, women may not be able to have spontaneous labor as this increases their chances of a uterine rupture along the scar tissue lines. Caesarean section is recommended before the onset of labor.

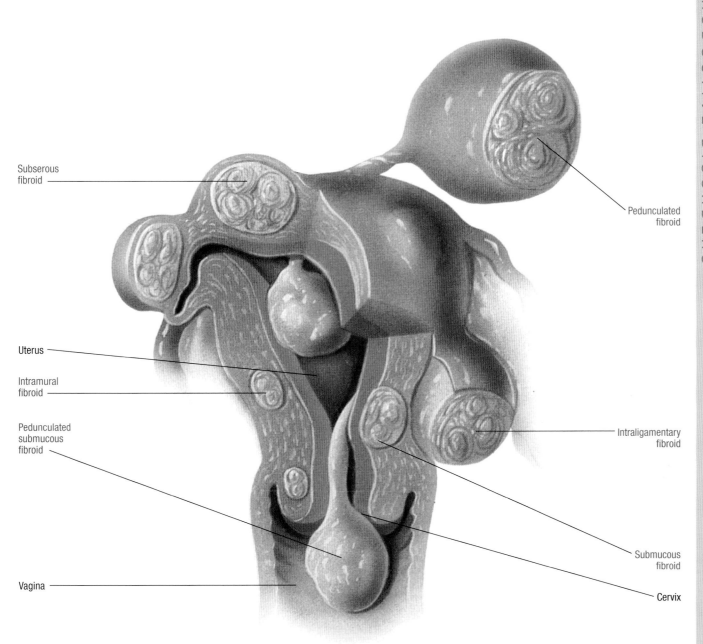

Subserous
fibroid

Pedunculated
fibroid

Uterus

Intramural
fibroid

Pedunculated
submucous
fibroid

Intraligamentary
fibroid

Submucous
fibroid

Vagina

Cervix

HYDROCELE

A hydrocele is a collection of fluid between the visceral and parietal layers of the tunica vaginalis of the testicle or along the spermatic cord. It's the most common cause of scrotal swelling.

AGE ALERT
Congenital hydrocele commonly resolves spontaneously during the first year of life. Usually, no treatment is indicated.

Causes

- Congenital malformation (infants)
- Trauma to the testes or epididymis
- Infection of the testes or epididymis
- Testicular tumor

Pathophysiology

Congenital hydrocele occurs when an opening between the scrotal sac and the peritoneal cavity allows peritoneal fluids to collect in the scrotum. The exact mechanism is unknown.

In adults, the fluid accumulation may be caused by infection, trauma, tumor, an imbalance between the secreting and absorptive capacities of scrotal tissue, or an obstruction of lymphatic or venous drainage in the spermatic cord. Consequent swelling obstructs blood flow to the testes.

COMPLICATIONS
- Infection
- Inguinal hernia
- Tumor

Signs and Symptoms

- Scrotal swelling and feeling of heaviness
- Inguinal hernia (commonly accompanies congenital hydrocele)
- Fluid collection, presenting as flaccid or tense mass
- Pain with acute epididymal infection or testicular torsion
- Scrotal tenderness due to severe swelling

Diagnostic Test Results

- Transillumination distinguishes fluid-filled from solid mass; tumor doesn't transilluminate.
- Ultrasonography visualizes the testes and the presence of fluid.
- Tissue biopsy differentiates between normal cells and malignancy.

Treatment

- Inguinal hernia with bowel present in the sac: surgical repair
- Tense hydrocele that impedes blood circulation or causes pain: aspiration of fluid and injection of sclerosing drug
- Recurrent hydroceles: excision of tunica vaginalis
- Testicular tumor detected by ultrasound: suprainguinal excision

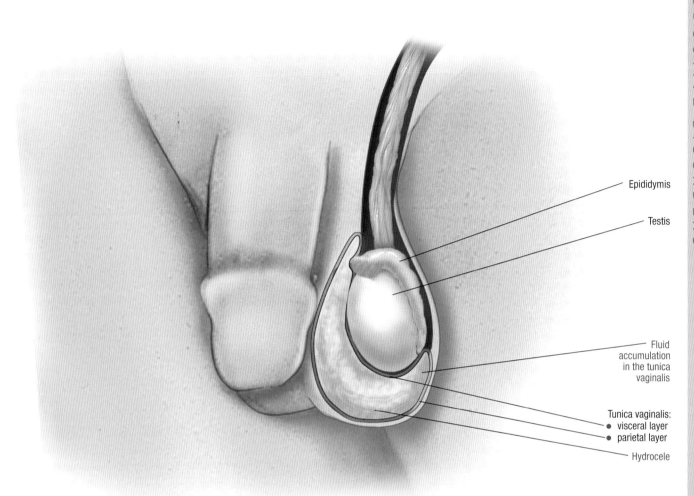

Epididymis

Testis

Fluid
accumulation
in the tunica
vaginalis

Tunica vaginalis:
• visceral layer
• parietal layer

Hydrocele

HYPOSPADIAS AND EPISPADIAS

Among the most common birth defects, congenital anomalies of the ureter, bladder, and urethra occur in about 5% of all births. The abnormality may be obvious at birth or may go unrecognized until symptoms appear.

Hypospadias is a congenital abnormality in which the urethral meatus is located on the ventral side, or undersurface of the penis. It may be on the glans, the base of the penis, the penoscrotal sac, or the perineum. The defect may be slight to extreme, and it occurs in 1 of 300 live male births. Epispadias occurs in 1 in 200,000 infant boys and 1 in 400,000 infant girls. In males, the urethral opening is on the dorsal aspect of the penis; in females, a cleft along the ventral urethral opening extends to the bladder neck.

Causes

- Congenital malformation
- Genetic factors
- Hormonal variations

Pathophysiology

In *hypospadias*, the urethral opening is on the ventral surface of the penis. A genetic factor is suspected in less severe cases. It's usually associated with a downward bowing of the penis (chordee), making normal urination with the penis elevated impossible. The ventral prepuce may be absent or defective, and the genitalia may be ambiguous. In the rare case of hypospadias in a female, the urethral opening is in the vagina, and abnormal vaginal discharge may be present.

Epispadias occurs more commonly in males than in females and often accompanies bladder exstrophy, in which a portion of posterior bladder wall protrudes through a defect in the lower abdominal and anterior bladder wall. In mild cases, the orifice is on the dorsum of the glans and in severe cases, on the dorsum of the penis. Affected females have a bifid (cleft into two parts) clitoris and a short, wide urethra. Total urinary incontinence occurs when the urethral opening is proximal to the sphincter.

COMPLICATIONS
- Infections
- Hematuria
- Calculi

Signs and Symptoms

- Displaced urethral opening
- Altered voiding patterns due to displaced opening of the urethra
- Urinary incontinence
- Chordee, or bending of the penis (in hypospadias)
- Ejaculatory dysfunction due to displaced penile opening

Diagnostic Test Results

- None are necessary if sexual identification is clear.
- If sexual identification is unclear, buccal smears or karyotyping determines gender.

Treatment

- Mild, asymptomatic hypospadias: no treatment
- Severe hypospadias: surgery, preferably before child reaches school age
- Epispadias: multistage surgical repair, almost always necessary

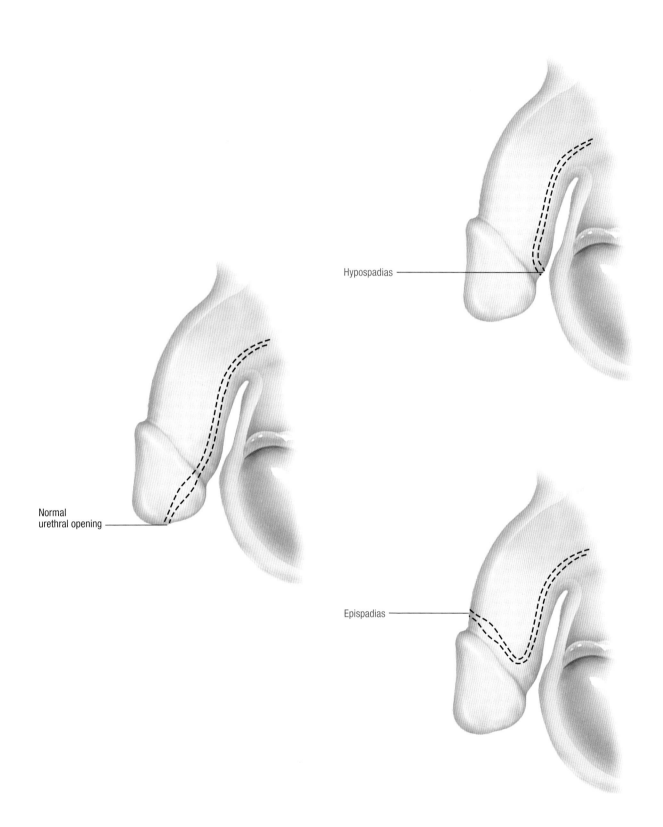

Hypospadias

Normal
urethral opening

Epispadias

OVARIAN CANCER

Ovarian cancer is the fifth leading cause of cancer death among U.S. women and has the highest mortality rate of all gynecologic cancers. In women with previously treated breast cancer, metastatic ovarian cancer is more common than is cancer at any other site.

AGE ALERT
More than half of all deaths from ovarian cancer occur in women between ages 65 and 84, and more than one-quarter of ovarian cancer deaths occur between ages 45 and 64.

The prognosis varies with the histologic type and stage of the disease. It is generally poor because ovarian tumors produce few early signs and are usually advanced at diagnosis. With early detection, about 90% of women with ovarian cancer at the localized stage survive for 5 years. The overall survival rate is about 45%.

Causes

Exact cause unknown

Associated Factors

- Infertility, nulliparity
- Familial tendency
- Ovarian dysfunction, irregular menses, ovarian cysts
- Exposure to asbestos, talc, industrial pollutants
- History of the use of fertility drugs
- Diet high in saturated fat, obesity by age 18
- Hormone replacement therapy
- Breast cancer genes (BRCA1 or BRCA2)

Pathophysiology

Primary epithelial tumors (account for 90% of all ovarian cancers) arise in the Müllerian epithelium; germ cell tumors, in the ovum itself; and sex cord tumors, in the ovarian stroma. Ovarian tumors spread rapidly intraperitoneally by local extension or surface seeding and, occasionally, through the lymphatics and the bloodstream. Generally, extraperitoneal spread travels through the diaphragm into the chest cavity, where the tumor may cause pleural effusions. Other metastasis is rare.

COMPLICATIONS
- Fluid and electrolyte imbalances
- Leg edema
- Intestinal obstruction
- Cachexia
- Malignant effusions

Signs and Symptoms

- May grow to considerable size before overt symptoms appear

Occasionally, in the Early Stages

- Vague abdominal discomfort, distention
- Mild GI discomfort (nausea, vomiting, bloating)
- Urinary frequency, pelvic discomfort

- Constipation
- Vaginal bleeding
- Weight loss
- Dyspareunia

Later Stages

- Tumor rupture, torsion, or infection — pain, which, in young patients, may mimic appendicitis
- Granulosa cell tumors — effects of estrogen excess such as bleeding between periods in premenopausal women
- Arrhenoblastomas (seen rarely) — virilizing effects

Advanced Ovarian Cancer

- Ascites
- Postmenopausal bleeding and pain (rarely)
- Symptoms of metastatic tumors, most commonly pleural effusion

Diagnostic Test Results

- Exploratory laparotomy, including lymph node evaluation and tumor resection, is required for accurate diagnosis and staging.
- Laboratory tumor marker studies (such as ovarian carcinoma antigen, carcinoembryonic antigen, and human chorionic gonadotropin) show abnormalities that may indicate complications.
- Abdominal ultrasonography, computed tomography scan, or X-rays delineate tumor size.
- Aspiration of ascitic fluid reveals atypical cells.

Treatment

- Varying combinations of surgery, chemotherapy, and radiation

Conservative Treatment for Unilateral Encapsulated Tumor in Young Girl or Young Woman

- Resection of the involved ovary
- Careful follow-up, including periodic chest X-rays to rule out lung metastasis

More Aggressive Treatment

- Total abdominal hysterectomy and bilateral salpingo-oophorectomy with tumor resection, omentectomy, possible appendectomy, lymphadenectomy, tissue biopsies, and peritoneal washings

If Tumor has Matted around Other Organs or Involves Organs that Cannot be Resected

- Surgically debulk tumor implants to less than 2 cm (or smaller) in greatest diameter.

Chemotherapy

- May be curative; extends survival time in most patients; largely palliative in advanced disease
- Current standard is combination paclitaxel and platinum-based chemotherapy

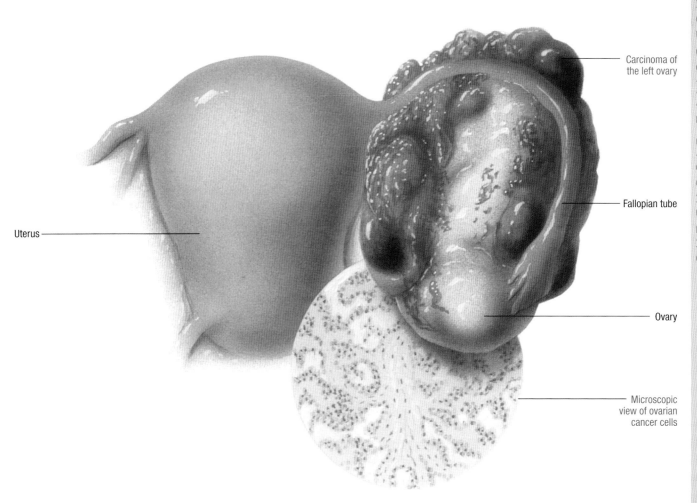

Uterus

Carcinoma of
the left ovary

Fallopian tube

Ovary

Microscopic
view of ovarian
cancer cells

CLINICAL TIP

METASTATIC SITES FOR OVARIAN CANCER

Ovarian cancer can metastasize to almost any site. Illustrated here are the most common sites.

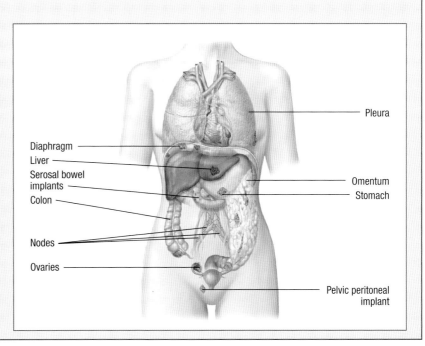

Pleura

Diaphragm

Liver

Serosal bowel
implants

Colon

Nodes

Ovaries

Omentum

Stomach

Pelvic peritoneal
implant

OVARIAN CYSTS

Ovarian cysts are usually benign sacs that contain fluid or semisolid material. Although these cysts are usually small and produce no symptoms, they may require thorough investigation as possible sites of malignant change. Cysts may be single or multiple (polycystic ovarian disease). Most ovarian cysts are physiologic, or functional; that is, they arise during the normal ovulatory process. Physiologic ovarian cysts include *follicular* cysts, *theca lutein* cysts, which are commonly bilateral and filled with clear, straw-colored liquid, and *corpus luteum* cysts. Ovarian cysts can develop any time between puberty and menopause, including during pregnancy. The prognosis for benign ovarian cysts is excellent. The presence of a functional ovarian cyst doesn't increase the risk for malignancy.

CLINICAL TIP
Polycystic ovarian syndrome is a metabolic disorder characterized by multiple ovarian cysts. About 22% of the women in the United States have the disorder, and about 50% to 80% of these women are obese and hirsute. Among those who seek treatment for infertility, more than 75% have some degree of polycystic ovarian syndrome, usually manifested by anovulation alone.

Causes

- Granulosa lutein cysts (occur within the corpus luteum): excessive accumulation of blood during hemorrhagic phase of menstrual cycle
- Theca lutein cysts:
  - hydatidiform mole, choriocarcinoma
  - hormone therapy (human chorionic gonadotropin [HCG] or clomiphene citrate).

Pathophysiology

Follicular cysts are generally very small and arise from follicles that either have not ruptured or have ruptured and resealed before their fluid is reabsorbed. *Luteal cysts* develop if a mature corpus luteum persists abnormally and continues to secrete progesterone. They consist of blood or fluid that accumulates in the cavity of the corpus luteum and are typically more symptomatic than follicular cysts. When such cysts persist into menopause, they secrete excessive amounts of estrogen in response to the hypersecretion of follicle-stimulating hormone and luteinizing hormone that normally occurs during menopause.

COMPLICATIONS
- Amenorrhea
- Oligomenorrhea
- Secondary dysmenorrhea
- Infertility
- Rupture of the cyst, peritonitis, intraperitoneal hemorrhage, shock, and death

Signs and Symptoms

- Large or multiple cysts:
  - mild pelvic discomfort, low back pain, or dyspareunia
  - abnormal uterine bleeding
- Ovarian cysts with torsion: acute abdominal pain similar to that of appendicitis
- Granulosa lutein cysts:
  - in pregnancy: unilateral pelvic discomfort
  - in nonpregnant women: delayed menses, followed by prolonged or irregular bleeding.

Diagnostic Test Results

- Ultrasound, laparoscopy, or surgery confirms the presence of ovarian cysts.

Treatment

- If cyst disappears spontaneously within one to two menstrual cycles — only symptomatic treatment
- Persisting cyst indicates excision to rule out malignancy
- Functional cysts that appear during pregnancy — analgesics
- Theca lutein cysts:
  - elimination of hydatidiform mole
  - destruction of choriocarcinoma
  - discontinuation of HCG or clomiphene therapy.
- Persistent or suspicious ovarian cyst:
  - laparoscopy or exploratory laparotomy with possible ovarian cystectomy or oophorectomy
  - if treatment is necessary during pregnancy, optimal time is second trimester.
- Ruptured corpus luteum cyst:
  - culdocentesis to drain intraperitoneal fluid
  - surgery for ongoing hemorrhage.

OVARIAN CYSTS

Follicular cyst

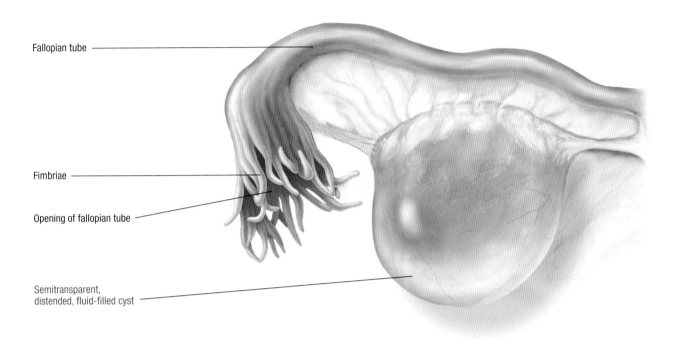

Fallopian tube

Fimbriae

Opening of fallopian tube

Semitransparent,
distended, fluid-filled cyst

Dermoid cyst

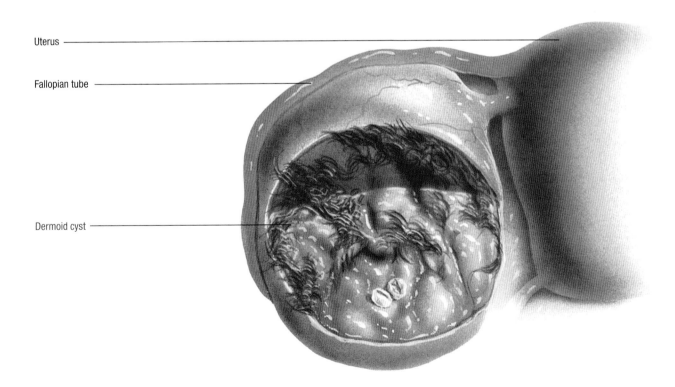

Uterus

Fallopian tube

Dermoid cyst

PELVIC INFLAMMATORY DISEASE

Pelvic inflammatory disease (PID) is infection of the uterus, fallopian tubes, or ovaries or combinations of these structures. About 1 million women are treated for PID each year in the United States, and about 1 in 7 women are treated for the disease at some point in their lives. Early diagnosis and treatment prevent damage to the reproductive system. Untreated PID may cause infertility and may lead to potentially fatal septicemia and shock.

Causes

- Infection with aerobic or anaerobic organisms, such as:
  - *Neisseria gonorrhoeae* and *Chlamydia trachomatis* (most common)
  - staphylococci, streptococci, diphtheroids, *Pseudomonas*, *Escherichia coli*

Predisposing Conditions

- Conization or cauterization of the cervix
- Insertion of an intrauterine device
- Use of a biopsy curette or an irrigation catheter
- Tubal insufflation
- Abortion, pelvic surgery, infection during or after pregnancy

Pathophysiology

Normally, cervical secretions have a protective and defensive function. Conditions or procedures that alter or destroy cervical mucus impair this bacteriostatic mechanism and allow bacteria present in the cervix or vagina to ascend into the uterine cavity, fallopian tubes, and pelvic cavity. Uterine infection can also follow the transfer of contaminated cervical mucus into the endometrial cavity by instrumentation. Bacteria may also enter the uterine cavity through the bloodstream or from drainage from a chronically infected fallopian tube, a pelvic abscess, a ruptured appendix, diverticulitis of the sigmoid colon, or other infectious foci.

Uterine infection can result from contamination by one or several common pathogens or may follow the multiplication of normally nonpathogenic bacteria in an altered endometrial environment. Bacterial multiplication is most common during parturition because the endometrium is atrophic, quiescent, and not stimulated by estrogen.

COMPLICATIONS
- Chronic pelvic pain
- Formation of adhesions
- Septicemia
- Pulmonary emboli
- Infertility
- Shock

Signs and Symptoms

- Profuse, purulent vaginal discharge
- Low-grade fever, malaise
- Lower abdominal pain
- Severe pain on movement of cervix or palpation of adnexa
- Vaginal bleeding
- Chills
- Nausea and vomiting
- Dysuria
- Dyspareunia

Diagnostic Test Results

- Culture and sensitivity and Gram stain testing of endocervix or cul-de-sac secretions show the causative agent.
- Urethral and rectal secretions reveal the causative agent.
- Blood test reveals elevated C-reactive protein level.
- Transvaginal ultrasonography shows the presence of thickened, fluid-filled fallopian tubes.
- Computed tomography scan shows complex tuboovarian abscesses.
- Magnetic resonance imaging provides images of soft tissue; useful not only for establishing the diagnosis of PID, but also for detecting other processes responsible for symptoms.
- Culdocentesis obtains peritoneal fluid or pus for culture and sensitivity testing.
- Diagnostic laparoscopy identifies cul-de-sac fluid, tubal distention, and masses in pelvic abscess.

Treatment

Antibiotic therapy beginning immediately after culture specimens are obtained and reevaluated as soon as laboratory results are available (usually after 24 to 48 hours); infection may become chronic if treated inadequately; PID therapy regimens should provide broad-spectrum coverage of likely etiologic pathogens: *C. trachomatis*, *N. gonorrhoeae*, anaerobes, gram-negative rods, and streptococci.

- Adequate treatment of partner(s)
- Analgesics
- I.V. fluids
- Adequate drainage if pelvic abscess forms
- Ruptured abscess (life-threatening complication):
  - total abdominal hysterectomy with bilateral salpingo-oophorectomy
  - laparoscopic drainage with preservation of the ovaries and uterus appears to hold promise

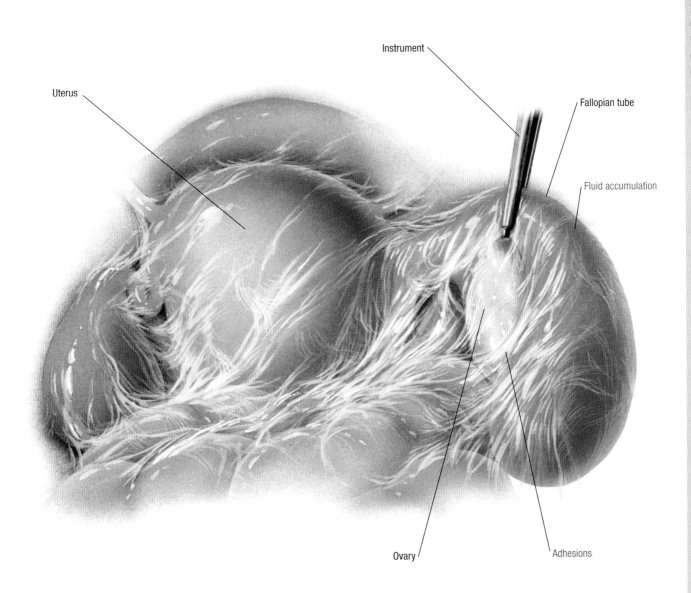

Instrument

Uterus

Fallopian tube

Fluid accumulation

Ovary

Adhesions

PROSTATE CANCER

Prostate cancer is the most common cancer in men over age 50. Adenocarcinoma is its most common form; sarcoma occurs only rarely. Most prostatic carcinomas originate in the posterior prostate gland; the rest originate near the urethra. Malignant prostatic tumors seldom result from the benign hyperplastic enlargement that commonly develops around the prostatic urethra in elderly men. Prostatic cancer seldom produces symptoms until it is advanced.

AGE ALERT
The incidence of prostate cancer increases with age more rapidly than the incidence of any other cancer.

Causes

Exact cause unknown

Implicated Contributing Factors

- Familial or ethnic predisposition
- Exposure to environmental toxins (radiation, air pollution: arsenic, benzene, hydrocarbons, polyvinyl chlorides)
- Sexually transmitted infections
- Endogenous hormonal influence
- Diet containing fat from animal products

Pathophysiology

Typically, when a primary prostatic lesion spreads beyond the prostate gland, it invades the prostatic capsule and spreads along ejaculatory ducts in the space between the seminal vesicles or perivesicular fascia. Endocrine factors may play a role, leading researchers to suspect that androgens speed tumor growth.

COMPLICATIONS
- Spinal cord compression
- Deep vein thrombosis
- Pulmonary emboli
- Myelophthisis

Signs and Symptoms

Early Stages

- Nonraised, firm, nodular mass with a sharp edge

Advanced Disease

- Blood in the seminal fluid
- New onset of erectile dysfunction
- Difficulty initiating a urine stream
- Dribbling, urine retention, urinary frequency especially at night
- Unexplained cystitis
- Hematuria
- Edema of the scrotum or leg
- Hard lump in the prostate region
- Pain

Diagnostic Test Results

- Serum prostate-specific antigen test reveals elevated levels indicating cancer with or without metastases.
- Transrectal prostatic ultrasonography shows prostate size and presence of abnormal growths.
- Bone scan and excretory urography determine the extent of disease.
- Magnetic resonance imaging and computed tomography scan define the extent of the tumor.
- Standard screening test of a digital rectal examination is recommended yearly by the American Cancer Society for men over age 40.

Treatment

- Prostatectomy
- Orchiectomy
- Radiation by external beam radiation or radioactive implants
- Hormonal manipulation
- Luteinizing hormone–releasing hormone agonists, such as Lupron or Zoladex
- Androgen-blocking agents
- Chemotherapy

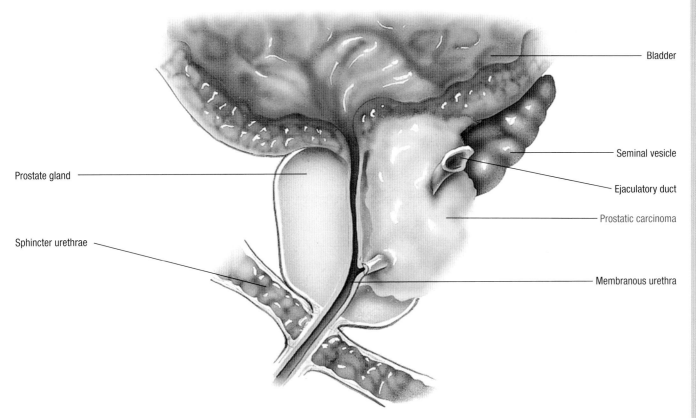

Prostate gland

Sphincter urethrae

Bladder

Seminal vesicle

Ejaculatory duct

Prostatic carcinoma

Membranous urethra

BENIGN PROSTATIC HYPERPLASIA

In benign prostatic hyperplasia (BPH), also known as *benign prostatic hypertrophy*, the prostate gland enlarges enough to compress the urethra and cause overt urinary obstruction. Depending on the size of the enlarged prostate, the age and health of the patient, and the extent of obstruction, BPH is treated symptomatically or surgically.

AGE ALERT
BPH is common, affecting more than 90% of men over age 80.

Causes

- Age-associated changes in hormone activity
- Arteriosclerosis
- Inflammation
- Metabolic or nutritional disturbances

Pathophysiology

Androgenic hormone production decreases with age, causing imbalance in androgen and estrogen levels and high levels of dihydrotestosterone, the main prostatic intracellular androgen. The shift in hormone balance induces the early, nonmalignant changes of BPH in periurethral glandular tissue. The growth of the fibroadenomatous nodules (masses of fibrous glandular tissue) progresses to compress the remaining normal gland (nodular hyperplasia). The hyperplastic tissue is mostly glandular, with some fibrous stroma and smooth muscle. As the prostate enlarges, it may extend into the bladder and obstruct urinary outflow by compressing or distorting the prostatic urethra. Progressive bladder distention may lead to formation of a pouch that retains urine when the rest of the bladder empties. This retained urine may lead to calculus formation or cystitis.

COMPLICATIONS
- Urinary stasis, urinary tract infection (UTI), or calculi
- Bladder wall trabeculation
- Detrusor muscle hypertrophy
- Bladder diverticula and saccules
- Urethral stenosis
- Hydronephrosis
- Paradoxical (overflow) incontinence
- Acute or chronic renal failure
- Acute postobstructive diuresis
- Pyelonephritis

Signs and Symptoms

Presenting Signs and Symptoms

- Reduced urinary stream caliber and force
- Urinary hesitancy
- Feeling of incomplete voiding, interrupted stream

As Obstruction Increases

- Frequent urination with nocturia and incomplete emptying
- Sense of urgency
- Retention, dribbling, incontinence
- Possible hematuria

Diagnostic Test Results

- Excretory urography rules out urinary tract obstruction, hydronephrosis (distention of the renal pelvis and calices due to obstruction of the ureter and consequent retention of urine), calculi or tumors, and filling and emptying defects in the bladder.
- Cystoscopy rules out other causes of urinary tract obstruction (neoplasm, calculi).
- Elevated blood urea nitrogen and serum creatinine levels (suggest renal dysfunction).
- Laboratory studies reveal elevated prostate-specific antigen; however, prostatic carcinoma must be ruled out.
- Urinalysis and urine cultures show hematuria, pyuria, and, with bacterial count more than 100,000/µL, revealing UTI.
- Cystourethroscopy for severe symptoms (definitive diagnosis) shows prostate enlargement, bladder wall changes, and a raised bladder. (Cystourethroscopy is only done immediately before surgery to determine the next course of therapy.)

Treatment

Conservative Therapy

- Prostate massages
- Sitz baths
- Fluid restriction for bladder distention
- Antimicrobials for infection
- Regular ejaculation
- Alpha-adrenergic blockers (terazosin, prazosin)
- Medical management to reduce risk of urinary retention (finasteride)
- Continuous drainage with a urinary catheter to alleviate urine retention (high-risk patients)

Surgical Procedures (To Relieve Intolerable Symptoms)

- Suprapubic (transvesical) resection
- Transurethral resection
- Retropubic (extravesical) resection allowing direct visualization; usually maintains potency and continence
- Suprapubic cystostomy under local anesthetic if indwelling urinary catheter can't be passed transurethrally
- Laser excision to relieve prostatic enlargement
- Nerve-sparing surgery to reduce common complications
- Indwelling urinary catheter for urine retention
- Balloon dilation of urethra and prostatic stents to maintain urethral patency

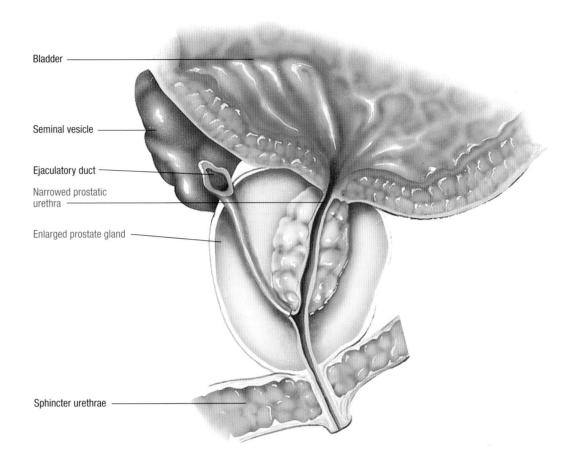

Bladder

Seminal vesicle

Ejaculatory duct

Narrowed prostatic urethra

Enlarged prostate gland

Sphincter urethrae

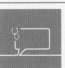

CLINICAL TIP

PALPATING THE PROSTATE GLAND

To detect early signs of prostate enlargement, follow these steps:

- Have the patient stand and lean over the examination table; if he can't do this, have him lie on his left side with his right knee and hip flexed or with both knees drawn to his chest.
- Inspect the skin of the perineal, anal, and posterior scrotal walls.
- Insert a lubricated gloved finger into the rectum.
- Palpate the prostate through the anterior rectal wall.
- The gland should feel smooth and rubbery, about the size of a walnut.

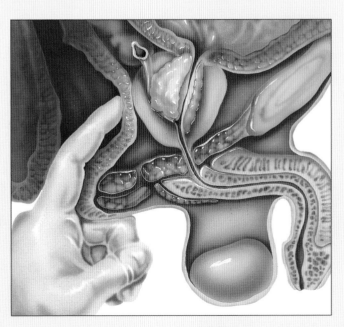

PROSTATITIS

Prostatitis, or inflammation of the prostate gland, may be classified according to four categories:
- acute bacterial prostatitis
- chronic bacterial prostatitis
- chronic nonbacterial prostatitis and chronic pelvic pain syndrome
- asymptomatic inflammatory prostatitis.

Causes

Acute Bacterial

- Previous bladder or urethral infection
- Gram-negative organisms, such as *Escherichia coli, Enterobacter, Serratia, Pseudomonas,* and *Proteus* species, and enterococci (account for 80% of cases)

Chronic Bacterial

- Cytomegalovirus
- Chlamydia
- Human immunodeficiency virus
- Urinary catheter tube use
- Acute prostatitis

Chronic Nonbacterial

- Ejaculatory duct obstruction
- Interstitial cystitis and other infectious agents
- Pelvic muscle spasm
- Structural abnormalities of the urinary tract such as strictures
- Heavy lifting when the bladder is full

Asymptomatic Inflammatory

- Similar to chronic inflammatory form but without symptoms

Pathophysiology

Spasms in the genitourinary tract or tension in the pelvic floor muscles may cause inflammation in nonbacterial prostatitis.

Bacterial prostatic infection can be a result of previous or recurrent infection, which stimulates an inflammatory response in the prostate. Inflammation is usually limited to a few of the gland's ducts.

COMPLICATIONS
- Infertility
- Bacteremia
- Pyelonephritis
- Prostatic abscess
- Epididymitis

Signs and Symptoms

Acute Bacterial

- Fever, chills
- Low back pain, especially when standing

- Frequent and urgent urination, difficulty with urine stream
- Dysuria, nocturia, urinary obstruction, blood-tinged urine

Chronic Bacterial

- Same urinary symptoms as in acute form but to a lesser degree
- Painful ejaculation
- Recurrent symptomatic cystitis

Chronic Nonbacterial

- Same as chronic bacterial form but afebrile
- Pelvic pain
- Painful ejaculation
- Erectile dysfunction
- Incomplete voiding

Diagnostic Test Results

- Elevated PSA level supports diagnosis of chronic bacterial prostatitis.
- Transrectal ultrasound reveals enlarged, thickened seminal vesicles.
- Computed tomography scan of the prostate may reveal abscess or a suspected neoplasm.
- Urine culture identifies the causative agent; must be performed when the patient starts voiding, then during midstream, after the patient stops voiding, and after the physician/HCP massages the prostate to express prostate secretions along with the voiding.

Treatment

General

- Muscle relaxants to relieve muscle spasms
- Alpha-adrenergic blockers (terazosin, tamsulosin) to relax the bladder
- Pain relievers
- Finasteride
- Limiting alcohol and caffeine and increasing water intake
- Regular ejaculation and urination (helps promote drainage of prostate secretions) and careful massage of the prostate (to relieve discomfort); vigorous massage may cause secondary epididymitis or septicemia

Acute Bacterial

- Broad-spectrum antibiotics

Chronic Bacterial

- Antibiotics (such as co-trimethoprim), fluoroquinolones (such as ofloxacin, ciprofloxacin, or levofloxacin), alpha-adrenergic blockers, or diazepam
- Sitz baths for symptomatic relief

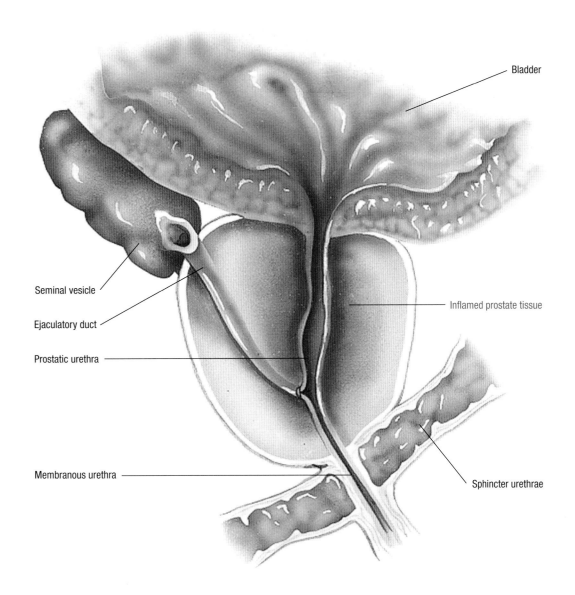

Bladder

Seminal vesicle

Ejaculatory duct

Inflamed prostate tissue

Prostatic urethra

Sphincter urethrae

Membranous urethra

SEXUALLY TRANSMITTED INFECTIONS

CHLAMYDIA

Chlamydial infections are transmitted by orogenital contact or vaginal or rectal intercourse with an infected person. It is the most common sexually transmitted infection in the United States. An infected mother can transmit it to the neonate during delivery.

COMPLICATIONS
- Epididymitis and prostatitis
- Salpingitis with subsequent tubal scarring, pelvic inflammatory disease (PID), and sterility
- Spontaneous abortion, premature delivery, and neonatal death

Causes

Chlamydia trachomatis

Signs and Symptoms

- Commonly asymptomatic
- Dysuria, urinary frequency, pyuria, pelvic or abdominal pain
- Chills, fever
- Genital discharge, genital pain
- Vaginal bleeding after intercourse; painful scrotal swelling

Diagnostic Test Results

- Swab culture of the infection site shows *C. trachomatis*.
- Serologic studies reveal previous exposure.
- Enzyme-linked immunosorbent assay shows *C. trachomatis* antibody.

Treatment

- Azithromycin, erythromycin, or doxycycline

GONORRHEA

Gonorrhea of the genitourinary tract (most commonly the urethra or cervix), or, occasionally, the rectum, pharynx, or eyes, almost always follows sexual contact with an infected person. An infected mother can transmit it to the neonate during delivery.

COMPLICATIONS
- Epididymitis and prostatitis
- PID and salpingitis
- Septic arthritis, dermatitis, and perihepatitis
- Conjunctivitis, corneal ulceration, and blindness (ophthalmia neonatorum) in the neonate

Causes

Neisseria gonorrhoeae

Signs and Symptoms

- May be asymptomatic
- In sexually active males, 3 to 6 days after contact, urethritis, dysuria, purulent discharge, redness, and swelling at the site
- Occasionally, vaginal inflammation, burning, itching, or greenish-yellow vaginal discharge
- Urinary frequency, incontinence, pelvic and lower abdominal pain or distention
- Nausea, vomiting, fever, tachycardia, polyarthritis (advanced disease)

Gonococcal Ophthalmia Neonatorum

- Lid edema, redness, abundant purulent discharge in the neonate appearing 2 or 3 days postpartum

Diagnostic Test Results

- Positive culture of *N. gonorrhoeae* from site confirms infection.
- Conjunctival scrapings confirm gonococcal conjunctivitis.
- Gonococcal arthritis is confirmed by Gram stain of smears from joint fluid and skin lesions.

Treatment

- Ceftriaxone plus doxycycline
- Alternative agents given with doxycycline: cefixime, ofloxacin, spectinomycin, ciprofloxacin, erythromycin
- Erythromycin ophthalmic ointment after delivery of the neonate

GENITAL HERPES

Genital herpes is an acute inflammatory disease of the genitalia. It's typically transmitted through sexual intercourse, orogenital sexual activity, kissing, and hand-to-body contact. Pregnant women may transmit the infection to neonates during vaginal delivery if an active infection is present.

COMPLICATIONS
- Chronic herpetic outbreaks
- Neonatal infections
- Secondary dermatologic infection from open vesicles

Causes

- Herpes simplex virus (HSV) type 2 — most common
- HSV type 1 — increasing incidence

Signs and Symptoms

After a 3- to 7-Day Incubation Period

- Appearance of genital vesicles
- Fever, malaise, dysuria, possible lesions on mouth or anus
- Leukorrhea

Diagnostic Test Results

- Staining of lesion scrapings shows characteristic giant cells or intranuclear inclusion of herpes virus infection.
- Tissue culture shows isolation of virus.
- Tissue analysis shows HSV antigens or deoxyribonucleic acid.

Treatment

- Acyclovir or other antiviral agents. Frequency of these treatments generally with first outbreak and then either as intermittent treatment or suppressive treatment

Genital herpes

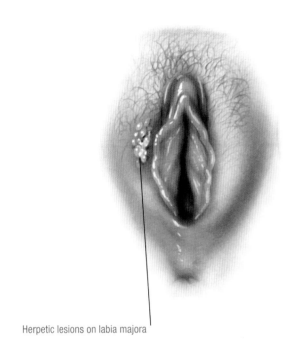

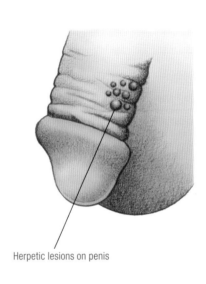

Herpetic lesions on labia majora

Herpetic lesions on penis

Genital warts

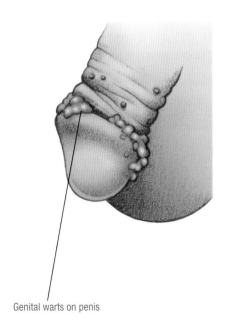

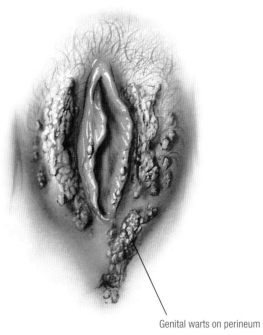

Genital warts on penis

Genital warts on perineum

GENITAL WARTS

Genital warts, also known as *venereal warts* or *condylomata acuminata*, grow rapidly in the presence of immune suppression or pregnancy and can accompany other genital infections.

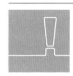

COMPLICATIONS
- Genital tract dysplasia or cancer
- Vaginal delivery problems from growths that become occlusive

Causes

Human papillomavirus

Signs and Symptoms

- After a 1- to 6-month incubation period (usually 2 months), tiny, red or pink, painless swellings on moist surfaces:
  - subpreputial sac, in urethral meatus and, less commonly, on penile shaft
  - vulva and on vaginal and cervical walls.
- Progressive disease:
  - spread to perineum and perianal area
  - large warts up to about 4 inches (10 cm) in diameter
  - pedunculated; typical cauliflowerlike appearance.

Diagnostic Test Results

- Dark-field microscopy of wart cell scrapings shows marked epidermal cell vascularization.
- Application of 5% acetic acid turns warts white if they're papillomas.

Treatment

- None to eradicate virus; relapse is common
- Small warts: topical 10% to 25% podophyllum in tincture of benzoin, trichloroacetic acid, or bichloroacetic acid
- Warts larger than 1 inch (2.5 cm): carbon dioxide laser treatment, cryosurgery, or electrocautery
- Podofilox, imiquimod, interferon, combined laser, and interferon therapy

SYPHILIS

Syphilis is a contagious, systemic venereal or congenital disease caused by a spirochete. It begins in the mucous membranes and quickly spreads to nearby lymph nodes and the bloodstream. Transmission occurs primarily through sexual contact during the primary, secondary, and early latent stages of infection. Transmission from a mother to her fetus is possible.

Causes

The spirochete *Treponema pallidum*

COMPLICATIONS
- Aortic regurgitation or aneurysm
- Meningitis and central nervous system damage
- Neonatal syphilis if mother is infected during pregnancy

Signs and Symptoms

Primary Syphilis

- Develops after a 3-week incubation period

- One or more chancres erupt at site of infection, usually genitalia or, possibly, on anus, fingers, lips, tongue, nipples, tonsils, eyelids

Secondary Syphilis

- Symptoms develop within a few days or up to 8 weeks after onset of primary chancres
- Symmetrical mucocutaneous lesions — of uniform size; well defined; macular, papular, pustular, or nodular:
  - commonly between rolls of fat on the trunk and, proximally, on the arms, palms, soles, face, and scalp
  - in warm, moist areas, lesions enlarge and erode, becoming highly contagious, pink or grayish-white lesions (*condylomata lata*).
- Headache, malaise, anorexia, weight loss, nausea, vomiting, sore throat and, possibly, slight fever; lymphadenopathy
- Alopecia, usually temporary; brittle, pitted nails

Latent Tertiary Syphilis

- Absence of clinical symptoms
- Reactive serologic test for syphilis

Late Syphilis

- Final, destructive but noninfectious stage of the disease
- Any or all of three subtypes: late benign syphilis, cardiovascular syphilis, and neurosyphilis

Diagnostic Test Results

- Dark-field microscopy identifies *T. pallidum* from lesion exudate.
- Nontreponemal serologic tests include the Venereal Disease Research Laboratory (VDRL) slide test, the rapid plasma reagin (RPR) test, and the automated reagin test, detecting nonspecific antibodies.
- Treponemal serologic studies include the fluorescent treponemal antibody absorption test, the *T. pallidum* hemagglutination assay, and the microhemagglutination assay that detect the specific antitreponemal antibody and confirm positive screening results.
- Cerebrospinal fluid examination identifies neurosyphilis when the total protein level is above 40 mg/dL, the VDRL slide test is reactive, and the white blood cell count exceeds 5 mononuclear cells/mm.

Treatment

- Penicillin G benzathine I.M.
- Nonpregnant patients allergic to penicillin: oral tetracycline or doxycycline
- For pregnant patients with history of anaphylaxis to penicillin, follow-up for allergy reactions per CDC standards is recommended
- Neonate may need to be treated within 4 weeks of birth

TRICHOMONIASIS

A protozoal infection, trichomoniasis affects about 15% of sexually active females and 10% of sexually active males. Common sites of infection in females include the vagina, urethra, and, possibly, the endocervix, bladder, Bartholin's glands, or Skene's glands and in males the lower urethra and, possibly, the prostate gland, seminal vesicles, or epididymis.

COMPLICATIONS
- Vaginal infection and PID
- Epididymitis

Causes

Trichomonas vaginalis, a tetraflagellated, motile protozoan

Signs and Symptoms

- None in approximately 70% of females and most males
- In females: gray or greenish-yellow and possibly profuse and frothy, malodorous vaginal discharge; severe itching, redness, swelling, dyspareunia, dysuria; occasionally, postcoital spotting, menorrhagia, dysmenorrhea
- In males: itching or irritation inside penis, some penile discharge, burning on urination and/or ejaculation

Diagnostic Tests

- Microscopic examination of vaginal or seminal discharge or urine specimen is positive for *T. vaginalis*.

Treatment

- Metronidazole

MANIFESTATIONS OF SEXUALLY TRANSMITTED INFECTIONS *(continued)*

Syphilis

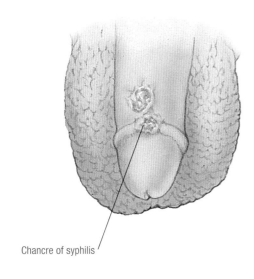

Chancre of syphilis

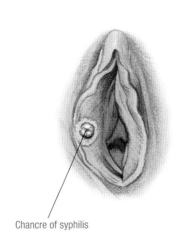

Chancre of syphilis

Mucopurulent cervicitis with chlamydia and gonorrhea

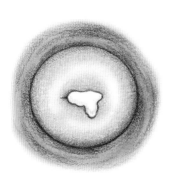

Trichomoniasis

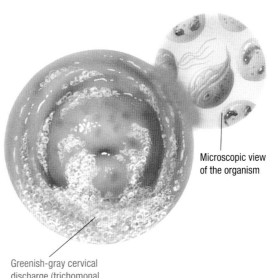

Microscopic view of the organism

Greenish-gray cervical discharge (trichomonal vaginitis)

TESTICULAR CANCER

Most testicular tumors originate in gonadal cells. About 40% are seminomas — uniform, undifferentiated cells resembling primitive gonadal cells. The remainder are non-seminomas — tumor cells showing various degrees of differentiation. The prognosis varies with the cell type and disease stage. When treated with surgery and radiation, almost all patients with localized disease survive beyond 5 years.

AGE ALERT
Malignant testicular tumors primarily affect young to middle-aged men and are the most common solid tumor in these age-groups. Incidence peaks between ages 20 and 40. Testicular tumors seldom occur in children.

Testicular cancer is rare in nonwhite males and accounts for fewer than 1% of male cancer deaths.

Causes

Primary cause unknown

Associated Conditions

- Cryptorchidism (even if surgically corrected)
- Maternal use of diethylstilbestrol during pregnancy

Pathophysiology

Testicular cancer may metastasize to the lungs, liver, viscera, or bone. It spreads through the lymphatic system to the iliac, para-aortic, and mediastinal lymph nodes.

COMPLICATIONS
- Back or abdominal pain
- Lung metastasis
- Ureteral obstruction

Signs and Symptoms

- Firm, painless, smooth testicular mass, varying in size and sometimes producing a sense of testicular heaviness
- Gynecomastia and nipple tenderness may result if tumor produces chorionic gonadotropin or estrogen.
- Dull ache in the lower abdomen or back
- Lump or swelling in either testicle

In Advanced Stages

- Ureteral obstruction
- Abdominal mass
- Cough, hemoptysis, shortness of breath
- Weight loss
- Fatigue, pallor, lethargy

Diagnostic Test Results

- Scrotal ultrasound confirms the presence of a solid mass.
- Laboratory studies show elevated human corticotropin, human chorionic gonadotropin (HCG), and alfa fetoprotein (AFP) (nonseminoma) or elevated HCG and normal AFP (seminoma).
- Tissue biopsy confirms the diagnosis and stages the disease.

Treatment

Surgery

- Orchiectomy and retroperitoneal node dissection
- Hormone replacement therapy after bilateral orchiectomy

Postoperative Radiation

- Seminoma — retroperitoneal and homolateral iliac nodes
- Nonseminoma — all positive nodes
- Retroperitoneal extension — mediastinal and supraclavicular nodes prophylactically

Combination Chemotherapy

- Essential for tumors beyond stage 0
- Agents include bleomycin with etoposide and cisplatin; cisplatin, vindesine, and bleomycin; cisplatin, vinblastine, and bleomycin; cisplatin, vincristine, methotrexate, bleomycin, and leucovorin

Unresponsive Malignancy

- Chemotherapy and radiation
- Autologous bone marrow transplantation

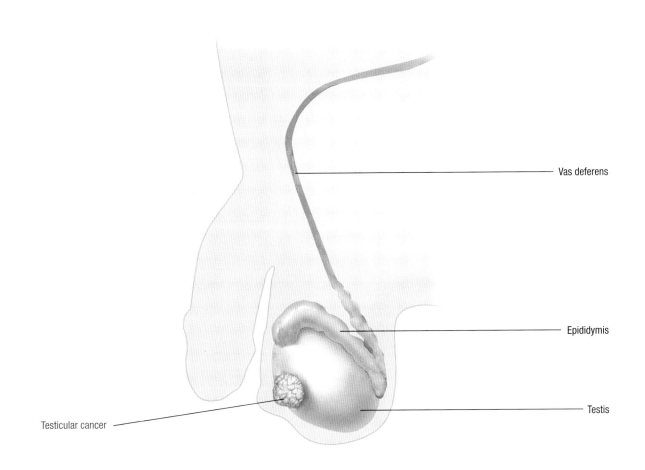

Vas deferens

Epididymis

Testis

Testicular cancer

CLINICAL TIP

STAGING TESTICULAR CANCER
The extent of metastasis determines the stage of testicular cancer.

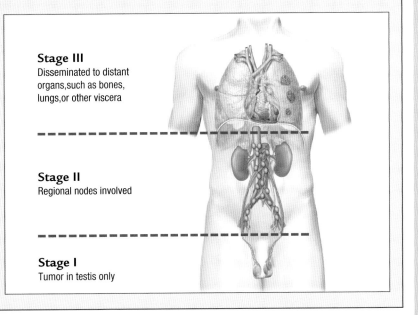

Stage III
Disseminated to distant organs,such as bones, lungs,or other viscera

Stage II
Regional nodes involved

Stage I
Tumor in testis only

TESTICULAR TORSION

Testicular torsion is an abnormal twisting of the spermatic cord due to rotation of a testis or the mesorchium; it may occur inside or outside the tunica vaginalis. Intravaginal torsion is most common in adolescents; extravaginal torsion is most common in neonates. Onset may be spontaneous or follow physical exertion or trauma. Potential outcomes range from strangulation to eventual infarction of the testis without treatment. This condition is almost always (90%) unilateral.

AGE ALERT
The greatest risk of testicular torsion occurs during the neonatal period and again between ages 12 and 18 (puberty), but it may occur at any age. Infants with torsion of one testis have a greater incidence of torsion of the other testis later in life than do males in the general population. The prognosis is good with early detection and prompt treatment.

Causes

Intravaginal Torsion

- Abnormality of the coverings of the testis and abnormally positioned testis
- Incomplete attachment of the testis and spermatic fascia to the scrotal wall, leaving the testis free to rotate around its vascular pedicle

Extravaginal Torsion

- Loose attachment of the tunica vaginalis to the scrotal lining causing spermatic cord rotation above the testis
- Sudden forceful contraction of the cremaster muscle due to physical exertion or irritation of the muscle

Pathophysiology

Normally, the tunica vaginalis envelops the testis and attaches to the epididymis and spermatic cord. Normal contraction of the cremaster muscle causes the left testis to rotate counterclockwise and the right, clockwise. In testicular torsion, the testis rotates on its vascular pedicle and twists the arteries and vein in the spermatic cord, interrupting blood flow to the testis. Vascular engorgement and ischemia ensue, causing scrotal swelling unrelieved by rest or elevation of the scrotum. If manual reduction is unsuccessful, torsion must be surgically corrected within 6 hours after the onset of symptoms to preserve testicular function (70% salvage rate). After 12 hours, the testis becomes dysfunctional and necrotic.

COMPLICATIONS
- Complete testicular infarction
- Testicular atrophy
- Potential infertility

Signs and Symptoms

- Excruciating pain in the affected testis or iliac fossa of the pelvis
- Edematous, elevated, and ecchymotic scrotum
- Loss of the cremasteric reflex (stimulation of the skin on the inner thigh retracts the testis on the same side) on the affected side
- Abdominal pain; nausea and vomiting
- Light-headedness

Diagnostic Test Results

Doppler ultrasonography distinguishes testicular torsion from strangulated hernia, undescended testes, or epididymitis (absent blood flow and avascular testis in torsion).

Treatment

- Manual manipulation of the testis counterclockwise to improve blood flow before surgery (not always possible)
- Immediate surgical repair by:
  - *orchiopexy* — fixation of a viable testis to the scrotum and prophylactic fixation of the contralateral testis
  - *orchiectomy* — excision of a nonviable testis to limit risk for autoimmune response to necrotic testis and its contents, damage to unaffected testis, and subsequent infertility.

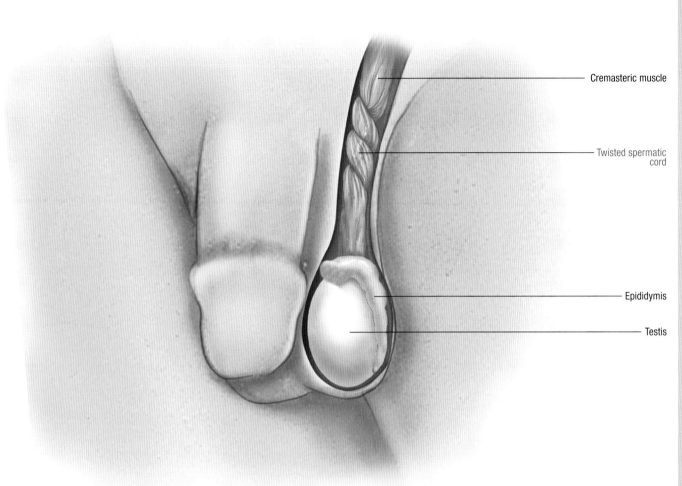

Cremasteric muscle

Twisted spermatic cord

Epididymis

Testis

DYSFUNCTIONAL UTERINE BLEEDING

Dysfunctional uterine bleeding refers to endometrial bleeding without recognizable organic lesions. It is the indication for almost 25% of gynecologic surgical procedures. The prognosis varies with the cause. Correction of hormonal imbalance or structural abnormality yields a good prognosis.

AGE ALERT
Approximately 20% of dysfunctional uterine bleeding cases occur in adolescents and 40% in women over age 40.

Causes

- Polycystic ovarian syndrome
- Obesity — enzymes in peripheral adipose tissue convert the androgen androstenedione to estrogens
- Immaturity of the hypothalamic-pituitary-ovarian mechanism (postpubertal teenagers)
- Anovulation (women in their late 30s or early 40s)
- Hormone-producing ovarian tumor
- Endometriosis
- Sexual assault
- Trauma
- Pelvic inflammatory disease
- Coagulopathy

Pathophysiology

Irregular bleeding is associated with hormonal imbalance and absence of ovulation (anovulation). When progesterone secretion is absent but estrogen secretion continues, the endometrium proliferates and becomes hypervascular. When ovulation doesn't occur, the endometrium randomly breaks down, and exposed vascular channels cause prolonged and excessive bleeding. In the absence of adequate progesterone levels, the usual endometrial control mechanisms are missing, such as vasoconstrictive rhythmicity, tight coiling of spiral vessels, and orderly collapse, and stasis doesn't occur. Unopposed estrogen induces a progression of endometrial responses beginning with proliferation, hyperplasia, and adenomatous hyperplasia; over a course of years, unopposed estrogen may lead to atypia and carcinoma.

COMPLICATIONS
- Anemia
- Atypia
- Carcinoma

Signs and Symptoms

- Metrorrhagia — episodes of vaginal bleeding between menses
- Hypermenorrhea — heavy or prolonged menses, longer than 8 days
- Chronic polymenorrhea (menstrual cycle less than 18 days) or oligomenorrhea (infrequent menses)
- Fatigue due to anemia
- Oligomenorrhea and infertility due to anovulation

Diagnostic Test Results

- Laboratory studies reveal decreased progesterone levels.
- Complete blood count test reveals anemia if excessive bleeding is present.
- Coagulation profile detects prolonged bleeding times in the presence of a coagulation disorder.
- Thyroid studies detect abnormal thyroid hormone levels.
- Dilation and curettage and endometrial biopsy detect endometrial hyperplasia or carcinoma.

Treatment

- High-dose estrogen-progestogen combination therapy (oral contraceptives) to control endometrial growth and reestablish a normal cyclic pattern of menstruation (usually given four times daily for 5 to 7 days even though bleeding usually stops in 12 to 24 hours; drug choice and dosage determined by patient's age and cause of bleeding); maintenance therapy with lower-dose combination oral contraceptives
- Progestogen therapy — alternative in many women, especially those susceptible to adverse effects of estrogen such as thrombophlebitis
- I.V. estrogen followed by progesterone or combination oral contraceptives if the patient is young (more likely to be anovulatory) and severely anemic (if oral drug therapy is ineffective)
- Iron replacement or transfusions of packed cells or whole blood, as indicated, due to anemia caused by recurrent bleeding
- Dilatation and curettage
- Endometrial oblation
- Hysterectomy

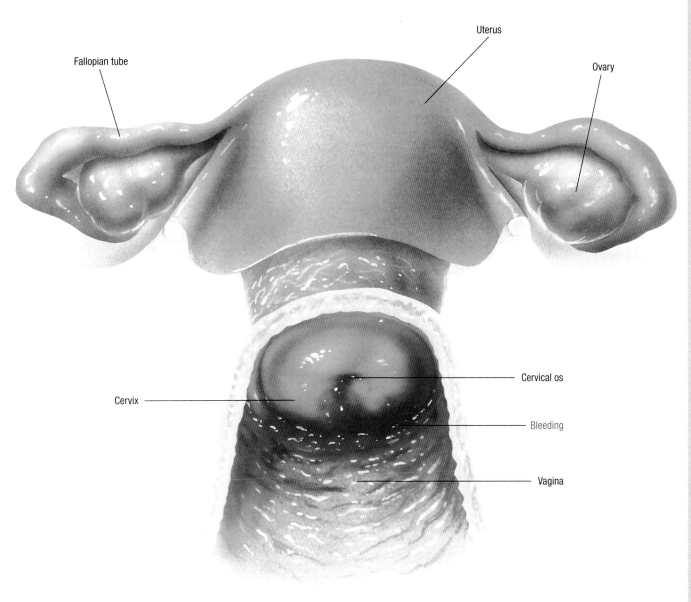

Fallopian tube

Uterus

Ovary

Cervical os

Cervix

Bleeding

Vagina

VAGINITIS

Vaginitis is inflammation of the vulva (vulvitis) and vagina (vaginitis). Because of the proximity of these two structures, inflammation of one occasionally causes inflammation of the other. Vaginitis may occur at any age and affects most females at some time. The prognosis is excellent with treatment.

Causes

Vaginitis (With or Without Consequent Vulvitis)

- *Trichomonas vaginalis*, a protozoan flagellate, usually transmitted through sexual intercourse
- *Candida albicans*, a fungus that requires glucose for growth

CLINICAL TIP

Some women are at particular risk of infection with *C. albicans*. The incidence of candidal vaginitis rises during the secretory phase of the menstrual cycle and doubles during pregnancy. The infection is also common in women with diabetes and in those who use oral contraceptives. Incidence may reach 75% in patients receiving systemic therapy with broad-spectrum antibiotics.

- *Gardnerella vaginalis*, a gram-negative bacillus

Vulvitis

- Parasite infestation, as with *Phthirus pubis* (crab louse)
- Trauma
- Poor personal hygiene
- Chemical irritants, or allergic reactions to hygiene sprays, douches, detergents, clothing, or toilet paper
- Vulvar atrophy in menopausal women due to decreasing estrogen levels
- Retention of a foreign body, such as a tampon or diaphragm

Pathophysiology

Bacterial vaginosis is caused by a disturbance of the normal vaginal flora. There's an overgrowth of anaerobic bacteria and of an organism, *Gardnerella*, with an associated loss of the normally dominant *Lactobacillus* species.

Candida albicans (yeast infection) is normally found in small amounts in the vagina, mouth, digestive tract, and on the skin, without causing disease or symptoms. Symptoms appear when the balance between normal microorganisms of the vagina is lost; the *C. albicans* population then becomes larger in relation to other microorganism populations. This happens when the environment (vagina) has certain favorable conditions that allow for growth and nourishment of *C. albicans*. An environment that makes it difficult for other microorganisms to survive may also cause an imbalance and lead to yeast infection.

Yeast infection may develop in reaction to antibiotics prescribed for another purpose. The antibiotics change the normal flora in the vagina and suppress the growth of the protective bacteria, *Lactobacillus*. Infection is common among women who use estrogen-containing birth control pills and among women

who are pregnant. This is due to the increased level of estrogen in the body, causing changes in the environment that make it perfect for fungal growth and nourishment.

COMPLICATIONS
- Secondary infections
- Skin breakdown
- Edema of the perineum
- Preterm delivery and low-birth-weight babies

Signs and Symptoms

T. vaginitis

- Thin, bubbly, green-tinged, malodorous discharge
- Irritation, itching; urinary symptoms, such as burning and frequency

C. albicans

- Thick, white, cottage cheeselike discharge
- Red, edematous mucous membranes, with white flecks adhering to the vaginal wall
- Intense itching

G. vaginalis

- Gray, foul, "fishy" smelling discharge

Acute Vulvitis

- Mild to severe inflammatory reaction, including edema, erythema, burning, and pruritus
- Severe pain on urination, dyspareunia

Chronic Vulvitis

- Relatively mild inflammation

Diagnostic Test Results

Microscopic examination of vaginal exudate on a wet slide preparation (a drop of vaginal exudate placed in normal saline solution) reveals the infectious organism.

Treatment

- Trichomonal vaginitis: oral metronidazole
- Candidal infection:
    - topical miconazole or clotrimazole
    - single dose of oral fluconazole
- *Gardnerella* infection: oral or vaginal metronidazole
- Acute vulvitis:
    - cold compresses or cool sitz baths for pruritus
    - warm compresses for severe inflammation
    - topical corticosteroids to reduce inflammation
- Chronic vulvitis:
    - topical hydrocortisone or antipruritics
    - good hygiene, especially in elderly or incontinent patients
- Atrophic vulvovaginitis: topical estrogen ointment

Candida infection

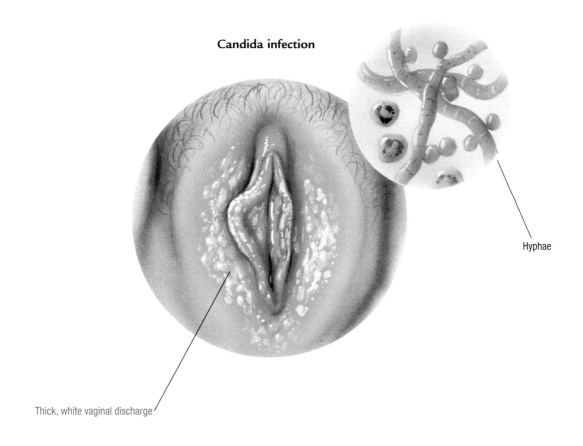

Hyphae

Thick, white vaginal discharge

Bacterial vaginosis

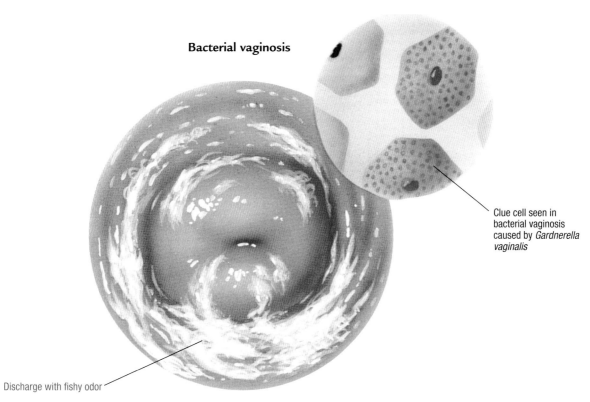

Clue cell seen in bacterial vaginosis caused by *Gardnerella vaginalis*

Discharge with fishy odor

VARICOCELE

A mass of dilated and tortuous varicose veins in the spermatic cord is called a *varicocele*. It's classically described as a "bag of worms." Thirty percent of all men diagnosed with infertility have a varicocele; 95% of cases affect the left spermatic cord.

AGE ALERT
Varicoceles are more common in men between ages 15 and 25.

Causes

- Incompetent or congenitally absent valves in spermatic veins
- Tumor or thrombus obstructing inferior vena cava (unilateral left-sided varicocele)

CLINICAL TIP
Sudden development of a varicocele in an older man may be caused by a renal tumor that has affected the renal vein and altered blood flow into the spermatic vein.

Pathophysiology

As a result of a valvular disorder in the spermatic vein, blood pools in the pampiniform plexus of veins that drain each testis rather than flowing into the venous system. One function of the pampiniform plexus is to keep the testes slightly cooler than the body temperature, which is the optimum temperature for sperm production.

COMPLICATIONS
- Testicular atrophy
- Infertility

Signs and Symptoms

- Usually asymptomatic
- Feeling of heaviness on the affected side
- Testicular pain and tenderness on palpation

Diagnostic Test Results

None exist. A physical examination is performed.

Treatment

- Mild varicocele (fertility not a concern): scrotal support to relieve discomfort
- To retain or restore fertility, surgical repair or removal by ligation of the spermatic cord at the internal inguinal ring

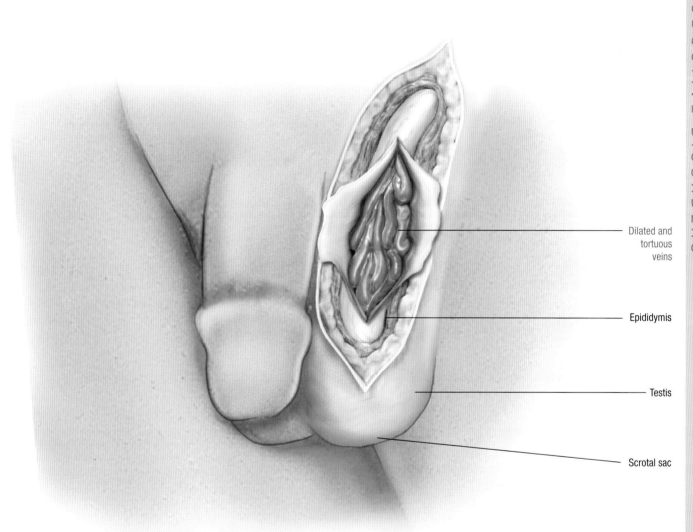

Dilated and tortuous veins

Epididymis

Testis

Scrotal sac

VULVAR CANCER

Cancer of the vulva accounts for approximately 4% of all gynecologic malignancies.

AGE ALERT
Vulvar cancer can occur at any age, even in infants, but its peak incidence is after age 60.

The most common vulvar cancer is squamous cell carcinoma. Early diagnosis increases the chance of effective treatment and survival. If lymph node dissection reveals no positive nodes, 5-year survival rate is 90%; otherwise, it is 50% to 60%.

Causes

Primary cause unknown

Predisposing Factors

- Leukoplakia (white epithelial hyperplasia), in about 25% of patients
- Chronic vulvar granulomatous disease
- Chronic pruritus of the vulva, with friction, swelling, and dryness
- Pigmented moles that are constantly irritated by clothing or perineal pads
- Irradiation of the skin such as nonspecific treatment for pelvic cancer
- Infection with human papilloma virus
- Obesity, hypertension, diabetes

Pathophysiology

Vulvar neoplasms may arise from varying cell origins. Because much of the vulva is made of skin, any type of skin cancer can develop there. The majority of vulvar cancers arise from squamous epithelial cells.

COMPLICATIONS
- Metastasis

Signs and Symptoms

In 50% of Patients

- Vulvar pruritus, bleeding
- Small vulvar mass — may begin as small ulcer on the surface, which eventually becomes infected and painful

Less Common

- Mass in the groin
- Abnormal urination or defecation

Diagnostic Test Results

- Colposcopy and toluidine blue staining identify biopsy sites.
- Histologic examination of biopsy samples confirm diagnosis and identify the type of cancer.

Treatment

Small, Confined Lesions with No Lymph Node Involvement

- Simple vulvectomy or hemivulvectomy (without pelvic node dissection):
  - Personal considerations (young age of patient, active sexual life) may mandate such conservative management.
  - It requires careful postoperative follow-up because it leaves the patient at risk for developing a new lesion.

For Widespread Tumor

- Radical vulvectomy
- Radical wide local excision — can be as effective as more radical resection, but with much less morbidity
- Depending on extent of metastasis, resection may include the urethra, vagina, and bowel, leaving an open perineal wound until healing — about 2 to 3 months.
- Plastic surgery, including mucocutaneous graft to reconstruct pelvic structures
- Radiation therapy

Extensive Metastasis, Advanced Age, or Fragile Health

- Rules out surgery
- Palliative treatment with irradiation of the primary lesion or chemotherapy

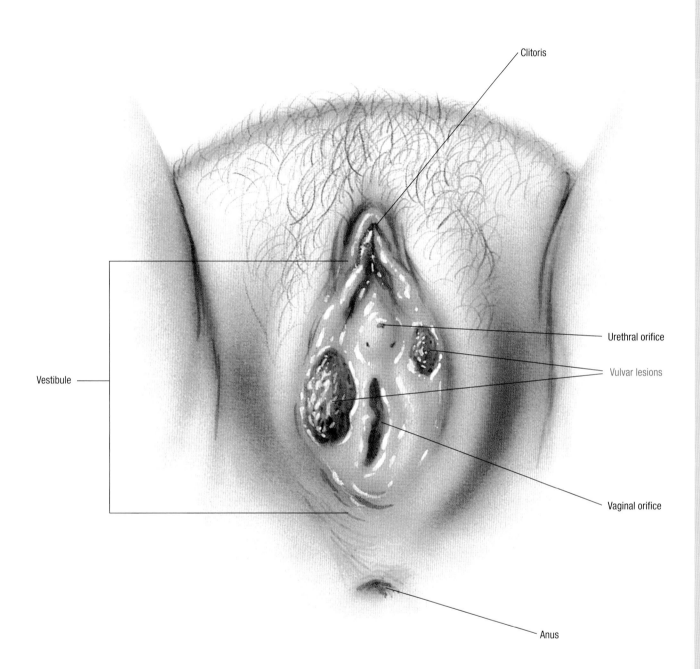

Clitoris

Urethral orifice

Vulvar lesions

Vaginal orifice

Vestibule

Anus

RENAL DISORDERS

ACUTE KIDNEY INJURY (ACUTE RENAL FAILURE)

Acute kidney injury, formerly known as acute renal failure, is the sudden interruption of renal function. Acute kidney injury can be caused by obstruction, poor circulation, or underlying kidney disease. It may be prerenal, intrarenal, or postrenal in origin; it usually passes through three distinct phases: oliguric, diuretic, and recovery.

Causes

Prerenal Kidney Injury

- Arrhythmias, cardiac tamponade, cardiogenic shock, heart failure, and myocardial infarction
- Prolonged hypotension
- Burns, trauma, sepsis, and tumor
- Dehydration and hypovolemic shock
- Diuretic overuse and antihypertensive drugs
- Hemorrhage, arterial embolism, arterial or venous thrombosis, and vasculitis
- Disseminated intravascular coagulation
- Eclampsia and malignant hypertension

Intrarenal Kidney Injury

- Poorly treated prerenal failure
- Nephrotoxins
- Obstetric complications
- Crush injuries
- Myopathy
- Transfusion reaction
- Acute glomerulonephritis, acute interstitial nephritis, acute pyelonephritis, bilateral renal vein thrombosis, malignant nephrosclerosis, and papillary necrosis
- Polyarteritis nodosa
- Renal myeloma
- Sickle cell disease
- Systemic lupus erythematosus
- Vasculitis

Postrenal Kidney Injury

- Bladder, ureteral, or urethral obstruction

Pathophysiology

Prerenal kidney injury is caused by a condition that diminishes blood flow to the kidneys, leading to hypoperfusion.

Hypoperfusion leads to hypoxemia, which can rapidly damage the kidney. The tubules are most susceptible to hypoxemia's effect. The impaired blood flow results in decreased glomerular filtration rate (GFR) and increased tubular reabsorption of sodium and water. Life-threatening consequences include volume overload, hyperkalemia, and metabolic acidosis.

Intrarenal kidney injury, also called *intrinsic* or *parenchymal renal failure,* results from damage to the filtering structures of the kidneys. Nephrotoxicity or inflammation irreparably damages the delicate layer under the epithelium (basement membrane). Use of nephrotoxins also causes acute kidney injury because they accumulate in the renal cortex.

Postrenal kidney injury is a consequence of bilateral obstruction of urine outflow. The cause may be in the bladder, ureters, or urethra. Common causes include stones, blood clots, bladder tumors, pelvic malignancy, and prostatic hypertrophy.

COMPLICATIONS

- Volume overload
- Acute pulmonary edema
- Hypertensive crisis
- Hyperkalemia
- Infection

Signs and Symptoms

- Oliguria or anuria
- Tachycardia and hypotension
- Dry mucous membranes and flat neck veins
- Lethargy
- Cool, clammy skin

Progressive Disease

- Edema
- Confusion
- GI symptoms
- Crackles
- Infection
- Seizures and coma
- Hematuria, petechiae, and ecchymosis

Diagnostic Test Results

- Blood studies show elevated blood urea nitrogen, serum creatinine, and potassium levels; decreased bicarbonate level, hematocrit, and hemoglobin levels; and low blood pH.
- Urine studies show casts, cellular debris, and decreased specific gravity; in glomerular diseases, proteinuria and urine osmolality close to serum osmolality; urine sodium level less than 20 mEq/L if oliguria results from decreased perfusion and more than 40 mEq/L if the cause is intrarenal.
- Creatinine clearance test measures GFR and reflects the number of remaining functioning nephrons.
- Electrocardiogram (ECG) shows tall, peaked T waves, widening QRS complex, and disappearing P waves if hyperkalemia is present.
- Ultrasonography, plain films of the abdomen, kidney-ureter-bladder (KUB) radiography, excretory urography, renal scan, retrograde pyelography, computed tomography scans, and nephrotomography are used to investigate the cause of renal failure.

Treatment

- High-calorie diet low in protein, sodium, and potassium
- Electrolyte imbalance: I.V. fluids and electrolytes; hemodialysis or peritoneal dialysis if needed; continuous renal replacement therapies
- Edema: fluid restriction
- Oliguria: diuretic therapy

- With mild hyperkalemic symptoms (malaise, anorexia, muscle weakness): sodium polystyrene sulfonate by mouth or enema
- With severe hyperkalemic symptoms (numbness and tingling and ECG changes): hypertonic glucose, insulin, and sodium bicarbonate I.V.
- Short-term dialysis

MECHANISM OF ACUTE KIDNEY INJURY

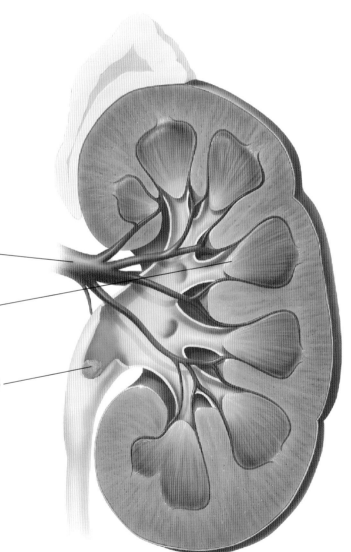

Prerenal (marked decrease in renal blood flow)

Intrinsic (damage to structures within the kidney)

Postrenal (obstruction of urine outflow from kidney [renal calculi])

ACUTE TUBULAR NECROSIS

Acute tubular necrosis, also known as *acute tubulointerstitial nephritis,* accounts for about 75% of all cases of acute renal failure and is the most common cause of acute renal failure in hospitalized patients. Acute tubular necrosis injures the tubular segment of the nephron, causing renal failure and uremic syndrome. Mortality ranges from 40% to 70%, depending on complications from underlying diseases. Nonoliguric forms of acute tubular necrosis have a better prognosis.

Causes

Acute tubular necrosis results from ischemic or nephrotoxic injury, most commonly in debilitated patients, such as the critically ill or those who have undergone extensive surgery.

Ischemic Injury

- Sepsis
- Severe hypotension
- Dehydration
- Heart failure
- Surgery
- Anesthetics
- Transfusion reactions
- Burns

Nephrotoxic Injury

- Certain medications such as aminoglycosides
- Contrast media

Pathophysiology

When ischemic injury occurs, the tubular cells of the kidney suffer from cellular energy depletion, intracellular accumulation of calcium, and damage to the cell membranes. Patch necrosis results at multiple points in the tubules, the basement membrane may be ruptured, and the tubular lumen may become occluded by casts and debris. The occlusion is worsened by the inflammatory cells that produce casts and debris, contributing further to the urinary occlusion. Obstructed urine flow causes an increase tubular intraluminal pressure in the nephron, resulting in a decrease GFR. If the basement membrane is not severely destroyed or if the episode of acute tubular necrosis is not fatal, regeneration eventually will completely reverse the damage.

When nephrotoxic injury occurs, hemoglobin or myoglobin precipitates in the urine. Tubular cells are destroyed by direct toxic effects, lysis of red blood cells (RBCs), activating the cascade of the inflammatory mediators, intravascular coagulation, occlusion of tubules, and tissue hypoxia. In this form of acute tubular necrosis, most necrosis occurs in the proximal tubules.

COMPLICATIONS
- Infections
- GI hemorrhage
- Fluid and electrolyte imbalances
- Cardiovascular dysfunction
- Neurologic complications

Signs and Symptoms

- Early stages: effects of primary disease may mask symptoms of acute tubular necrosis
- Decreased urine output may be first recognizable effect
- Hyperkalemia
- Uremic syndrome, with oliguria (or, rarely, anuria) and confusion, which may progress to uremic coma
- Heart failure and uremic pericarditis
- Pulmonary edema and uremic lung
- Anemia
- Anorexia
- Intractable vomiting
- Poor wound healing

CLINICAL TIP
Fever and chills may signal the onset of an infection, the leading cause of death in acute tubular necrosis.

Diagnostic Test Results

- Urine analysis shows sediment containing RBCs and casts, low specific gravity (1.010), osmolality less than 400 mOsm/kg, and high sodium level (40 to 60 mEq/L).
- Blood studies reveal elevated blood urea nitrogen and creatinine levels, anemia, defects in platelet adherence, metabolic acidosis, and hyperkalemia.
- ECG shows arrhythmias and, with hyperkalemia, widening QRS segment, disappearing P waves, and tall, peaked T waves.

Treatment

Acute Phase

- Vigorous supportive measures until normal kidney function resumes; initial treatment may include:
  - diuretics
  - I.V. fluids to flush tubules of cellular casts and debris and to replace fluid loss.
- Give vasopressors and/or inotropes.

Long-Term Fluid Management

- Daily replacement of projected and calculated losses (including insensible loss)

Other Measures to Control Complications

- Epoetin alfa to stimulate RBC production; packed RBCs for anemia
- Stop all possible nephrotoxic drugs
- Antibiotics for infection
- Emergency I.V. administration of 50% glucose, regular insulin, and sodium bicarbonate for hyperkalemia
- Sodium polystyrene sulfonate with sorbitol by mouth or by enema to reduce extracellular potassium levels
- Hemodialysis
- Continuous renal replacement therapies

ISCHEMIC NECROSIS

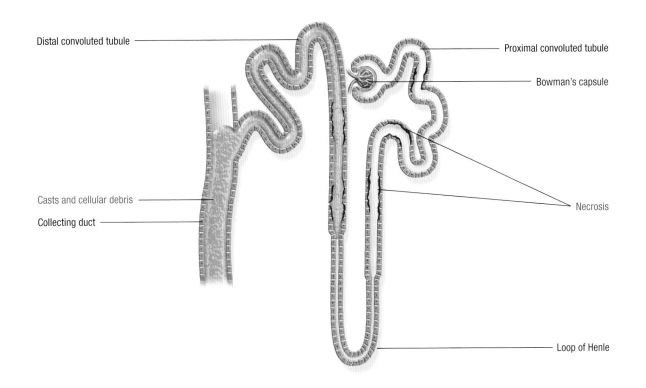

Distal convoluted tubule

Proximal convoluted tubule

Bowman's capsule

Casts and cellular debris

Collecting duct

Necrosis

Loop of Henle

NEPHROTOXIC INJURY

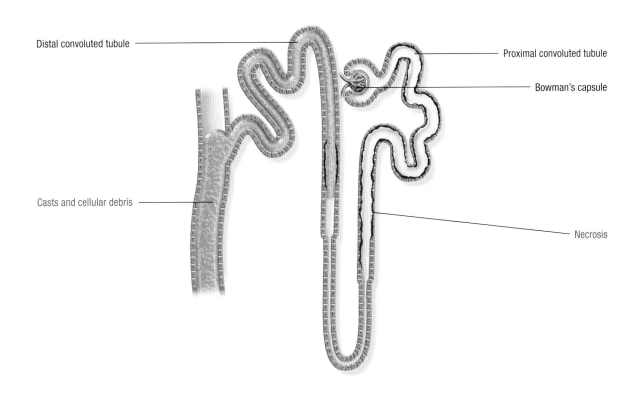

Distal convoluted tubule

Proximal convoluted tubule

Bowman's capsule

Casts and cellular debris

Necrosis

BLADDER CANCER

Cancer of the bladder is the most common cancer of the urinary tract.

Workers in certain industries (rubber workers, weavers and leather finishers, aniline dye workers, hairdressers, petroleum workers, and spray painters) are at high risk for bladder cancer. The period between exposure to the carcinogen and development of symptoms is about 18 years.

AGE ALERT
Bladder tumors are most prevalent in men over age 50 and are most common in densely populated industrial areas.

Causes

Primary cause unknown

Predisposing Factors

- Smoking is most common causative factor
- Transitional cell tumors — certain environmental carcinogens, including 2-naphthylamine, benzidine, tobacco, and nitrates
- Squamous cell carcinoma of the bladder:
  - chronic bladder irritation or infection; for example, from kidney stones, indwelling urinary catheters, and cystitis from cyclophosphamide
  - schistosomiasis.

Pathophysiology

Carcinogens are excreted in the urine, creating a medium for prolonged exposure to mucous membranes of the bladder. Bladder tumors can develop on the surface of the bladder wall (benign or malignant papillomas) or grow within the bladder wall (generally more virulent) and quickly invade underlying muscles. Ninety percent of bladder tumors are transitional cell carcinomas, arising from the transitional epithelium of mucous membranes. Less common are adenocarcinomas, epidermoid carcinomas, squamous cell carcinomas, sarcomas, tumors in bladder diverticula, and carcinoma in situ.

COMPLICATIONS
- Metastasis to the bone
- Tumor invasion of contiguous viscera

Signs and Symptoms

- In early stages, no symptoms in approximately 25% of patients
- First sign: gross, painless, intermittent hematuria (in many cases with clots in the urine)
- Invasive lesions: suprapubic pain after voiding
- Other signs and symptoms:
  - bladder irritability and urinary frequency
  - nocturia
  - dribbling.

Diagnostic Test Results

- Cystoscopy and biopsy confirm bladder cancer diagnosis.
- Excretory urography identifies a large, early-stage tumor or an infiltrating tumor, delineates functional problems in the upper urinary tract, assesses hydronephrosis, and detects rigid deformity of the bladder wall.
- Retrograde cystography evaluates bladder structure and integrity and also helps confirm bladder cancer diagnosis.
- Bone scan detects metastases.
- Computed tomography scan defines the thickness of the involved bladder wall and discloses enlarged retroperitoneal lymph nodes.
- Ultrasonography finds metastases in tissues beyond the bladder and distinguishes a bladder cyst from a bladder tumor.
- Complete blood count detects anemia.
- Urinalysis detects blood in the urine.

Treatment

Superficial Bladder Tumors

- Transurethral cystoscopic resection and fulguration (electrical destruction); adequate when the tumor has not invaded the muscle
- Intravesicular chemotherapy; useful for multiple tumors (especially those that occur in many sites) and to prevent tumor recurrence
- Transurethral resection of the prostate (TURP) as adjunctive therapy
- If additional tumors develop:
  - fulguration every 3 months
  - more radical therapy if tumors penetrate the muscle layer or recur frequently.

Larger Tumors

- Segmental bladder resection to remove a full-thickness section of the bladder; only if tumor is not near the bladder neck or ureteral orifices
- Instillation of thiotepa after transurethral resection

Infiltrating Bladder Tumors

- Radical cystectomy — removal of the bladder with perivesical fat, lymph nodes, urethra, and prostate and seminal vesicles or uterus and adnexa
- Possibly, preoperative external beam therapy to bladder
- Urinary diversion, usually an ileal conduit (patient must then wear an external pouch continuously)
- Possible later penile implant

Advanced Bladder Cancer

- Cystectomy to remove tumor
- Radiation therapy
- Systemic chemotherapy:

- cyclophosphamide, fluorouracil, doxorubicin, and cisplatin combination may arrest bladder cancer
- cisplatin most effective single agent.

Investigational Treatments

- Photodynamic therapy:
  - I.V. injection of a photosensitizing agent such as hematoporphyrin ether, which malignant cells readily absorb, followed by cystoscopic laser treatment to kill malignant cells
  - treatment also renders normal cells photosensitive (patient must totally avoid sunlight for about 30 days)
- Intravesicular administration of interferon alfa and tumor necrosis factor

BLADDER TUMOR

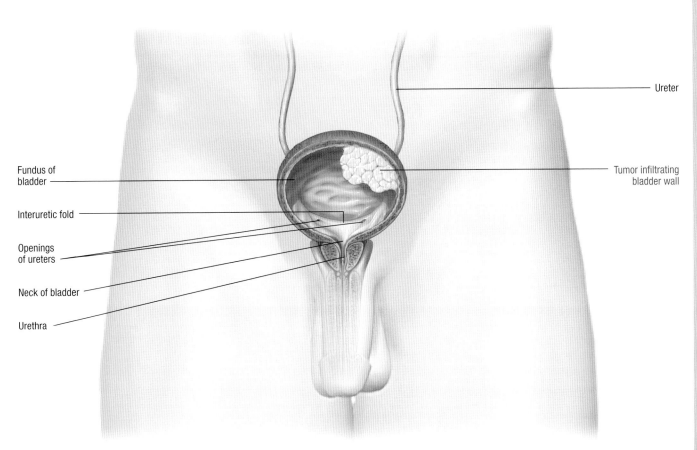

Ureter

Fundus of bladder

Interuretic fold

Openings of ureters

Neck of bladder

Urethra

Tumor infiltrating bladder wall

CYSTITIS

Cystitis and urethritis, the two forms of lower urinary tract infection (UTI), are nearly 10 times more common in women than in men and affect about 10% to 20% of all women at least once. Lower UTI is also a prevalent bacterial disease in children, most commonly in girls. Men are less vulnerable because their urethras are longer and their prostatic fluid serves as an antibacterial shield. In both men and women, infection usually ascends from the urethra to the bladder. UTIs generally respond readily to treatment, but recurrence and resistant bacterial flare-up during therapy are possible.

CLINICAL TIP
All children with a proven UTI should receive a workup to exclude an abnormality of the urinary tract that would predispose them to renal damage.

Causes

Ascending infection by a single, gram-negative, enteric species of bacteria, the most common being Escherichia (commonly *Escherichia coli*). Other less common organisms include *Klebsiella, Proteus, Enterobacter, Pseudomonas, Staphylococcus saprophyticus,* or *Serratia.*

In Women

- Predisposition to infection by bacteria from vagina, perineum, rectum, or a sexual partner, a possible result of a short urethra

In Men and Children

- Commonly related to anatomic or physiologic abnormalities

Recurrence

- In 99% of patients, reinfection by the same organism or a new pathogen
- Persistent infection — usually from renal calculi, chronic bacterial prostatitis, or a structural anomaly that harbors bacteria

AGE ALERT
As a person ages, progressive weakening of bladder muscles may result in incomplete bladder emptying and chronic urine retention — factors that predispose the older person to bladder infections.

Pathophysiology

Infection results from a breakdown in local defense mechanisms in the bladder that allow bacteria to invade the bladder mucosa and multiply. The antibacterial features in the urine that aid in the prevention of bacterial growth are pH less than 5.5, urea concentration, and presence of organic acids. These factors create an unfavorable medium for bacterial growth due to the acidity. When the local defenses are changed, bacteria quickly grows if present.

Normally, a small amount of urine remains in the bladder after emptying without incident if the natural defenses are present. In cases when the urine is more alkanine, bacteria is allowed to germinate.

Another defense is the unidirectional flow of the urine. If the urine flow is decreased, a catheter or other instrumentation is inserted, or post sexual intercourse, bacteria travels more readily into the bladder. Without the natural defense mechanisms, bacteria can flourish resulting in a local infection.

COMPLICATIONS
- Chronic UTIs
- Damage to the urinary tract lining
- Infection of adjacent organs such as the kidneys (pyelonephritis)

Signs and Symptoms

- Urgency, frequency, and dysuria
- Cramps or spasms of the bladder
- Itching and feeling of warmth or burning during urination
- Nocturia
- Urethral discharge in males
- Hematuria
- Fever and chills
- Other common features:
  - malaise
  - nausea and vomiting
  - low back pain and flank pain
  - abdominal pain and tenderness over the bladder area.

Diagnostic Test Results

- Microscopic urinalysis is positive for pyuria, hematuria, or bacteriuria.
- Bacterial count in clean-catch midstream urine specimen reveals more than 100,000 bacteria per milliliter.
- Sensitivity testing determines the appropriate therapeutic antimicrobial agent.
- Blood test or stained smear of the discharge rules out sexually transmitted disease.
- Voiding cystoureterography or excretory urography detects congenital anomalies that predispose the patient to recurrent UTIs.

Treatment

- Appropriate antimicrobials:
  - Single-dose therapy with trimethoprim and sulfamethoxazole for 3 to 5 days or nitrofurantoin for 7 days may be effective in women with acute noncomplicated UTI.
- If urine is not sterile after 3 days:
  - bacterial resistance likely
  - use of a different antimicrobial necessary.
- Sitz baths or warm compresses
- Increased fluid intake
- Phenazopyridine hydrochloride (Pyridium) — a urinary analgesic

Recurrent Infections

- Infected renal calculi, chronic prostatitis, or structural abnormality — possible surgery
- Prostatitis — long-term antibiotic therapy
- In absence of predisposing conditions — long-term, low-dose antibiotic therapy

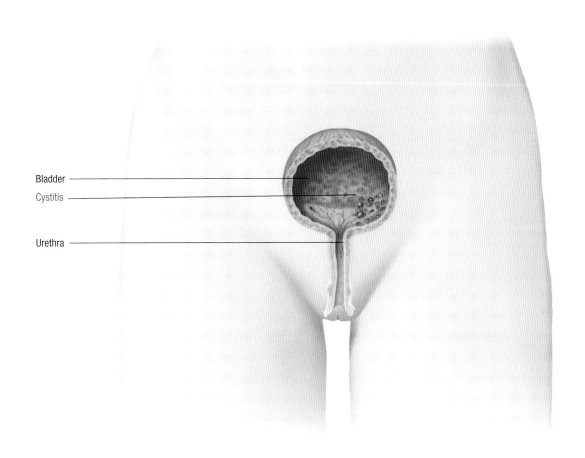

Bladder

Cystitis

Urethra

CLINICAL TIP

ROUTES OF INFECTION IN THE URINARY TRACT

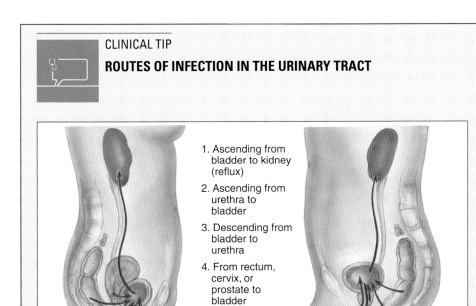

1. Ascending from bladder to kidney (reflux)

2. Ascending from urethra to bladder

3. Descending from bladder to urethra

4. From rectum, cervix, or prostate to bladder

5. From bowel to bladder

Bladder wall — Endoscopic view

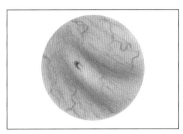

Normal wall

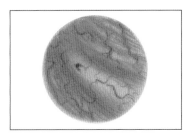

Acute cystitis

GLOMERULONEPHRITIS

Glomerulonephritis is a bilateral inflammation of the glomeruli, commonly following a streptococcal infection. Acute glomerulonephritis is also called *acute poststreptococcal glomerulonephritis.*

AGE ALERT
Although the incidence rate of acute glomerulonephritis has been on the decline for the past few decades in most developed countries, acute glomerulonephritis is most common in boys ages 3 to 7 but can occur at any age. Rapidly progressive glomerulonephritis most commonly occurs between ages 50 and 60. Up to 95% of children and 70% of adults recover fully. Elderly patients may progress to chronic renal failure within months.

Rapidly progressive glomerulonephritis — also called subacute, crescentic, or extracapillary glomerulonephritis — may be idiopathic or associated with a proliferative glomerular disease such as poststreptococcal glomerulonephritis.

Chronic glomerulonephritis is a slowly progressive disease characterized by inflammation, sclerosis, scarring, and, eventually, renal failure. It usually remains undetected until the progressive (irreversible) phase.

Causes

Acute or Rapidly Progressive Glomerulonephritis

- Streptococcal infection of the respiratory tract (1 to 3 weeks prior)
- Immunoglobulin A nephropathy (Berger's disease)
- Impetigo
- Lipoid nephrosis

Chronic Glomerulonephritis

- Membranoproliferative glomerulonephritis
- Membranous glomerulopathy
- Focal glomerulosclerosis
- Rapidly progressive glomerulonephritis and poststreptococcal glomerulonephritis
- Systemic lupus erythematosus and Goodpasture's syndrome
- Hemolytic uremic syndrome

Pathophysiology

In nearly all types of glomerulonephritis, the epithelial or podocyte layer of the glomerular membrane is damaged.

Acute poststreptococcal glomerulonephritis results from the entrapment and collection of antigen-antibody complexes, also known as immune complexes, in the glomerular capillary membranes, after infection with a group A beta-hemolytic streptococcus. The antigens, which are endogenous or exogenous, stimulate the formation of antibodies, which form immune complexes. Circulating immune complexes become lodged in the glomerular capillaries. The severity of glomerular damage and consequent renal insufficiency is related to the size, number, location (focal or diffuse), duration of exposure, and type of immune complexes. The decreased GFR leads to activating the renin-aldosterone system, causing salt and water retention. The consequence of this action is edema and hypertension, hallmark signs and symptoms of glomerulonephritis.

In the glomerular capillary wall, immune complexes activate biochemical mediators of inflammation — complement, leukocytes, and fibrin. Activated complement attracts neutrophils and monocytes, which release lysosomal enzymes that damage the cell walls and cause a proliferation of the extracellular matrix, affecting glomerular blood flow. Those events increase membrane permeability, which causes a loss of negative charge across the glomerular membrane and enhanced protein filtration. Membrane damage also leads to platelet aggregation, and platelet degranulation releases substances that increase glomerular permeability.

Protein molecules and RBCs can now pass into the urine, resulting in proteinuria or hematuria. Activation of the coagulation system leads to fibrin deposits in Bowman's space. The result is formation of crescent-shaped blood cells and diminished renal blood flow and GFR. The presence of crescents signifies severe, often irreversible kidney damage. Glomerular bleeding acidifies the urine and thereby transforms hemoglobin to methemoglobin; the result is brown urine without clots.

COMPLICATIONS
- End-stage renal failure
- Cardiac hypertrophy
- Heart failure

Signs and Symptoms

- Decreased urination; smoky or coffee-colored urine
- Sudden onset of hematuria and proteinuria
- Shortness of breath, dyspnea, orthopnea, and bibasilar crackles
- Periorbital and peripheral edema
- Mild to severe hypertension

Diagnostic Test Results

- Blood studies reveal elevated blood urea nitrogen and creatinine levels, decreased serum protein levels, decreased hemoglobin, elevated antistreptolysin-O titers in 80% of patients, elevated streptozyme (a hemagglutination test that detects antibodies to several streptococcal antigens) and anti-DNase B (a test to determine a previous infection of group A beta-hemolytic streptococcus) titers, and low serum complement levels indicate recent streptococcal infection.
- Urinalysis reveals RBCs, white blood cells, mixed cells casts, and protein.
- Throat culture detects group A beta-hemolytic streptococcus.
- KUB X-ray shows bilateral kidney enlargement (acute glomerulonephritis).
- Renal biopsy confirms the diagnosis or assesses renal tissue.

Treatment

- Treatment for primary disease and antibiotics for infections
- Bed rest to reduce metabolic demands

- Fluid and dietary sodium restriction and correction of electrolyte imbalances
- Loop diuretics for extracellular fluid overload
- Vasodilators for hypertension
- Corticosteroids to decrease antibody synthesis and suppress inflammatory response

- In rapidly progressive glomerulonephritis, plasmapheresis to suppress rebound antibody production, possibly combined with corticosteroids and cyclophosphamide
- In chronic glomerulonephritis, dialysis or kidney transplantation

IMMUNE COMPLEX DEPOSITS ON GLOMERULUS

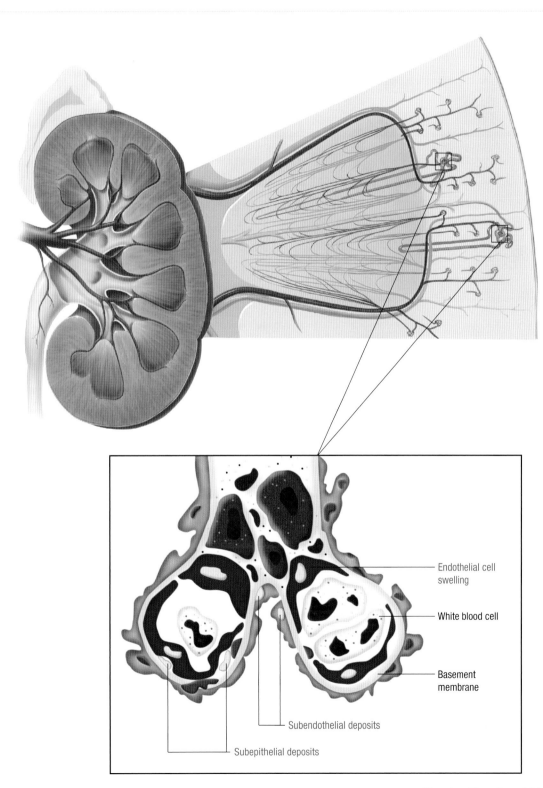

Endothelial cell swelling

White blood cell

Basement membrane

Subendothelial deposits

Subepithelial deposits

HYDRONEPHROSIS

Hydronephrosis is an abnormal dilation of the renal pelvis and the calyces of one or both kidneys, caused by an obstruction of urine flow distal to the renal pelvis in the genitourinary tract. Although partial obstruction and hydronephrosis may not produce symptoms initially, the pressure built up behind the area of obstruction eventually results in symptomatic renal dysfunction.

AGE ALERT
Hydronephrosis is a normal finding in pregnant women and may be detected by prenatal ultrasound. The dilation of the ureters and renal pelvis should resolve between 6 and 12 weeks postpartum; however, if postnatal, follow-up is critical.

Causes

- Obstructive uropathy
- Most common:
  - benign prostatic hyperplasia
  - urethral strictures
  - calculi (most common in adults).
- Less common:
  - strictures or stenosis of the ureter or bladder outlet (more common in children)
  - congenital abnormalities (more common in children)
  - trauma
  - retroperitoneal or pelvic tumors
  - blood clots
  - neurogenic bladder.

Pathophysiology

If obstruction of the flow of urine is in the urethra or bladder, hydronephrosis is usually bilateral; if obstruction is in a ureter, only one kidney is affected. Obstructions distal to the bladder cause the bladder to dilate and act as a buffer zone, delaying hydronephrosis. Total obstruction of urine flow with dilation of the collecting system quickly leads to decrease in glomerular filtration function, tubular function, and renal blood flow. Ultimately, the marked decline in the kidney function causes complete cortical atrophy and cessation of glomerular filtration.

In acute hydronephrosis, when the obstruction is cleared and urine flow is restored, the decreased GFR and tubular dysfunction persist for weeks. When the obstruction occurred over a short time span, the functions of the kidneys are eventually restored. In more chronic obstructions, irreversible damage has been seen.

COMPLICATIONS
- Pyelonephritis
- Paralytic ileus
- Renal failure

Signs and Symptoms

Clinical features of hydronephrosis vary with the cause of the obstruction.

- No symptoms or mild pain and slightly decreased urinary flow
- Severe, colicky renal pain or dull flank pain that may radiate to the groin
- Gross urinary abnormalities, such as hematuria, pyuria, dysuria, alternating oliguria and polyuria, or complete anuria
- Nausea, vomiting, abdominal fullness, pain on urination, dribbling, and hesitancy

Diagnostic Test Results

- Renal function blood studies are abnormal.
- Urine studies confirm the inability to concentrate urine, decreased GFR, and pyuria if infection is present.
- Excretory urography, retrograde pyelography, and renal ultrasound confirm the diagnosis.
- I.V. urogram detects the site of obstruction.
- Nephrogram shows delayed appearance time.
- Radionuclide scan shows the site of obstruction.

Treatment

- Ureteral stent or nephrostomy tube
- Surgical removal of the obstruction:
  - dilation for stricture of the urethra
  - prostatectomy for benign prostatic hyperplasia.
- With renal damage: diet low in protein, sodium, and potassium to slow progression before surgery
- Inoperable obstructions: decompression and drainage of kidney through temporary or permanent nephrostomy tube in the renal pelvis
- Concurrent infection: appropriate antibiotic therapy

Hydronephrotic kidney

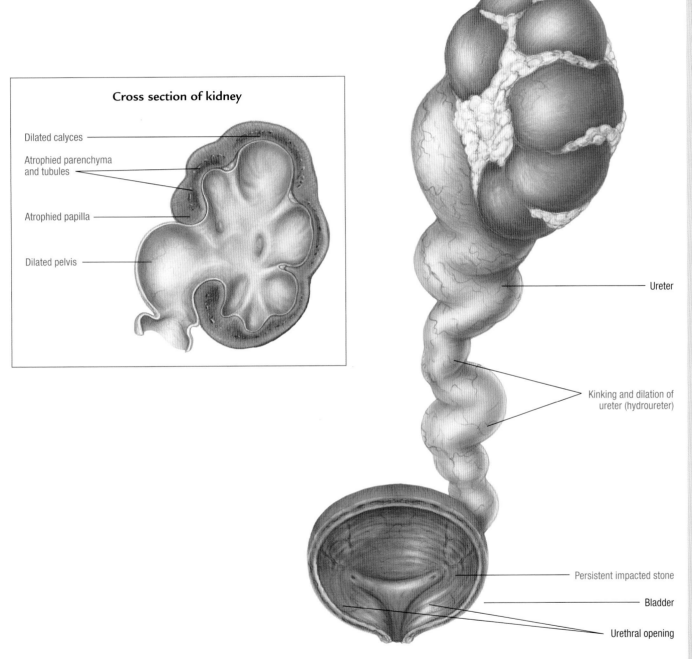

Cross section of kidney

Dilated calyces

Atrophied parenchyma
and tubules

Atrophied papilla

Dilated pelvis

Ureter

Kinking and dilation of
ureter (hydroureter)

Persistent impacted stone

Bladder

Urethral opening

NEUROGENIC BLADDER

Neurogenic bladder is any type of bladder dysfunction caused by an interruption of normal bladder innervation by the nervous system. It can be hyperreflexic (hypertonic, spastic, or automatic) or flaccid (hypotonic, atonic, or autonomous).

Causes

Once thought to result primarily from spinal cord injury; now appears to stem from several underlying conditions:

- cerebral disorders, such as stroke, brain tumor, Parkinson's disease, multiple sclerosis, dementia, and incontinence associated with aging
- spinal cord disease or trauma, such as spinal stenosis or arachnoiditis
- disorders of peripheral innervation, including autonomic neuropathies resulting from endocrine disturbances such as diabetes mellitus
- metabolic disturbances such as hypothyroidism
- acute inflammatory demyelinating diseases such as Guillain-Barré syndrome
- heavy metal toxicity
- chronic alcoholism
- collagen diseases such as systemic lupus erythematosus
- vascular diseases such as atherosclerosis
- distant effects of certain cancers such as primary oat cell carcinoma of the lung
- herpes zoster
- sacral agenesis.

Pathophysiology

Bladder function is controlled by the brain and automatic. In the brain stem, the pons area, the pontine micturition center (PMC) coordinates through receptors in the bladder the urethral sphincter relaxation and contraction of the detrusor muscle. The receptors in the bladder signal to the brain when voiding is necessary as the bladder stretches. When a disruption of the brain stem or spinal cord occurs, the bladder no longer receives a signal when to void in a socially acceptable time or place, resulting in incontinence.

Lesions of the brains in the pons area causes complete dysfunction of the PMC system, causing complete loss of controlling urination. The bladder is then controlled by the voiding reflex found in the lower spinal cord. This loss causes overflow incontinence and dribbling of urine.

An upper motor neuron lesion (at or above T12) causes spastic neurogenic bladder, with spontaneous contraction of the detrusor muscles, increased intravesical voiding pressure, bladder wall hypertrophy with trabeculation, and urinary sphincter spasms. The patient may experience incomplete emptying and loss of voluntary control of voiding. Urine retention can also lead to UTI.

A lower motor neuron lesion (at or below S2 to S4) affects the spinal reflex that controls micturition. The result is a flaccid neurogenic bladder with decreased intravesical pressure, increased bladder capacity and residual urine retention, and poor detrusor contraction. The bladder may not empty spontaneously. The patient experiences loss of voluntary and involuntary control of urination. Lower motor neuron lesions lead to overflow incontinence. When sensory neurons are interrupted, the patient cannot perceive the need to void.

The lack of bladder control causes urine retention, which contributes to renal calculi and infection. If not promptly diagnosed and treated, neurogenic bladder can lead to the deterioration of renal function.

COMPLICATIONS
- Incontinence
- Residual urine retention
- UTI
- Calculus formation
- Renal failure

Signs and Symptoms

General

- Some degree of incontinence
- Interruption or changes in initiation of micturition
- Inability to completely empty the bladder
- History of frequent UTIs
- Vesicoureteral reflux
- Hydroureteral nephrosis

Spastic Neurogenic Bladder

- Involuntary or frequent scanty urination without a feeling of bladder fullness
- Increased anal sphincter tone
- Increased tactile stimulation of the abdomen, thighs, or genitalia possibly precipitating voiding

Flaccid Neurogenic Bladder

- Overflow incontinence
- Diminished anal sphincter tone
- Greatly distended bladder (evident on palpation or percussion) but with the patient possibly not experiencing the feeling of bladder fullness because of sensory impairment

Diagnostic Test Results

- Uroflow shows diminished or impaired flow.
- Cystometry evaluates the bladder's nerve supply, detrusor muscle tone, and intravesical pressures during bladder filling and contraction.
- Urethral pressure profile determines urethral function by examining urethral length and outlet pressure resistance.
- Sphincter electromyography correlates the neuromuscular function of the external sphincter with bladder muscle function during bladder filling and contraction, indicating how well the bladder and urinary sphincter muscles work together.
- Video urodynamic studies correlate visual documentation of bladder function with pressure studies.

Treatment

- Treatment goals: maintain the integrity of the upper urinary tract, control infection, and prevent urinary incontinence through evacuation of the bladder, drug therapy, surgery, or, less often, nerve blocks and electrical stimulation
- Bladder evacuation techniques, such as Credé's method, Valsalva's maneuver, and intermittent self-catheterization

- Bethanechol or phenoxybenzamine to promote bladder emptying; propantheline, methantheline, flavoxate, dicyclomine, imipramine, or pseudoephedrine to aid urine storage
- Botulinum toxin injection
- When conservative treatment fails, surgery to correct structural impairment: transurethral resection of the bladder neck, urethral dilation, external sphincterotomy, or urinary diversion procedures; if permanent incontinence follows surgery, possible implantation of an artificial urinary sphincter

LOOKING AT NEUROGENIC BLADDER

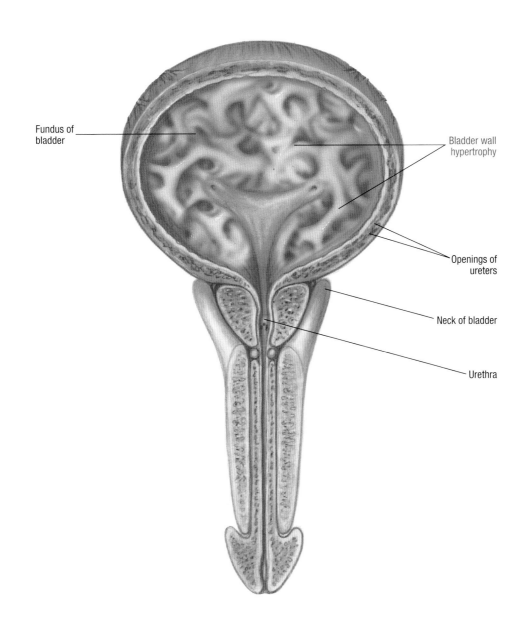

Fundus of bladder

Bladder wall hypertrophy

Openings of ureters

Neck of bladder

Urethra

POLYCYSTIC KIDNEY DISEASE

Polycystic kidney disease is an autosomal dominant inherited disorder characterized by multiple, bilateral, grapelike clusters of fluid-filled cysts that enlarge the kidneys, compressing and eventually replacing functioning renal tissue. The disease affects males and females equally and appears in distinct infantile and adult-onset forms. The adult form, autosomal dominant polycystic kidney disease, occurs in nearly 1 in 1,000 persons and accounts for about 6% to 10% of end-stage renal disease in the United States. Autosomal recessive polycystic kidney disease occurs in 1 in 10,000 to 1 in 40,000 live births. Renal deterioration is more gradual in adults than infants, but in both age-groups, the disease progresses relentlessly to fatal uremia.

AGE ALERT

The rare infantile form of polycystic kidney disease causes stillbirth or early neonatal death due to pulmonary hypoplasia. The adult form has an insidious onset. It usually becomes obvious between ages 30 and 50; rarely, it remains asymptomatic until the patient is in his 60s.

The prognosis in adults is extremely variable. Progression may be slow, even after symptoms of renal insufficiency appear. After uremia symptoms develop, polycystic disease usually is fatal within 4 years, unless the patient receives dialysis.

Causes

- Autosomal dominant trait (adult type); three genetic variants identified
- Autosomal recessive trait (infantile type)

Pathophysiology

The Autosomal Dominant

Grossly enlarged kidneys are caused by multiple spherical cysts, a few millimeters to centimeters in diameter that contain straw-colored or hemorrhagic fluid. The cysts are distributed evenly throughout the cortex and medulla. The cysts may also be found in the liver and spleen. Hyperplastic polyps and renal adenomas are common. Renal parenchyma may have varying degrees of tubular atrophy, interstitial fibrosis, and nephrosclerosis. The cysts cause elongation of the pelvis, flattening of the calyces, and indentations in the kidney. The cells that cause the cyst are mutuated and continue to proliferate, resulting in a progressive disease that continues to have more cysts. Although the nephrons are not significantly affected, between 1% and 5% only, the kidneys remain dysfunctional due to the changes elicited by the cysts, including tubule base membrane thickening, and new vacularization.

Accompanying hepatic fibrosis and intrahepatic bile duct abnormalities may cause portal hypertension and bleeding varices. In most cases, about 10 years after symptoms appear, progressive compression of kidney structures by the enlarging mass causes renal failure.

Cysts also form on the liver, spleen, pancreas, or ovaries. Intracranial aneurysms, colonic diverticula, and mitral valve prolapse also occur.

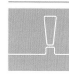

COMPLICATIONS

In Neonates
- Renal failure
- Respiratory failure
- Heart failure

In Adults
- Hematuria
- Retroperitoneal bleeding from cyst rupture
- Proteinuria
- Abdominal and flank pain from passage of clots or calculi
- Mitral valve prolapse
- Colonic diverticuli
- Subarachnoid hemorrhage

Signs and Symptoms

In Neonates

- Potter facies — pronounced epicanthic folds; pointed nose; small chin; floppy, low-set ears
- Huge, bilateral, symmetrical masses on the flanks that are tense and can't be transilluminated
- Signs of respiratory distress, heart failure, and, eventually, uremia and renal failure

In Adults

- Hypertension
- Headache
- Lumbar pain
- Widening abdominal girth
- Swollen or tender abdomen, worsened by exertion and relieved by lying down
- Grossly enlarged kidneys on palpation

Diagnostic Test Results

- Excretory or retrograde urography shows enlarged kidneys, with elongation of the pelvis, flattening of the calyces, and indentations in the kidney caused by cysts.
- Excretory urography of the neonate shows poor excretion of contrast medium.
- Ultrasonography, tomography, and radioisotope scans show kidney enlargement and cysts; tomography, computed tomography, and magnetic resonance imaging show multiple areas of cystic damage.
- Urinalysis detects hematuria, bacteriuria, or proteinuria.
- Creatinine clearance tests show renal insufficiency or failure.

Treatment

- Antibiotics for infections
- Analgesics for abdominal pain
- Adequate hydration to maintain fluid balance
- Antihypertensives and diuretics to control blood pressure
- Changes in diet and exercise (no contact sports to protect the kidney)

- Surgical drainage of cystic abscess or retroperitoneal bleeding
- Nephrectomy not recommended (polycystic kidney disease occurs bilaterally, and infection could recur in the remaining kidney)
- Dialysis or kidney transplantation for progressive renal failure

POLYCYSTIC KIDNEY

Cross section

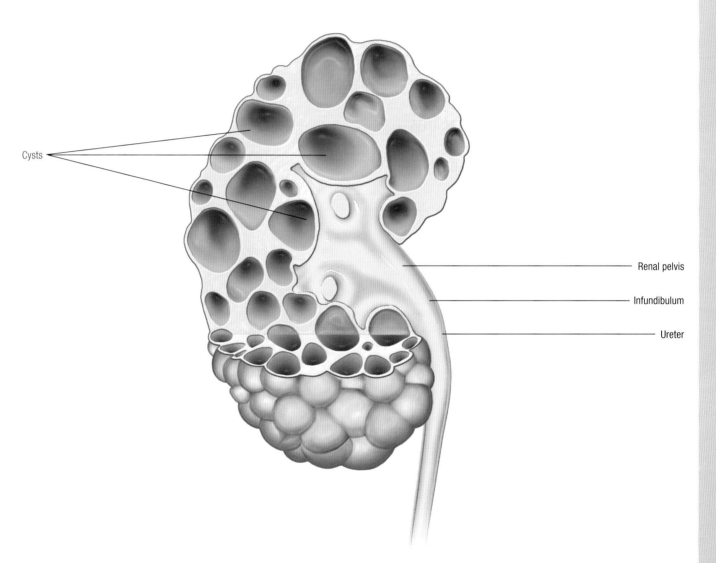

Cysts

Renal pelvis

Infundibulum

Ureter

PYELONEPHRITIS

Acute pyelonephritis (also known as *acute infective tubulointerstitial nephritis*) is a sudden inflammation caused by bacterial infection; it primarily affects the interstitial area and the renal pelvis or, less often, the renal tubules. Pyelonephritis is one of the most common renal diseases. Symptoms characteristically develop rapidly over a few hours or days and may disappear within days, even without treatment. However, residual bacterial infection is likely and may cause symptoms to recur later. With treatment and continued follow-up care, the prognosis is good and extensive permanent damage is rare.

Causes

Acute pyelonephritis results from bacterial infection of the kidneys. Infecting bacteria usually are normal intestinal and fecal flora that grow readily in urine. The most common causative organism is *E. coli*, but *Proteus* or *Pseudomonas* species, *Staphylococcus aureus*, or *Enterococcus faecalis* (formerly *Streptococcus faecalis*) may also cause this infection.

CLINICAL TIP
Emphysematous pyelonephritis is an uncommon disorder seen in patients with diabetes or those who are immunocompromised. It's caused by a gas-forming organism such as *E. coli*, which produces gas that forms in the renal parenchyma or perirenal space. This life-threatening condition requires aggressive medical management or nephrectomy.

CLINICAL TIP
Pyelonephritis occurs more commonly in females, probably because bacteria reach the bladder more easily through the short female urethra; the urinary meatus is in close proximity to the vagina and the rectum, and women lack the male's antibacterial prostatic secretions.

Pathophysiology

Typically, the infection spreads from the bladder to the ureters, then to the kidneys, as in vesicoureteral reflux. Vesicoureteral reflux may result from congenital weakness at the junction of the ureter and the bladder. Bacteria refluxed to intrarenal tissues may create colonies of infection within 24 to 48 hours. Infection may also result from instrumentation (such as catheterization, cystoscopy, or urologic surgery), a hematogenic infection (as in septicemia or endocarditis), or possibly lymphatic infection.

Pyelonephritis may also result from an inability to empty the bladder (for example, in patients with neurogenic bladder), urinary stasis, or urinary obstruction due to tumors, strictures, or benign prostatic hyperplasia.

COMPLICATIONS
- Chronic pyelonephritis
- Acute renal failure
- Sepsis

Signs and Symptoms

- Urgency, frequency, and nocturia
- Burning during urination and dysuria
- Hematuria, usually microscopic but may be gross
- Cloudy urine and ammonialike or fishy odor
- Fever of 102°F (38.9°C) or higher and shaking chills
- Costovertebral angle pain/flank pain (unilateral but discomfort in both)
- Nausea and vomiting
- Anorexia
- General fatigue

AGE ALERT
Elderly patients may exhibit GI or pulmonary symptoms rather than the usual febrile responses to pyelonephritis.

In children younger than age 2, fever, vomiting, nonspecific abdominal complaints, or failure to thrive may be the only signs of acute pyelonephritis.

Diagnostic Test Results

- Urine sediment reveals the presence of leukocytes singly, in clumps, and in casts and, possibly, a few RBCs.
- Urine culture reveals more than 100,000 organisms/µL of urine.
- Urinalysis reveals low specific gravity and osmolality, proteinuria, glycosuria, and ketonuria.
- Urine pH testing shows a slightly alkaline pH.
- Computed tomography scan of the kidneys, ureters, and bladder reveals calculi, tumors, or cysts in the kidneys and the urinary tract.
- Excretory urography shows asymmetrical kidneys.

Treatment

Antibiotic therapy appropriate to the specific infecting organism after identification by urine culture and sensitivity studies:

- *Enterococcus* — ampicillin, penicillin G, and vancomycin
- *Staphylococcus* — penicillin G; if resistance develops, a semisynthetic penicillin, such as nafcillin, or a cephalosporin
- *E. coli* — sulfisoxazole, nalidixic acid, and nitrofurantoin
- *Proteus* — ampicillin, sulfisoxazole, nalidixic acid, and a cephalosporin
- *Pseudomonas* — gentamicin, tobramycin, and carbenicillin
- Not identified — broad-spectrum antibiotic, such as ampicillin or cephalexin
- Pregnancy or renal insufficiency — antibiotics prescribed cautiously

Follow-up

- Urine culture repeated 1 week after drug therapy stops and then periodically for the next year

Infection from Obstruction or Vesicoureteral Reflux
- Antibiotics possibly less effective
- Surgery to relieve the obstruction or correct the anomaly

Patients at High Risk for Recurring Urinary Tract and Kidney Infections
- Prolonged use of an indwelling catheter or maintenance antibiotic therapy
- Long-term follow-up to prevent chronic pyelonephritis

PHASES OF PYELONEPHRITIS

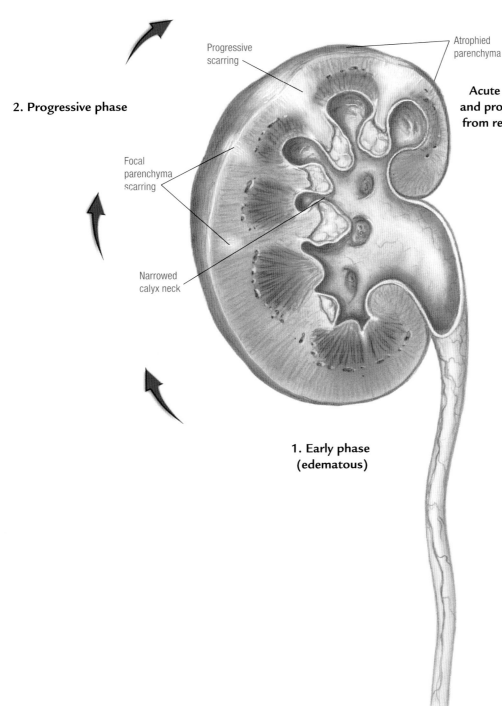

3. End phase

Progressive scarring

Atrophied parenchyma

Acute pyelonephritis and progressive scarring from repeated infection

2. Progressive phase

Focal parenchyma scarring

Narrowed calyx neck

1. Early phase (edematous)

RENAL CALCULI

Renal calculi, or stones (nephrolithiasis), can form any-where in the urinary tract, although they most commonly develop on the renal pelves or calyces. They may vary in size and may be single or multiple.

AGE ALERT
Renal calculi are more common in men than in women and rarely occur in children. Calcium stones generally occur in men between the ages of 35 to 45 years old with a familial history of stone formation.

Causes

Exact cause unknown

Predisposing Factors

- Dehydration
- Infection
- Changes in urine pH (calcium carbonate stones, high pH; uric acid stones, lower pH)
- Obstruction to urine flow leading to stasis in the urinary tract
- Immobilization causing bone reabsorption
- Metabolic factors, such as hyperparathyroidism, renal tubular acidosis, elevated uric acid, and defective oxalate metabolism
- Dietary factors such as increased intake of calcium or of oxalate-rich foods
- Renal disease

Pathophysiology

Calculi form when substances that are normally dissolved in the urine, such as calcium oxalate and calcium phosphate, precipi-tate. Dehydration may lead to renal calculi as calculus-forming substances concentrate in urine when urine flow is decreased.

Stones form around a nucleus or nidus in the appropriate environment. A stone-forming substance (calcium oxalate, cal-cium carbonate, magnesium, ammonium, phosphate, uric acid, or cystine) forms a crystal that becomes trapped in the urinary tract, where it attracts other crystals to form a stone. The ure-ters subsequently dilate from the obstruction, resulting in a high urine saturation of the crystal-forming substances, which contin-ues the growth of the stone, encourages crystal formation, and results in stone growth. The pH of the urine affects the solubility of many stone-forming substances. Formation of calcium oxa-late and cystine stones is independent of urine pH. Most stones are calcium oxalate or a combination of oxalate and phosphate.

Stones may form in the papillae, renal tubules, calyces, renal pelves, ureter, or bladder. Most are less than 5 mm in diameter and are usually passed in the urine. Staghorn calculi (casts of the calyceal and pelvic collecting system) can continue to grow in the pelvis, extending to the calyces, forming a branching stone, and ultimately resulting in renal failure if not surgically removed.

Calcium stones are the smallest. Although 80% are idio-pathic, they frequently occur in patients with hyperuricosuria. Prolonged immobilization can lead to bone demineralization,

hypercalciuria, and stone formation. In addition, hyperparathy-roidism, renal tubular acidosis, and excessive intake of vitamin D or dietary calcium may predispose a person to renal calculi.

Struvite (magnesium, ammonium, and phosphate) stones are often precipitated by an infection, particularly with *Pseudomonas* or *Proteus* species. These urea-splitting organisms are more common in women. Struvite calculi can destroy renal parenchyma.

COMPLICATIONS
- Hydronephrosis
- Damage to renal parenchyma

Signs and Symptoms

- Severe pain caused by inflammation, stretching, and spasm of ureteral obstruction
- Nausea and vomiting
- Fever and chills from infection
- Hematuria when calculi abrade a ureter
- Abdominal distention
- Anuria from bilateral obstruction or obstruction of only kidney

Diagnostic Test Results

- KUB radiography shows most renal calculi.
- Excretory urography confirms the diagnosis and deter-mines the size and location of calculi.
- Kidney ultrasonography detects such obstructive changes as unilateral or bilateral hydronephrosis and radiolucent cal-culi not seen on KUB radiography.
- Urine culture shows pyuria.
- A 24-hour urine collection determines levels of calcium oxa-late, phosphorus, and uric acid excretion.
- Calculus analysis determines mineral content.
- Serial blood calcium and phosphorus levels diagnose hyperparathyroidism.
- Blood protein levels determine the level of free calcium unbound to protein.

Treatment

- Fluid intake greater than 3 L/d to promote hydration
- Antimicrobial agents; vary with the cultured organism
- Narcotic analgesics or nonsteroidal anti-inflammatory drugs
- Diuretics to prevent urinary stasis and further calculus for-mation; thiazides to decrease calcium excretion
- Acetohydroxamic acid to suppress calculus formation when infection is present
- Cystoscopy and manipulation of calculus to remove stones too large for natural passage
- Percutaneous ultrasonic lithotripsy and extracorporeal shock wave lithotripsy or laser therapy to shatter the calcu-lus into fragments for removal by suction or natural passage
- Surgical removal of cystine calculi or large stones
- Placement of urinary diversion around the stone

Type-Specific Treatment

- Low-calcium diet (new evidence says low-protein and low-sodium may be more beneficial)

- Oxalate-binding cholestyramine
- Allopurinol for uric acid calculi
- Daily small doses of ascorbic acid to acidify urine

TYPES OF RENAL CALCULI

Uric acid stones

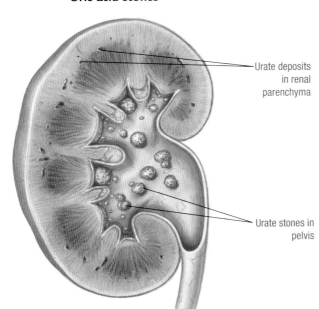

Urate deposits in renal parenchyma

Urate stones in pelvis

Ammoniomagnesium phosphate (struvite) stones

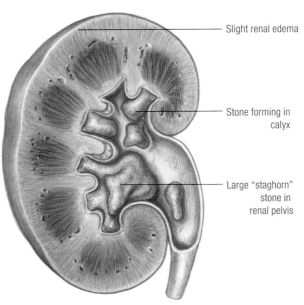

Slight renal edema

Stone forming in calyx

Large "staghorn" stone in renal pelvis

Calcium stones

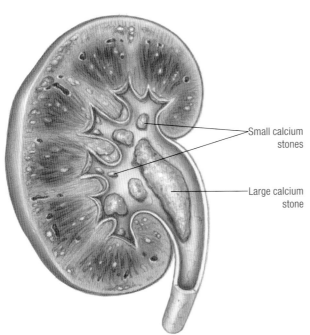

Small calcium stones

Large calcium stone

RENAL CANCER

Renal cancer (nephrocarcinoma, renal cell carcinoma, hypernephroma, or Grawitz's tumor) usually occurs in older adults. Although the incidence of this malignancy is rising, it accounts for only about 2% of all adult cancers. Most renal tumors are metastases from primary cancer sites. Renal pelvic tumors and Wilms' tumor occur primarily in children. Kidney tumors are large, firm, nodular, encapsulated, unilateral, and solitary; they're classified histologically as clear cell, granular, or spindle-cell tumors.

Causes

Primary cause unknown

Predisposing Factors

- Tobacco use
- Environmental toxins (cadmium, herbicides, trichloroethylene)
- Analgesic abuse
- Advancing age
- Obesity
- Genetics

AGE ALERT
Renal cancer is more common in men than in women and peaks in incidence between ages 50 and 70. Renal cancer is very uncommon in people under the age of 45.

Pathophysiology

Renal cancers arise from tubular epithelium and can occur anywhere in the kidney. The cells of the kidney change due to a catalyst, such as tobacco smoking or advanced age, resulting in the mutated cell to be cancerous. In the kidneys, the tumor margins are usually clearly defined, and the tumors can include areas of ischemia, necrosis, and focal hemorrhage. Tumor cells vary from well differentiated to very anaplastic. The focus of research is concentrating on understanding the role of specific genes to the change from normal cells to renal cell carcinoma.

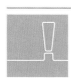

COMPLICATIONS
- Hemorrhage
- Metastases to the lungs, brain, and liver

Signs and Symptoms

Classic Clinical Triad

- Hematuria — microscopic or gross; may be intermittent; suggests spread to renal pelvis
- Pain — constant abdominal or flank pain (may be dull); if cancer causes bleeding or blood clots, acute and colicky
- Palpable mass — generally smooth, firm, and nontender
- All three present in only about 10% of patients

Other Signs

- Fever
- Hypertension
- Rapidly progressing hypercalcemia
- Urine retention and edema in the legs
- Nausea, vomiting, and weight loss

Diagnostic Test Results

- Computed tomography scan, I.V. and retrograde pyelography, ultrasound, cystoscopy (to rule out associated bladder cancer) and nephrotomography, and renal angiography identify the presence of the tumor and help differentiate it from a cyst.
- Liver function tests show increased levels of alkaline phosphatase, bilirubin, alanine aminotransferase, and aspartate aminotransferase.
- Prothrombin time is prolonged.
- Urinalysis reveals gross or microscopic hematuria.
- Complete blood count shows anemia, polycythemia, and increased erythrocyte sedimentation rate.
- Serum calcium levels are elevated.

Treatment

- Partial or radical nephrectomy, with or without regional lymph node dissection
- Thermal ablation for well-defined smaller tumors (requires needle biopsy preprocedure)
- High-dose radiation — used only if the cancer spreads to the perinephric region or the lymph nodes or if the primary tumor or metastatic sites can't be fully excised
- Chemotherapy — results usually poor against kidney cancer
- Biotherapy (interferon and interleukins) — commonly used in advanced disease; has produced few durable remissions
- Hormone therapy
- Pain control (analgesics)

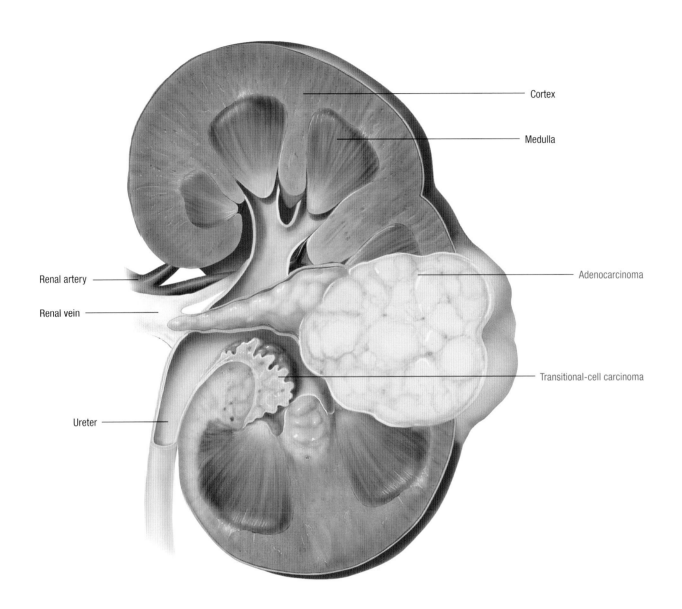

Cortex

Medulla

Adenocarcinoma

Renal artery

Renal vein

Transitional-cell carcinoma

Ureter

Renovascular hypertension is a rise in systemic blood pressure resulting from stenosis of the major renal arteries or their branches or from intrarenal atherosclerosis. Renovascular hypertension is most common type of secondary hypertension. The narrowing or sclerosis may be partial or complete, and the resulting blood pressure elevation may be benign or malignant. Approximately 5% to 10% of patients with high blood pressure display renovascular hypertension.

AGE ALERT

Renovascular hypertension is most common in persons under age 30 or over age 50. In children, if they are diagnosed with hypertension, they are more likely to have renovascular hypertension in young children than systemic hypertension.

Causes

In 95% of All Patients with Renovascular Hypertension

- Atherosclerosis (especially in older men)
- Fibromuscular diseases of the renal artery wall layers, such as medial fibroplasia and, less commonly, intimal or subadventitial fibroplasia or other congenital disorders

Other Causes

- Arteritis
- Anomalies of renal arteries
- Embolism
- Trauma
- Tumor
- Dissecting aneurysm

Pathophysiology

Stenosis or occlusion of the renal artery stimulates the affected kidney to release the enzyme renin, which converts the plasma protein angiotensinogen to angiotensin I. As angiotensin I circulates through the lungs and liver, angiotensin-converting enzyme (ACE) is released. ACE is the catalyst for angiotensin I to form angiotensin II, which causes vasoconstriction, increased arterial pressure, and aldosterone secretion. Angiotensin II's direct ability to cause vasoconstriction causes hypertension. Another function of angiotensin II is the release of aldosterone, which acts on the kidneys to stimulate reabsorption of sodium and water, creating retention of fluids and, subsequently, causing hypertension.

COMPLICATIONS

- Heart failure
- Myocardial infarction
- Stroke
- Renal failure

Signs and Symptoms

- Elevated systemic blood pressure
- Headache and light-headedness
- Palpitations and tachycardia
- Anxiety and mental sluggishness
- Decreased tolerance of temperature extremes
- Retinopathy
- Significant complications: heart failure, myocardial infarction, stroke, and renal failure

Diagnostic Test Results

- Renal scan testing that includes administration of an ACE inhibitor such as captopril, *renal angiography*, and renal ultrasound with Doppler evaluation shows evidence of renal stenosis.
- Excretory urography shows slow uptake in one or both kidneys.
- Complete blood count reveals anemia.
- Blood chemistries show abnormal electrolyte levels and elevated blood urea nitrogen and creatinine.

Treatment

- Symptomatic measures: antihypertensives, diuretics, and sodium-restricted diet
- Balloon catheter renal artery dilation in selected cases to correct renal artery stenosis without risks and morbidity of surgery
- Insertion of renal artery stents
- Surgery to restore adequate circulation and to control severe hypertension or severely impaired renal function:
  - renal artery bypass, endarterectomy, and arterioplasty
  - as a last resort, nephrectomy.

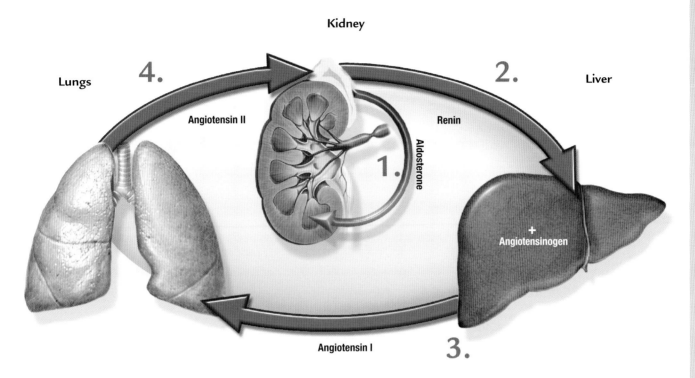

Mechanism of renovascular hypertension

1. Renal artery stenosis causes reduction of blood flow to the kidneys.
2. Kidneys secrete renin in response.
3. Renin combines with angiotensinogen in the liver to form angiotensin I.
4. In the lungs, angiotensin I releases the angiotensin-converting enzyme (ACE).
5. ACE acts on angiotensin I to produce angiotensin II, which is a vasoconstrictor.
6. Angiotension II also acts on the adrenal gland to release aldosterone.
7. Aldosterone acts on the kidneys to reabsorb sodium and water.

Suggested References

Borghi, L., Schianchi, T., Meschi, T., Guerra, A., Allegri, F., Maggiore, U., & Novarini, A. (2002). Comparison of two diets for the prevention of recurrent stones in idiopathic hypercalciuria. *New England Journal of Medicine, 346*(2), 77–84.

Bowen, B. J., & Dronen, S. C. (2016). Emergent management of acute glomerulonephritis. Retrieved from http://emedicine.medscape.com/article/777272

Brusch, J. L., & Bronze, M. S. (2016). Cystitis in females: Practice essentials, background, and pathophysiology. *Medscape.* Retrieved from http://emedicine.medscape.com/article/233101

Gupta, K., Hooton, T. M., Naber, K. G., Wultz, B., Colgan, R., Miller, L. G., … Soper, D. E. (2011). International clinical practice guidelines for the treatment of acute uncomplicated cystitis and pyelonephritis in women: A 2010 update by the Infectious Diseases Society of America and the European Society for Microbiology and Infectious Diseases. *Clinical Infectious Disease, 52*, 103–120.

Hilton, R. (2013). Acute kidney injury (formerly known as acute renal failure). In D. Goldsmith, S. Jayawardene, & P. Ackland (Eds.), *ABC series of ABC of kidney disease.* Hoboken, NJ: Wiley. Retrieved from http://0-literati.credoreference.com.shulsso.sacredheart.edu/content/entry/wileykidney/acute_kidney_injury_formerly_known_as_acute_renal_failure/0

Hogan, J., Mohan, P., & Appel, G. B. (2014). Diagnostic tests and treatment options in glomerular disease. *American Journal of Kidney Disease, 63*(4), 656–666.

Jamison, J., Maguire, S., & McCann, J. (2013). Catheter policies for management of long term voiding problems in adults with neurogenic bladder disorders. *Cochrane Database Systematic Review, 11*, CD004375.

Lamm, D. (2015). Bladder cancer. *BMJ Best Practice.* Retrieved from us.bestpractice.bmj.com

Lerma, E. V. (2016). Acute tubular necrosis. *Medscape.* Retrieved from http://emedicine.medscape.com

Lusaya D. G., & Schwartz, B. F. (2016). Hydronephrosis and hydroureter. *Medscape.* Retrieved from emedicine.medscape.com/article/436259

Ness, B., & Stovall, K. (2016). Current recommendations for treating autosomal dominant polycystic kidney disease. *Journal of the American Academy of Physician Assistants, 29*(12), 24–28. doi:10.1097/01.JAA.00000508201.79685.50

Penniston, K. L., Wertheim, M. L., & Jhagroo, R. A. (2016). Factors associated with patient recall of individualized dietary recommendations for kidney stones prevention. *European Journal of Clinical Nutrition, 70*(9), 1062–1067.

Qaseem, A., Dallas, P., Forciea, M. A., Starkey, M., & Denberg, T. D. (2014). Dietary and pharmacologic management to prevent recurrent nephrolithiasis in adults: A client practice guideline for the American College of Physicians. *Annals of Internal Medicine, 161*(9), 659–667. doi:10-7326/M13-2908

Qaseem, A., Dallas, P., Forciea, M. A., Starkey, M., Denberg, T. D., Shekelle, P.; Clinical Guidelines Committee of the American College of Physicians. (2014). Nonsurgical management of urinary incontinence in women: A clinical practice guideline from the American College of Physicians. *Annals of Internal Medicine, 161*(6), 429–440. doi:10.7326/M13-2410

Schmidt, R. J., & Batuman, V. (2016). Renovascular hypertension. *Medscape.* Retrieved from http://emedicine.medscapte/com/article/245140

Smith, C., & Chancellor, M. B. (2016). Botulinum toxin to treat neurogenic bladder. *Seminars in Neurology, 36*(1), 5–9.

Van De Voorde, R. G. (2015). Acute poststreptococcal glomerulonephritis: The most common acute glomerulonephritis. *Pediatric Review, 36*(1), 3–12.

SKIN DISORDERS

ACNE

Acne is an inflammatory disease of the pilosebaceous units (hair follicles). It occurs on areas of the body that have sebaceous glands, such as the face, neck, chest, back, and shoulders, and is associated with a high rate of sebum secretion. When sebum blocks a hair follicle, one of two types of acne develops. In inflammatory acne, bacterial growth in the blocked follicle leads to inflammation and eventual rupture of the follicle. In noninflammatory acne, the follicle remains dilated by accumulating secretions but does not rupture.

AGE ALERT
Acne occurs in both males and females. Acne vulgaris develops in 80% to 90% of adolescents or young adults, primarily between ages 15 and 18, although the lesions can appear as early as age 8 or into the late 20s.

Causes

- Multifactorial — diet not believed to be a factor

Predisposing Factors

- Heredity
- Androgen stimulation
- Certain drugs, including corticosteroids, corticotropin, androgens, iodides, bromides, trimethadione, phenytoin, isoniazid, lithium, and halothane
- Exposure to heavy oils, greases, tars, and cosmetics
- Cobalt irradiation
- Hyperalimentation
- Trauma, skin occlusion, or pressure
- Emotional stress
- Hormonal contraceptive use (may exacerbate acne in some women)

Pathophysiology

Androgens stimulate sebaceous gland growth, sebum production, and shedding of the epithelial cells that line sebaceous follicles. The stimulated follicles become dilated, and sebum and keratin from the epithelial cells form a plug that seals the follicle, creating a favorable environment for bacterial growth. The bacteria, usually *Propionibacterium acnes* or *Staphylococcus epidermidis*, are normal skin flora that secrete lipase. This enzyme converts sebum to free fatty acids, which provoke inflammation and formation of open or closed comedones that may rupture and cause a foreign body response resulting in the formation of papules, nodules, or pustules. Rupture and inflammation may lead to scarring.

COMPLICATIONS
- Infection
- Gross inflammation
- Abscess
- Scars
- Hyperpigmentation

Signs and Symptoms

- Closed comedo, or whitehead does not protrude from follicle, covered by epidermis
- Open comedo, or blackhead protrudes from the follicle, not covered by epidermis; black color caused by melanin or pigment of the follicle
- Rupture or leakage of comedo into the epidermis:
  - inflammation
  - pustules, papules
  - in severe forms, cysts or abscesses (chronic, recurring lesions producing acne scars)

Diagnostic Test Results

No test for acne vulgaris exists other than visualization of acne lesions to confirm diagnosis.

Treatment

- Gentle cleaning with a sponge to dislodge superficial comedones
- Recommend using the 2016 treatment regimen from American Academy of Dermatology (Zaenglein, A. L., Pathy, A. L., Schlosser, B. J., Alikhan, A., Baldwin, H. E., Berson D. S., … Bhushan, R. (2016). Guidelines of care for the management of acne vulgaris. *American Academy of Dermatology*, 74(5), 945.)

Topical Agents for Mild Acne

- Antibacterial agents, such as benzoyl peroxide gels (2%, 5%, or 10%), clindamycin, or erythromycin

Keratolytic Agents

- Dry and peel the skin to open blocked follicles and release sebum
- Benzoyl peroxide, tretinoin

Systemic Therapy for Moderate to Severe Acne

- Tetracycline or minocycline
- Oral isotretinoin to inhibit sebaceous gland function and abnormal keratinization; has severe adverse effects, which limit its use to patients with severe papulopustular or cystic acne not responding to conventional therapy
- For females, antiandrogens — birth control pills, such as norgestimate and ethinyl estradiol, or spironolactone

For Severe Acne

- For severe scarring — dermabrasion or laser resurfacing to smooth the skin
- Bovine collagen injections into dermis beneath scarred area to fill in pitted areas and smooth skin surface (not recommended by all dermatologists)

HOW ACNE DEVELOPS

Excessive sebum production

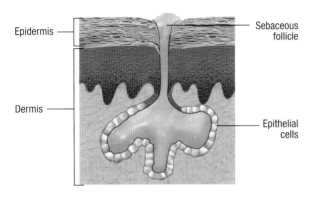

Epidermis

Dermis

Sebaceous follicle

Epithelial cells

Increased shedding of epithelial cells

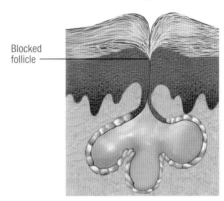

Blocked follicle

Inflammatory response in follicle

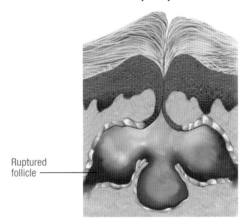

Ruptured follicle

COMEDONES OF ACNE

Closed comedo (whitehead)   ### Open comedo (blackhead)

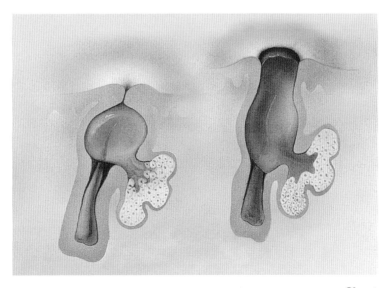

ATOPIC DERMATITIS

Atopic dermatitis (also called *atopic* or *infantile eczema*) is a chronic or recurrent inflammatory skin disease. It is commonly associated with other atopic diseases, such as bronchial asthma and allergic rhinitis. Atopic dermatitis is genetically transmitted.

AGE ALERT
Atopic dermatitis commonly develops in infants and toddlers between ages 1 month and 1 year, usually in those with a strong family history of atopic disease. These children can develop atopic dermatitis in infancy, then subsequent allergic rhinitis and asthma in later childhood is known as the atopic march.

Typically, atopic dermatitis flares and subsides repeatedly before finally resolving during adolescence, but it can persist into adulthood.

Causes

The exact etiology is unknown. A genetic predisposition is likely, with a complex relationship between genetic and environmental factors.

Possible Contributing Factors

- Studies are showing that second hand tobacco smoke exposure is a contributing factor
- Food allergy, especially eggs, peanuts, milk, or wheat
- Infection
- Chemical irritants
- Extremes of temperature and humidity
- Psychological stress or strong emotions

Pathophysiology

The allergic mechanism of hypersensitivity results in a release of inflammatory mediators through sensitized antibodies of the immunoglobulin IgE class. Histamine and other cytokines induce acute inflammation. Abnormally dry skin and a decreased threshold for itching set up the "itch-scratch-itch" cycle, which eventually causes lesions (excoriations, lichenification).

COMPLICATIONS
- Sleep difficulties
- Secondary infection
- Scars

Signs and Symptoms

- Erythematous areas on excessively dry skin; in children, typically on the forehead, cheeks, and extensor surfaces of the arms and legs; in adults, at flexion points (antecubital fossa, popliteal area, and neck), infants spares the diaper area (this is important to note as some parents confuse eczema and diaper rash)
- Edema, crusting, scaling caused by pruritus and scratching
- Multiple areas of dry, scaly skin, with white dermatographism, blanching, and lichenification with chronic atrophic lesions
- Infantile form presents as red skin with tiny vesicles, especially on the face (sparing the mouth); possible development of wet crusts and fissures
- In blacks, follicular eczema common, appearing as discrete follicular papules involving hair follicles in the affected area
- Pinkish, swollen upper eyelid and double fold under lower lid
- Viral, fungal, or bacterial infections and ocular disorders possible secondary conditions

Diagnostic Test Results

Blood tests reveal eosinophilia and elevated IgE levels.

Treatment

- Important to control the itch to promote healing and prevent infection
- Eliminating allergens and avoiding irritants (strong soaps, cleansers, and other chemicals), extreme temperature changes, and other precipitating factors
- Preventing excessive dryness of the skin (critical to successful therapy) by maintaining adequate fluid intake, taking tepid baths, and humidifying air recommend including bleach baths recommend including soak and seal therapy (wet wraps)
- Topical tar preparations in a lubricating base (contraindicated for intensely inflamed or open lesions)
- Topical corticosteroid ointment, hydrocortisone 1% especially after bathing, to alleviate inflammation; moisturizing cream between steroid doses to help retain moisture
- Topical doxepin hydrochloride
- Topical immunomodulators, such as tacrolimus and pimecrolimus
- Systemic antihistamines such as diphenhydramine
- Systemic corticosteroid therapy for severe disease only
- Ultraviolet B or psoralens plus ultraviolet A therapy
- In severe adult-onset disease, cyclosporine A, if other treatments fail
- Antibiotics, if skin culture positive for bacteria

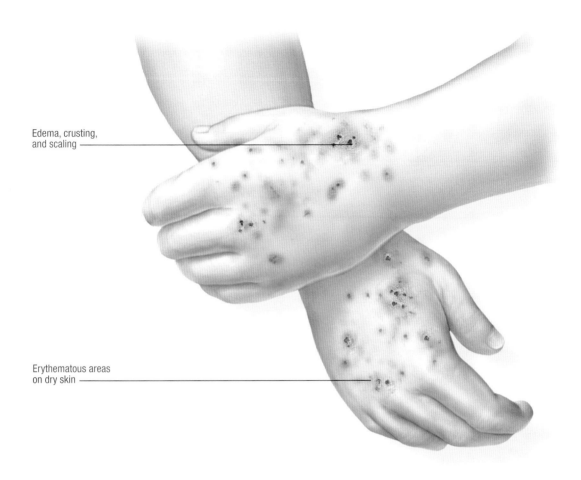

Edema, crusting, and scaling

Erythematous areas on dry skin

CLINICAL TIP
MORGAN'S LINE

In children with atopic dermatitis, severe pruritus with recurrent rubbing leads to characteristic pink pigmentation and swelling of the upper eyelid and a double fold under the lower lid (Morgan's line, Dennie's sign, or mongolian fold).

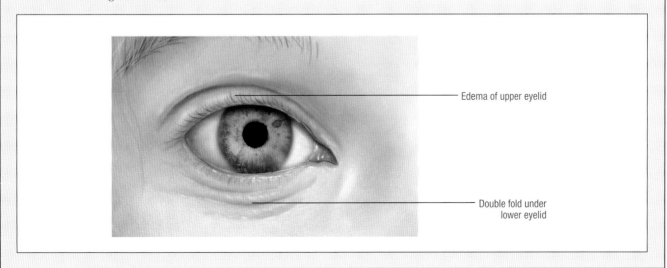

Edema of upper eyelid

Double fold under lower eyelid

BURNS

Burns are the third leading cause of accidental death in the United States.

Causes

- Thermal: residential fires, automobile accidents, playing with matches, improper handling of firecrackers, scalds caused by kitchen, or bathroom accidents
- Chemical: contact, ingestion, inhalation, or injection of acids, alkalis, or vesicants
- Electrical: contact with faulty electrical wiring, electrical cords, or high-voltage power lines
- Friction or abrasion
- Ultraviolet radiation: sunburn

Pathophysiology

The injuring agent denatures all cellular proteins. Some cells die because of traumatic or ischemic necrosis. Denaturation disrupts collagen cross-links in connective tissue. The consequent abnormal osmotic and hydrostatic pressure gradients force intravascular fluid into interstitial spaces. Cellular injury triggers the release of mediators of inflammation, further contributing to local or systemic increases in capillary permeability.

Burns are classified according to their depth and size.

First-degree burns. Localized injury to or destruction of epidermis by direct or indirect contact. The barrier function of the skin remains intact.

Second-degree superficial partial-thickness burns. Destruction of epidermis and some of the upper area of the dermis. The barrier function of the skin is lost.

Second-degree deep partial-thickness burns. Destruction of epidermis and more of the dermis.

Third- and fourth-degree burns. Affect every body system and organ. A third-degree burn extends through the epidermis and dermis and into the subcutaneous tissue layer; a fourth-degree burn damages muscle, bone, and interstitial tissues. Within hours, fluids and protein shift from capillary to interstitial spaces, causing edema.

COMPLICATIONS
- Sepsis
- Respiratory complications
- Hypovolemic shock and multisystem organ dysfunction
- Anemia
- Malnutrition
- Infection
- Deep burns can cause bone and joint limitations

Signs and Symptoms

- First-degree burn: localized pain and erythema, usually without blisters in the first 24 hours
- More severe first-degree burn: chills, headache, localized edema, nausea, and vomiting
- Second-degree superficial partial-thickness burn: thin-walled, fluid-filled blisters that appear within minutes of injury; mild to moderate edema; pain
- Second-degree deep partial-thickness burn: white, waxy appearance of damaged area, edema, and pain (or may be nonpainful)
- Third- and fourth-degree burns: white, brown, or black leathery tissue; visible thrombosed vessels; no blisters
- Electrical burn: silver-colored, raised area, usually at the site of electrical contact (damage to underlying tissue can occur even with intact epidermis)
- Smoke inhalation and pulmonary damage: singed nasal hairs, mucosal burns, voice changes, coughing, wheezing, soot in mouth or nose, darkened sputum

Total burn surface area (BSA) may be estimated quickly using the Rule of Nines, in which an adult patient's body parts are assigned percentages based on the number 9. The Lund-Browder classification reference allows more precise assessment by assigning specific percentages to an infant or child's body parts and accounts for burn thickness and age differences.

Minor Burns

- Third-degree burns on less than 2% of BSA
- Second-degree burns on less than 15% of adult BSA (less than 10% in children)
- All first-degree burns

Moderate Burns

- Third-degree burns on 2% to 10% of BSA
- Second-degree burns on 15% to 25% of adult BSA (10% to 20% in children)

Major Burns

- Third-degree burns on more than 10% of BSA
- Second-degree burns on more than 25% of adult BSA (more than 20% in children)
- Burns of hands, face, feet, or genitalia
- Burns complicated by fractures or respiratory damage
- Electrical burns and burns in poor-risk patients

Diagnostic Test Results

- Arterial blood gas levels show evidence of smoke inhalation; they may also show decreased alveolar function and hypoxia.
- Complete blood count reveals decreased hemoglobin level and hematocrit if blood loss occurs.
- Blood chemistries show abnormal electrolytes from fluid loss and shifts, increased blood urea nitrogen with fluid loss, and decreased glucose in children due to limited glycogen storage.
- Urinalysis shows myoglobinuria and hemoglobinuria.
- Other blood tests detect increased carboxyhemoglobin.
- Electrocardiogram shows ischemia, injury, or arrhythmias, especially in electrical burns.
- Fiber-optic bronchoscopy reveals edema of the airways.

Treatment

- Minor burns: immersion of burned area in cool water (55°F [12.8°C]) or application of cool compresses
- Immediate treatment for moderate and major burns: maintain an open airway, endotracheal intubation, 100% oxygen

- Immediate I.V. therapy to prevent hypovolemic shock and maintain cardiac output (lactated Ringer's solution or a fluid replacement formula; additional I.V. lines may be needed)
- Partial-thickness burns over 30% of BSA or full-thickness burns over 5% of BSA: cover patient with a clean, dry, sterile bed sheet to help preserve body temperature; don't cover large burns with saline-soaked dressings

- Debridement followed by application of antimicrobial and nonstick bulky dressing; tetanus prophylaxis if needed
- Fragments of necrotic blisters may increase the risk of infection and limit the contact of topical antimicrobial agents to the burn wound
- Pain or anti-inflammatory medication as needed
- Major burns: systemic antimicrobial therapy

CLASSIFICATION OF BURNS BY DEPTH OF INJURY

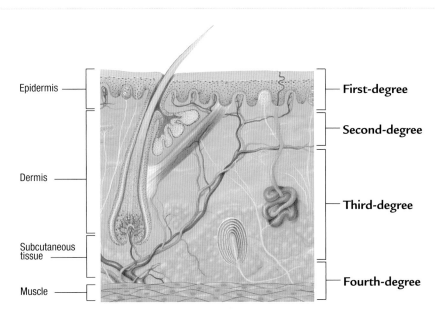

CLINICAL TIP

ESTIMATING THE EXTENT OF BURNS

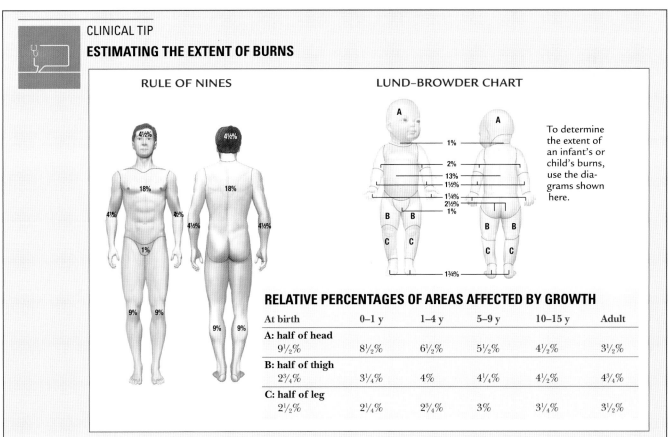

RELATIVE PERCENTAGES OF AREAS AFFECTED BY GROWTH

	At birth	0–1 y	1–4 y	5–9 y	10–15 y	Adult
A: half of head	$9\frac{1}{2}\%$	$8\frac{1}{2}\%$	$6\frac{1}{2}\%$	$5\frac{1}{2}\%$	$4\frac{1}{2}\%$	$3\frac{1}{2}\%$
B: half of thigh	$2\frac{3}{4}\%$	$3\frac{1}{4}\%$	4%	$4\frac{1}{4}\%$	$4\frac{1}{2}\%$	$4\frac{3}{4}\%$
C: half of leg	$2\frac{1}{2}\%$	$2\frac{1}{4}\%$	$2\frac{3}{4}\%$	3%	$3\frac{1}{4}\%$	$3\frac{1}{2}\%$

CELLULITIS

Cellulitis is an acute, spreading infection of the dermis or subcutaneous layer of the skin. It may follow damage to the skin, such as a bite or wound. As the cellulitis spreads, fever, erythema, and lymphangitis may occur. Persons with a chronic illness, such as diabetes mellitus immunodeficiency, or Peripheral artery disease contributing health problems, such as diabetes, immunodeficiency, or impaired circulation, have an increased risk for cellulitis. If treated promptly, the prognosis is usually good.

AGE ALERT
Cellulitis of the lower extremity is more likely to develop into thrombophlebitis in an elderly patient. Orbital cellulitis, especially in children, may require hospitalization and I.V. antibiotics because of the increased risk of spread to intracranial structures, such as in thin bones and numerous openings in the bone.

Causes

- Bacterial infections, commonly with group A beta-hemolytic streptococcus or *Staphylococcus aureus*
- In patients with diabetes or decreased immune function: *Escherichia coli*, *Proteus mirabilis*, *Acinetobacter*, *Enterobacter*, *Pseudomonas aeruginosa*, *Pasteurella multocida*, *Vibrio vulnificus*, *Mycobacterium fortuitum complex*, and *Cryptococcus neoformans*
- In children, less commonly caused by pneumococci and *Neisseria meningitidis* group B (periorbital)

Pathophysiology

After the organisms enter the tissue spaces and planes of cleavage, hyaluronidases break down the ground substances composed of polysaccharides, while fibrinolysins digest fibrin barriers and lecithinases destroy cell membranes. This overwhelms the normal cells of defense (neutrophils, eosinophils, basophils, and mast cells) that normally contain and localize inflammation, and cellular debris accumulates.

COMPLICATIONS
- Bacteremia
- Necrotizing fasciitis
- Lymphangitis
- Meningitis (in facial cellulitis)

Signs and Symptoms

- Classic signs: erythema and edema due to inflammatory response, usually well-demarcated
- Pain at site and possibly in surrounding area
- Fever and warmth
- Regional lymphadenopathy or lymphangitis

Diagnostic Test Results

- The diagnosis of cellulitis is based upon clinical manifestations. White blood cell count shows mild leukocytosis with a shift to the left.
- Erythrocyte sedimentation rate is mildly elevated.
- Culture and gram stain results of fluid from abscesses and bulla are positive for the offending organism.
- Using the "Touch" preparation, potassium hydroxide is applied to a microscope slide containing a skin lesion specimen that detects the presence of yeast or mycelial forms of fungus.

Treatment

- Oral or I.V. penicillinase-resistant penicillin (drug of choice for initial treatment) unless the patient has known penicillin allergy; antifungal medications if needed
- Antibiotic selection for treatment depends on the clinical presentation of purulent or nonpurulent cellulitis.
- Alternative antibiotics based on culture and sensitivity results
- Warm soaks to the site to help relieve pain and decrease edema by increasing vasodilation
- Pain medication as needed
- Elevation of infected extremity
- Surgical drainage or debridement for abscess formation

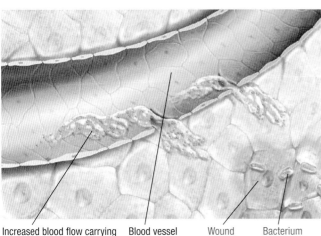

Increased blood flow carrying plasma proteins and fluid to injured tissue

Blood vessel

Wound

Bacterium

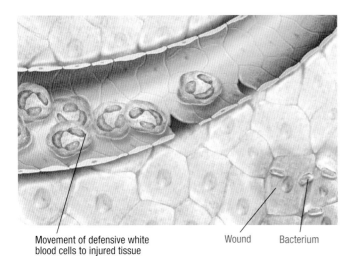

Movement of defensive white blood cells to injured tissue

Wound

Bacterium

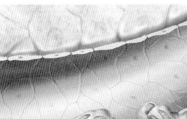

Phagocyte engulfing bacterium

Wound

CLINICAL TIP

RECOGNIZING CELLULITIS

The classic signs of cellulitis, a spreading soft tissue infection, are erythema and edema surrounding the initial wound. The tissue is warm to the touch.

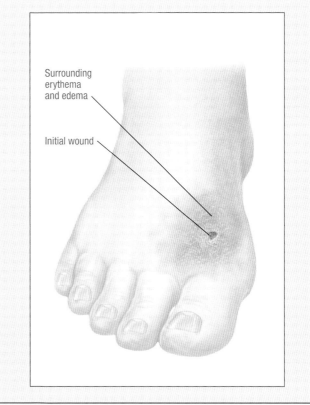

Surrounding erythema and edema

Initial wound

CONTACT DERMATITIS

Contact dermatitis commonly appears as a sharply demarcated inflammation of the skin that results from contact with an irritating chemical or atopic allergen (a substance that produces an allergic reaction in the skin). It can also appear as an irritation of the skin that results from contact with concentrated substances to which the skin is sensitized, such as perfumes, soaps, chemicals, or metals and alloys (such as nickel used in jewelry). Localized inflammatory skin resulting from exposure of a wide range of chemical or physical agents.

Causes

Mild Irritants

- Chronic exposure to detergents or solvents

Strong Irritants

- Damage on contact with acids or alkalis

Allergens

- Sensitization after repeated exposure

Pathophysiology

Irritant contact dermatitis is not immune mediated. The allergic mechanism of hypersensitivity results in a release of inflammatory mediators through sensitized antibodies of immunoglobulin E. Histamine and other cytokines induce an inflammatory response, resulting in edema, skin breakdown, and pruritus.

COMPLICATIONS
- Altered pigmentation
- Lichenification
- Scarring

Signs and Symptoms

Mild Irritants and Allergens

- Erythema
- Small vesicles that ooze, scale, and itch

Strong Irritants

- Blisters
- Ulcerations

Classic Allergic Response

- Clearly defined lesions with straight lines following points of contact

Severe Allergic Reaction

- Marked erythema
- Blistering
- Edema of the affected site

Diagnostic Test Results

- Patch test identifies allergens.

Treatment

- Eliminating known allergens
- Decreasing exposure to irritants
- Wearing protective clothing, such as gloves
- Washing immediately after contact with irritants or allergens
- Topical anti-inflammatory (including a corticosteroid)
- Systemic corticosteroids for edema and bullae
- Antihistamine
- Local application of Burrow's solution (for blisters)

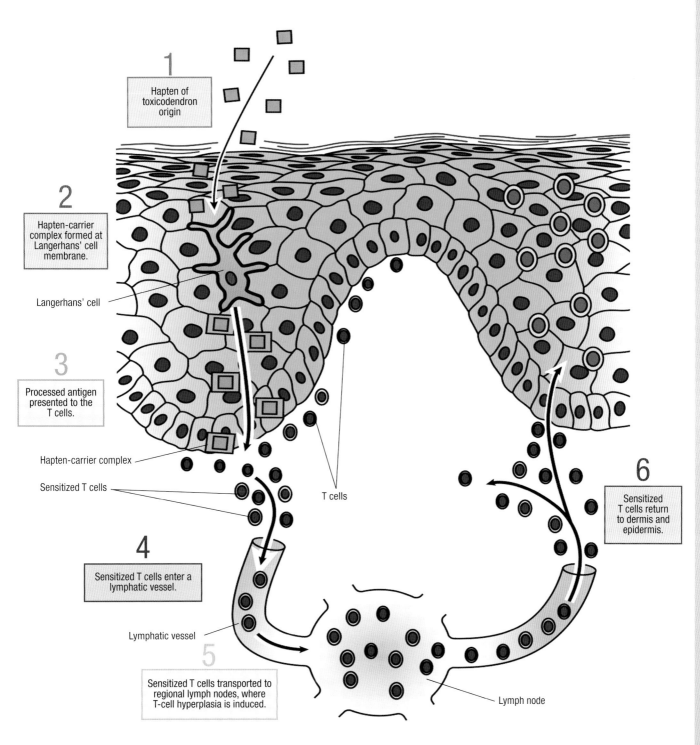

1

Hapten of toxicodendron origin

2

Hapten-carrier complex formed at Langerhans' cell membrane.

Langerhans' cell

3

Processed antigen presented to the T cells.

Hapten-carrier complex

Sensitized T cells

T cells

4

Sensitized T cells enter a lymphatic vessel.

Lymphatic vessel

5

Sensitized T cells transported to regional lymph nodes, where T-cell hyperplasia is induced.

Lymph node

6

Sensitized T cells return to dermis and epidermis.

FOLLICULITIS, FURUNCLES, CARBUNCLES

Folliculitis is a bacterial infection in the upper portion of a hair follicle that causes a papule, pustule, or erosion. The infection can be superficial (follicular impetigo or Bockhart's impetigo) or deep (sycosis barbae). Furuncles, also known as *boils*, affect the entire hair follicle and the adjacent subcutaneous tissue. Carbuncles are a group of interconnected furuncles.

With appropriate treatment, the prognosis for patients with folliculitis is good. The disorder usually resolves within 2 to 3 weeks. The prognosis for patients with carbuncles depends on the severity of the infection and the patient's physical condition and ability to resist infection.

Causes

- Coagulase-positive *S. aureus* (most common) *S. aureus* is the most common cause of bacterial folliculitis
- *Klebsiella*, *Enterobacter*, or *Proteus* organisms (gram-negative folliculitis in patients on long-term antibiotic therapy such as for acne)
- *P. aeruginosa* (thrives in warm environment with high pH and low chlorine content: "hot-tub folliculitis")

Predisposing Risk Factors

- Shaving, plucking, or waxing
- Infected wound, poor hygiene
- Chronic staphylococcus carrier state in nares, axillae, perineum, or bowel
- Diabetes
- Debilitation
- Immunosuppressive therapy, defects in chemotaxis, hyper-immunoglobulinemia E syndrome
- Tight clothes, friction
- Living in a tropical climate

Pathophysiology

The affecting organism enters the body, usually at a break in the skin barrier, such as a wound site. The organism then causes an inflammatory reaction within the hair follicle.

Staphylococcal infection commonly causes the abscess, which consists of a fibrin wall with surrounding inflamed tissues. This encloses a core of pus containing organisms and leukocytes.

Hematologic spread of infection is possible even from the smallest abscess and is enhanced by proteolytic enzymes produced by the staphylococcal organisms.

COMPLICATIONS
- Sepsis
- Cellulitis
- Scarring
- Pneumonia
- Endocarditis
- Infection of bones and joints

Signs and Symptoms

Folliculitis

- In children — papule or pustules on scalp, arms, or legs
- In adults — papule or pustules on trunk, buttocks, legs, or face

Furuncles

- Firm or fluctuant, painful nodules, commonly on neck, face, axillae, or buttocks
- Nodules enlarge for several days, then rupture, discharging pus and necrotic material
- After rupture, pain subsides (erythema and edema persist for days or weeks)

Carbuncles

- Extremely painful, deep abscesses draining through multiple openings onto the skin surface, around several hair follicles
- Fever and malaise

Diagnostic Test Results

- Wound culture and sensitivity test results show the offending organism.
- Blood chemistry reveals elevated white blood cell count.

Bacterial folliculitis is usually diagnosed by patient history and physical examination.

Treatment

- Thorough cleaning of the infected area with antibacterial soap and water several times per day
- Warm, wet compresses to promote vasodilation and drainage
- Topical antibiotics, such as mupirocin ointment or clindamycin or erythromycin solution

Specific Treatments

- Extensive folliculitis: systemic antibiotics, such as a cephalosporin or dicloxacillin
- Furuncles (ripe lesions):
  - warm, wet compresses
  - incision and drainage
  - systemic antibiotic therapy
- Carbuncles:
  - incision and drainage
  - systemic antibiotic therapy

DISTINGUISHING FOLLICULITIS, FURUNCLES, AND CARBUNCLES

Superficial folliculitis
- Erythema
- Pustule
- Single-follicle involvement

Deep folliculitis
- Extensive follicular involvement

Furuncle
- Red, tender nodule surrounding a follicle
- Single draining point

Carbuncle
- Deep follicular abscesses of several follicles
- Several draining points

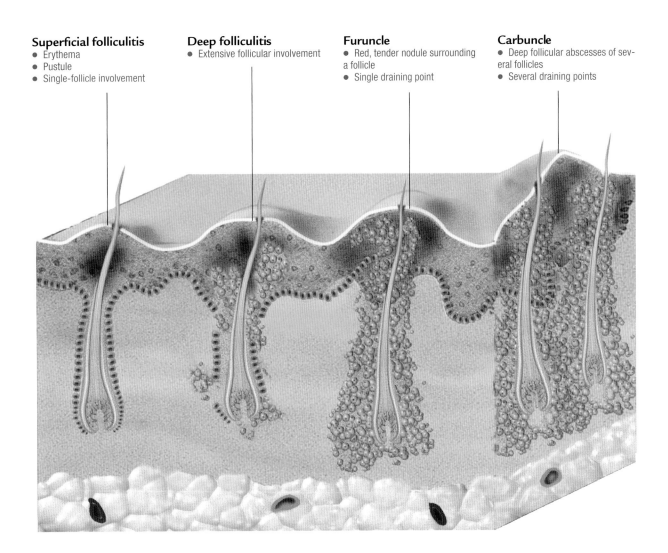

FUNGAL INFECTIONS

Fungal infections of the skin are often regarded as superficial infections affecting the hair, nails, and stratum corneum; the outermost layer of the epidermis consisting of the corneocytes or dead cells (the dead top layer of the skin). Fungi infect and survive only on the nonviable keratin within these structures. The most common fungal infections are dermatophyte infections (tineas) and candidiasis (moniliasis).

Tinea infections are classified by the body location in which they occur — for example:

- *capitis*, scalp
- *corporis*, body
- *pedis*, foot
- *cruris*, groin.

Some forms infect one gender more commonly than the other. For example, tinea cruris is more common in males. Obesity and diabetes predispose to tinea and candida infection.

AGE ALERT
Children develop tinea scalp infections, young adults more commonly develop infection in the intertriginous areas, and older adults develop onychomycosis.

Candidiasis of the skin or mucous membranes is also classified according to the infected site or area:

- intertrigo — axilla or inner aspect of thigh
- balanoposthitis — glans penis and prepuce
- vulvitis
- diaper dermatitis
- paronychia — folds of skin at the margin of a nail
- onychia — nail bed
- thrush — mouth.

Candida organisms may be normal flora of the skin, mouth, GI tract, or genitalia.

Causes

Tinea Infection

- *Microsporum*, *Trichophyton*, or *Epidermophyton* organisms
- Contact with contaminated objects or surfaces

Risk Factors for Tinea Infection

- Obesity
- Atopy, immunosuppression
- Antibiotic therapy with suppression of normal flora
- Softened skin from prolonged water contact, such as with water sports or diaphoresis

Candidiasis

- Overgrowth of *Candida* organisms and infection due to depletion of the normal flora (such as with antibiotic therapy)
- Neutropenia and bone marrow suppression in immunocompromised patients (at greater risk for the disseminating form)
- *Candida albicans*, normal GI flora (causes candidiasis in susceptible patients)
- *Candida* overgrowth in the mouth (thrush)

Pathophysiology

Dermatophytes, which grow only on or within keratinized structures, make keratinases that digest keratin and maintain the existence of fungi in keratinized tissue. The pathogenicity of dermatophytes is restricted by the cell-mediated immunity and antimicrobial activity of the polymorphonuclear leukocytes. Clinical presentation depends on fungal species, site of infection, and host susceptibility and immune response.

In candidiasis, the organism penetrates the epidermis after binding to integrin receptors and adhesion molecules and then secretes proteolytic enzymes, which facilitate tissue invasion. An inflammatory response results from the attraction of neutrophils to the area and from activation of the complement cascade.

COMPLICATIONS
Tinea Infection

- Hair or nail loss
- Secondary bacterial or candidal infection

Candidiasis

- *Candida* dissemination
- Organ failure: kidneys, brain, GI tract, eyes, lungs, heart

Signs and Symptoms

Tinea Infection

- Erythema, scaling, pustules, vesicles, bullae, maceration
- Itching, stinging, burning
- Circular lesions with erythema and a collarette of scale (central clearing)

Candidiasis

- Superficial papules and pustules; later, erosions
- Erythema and edema of epidermis or mucous membrane
- As inflammation progresses, a white-yellow, curdlike material over the infected area
- In thrush — white coating of tongue, buccal mucosa, and lips, which can be wiped off to reveal a red base
- Severe pruritus and pain at the lesion sites (common)

Diagnostic Test Results

- Microscopic examination of a potassium hydroxide–treated skin scraping reveals the offending organism.
- Culture determines the causative organism and suggests the mode of transmission.
- Wood's lamp examination in a darkened room demonstrates fluorescence.

Treatment

Tinea Infection

Tinea Pedis usually responds to topical antifungal agents such as ketoconazole, terbinafine, econazole, or ciclopirox creams.

- Topical fungicidal agents, such as imidazole or an allylamine product

- If no response to topical treatment — oral agents, such as allylamines or azoles

Candidiasis

- Intertrigo, balanitis, vulvitis, diaper dermatitis, paronychia — nystatin or imidazoles

- Oral candidiasis (thrush) — azoles, imidazoles
- Systemic infections — I.V. amphotericin B or oral ketoconazole

SKIN SCRAPINGS FROM FUNGAL SKIN INFECTION

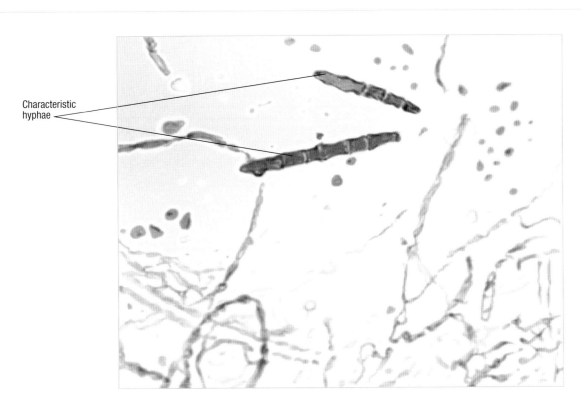

Characteristic hyphae

FUNGAL INFECTION OF NAIL

Onycholysis

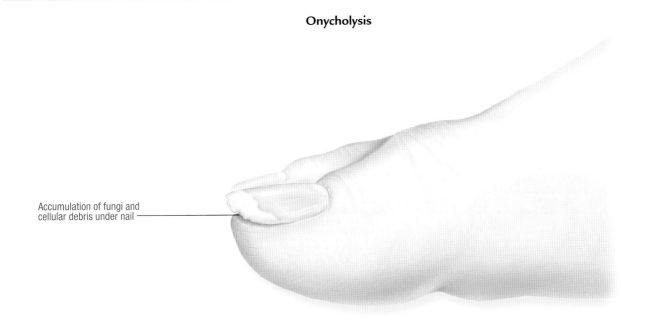

Accumulation of fungi and cellular debris under nail

LYME DISEASE

A multisystemic disorder, Lyme disease, is caused by the spirochete *Borrelia burgdorferi*, which is carried by the minute tick *Ixodes dammini* (also known as *Ixodes scapularis*) or another tick in the Ixodidae family. It commonly begins in the summer months with a papule that becomes red and warm but isn't painful. This classic skin lesion is called erythema migrans. Weeks or months later, cardiac or neurologic abnormalities sometimes develop, possibly followed by arthritis of the large joints.

Causes

B. burgdorferi is transmitted to humans through the bite of infected blacklegged ticks.

Pathophysiology

Lyme disease begins when a tick injects spirochete-laden saliva into the bloodstream or deposits fecal matter on the skin. After incubating for 3 to 32 days, the spirochetes migrate out to the skin, causing erythema migrans. Then they disseminate to other skin sites or organs by the bloodstream or lymph system. The spirochetes' life cycle isn't completely clear. They may survive for years in the joints, or they may trigger an inflammatory response in the host and then die.

COMPLICATIONS
- Myocarditis
- Pericarditis
- Arrhythmias
- Heart block
- Meningitis
- Encephalitis
- Cranial or peripheral neuropathies
- Arthritis
- Memory loss
- Difficulty concentrating

Signs and Symptoms

Prodrome

- Malaise
- Fatigue
- Headache
- Fever
- Lethargy
- Chills
- Arthralgia
- Myalgia
- Anorexia
- Sore throat
- Nausea
- Vomiting
- Abdominal pain
- Photophobia

Stage I

- Initial red macule or papule that enlarges within days, forming an expanding annular lesion with a well-defined red border and central clearing (erythema migrans) with an average maximum diameter of 15 to 20 cm; center of lesion may become vesicular, indurated, or necrotic, or concentric rings may occur (when occurring on the face, neck, or scalp, only a linear streak may be noted)
- Multiple tick bites producing multiple erythema migrans lesions
- Erythema migrans lesions most commonly occurring in the proximal extremities, especially the axillae and groin
- As erythema migrans lesion evolves, possible development of postinflammatory erythema or hyperpigmentation, alopecia, or desquamation
- Additionally, a malar rash, diffuse urticaria, or subcutaneous nodules possible

Stage II

- Low-grade fever in adults, high persistent fever in children; adenopathy
- Neurologic involvement occurs in up to 20% of untreated cases — meningitis, encephalitic signs (poor concentration, memory, and sleep, or irritability), cranial neuritis, radiculoneuropathy, and myelitis
- Cardiac involvement in up to 10% of untreated cases — atrioventricular block, myopericarditis, left ventricular dysfunction
- Migratory pain in joints, bursae, tendons, bones, or muscles

Stage III

- Fever and adenopathy
- Arthritis
- Chronic neurologic involvement

Diagnostic Test Results

- Assays for anti–*B. burgdorferi* show evidence of previous or current infection.
- Enzyme-linked immunosorbent technology or indirect immunofluorescence microscopy shows immunoglobulin (Ig) M levels that peak 3 to 6 weeks after infection; IgG antibodies detected several weeks after infection may continue to develop for several months and generally persist for years.
- Positive Western blot assay shows serologic evidence of past or current infection with *B. burgdorferi*.
- Lumbar puncture with analysis of cerebrospinal fluid reveals antibodies to *B. burgdorferi*.

Treatment

- Antibiotics, such as doxycycline, tetracycline, cefuroxime, ceftriaxone, and penicillin
- Anti-inflammatory medications such as ibuprofen

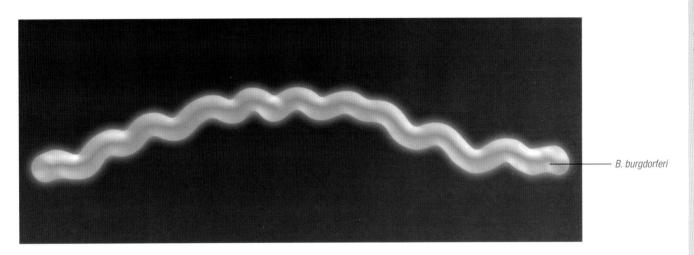

B. burgdorferi

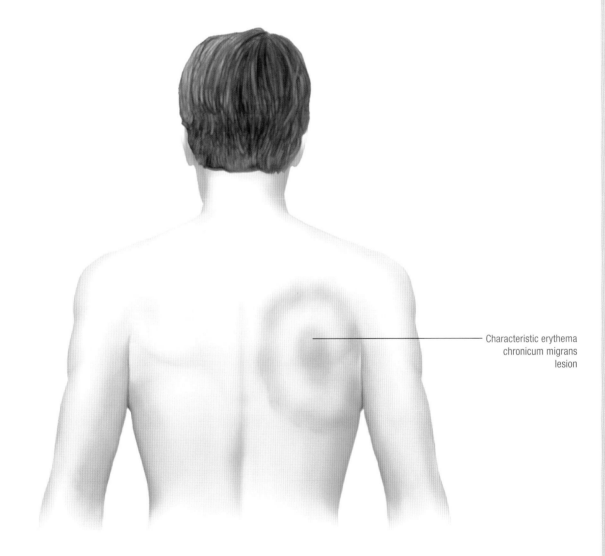

Characteristic erythema
chronicum migrans
lesion

PRESSURE ULCERS

Pressure ulcers are localized areas of cellular necrosis that occur most commonly in the skin and subcutaneous tissue over bony prominences. These ulcers may be superficial, caused by local skin irritation with subsequent surface maceration, or deep, originating in underlying tissue. Deep lesions commonly go undetected until they penetrate the skin; by then, they have usually caused subcutaneous damage.

Five body locations together account for 95% of all pressure ulcer sites: sacral area, greater trochanter, ischial tuberosity, heel, and lateral malleolus. Patients who have contractures are at an increased risk for developing pressure ulcers because the abnormal position adds pressure on the tissue and the alignment of the bones.

AGE ALERT
Age also has a role in the incidence of pressure ulcers. Muscle and subcutaneous tissue is lost with aging, and skin elasticity decreases. Both factors increase the risk of developing pressure ulcers.

A *stage I* pressure ulcer is characterized by intact skin with nonblanchable redness of a localized area, usually over a bony prominence. In darker skin, the ulcer may appear with persistent red, blue, or purple hues.

A *suspected deep tissue injury* is characterized by a purple or maroon localized intact area or blood-filled blister caused by damage to underlying soft tissue from pressure or shear. Preceding the injury, the tissue may be painful, firm, mushy, boggy, or warm or cool compared to adjacent tissue. It may be hard to detect in dark-skinned patients.

A *stage II* pressure ulcer is characterized by partial-thickness skin loss involving the dermis. The ulcer is shallow and has a red-pink wound bed without slough. It may also appear as an intact or open serum-filled blister.

A *stage III* pressure ulcer is characterized by full-thickness skin loss involving damage or necrosis of subcutaneous tissue, which may extend down to, but not through, the underlying fascia. The ulcer appears as a deep crater with or without undermining of adjacent tissue.

Stage IV is characterized by full-thickness skin and tissue loss with exposed or directly palpable fascia, muscle, tendon, ligament, cartilage, or bone in the ulcer.

Full-thickness skin loss with extensive destruction, tissue necrosis, or damage to muscle, bone, or support structures (tendon or joint capsule) characterizes a *stage IV* pressure ulcer. Tunneling and sinus tracts may also occur.

An *unstageable* ulcer is characterized by full-thickness tissue loss in which the base of the ulcer in the wound bed is covered by slough (yellow, tan, gray, green, or brown) or eschar (tan, brown, or black), or both. Until enough slough is removed to expose the base of the wound, the true depth and staging cannot be determined — and therefore, stage — can't be determined.

Causes

- Immobility and decreased level of activity
- Friction and shear, causing damage to the epidermal and upper dermal skin layers

- Tissue maceration
- Skin breakdown

Contributing Conditions

- Malnutrition, hypoalbuminemia
- Medical conditions such as diabetes; orthopedic injuries
- Depression, chronic emotional stress

Pathophysiology

A pressure ulcer is caused by an injury to the skin and its underlying tissues. The pressure exerted on the area restricts blood flow to the site and causes ischemia and hypoxemia. As the capillaries collapse, thrombosis occurs and leads to tissue edema and necrosis. Ischemia also contributes to an accumulation of toxins. The toxins further break down the tissue and also contribute to tissue necrosis.

COMPLICATIONS
- Bacteremia and septicemia
- Necrotizing fasciitis
- Osteomyelitis

Signs and Symptoms

- First clinical sign: blanching erythema, varying from pink to bright red depending on the patient's skin color; in dark skin, purple discoloration or a darkening of normal skin color
- Pain at the site and surrounding area
- Localized edema and increased body temperature due to initial inflammatory response; in more severe cases, cool skin due to severe damage or necrosis
- In more severe cases with deeper dermal involvement: non-blanching erythema, ranging from dark red to cyanotic
- As ulcer progresses: skin deterioration, blisters, crusts, or scaling
- Deep ulcer originating at or extending to the bony prominence below the skin surface: usually dusky red, possibly mottled appearance, doesn't bleed easily, warm to the touch

Diagnostic Test Results

- Wound culture and sensitivity tests detect infectious organisms.
- Blood testing reveals elevated white blood cells, elevated erythrocyte sedimentation rate, and hypoproteinemia.

Treatment

Wound management includes debridement of necrotic tissue, and appropriate dressings or wound packing to promote healing of the wound bed, and wound coverage as appropriate. Treatment is based on the stage and may include the following:

- For immobile patients, repositioning at least every 2 hours with support of pillows; for those able to move, a pillow and encouragement to change position
- Foam, gel, or air mattress to aid in healing by reducing pressure on the ulcer site and reducing the risk of more ulcers

- Nutritional supplements, such as vitamin C and zinc, for the malnourished patient; adequate protein intake
- Adequate fluid intake to prevent dehydration
- Meticulous skin care and hygiene practices, particularly for incontinent patients

- Transparent film, polyurethane foam, or hydrocolloid dressing
- Wound loosely filled with saline- or gel-moistened gauze; exudate managed with absorbent dressing (moist gauze or foam); covered with secondary dressing
- Surgical debridement

STAGING PRESSURE ULCERS

Stage I

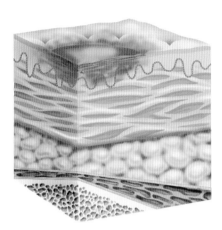

Suspected deep tissue injury

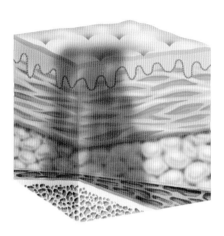

Stage II

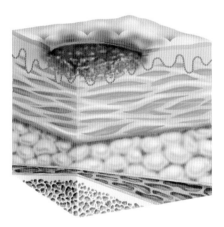

Stage III

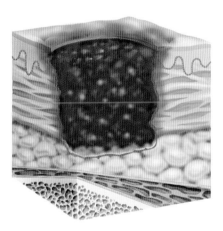

Stage IV

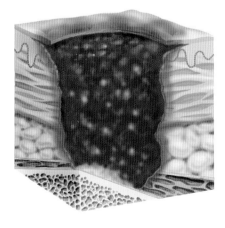

Unstageable

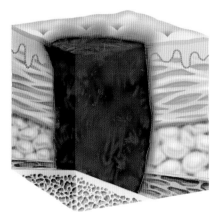

PSORIASIS

Psoriasis is a chronic, recurrent disease marked by epidermal proliferation and characterized by remissions and exacerbations. Flare-ups are commonly related to specific systemic and environmental factors but may be unpredictable. Widespread involvement is called *exfoliative* or *erythrodermic psoriasis*. The most common presentation of psoriasis is chronic plaque psoriasis.

Although this disorder commonly affects young adults, it may strike at any age, including infancy. Genetic factors predetermine the incidence of psoriasis; affected families have a significantly greater incidence of human leukocyte antigens (HLA) B13, B17, and CW6.

Flare-ups can usually be controlled with therapy. Appropriate treatment depends on the type of psoriasis, the extent of the disease, the patient's response, and the effect of the disease on the patient's lifestyle. No permanent cure exists, and all methods of treatment are palliative.

Causes

- Genetically determined tendency to develop psoriasis
- Possible immune disorder, as suggested by HLA type in families
- Flare-up of guttate (drop-shaped) lesions from infections, especially beta-hemolytic streptococci

Other Contributing Factors

- Pregnancy
- Endocrine changes
- Climate (cold weather tends to exacerbate psoriasis)
- Emotional stress or physical illness
- Infection
- Certain medications, such as systemic glucocorticoids and lithium

Pathophysiology

A skin cell normally takes 14 days to move from the basal layer to the stratum corneum, where it's sloughed off after 14 days of normal wear and tear. Thus, the life cycle of a normal skin cell is 28 days.

In psoriasis, the immune system sends signals that speed up the normal process from 28 days to just 4 days. This markedly shortened cycle doesn't allow time for the cell to mature. Consequently, the stratum corneum becomes thick with extra skin cells. On the surface, the skin cells pile up, and the dead cells create a white, flaky layer, the cardinal manifestation of psoriasis.

COMPLICATIONS
- Infection
- Altered self-image, depression, and isolation

Signs and Symptoms

- Erythematous papules and plaques with thick silver scales, most commonly on the scalp, chest, elbows, knees, back, and buttocks
- Plaques with characteristic silver scales that either flake off easily or thicken, covering the lesion (scale removal can produce fine bleeding [Auspitz's sign])
- Itching and occasional pain from dry, cracked, encrusted lesions
- Occasional small guttate lesions (usually thin and erythematous, with few scales), either alone or with plaques

Diagnostic Test Results

Diagnosis is based on patient history, appearance of the lesions and, if needed, the results of skin biopsy. Blood chemistry reveals elevated serum uric acid level.

Treatment

- Topical fluorinated glucocorticoids
- Low-dose antihistamines, oatmeal baths, emollients, and open wet dressings to help relieve pruritus
- Aspirin and local heat to help alleviate the pain of psoriatic arthritis; nonsteroidal anti-inflammatory drugs in severe cases
- Ultraviolet B (UVB) or natural sunlight exposure to retard rapid cell production to the point of minimal erythema
- Tar preparations or crude coal tar applications to the affected areas about 15 minutes before exposure to UVB or at bedtime and wiped off the next morning
- Intralesional steroid injection for small, stubborn plaques
- Anthralin ointment or paste mixture for well-defined plaques (because anthralin injures and stains normal skin, apply petroleum jelly around the affected skin before applying it)
- Calcipotriene ointment, a vitamin D analogue; best when alternated with a topical steroid
- Tazarotene, a topical retinoid
- Topical administration of psoralens (plant extracts that accelerate exfoliation) followed by exposure to high-intensity UVA
- Extensive psoriasis: acitretin, a retinoid compound
- Resistant disease: cyclosporine
- Last-resort treatment for refractory psoriasis: cytotoxin, usually methotrexate
- Psoriasis of scalp: tar shampoo followed by a steroid lotion
- Management of psoriasis includes psychosocial and physical aspects of the disease.

PSORIATIC LESION

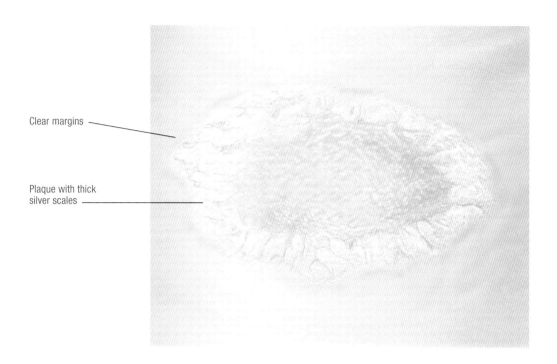

Clear margins

Plaque with thick silver scales

DIFFUSE PSORIATIC PLAQUES

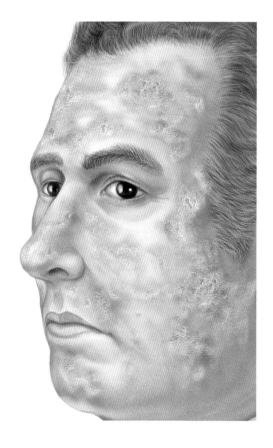

SKIN CANCERS

BASAL CELL CARCINOMA

Basal cell carcinoma, also known as *basal cell epithelioma*, is a slow-growing, destructive skin tumor. The most common form of skin cancer, which rarely metastasizes.

Causes

- Both environmental and genetic factors contribute to the development of basal cell carcinoma

Prolonged sun exposure (most common)

- Extensive sunburns or sun exposure in childhood
- Arsenic, radiation, burns, immunosuppression
- Previous X-ray therapy for acne

Pathophysiology

The pathogenesis is uncertain, but it's thought to originate when undifferentiated basal cells become carcinomatous instead of differentiating into sweat glands, sebum, and hair.

COMPLICATIONS
- Disfiguring lesions

Signs and Symptoms

Noduloulcerative Lesions

- Usually occur on the face, particularly the forehead, eyelid margins, nasolabial folds
- Lesions small, smooth, pinkish, and translucent papules with telangiectatic vessels crossing the surface; occasionally pigmented
- When lesions enlarge, centers possibly depressed and borders firm and elevated
- Eventual local invasion and ulceration, or "rodent ulcers" (these rarely metastasize but can spread to vital areas and become infected or cause massive hemorrhage)

Superficial Basal Cell Carcinoma

- Commonly multiple; usually occur on the chest and back
- Oval or irregularly shaped, lightly pigmented plaques, with sharply defined, slightly elevated threadlike borders:
  - superficial erosion scaly in appearance; small, atrophic areas in center resembling psoriasis or eczema
  - usually chronic and *unlikely* to invade other areas

Sclerosing Basal Cell Carcinoma (Morphea-Like Carcinoma)

- Waxy, sclerotic, yellow to white plaques; no distinct borders
- Occur on the head and neck

Diagnostic Test Results

Incisional or excisional biopsy and histologic study determine the tumor type.
  Confirmation of the diagnosis.

Treatment

- Surgical excision
- Curettage and electrodesiccation
- Topical 5-fluorouracil, imiquimod
- Microscopically controlled surgical excision (Mohs' surgery)
- Irradiation
- Cryotherapy with liquid nitrogen
- Chemosurgery: for persistent or recurrent lesions

SQUAMOUS CELL CARCINOMA

Squamous cell carcinoma of the skin is an invasive tumor with metastatic potential. It usually occurs on sun-exposed areas but can occur elsewhere.

Causes

- Overexposure to the sun's ultraviolet rays
- Premalignant lesions, such as actinic keratosis or leukoplakia
- X-ray therapy
- Ingested herbicides, medications, or waxes containing arsenic
- Chronic skin irritation and inflammation
- Local carcinogens, such as tar and oil
- Hereditary diseases, such as xeroderma pigmentosum and albinism

Pathophysiology

Squamous cell carcinoma arises from keratinizing epidermal cells.

COMPLICATIONS
- Lymph node and visceral metastases
- Respiratory problems

Signs and Symptoms

- Induration and inflammation of a preexisting lesion
- Slowly growing nodule on a firm, indurated base; eventual ulceration and invasion of underlying tissues
- Metastasis to regional lymph nodes: characteristic systemic symptoms of pain, malaise, fatigue, weakness, and anorexia

Diagnostic Test Results

Excisional biopsy determines the tumor type.
  Clinical findings of cutaneous squamous cell carcinoma depend on the type of lesion and location of involvement.

Treatment

- Surgical excision
- Electrodesiccation and curettage
- Radiation therapy
- Chemosurgery

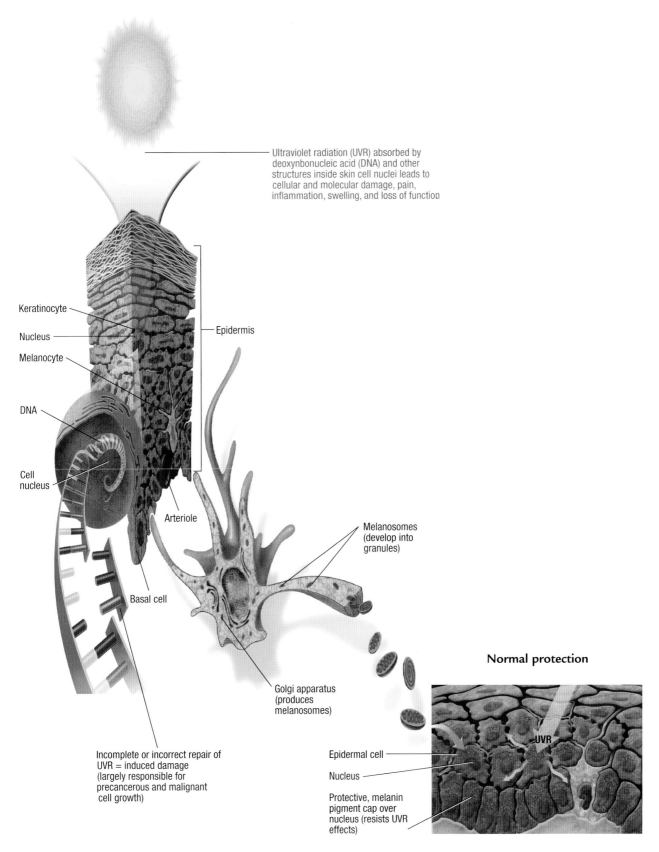

Ultraviolet radiation (UVR) absorbed by deoxynbonucleic acid (DNA) and other structures inside skin cell nuclei leads to cellular and molecular damage, pain, inflammation, swelling, and loss of function

Keratinocyte

Nucleus

Melanocyte

DNA

Cell nucleus

Epidermis

Arteriole

Basal cell

Melanosomes (develop into granules)

Golgi apparatus (produces melanosomes)

Incomplete or incorrect repair of UVR = induced damage (largely responsible for precancerous and malignant cell growth)

Normal protection

Epidermal cell

Nucleus

Protective, melanin pigment cap over nucleus (resists UVR effects)

UVR

MALIGNANT MELANOMA

A malignant neoplasm that arises from melanocytes, malignant melanoma is relatively rare and accounts for only 1% to 2% of all malignancies reference. The incidence is rapidly increasing, by 300% in the past 40 years. The four types of melanomas are *superficial spreading*, *nodular malignant*, *lentigo maligna*, and *acral lentiginous*.

Melanoma spreads through the lymphatic and vascular systems and metastasizes to the regional lymph nodes, skin, liver, lungs, and central nervous system. Its course is unpredictable, and recurrence and metastases may not appear for more than 5 years after resection of the primary lesion. The prognosis varies with tumor thickness. Generally, superficial lesions are curable, whereas deeper lesions tend to metastasize.

Causes

- Excessive exposure to sunlight

Contributing Factors

- Skin type: most common in persons with blonde or red hair, fair skin, and blue eyes; who are prone to sunburn; and who are of Celtic or Scandinavian ancestry; rare among people of African ancestry
- Hormonal factors: growth possibly exacerbated by pregnancy
- Family history: slightly more common within families
- Past history of melanoma

Pathophysiology

Malignant melanoma arises from melanocytes, the pigment-producing cells of the skin.

Up to 70% of patients with melanoma have a preexisting nevus (mole) at the tumor site.

COMPLICATIONS
- Metastases to the lungs, liver, or brain

Signs and Symptoms

Melanoma (If Any Skin Lesion or Nevus)

- Enlarges, becomes inflamed or sore, itches, ulcerates, bleeds, undergoes textural changes
- Changes color or shows signs of surrounding pigment regression (halo nevus or vitiligo)

Superficial Spreading Melanoma

- Arises on an area of chronic irritation
- In women, most common between the knees and ankles; in Blacks and Asians, on the toe webs and soles — lightly pigmented areas subject to trauma

- Red, white, and blue color over a brown or black background and an irregular, notched margin
- Irregular surface with small elevated tumor nodules that may ulcerate and bleed

Nodular Melanoma

- Usually a polypoidal nodule, with uniformly dark or grayish coloration — resembles a blackberry
- Occasionally, flesh-colored, with flecks of pigment around its base; possibly inflamed

Lentigo Maligna Melanoma

- Resembles a large (3- to 6-cm) flat freckle of tan, brown, black, whitish, or slate color
- Irregularly scattered black nodules on the surface
- Develops slowly, usually over many years, and eventually may ulcerate
- Commonly develops under fingernail, on face, or on back of the hand

CLINICAL TIP
Remember the ABCDEs of malignant melanoma when examining skin lesions:
A: ASYMMETRICAL lesion
B: BORDER is irregular
C: COLORS of lesion are multiple types
D: DIAMETER of the lesion is less than 0.5 cm
E: ELEVATED or ENLARGING lesion

Diagnostic Test Results

- Excisional biopsy and full-depth punch biopsy with histologic examination shows tumor thickness and disease stage.
- Complete blood count with differential reveals anemia.
- Other blood tests show elevated erythrocyte sedimentation rate, abnormal platelet count, and abnormal liver function tests.
- Chest X-ray assists with staging.
- Computed tomography scan of abdomen, pelvis, and neck; magnetic resonance imaging of the eye and brain; and bone scan detect metastasis.

Treatment

- Surgical resection to remove the tumor
- Regional lymphadenectomy
- Adjuvant chemotherapy and biotherapy
- Radiation therapy

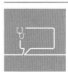

CLINICAL TIP VERY NICE!
Regardless of the treatment method, melanomas require close long-term follow-up to detect metastasis and recurrences. Statistics show that 13% of recurrences develop more than 5 years after primary surgery.

TYPES OF SKIN CANCER

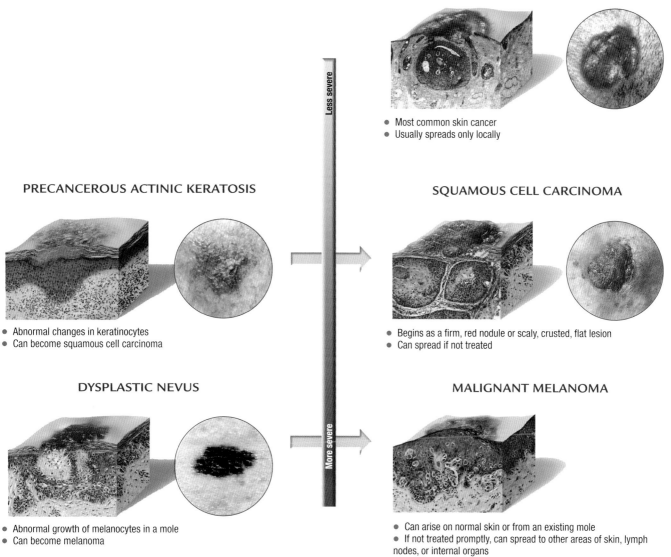

BASAL CELL CARCINOMA

- Most common skin cancer
- Usually spreads only locally

PRECANCEROUS ACTINIC KERATOSIS

- Abnormal changes in keratinocytes
- Can become squamous cell carcinoma

SQUAMOUS CELL CARCINOMA

- Begins as a firm, red nodule or scaly, crusted, flat lesion
- Can spread if not treated

DYSPLASTIC NEVUS

- Abnormal growth of melanocytes in a mole
- Can become melanoma

MALIGNANT MELANOMA

- Can arise on normal skin or from an existing mole
- If not treated promptly, can spread to other areas of skin, lymph nodes, or internal organs

Less severe

More severe

ABCDEs OF MALIGNANT MELANOMA

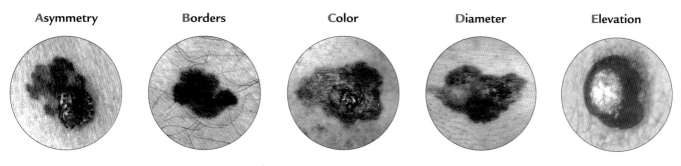

| Asymmetry | Borders | Color | Diameter | Elevation |

WARTS

Warts, also known as *verrucae*, are common, benign, skin growths that appear when a virus infects the skin. The prognosis varies as some warts disappear spontaneously, some readily with treatment, and others need vigorous and prolonged treatment. Warts are contagious and transmitted by direct contact.

AGE ALERT
Although their incidence is highest in children and young adults, warts may occur at any age.

Causes

- Human papilloma virus (HPV)
- Probably transmitted through direct contact; autoinoculation

Pathophysiology

HPV replicates in the epidermal cells, causing irregular thickening of the stratum corneum in the infected areas. People who lack virus-specific immunity are susceptible.

COMPLICATIONS
- Secondary infection
- Scarring

Signs and Symptoms

- Common (*verruca vulgaris*): rough, elevated, rounded surface; appears most frequently on extremities, particularly hands and fingers; most prevalent in children and young adults
- Filiform: single, thin, threadlike projection; commonly occurs around the face and neck
- Periungual: rough, irregularly shaped, elevated surface; occurs around edges of fingernails and toenails; when severe, may extend under the nail and lift it off the nail bed, causing pain
- Flat (juvenile): multiple groupings of up to several hundred slightly raised lesions with smooth, flat, or slightly rounded tops; common on the face, neck, chest, knees, dorsa of hands, wrists, and flexor surfaces of the forearms; usually occurs in children but can affect adults; distribution is often linear because these can spread from scratching or shaving
- Plantar: slightly elevated or flat; occurs singly or in large clusters (mosaic warts), primarily at pressure points of the feet; typically cause pain with weight bearing

- Digitate: fingerlike, horny projection arising from a pea-shaped base; occurs on scalp or near hairline
- Condyloma acuminatum (moist wart): usually small, flesh-colored pink to red, moist, soft; may occur singly or in large cauliflower-like clusters on penis, scrotum, vulva, or anus; may be transmitted through sexual contact; not always venereal in origin

Diagnostic Test Results

- Sigmoidoscopy when anal warts are recurrent rules out internal involvement necessitating surgery.
- Application of 5% acetic acid turns warts white if they are papillomas.

Treatment

Electrodesiccation and Curettage

- High-frequency electric current to destroy the wart, surgical removal of dead tissue at the base
- Effective for common, filiform and, occasionally, plantar warts
- More effective than cryosurgery

Cryotherapy

- Liquid nitrogen kills the wart; resulting dried blister peeled off several days later
- If initial treatment unsuccessful, can be repeated at 2- to 4-week intervals
- Useful for periungual warts or for common warts on face, extremities, penis, vagina, or anus

Acid Therapy (Primary or Adjunctive)

- Applications of plaster patches impregnated with acid (such as 40% salicylic acid plasters) or acid drops (such as 5% to 16.7% salicylic acid in flexible collodion) every 12 to 24 hours for 2 to 4 weeks
- Hyperthermia for *verruca plantaris*

For Genital Warts

- Cryotherapy
- Podophyllin in tincture of benzoin; may be repeated every 3 to 4 days (avoid using this drug on pregnant patients)
- 25% to 50% trichloroacetic acid applied to wart and neutralized with baking soda or water when wart turns white
- Carbon dioxide laser therapy

Other

- Antiviral drugs under investigation
- If immunity develops, possible resolution without treatment
- Imiquimod ointment

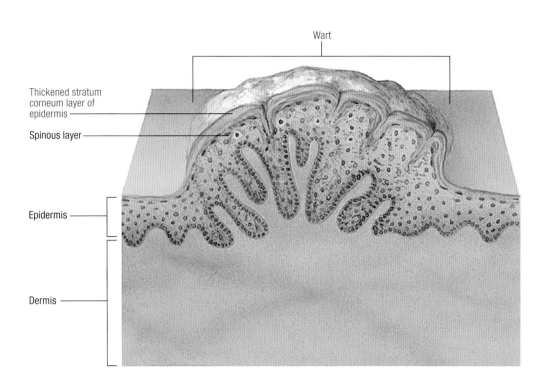

Wart

Thickened stratum corneum layer of epidermis

Spinous layer

Epidermis

Dermis

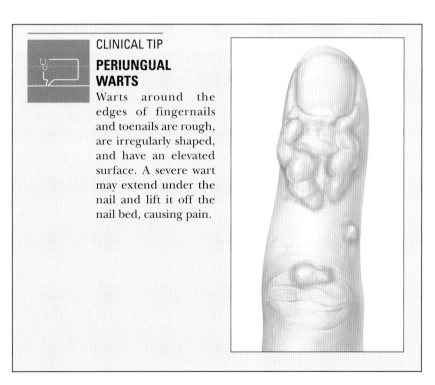

CLINICAL TIP

PERIUNGUAL WARTS

Warts around the edges of fingernails and toenails are rough, are irregularly shaped, and have an elevated surface. A severe wart may extend under the nail and lift it off the nail bed, causing pain.

A cataract is a gradually developing opacity of the lens or lens capsule. Light shining through the cornea is blocked by this opacity, and a blurred image is cast onto the retina. As a result, the brain interprets a hazy image. Cataracts commonly occur bilaterally, and each progresses independently. Exceptions are traumatic cataracts, which are usually unilateral, and congenital cataracts, which may remain stationary.

AGE ALERT
Cataracts are most prevalent in people older than age 70. The prognosis is generally good; surgery improves vision in 95% of affected people.

Causes

- Aging
- Trauma, foreign body injury
- Exposure to ionizing radiation or infrared rays
- Exposure to ultraviolet radiation
- Drugs that are toxic to the lens, such as prednisone, ergot alkaloids, dinitrophenol, naphthalene, phenothiazines, or pilocarpine
- Genetic abnormalities
- Infection such as maternal rubella during the first trimester of pregnancy
- Maternal malnutrition
- Metabolic disease, such as diabetes mellitus or hypothyroidism
- Myotonic dystrophy
- Uveitis, glaucoma, retinitis pigmentosa, or retinal detachment
- Atopic dermatitis

Pathophysiology

Pathophysiology varies with each form of cataract. Congenital cataracts are particularly challenging. They may result from chromosomal abnormalities, metabolic disease, intrauterine nutritional deficiencies, or infections during pregnancy (such as rubella). Senile cataracts show evidence of protein aggregation, oxidative injury, and increased pigmentation in the center of the lens. In traumatic cataracts, phagocytosis of the lens or inflammation may occur when a lens ruptures. The mechanism of a complicated cataract varies with the disease process — for example, in diabetes, increased glucose in the lens causes it to absorb water.

Typically, cataract development goes through these four stages:

- *immature* — partially opaque lens
- *mature* — completely opaque lens; significant vision loss

- *tumescent* — water-filled lens; may lead to glaucoma
- *hypermature* — lens proteins deteriorate; peptides leak through the lens capsule; glaucoma may develop if intraocular fluid outflow is obstructed.

COMPLICATIONS
- Vision loss

Signs and Symptoms

- Gradual painless blurring and loss of vision
- Milky white pupil
- Blinding glare from headlights at night
- Poor reading vision caused by reduced clarity of images
- In central opacity — vision improves in dim light; as pupils dilate, patients able to see around the opacity

AGE ALERT
Elderly patients with reduced vision may become depressed and withdraw from social activities rather than complain about reduced vision.

Diagnostic Test Results

- Indirect ophthalmoscopy and slit-lamp examination show a dark area in the normally homogeneous red reflex.
- Visual acuity test confirms vision loss.

Treatment

- Phacoemulsification cataract extraction to remove lens but leave capsule in place:
  - phacoemulsification to fragment the lens with ultrasonic vibrations
  - aspiration of pieces
  - implantation of intraocular lens.
- Extracapsular cataract extraction:
  - lens removed in one piece, capsule left intact
  - implantation of intraocular lens.
- Intracapsular cataract extraction of entire lens and capsule:
  - rarely performed; may be necessary in trauma cases
  - intraocular lens placed in front of iris.
- Laser surgery to restore visual acuity if a secondary membrane forms in the intact posterior lens capsule after an extracapsular cataract extraction
- Discission (an incision) and aspiration possibly still used in children with soft cataracts
- Contact lenses or lens implantation after surgery to improve visual acuity, binocular vision, and depth perception

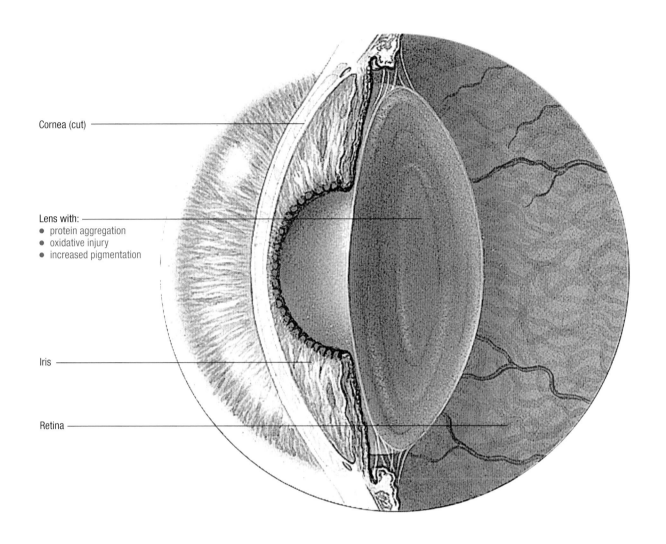

Cornea (cut)

Lens with:
- protein aggregation
- oxidative injury
- increased pigmentation

Iris

Retina

CLEFT LIP AND CLEFT PALATE

Cleft lip and cleft palate — an opening in the lip or palate — may occur separately or in combination. Cleft lip and cleft palate are twice as common in males as in females; isolated cleft palate is more common in females.

Causes

- Isolated birth defect: normal development of orofacial structures disrupted by a combination of genetic and environmental factors
- Part of a chromosomal or Mendelian syndrome (cleft defects are associated with over 300 syndromes)
- Exposures to specific teratogens during fetal development

CLINICAL TIP
A family history of cleft defects increases the risk that a couple may have a child with a cleft defect. Likewise, an individual with a cleft defect is at an increased risk to have a child with a cleft defect. Children with cleft defects and their parents or adult individuals should be referred for genetic counseling for accurate diagnosis of cleft type and recurrence risk counseling. Recurrence risk is based on family history, the presence or absence of other physical or cognitive traits within a family, and prenatal exposure information.

Pathophysiology

Cleft deformities originate in the 2nd month of pregnancy, when the front and sides of the face and the palatine shelves fuse imperfectly. Cleft deformities usually occur unilaterally or bilaterally, rarely midline.

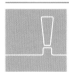

COMPLICATIONS
- Speech difficulties
- Failure to thrive related to feeding difficulties
- Dentition problems
- Otitis media
- Hearing defects
- Physical deformity and self-image issues

Signs and Symptoms

- *Cleft lip* may range from a simple notch in the upper lip to a complete cleft from the lip edge through the floor of the nostril.

- *Cleft palate* may be partial or complete, involving only the soft palate or extending from the soft palate completely through the hard palate into the upper jaw or nasal cavity.

CLINICAL TIP
The constellation of U-shaped cleft palate, mandibular hypoplasia, and glossoptosis (downward displacement and retraction of the tongue) is known as Pierre Robin sequence, or Robin sequence. It can occur as an isolated defect or one feature of many different syndromes; therefore, a comprehensive genetic evaluation is suggested for infants with Robin sequence. Because of the mandibular hypoplasia and glossoptosis, careful evaluation and management of the airway are mandatory for infants with Robin sequence.

Diagnostic Test Results

Prenatal ultrasonography reveals the defect.

Treatment

Surgical Correction (Timing Varies)

- Cleft lip:
  - within the first few days of life to make feeding easier
  - delay lip repairs for 2 to 8 months to minimize surgical and anesthesia risks, rule out associated congenital anomalies, and allow time for parental bonding.
- Cleft palate:
  - performed only after the infant is gaining weight and is infection-free
  - usually completed by age 12 to 18 months
  - two steps: soft palate between ages 6 and 18 months; hard palate as late as age 5 years.

Speech Therapy

- Palate is essential to speech formation (structural changes, even in a repaired cleft, can permanently affect speech patterns).
- Hearing difficulties are common in children with cleft palate because of middle ear damage or infections.

Other

- Orthodontic prosthesis
- Adequate nutrition
- Use of a large soft nipple with large holes

Cleft lip

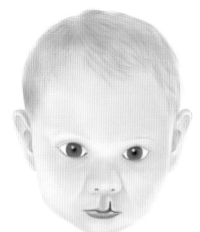

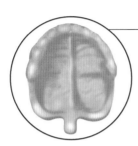

Front of palate

Unilateral cleft lip and cleft palate

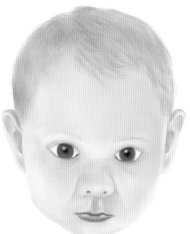

Bilateral cleft lip and cleft palate

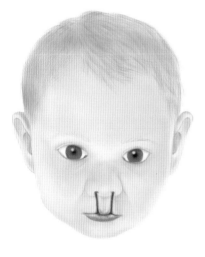

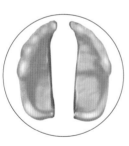

Cleft palate

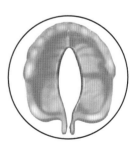

CONJUNCTIVITIS

Conjunctivitis (also known as *pinkeye*) is characterized by hyperemia of the conjunctiva. The three main types of conjunctivitis are infectious, allergic, and chemical. This disorder usually occurs as a benign, self-limiting condition; it may also be chronic, possibly indicating degenerative changes or damage from repeated acute attacks. Epidemic keratoconjunctivitis is an acute, highly contagious viral conjunctivitis. Careful handwashing is essential to prevent the spread of conjunctivitis.

Causes

Infectious Conjunctivitis

Most commonly by:

- bacterial — *Staphylococcus aureus, Streptococcus pneumoniae, Neisseria gonorrhoeae, Neisseria meningitidis*
- chlamydial — *Chlamydia trachomatis* (inclusion conjunctivitis)
- viral — adenovirus types 3, 7, and 8; herpes simplex 1; coxsackie; varicella zoster.

Allergic Conjunctivitis

Hypersensitivity to:

- pollen, grass, unknown seasonal allergens (vernal conjunctivitis), or animals
- topical medications, cosmetics, or fabrics
- air pollutants or smoke
- contact lenses or solutions

Chemical Conjunctivitis

Chemical reaction to:

- environmental irritants (wind, dust, smoke, swimming pool chlorine)
- occupational irritants (acids, alkalies)

Pathophysiology

Conjunctivitis is an inflammation of the conjunctiva, the transparent layer covering the surfaces in the inner eyelid (palpebral conjunctiva) and the front of the eyeball (bulbar conjunctiva). It usually begins in one eye and rapidly spreads to the other by contamination of towels, washcloths, or the patient's own unwashed hands.

Vernal conjunctivitis (so called because symptoms tend to be worse in the spring) is a severe form of immunoglobulin E–mediated mast cell hypersensitivity reaction. This form of conjunctivitis is bilateral. It usually begins between ages 3 and 5 years and persists until about 10 years or age. It's sometimes associated with other signs of allergy commonly related to pollens, asthma, or allergic rhinitis.

COMPLICATIONS
- Corneal infiltrates
- Corneal ulcers

Signs and Symptoms

- Hyperemia of the conjunctiva
- Discharge or tearing
- Pain or photophobia (red flags, may indicate more serious conditions such as iritis, keratitis)

Acute Bacterial Conjunctivitis (Pinkeye)

- Usually lasts only 2 weeks
- Itching, burning, and the sensation of a foreign body in the eye
- Crust of sticky, mucopurulent discharge (greenish) on the eyelids

N. gonorrhoeae Conjunctivitis

- Itching, burning, or foreign body sensation
- Profuse and purulent discharge

Viral Conjunctivitis

- Copious tearing (epiphora), minimal exudate
- Enlargement of the preauricular lymph node
- In children, sore throat or fever if the cause is an adenovirus
- Variable time course, depending on the virus:
    - some self-limiting, lasting 2 to 3 weeks
    - others chronic, producing a severe disabling disease

Diagnostic Test Results

- In stained smears of conjunctival scrapings, the predominance of lymphocytes indicates viral infection; of neutrophils, bacterial infection; and of eosinophils, allergy-related infection.
- Culture and sensitivity tests identify the causative organism (not routinely done).

Treatment

- Bacterial conjunctivitis: topical appropriate broad-spectrum antibiotic
- Viral conjunctivitis:
    - resist treatment; most important aspect of treatment is preventing transmission
    - herpes simplex infection generally responsive to treatment with trifluridine drops, vidarabine ointment, or oral acyclovir
    - secondary infection possibly prevented by sulfonamide or broad-spectrum antibiotic eyedrops
- Vernal (allergic) conjunctivitis:
    - corticosteroid drops followed by cromolyn sodium
    - cold compresses to relieve itching
    - occasionally, oral or ophthalmic antihistamines

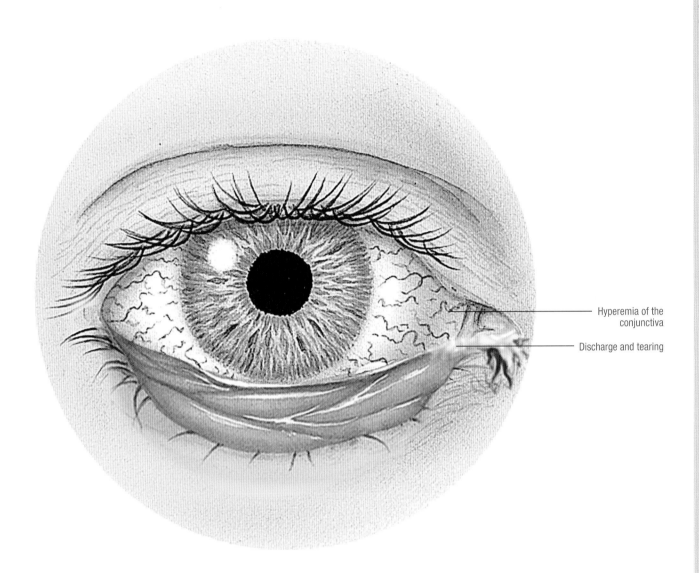

Hyperemia of the conjunctiva

Discharge and tearing

CORNEAL ULCER

Corneal ulcers produce corneal scarring or perforation and are a major cause of blindness worldwide. They occur in the central or marginal areas of the cornea, vary in shape and size, and may be singular or multiple. Marginal ulcers are the most common form. Prompt treatment (within hours of onset) and referral to an ophthalmologist are imperative to prevent visual impairment.

Causes

Protozoan Infection

- Acanthamoeba

Bacterial Infections

- *Staphylococcus aureus*
- *Pseudomonas aeruginosa*
- *Streptococcus viridans*
- *Streptococcus (Diplococcus) pneumoniae*
- *Moraxella liquefaciens*

Viral Infections

- Herpes simplex *1*
- Variola
- Vaccinia
- Varicella zoster

Fungal Infections

- *Candida*
- *Fusarium*
- *Acremonium*

Other

- Trauma
- Exposure reactions to bacterial infections, toxins, trichiasis, entropion, allergens, or contact lenses
- Vitamin A deficiency (xerophthalmia)
- Fifth cranial nerve lesions (neurotropic ulcers)

Pathophysiology

The introduction of a causative factor, such as bacterial or herpes virus infection, trauma, or misuse of contact lenses, starts the process. This leads to epithelial destruction of the stoma with inflammation and tearing. Superficial ulceration results in photophobia, epiphora, foreign body sensation, discomfort (eye pain), and decreased visual acuity.

Deep ulcerations penetrate the epithelial layers of the eye, leading to perforation and allowing infection of deeper eye structures and extrusion of eye contents. Fibrous tissue can form during healing of deep ulcerations, leading to scarring and eventual opacity of the cornea. These processes can lead to partial or total vision loss.

COMPLICATIONS

- Corneal scarring
- Loss of the *eye*
- Vision loss (permanent)

Signs and Symptoms

- Pain aggravated by blinking
- Foreign body sensation
- Increased tearing
- Photophobia
- Pronounced visual blurring
- Purulent discharge (with bacterial ulcer)

Diagnostic Test Results

- Flashlight examination reveals an irregular corneal surface.
- Fluorescein dye instilled in the conjunctival sac stains the outline of the ulcer and confirms the diagnosis.
- Culture and sensitivity testing of corneal scrapings may identify the causative bacteria or fungus.

Treatment

All Corneal Ulcers

- Prompt treatment and referral to ophthalmologist to prevent complications and permanent visual impairment
- Systemic and topical broad-spectrum antibiotics until culture results identify the causative organism
- Measures to eliminate the underlying cause of the ulcer and relieve pain

Fungal Infection

- Topical instillation of natamycin for *Fusarium, Acremonium,* and *Candida* infections

Infection with Herpes Simplex 1

- Topical application of trifluridine drops or vidarabine ointment
- Trifluridine for recurrence

Vitamin A Deficiency

- Correction of dietary deficiency or GI malabsorption of vitamin A

Infection with *P. aeruginosa*

- Polymyxin B and gentamicin administered topically and by subconjunctival injection
- Hospitalization and isolation and I.V. carbenicillin and tobramycin to stop the rapid spread of infection and prevent corneal perforation, which can occur within 48 hours

CLINICAL TIP

Treatment for a corneal ulcer caused by bacterial infection should never include an eye patch. Use of an eye patch creates the dark, warm, moist environment ideal for bacterial growth. Steroid drops should be utilized cautiously and only under the supervision of an ophthalmologist.

Neurotropic Ulcers or Exposure Keratitis

- Frequent instillation of artificial tears or lubricating ointments and use of a plastic bubble eye shield

Infection with Varicella Zoster

- Topical sulfonamide ointment applied three to four times daily to prevent secondary infection
- Analgesics for pain
- Cycloplegic eyedrops for associated anterior uveitis

LOOKING AT CORNEAL ULCERS

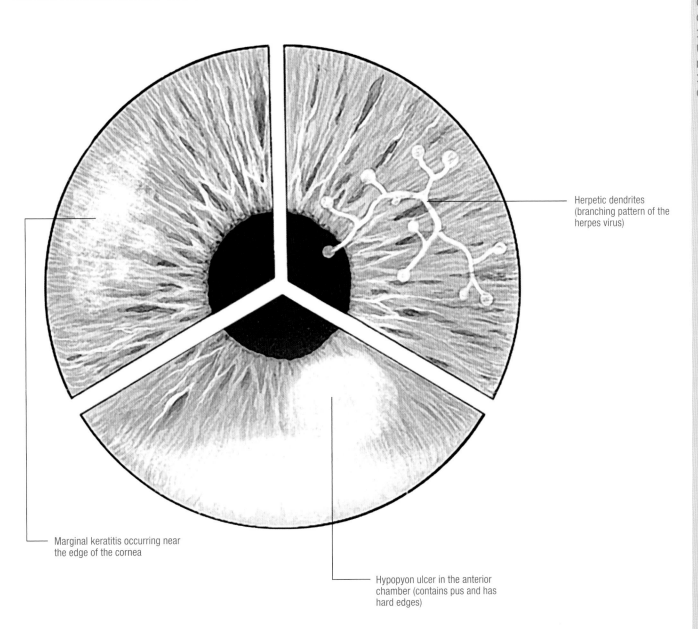

Herpetic dendrites (branching pattern of the herpes virus)

Marginal keratitis occurring near the edge of the cornea

Hypopyon ulcer in the anterior chamber (contains pus and has hard edges)

ECTROPION AND ENTROPION

Ectropion, the outward turning or eversion of the eyelid, may be congenital or acquired. Acquired ectropion may be involutional, paralytic, cicatricial, or mechanical. Involutional ectropion is the most common form and usually stems from age-related weakness in the lid. Paralytic ectropion may occur with seventh cranial nerve palsy from diverse causes, such as Bell's palsy, tumors, herpes zoster oticus, and infiltrations or tumors of the parotid gland. Cicatricial ectropion results from scarring of the anterior lamella from facial burns, trauma, chronic dermatitis, or excessive skin excision with blepharoplasty. Mechanical ectropion can occur with lid tumors that cause the lower eyelid to evert.

Entropion is the inward turning or inversion of the eyelid. It can be unilateral or bilateral and can occur in the upper or lower eyelid, although it occurs more commonly in the lower lid. Entropion can be congenital (rare), acute spastic, involutional, or cicatricial.

Although both ectropion and entropion can occur at any age, they're more common in adults over age 60.

Causes

Ectropion

- Deficiency of the anterior lamella (congenital)
- Genetic ocular syndromes
- Lack of tone of muscles that hold the eyelid taut (acquired)

Entropion

- Dysgenesis of the lower eyelid retractors (congenital)
- Ocular irritation from infection, inflammation, or trauma (acute spastic)
- Scarring of the palpebral conjunctiva and rotation of the eyelid margin (cicatricial)

Pathophysiology

Ectropion

Poor insertion of the muscles that pull the eyelid downward along with contraction of the orbicularis muscle allows the eyelid to turn one way or the other. Laxity of the canthal tendon can aggravate the problem. If both tendons become significantly lax, all of the horizontal support of the eyelid is weakened, resulting in an ectropion or eversion of the eyelid.

Entropion

In acute spastic entropion, the spastic closing of the orbicularis oculi muscle overtakes the opposing action of the lower eyelid retraction, resulting in an inward turning of the eyelid.

In acquired entropion, the brow and lower facial muscles are weak, which results in a drooping of the lower eyelid.

In involutional entropion, dehiscence of the lower lid retractors allows the inferior tarsal margin to move anteriorly. Horizontal eyelid laxity and overriding of the pretarsal and preseptal orbicularis muscles add to this, resulting in involutional entropion. Cicatricial entropion results from scarring of the palpebral conjunctiva and subsequent inward rotation of the eyelid margin.

COMPLICATIONS

- Corneal abrasions
- Corneal scarring
- Tearing
- Keratinization of the palpebral conjunctiva
- Vision loss

Signs and Symptoms

- Irritated or red eyes
- Tearing
- Watery eyes
- Discharge
- Crusting of the eyelid
- A sensation of something in the eye
- Eyelid eversion or inversion

Diagnostic Test Results

- Although laboratory studies don't show entropion, biopsy may help rule out antibasement membrane antibodies in cicatricial entropion.
- Exophthalmometry readings may reveal the presence of exophthalmos in involutional ectropion.
- Distraction and snapback tests reveal abnormal horizontal lid laxity in ectropion.

Treatment

- Ocular lubrication and artificial tear preparations for spastic entropion resulting from dry eye syndrome
- Antibiotics and corticosteroids for spastic entropion caused by blepharitis
- Botulinum (Botox) injection in small amounts for spastic entropion to weaken the pretarsal orbicularis oculi muscle
- Chemotherapy (dapsone) for cicatricial entropion secondary to pemphigus
- Surgical repair

ECTROPION

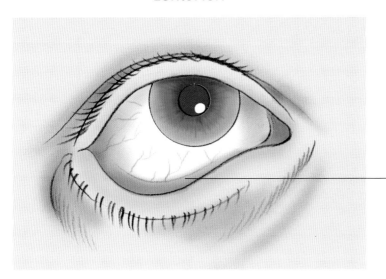

Weakness in the eyelid causes the outward turning of the eyelid.

ENTROPION

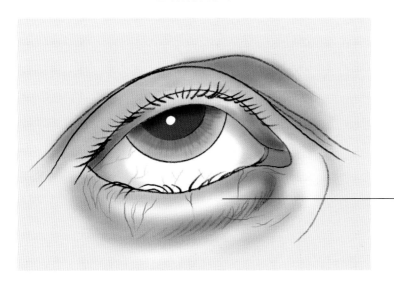

The eyelid turns inward.

GLAUCOMA

Glaucoma is a group of disorders characterized by an abnormally high intraocular pressure (IOP) that damages the optic nerve and other intraocular structures. Glaucoma occurs in several forms: chronic open angle (primary), acute angle closure, congenital (inherited as an autosomal recessive trait), and secondary to other causes. Chronic open-angle glaucoma is usually bilateral, with insidious onset and a slowly progressive course. Acute angle-closure glaucoma typically has a rapid onset, constituting an ophthalmic emergency. Unless treated promptly, this acute form of glaucoma causes blindness in 3 to 5 days.

Causes

Chronic Open-Angle Glaucoma

- Genetics
- Hypertension
- Diabetes mellitus
- Aging
- Black ethnicity
- Severe myopia

Acute Angle-Closure Glaucoma

- Drug-induced mydriasis (extreme dilation of the pupil)
- Excitement or stress, which can lead to hypertension

Secondary Glaucoma

- Uveitis
- Trauma
- Steroids
- Diabetes
- Infections
- Surgery

Pathophysiology

Chronic open-angle glaucoma results from overproduction or obstruction of the outflow of aqueous humor through the trabecular meshwork or the canal of Schlemm, causing increased IOP and damage to the optic nerve. In secondary glaucoma, conditions such as trauma and surgery increase the risk of obstruction of intraocular fluid outflow caused by edema or other abnormal processes.

Acute angle-closure glaucoma results from obstruction to the outflow of aqueous humor. Obstruction may be caused by anatomically narrow angles between the anterior iris and the posterior corneal surface, shallow anterior chamber, a thickened iris that causes angle closure on pupil dilation, or a bulging iris that presses on the trabeculae, closing the angle (peripheral anterior synechiae). Any of these may cause IOP to increase suddenly.

AGE ALERT
In older patients, partial closure of the angle also may occur, so that two forms of glaucoma may coexist.

COMPLICATIONS
- Vision loss and blindness

Signs and Symptoms

Chronic Open-Angle Glaucoma

- Typically bilateral
- Mild aching in the eyes
- Loss of peripheral vision
- Images of halos around lights
- Reduced visual acuity, especially at night, not correctable with glasses

Acute Angle-Closure Glaucoma

- Rapid onset; usually unilateral
- Inflammation; red, painful eye
- Sensation of pressure over the eye
- Moderate papillary dilation nonreactive to light
- Cloudy cornea
- Blurring and decreased visual acuity; halos around lights
- Photophobia
- Nausea and vomiting

Diagnostic Test Results

- Tonometry measurement shows increased IOP.
- Slit-lamp examination shows effects of glaucoma on anterior eye structures.
- Gonioscopy shows the angle of the eye's anterior chamber.
- Ophthalmoscopy aids visualization of the fundus.
- Perimetry or visual field tests show the extent of peripheral vision loss.
- Fundus photography shows optic disk changes.

Treatment

Chronic Open-Angle Glaucoma

- Beta-adrenergic blockers, such as timolol or betaxolol (a beta$_1$-preceptor antagonist)
- Alpha agonists, such as brimonidine or apraclonidine
- Carbonic anhydrase inhibitors, such as dorzolamide or acetazolamide
- Epinephrine
- Prostaglandins such as latanoprost
- Miotic eyedrops such as pilocarpine
- Surgical procedures if medical therapy fails to reduce IOP: argon laser trabeculoplasty of the trabecular meshwork of an open angle, to produce a thermal burn that changes the surface of the meshwork and increases the outflow of aqueous humor; trabeculectomy, to remove scleral tissue; and followed by a peripheral iridectomy, to produce an opening for aqueous outflow under the conjunctiva, creating a filtering bleb

Acute Angle-Closure Glaucoma

- Ocular emergency, requiring immediate intervention, including:
  - I.V. mannitol (20%) or oral glycerin (50%)
  - steroid drops
  - acetazolamide, a carbonic anhydrase inhibitor

- pilocarpine, to constrict the pupil, forcing the iris away from the trabeculae and allowing fluid to escape
- timolol, a beta-adrenergic blocker
- opioid analgesics

- laser iridotomy or surgical peripheral iridectomy
- cycloplegic drops, such as apraclonidine, in the affected eye (only after laser peripheral iridectomy).

OPTIC DISK CHANGES IN GLAUCOMA

Normal optic disk

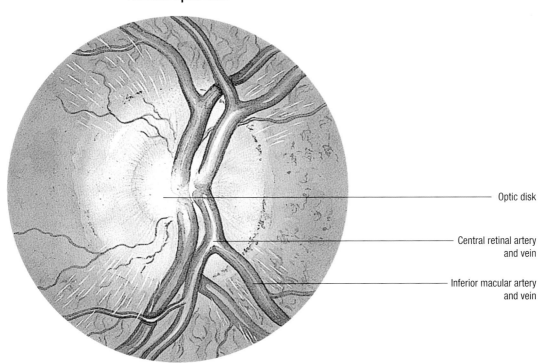

Optic disk

Central retinal artery and vein

Inferior macular artery and vein

Disk changes

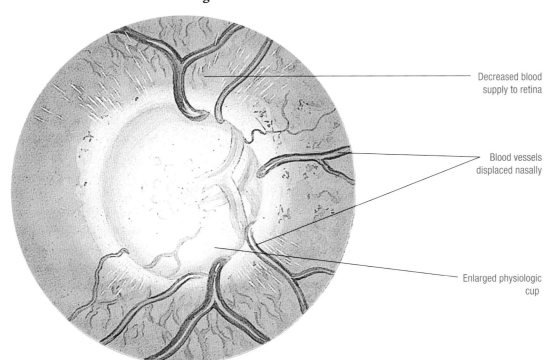

Decreased blood supply to retina

Blood vessels displaced nasally

Enlarged physiologic cup

HEARING LOSS

Hearing loss, or deafness, results from a mechanical or nervous impediment to the transmission of sound waves and is the most common pathologic process associated with hearing alteration. Hearing loss is further defined as an inability to perceive the normal range of sounds audible to an individual with normal hearing. Types of hearing loss include congenital hearing loss, sudden deafness, noise-induced hearing loss, and presbycusis.

Causes

Congenital Hearing Loss

- Dominant, autosomal dominant, autosomal recessive, or sex-linked recessive trait
- Maternal exposure to rubella, cytomegalovirus (CMV), or syphilis during pregnancy
- Use of ototoxic drugs during pregnancy
- Trauma or prolonged fetal anoxia during delivery
- Congenital abnormalities of ears, nose, or throat
- Prematurity or low birth weight
- Serum bilirubin levels above 20 mg/dL

Sudden Deafness

- Mumps — most common cause of unilateral sensorineural hearing loss in children
- Other bacterial and viral infections — rubella, rubeola, influenza, herpes zoster, infectious mononucleosis, mycoplasma, and CMV
- Metabolic disorders — diabetes mellitus, hypothyroidism, and hyperlipoproteinemia
- Vascular disorders — hypertension and arteriosclerosis
- Head trauma or brain tumors
- Ototoxic drugs — aminoglycosides such as tobramycin, streptomycin, quinine, and gentamicin; salicylates; loop diuretics such as furosemide, ethacrynic acid, and bumetanide; antineoplastic drugs such as cisplatin
- Neurologic disorders — multiple sclerosis and neurosyphilis
- Blood dyscrasias — leukemia and hypercoagulation

Noise-Induced Hearing Loss

- Prolonged exposure to loud noise (85 to 90 dB)
- Brief exposure to extremely loud noise (greater than 90 dB)

Presbycusis

- Loss of hair cells in the organ of Corti, can occur as a result of aging

Pathophysiology

The major forms of hearing loss are classified as conductive loss, interrupted passage of sound from the external ear to the junction of the stapes and oval window; sensorineural loss, impaired cochlea or acoustic (eighth cranial) nerve dysfunction, causing failure of transmission of sound impulses within the inner ear or brain; or mixed loss, combined dysfunction of conduction and sensorineural transmission.

COMPLICATIONS

- Difficulty communicating

Signs and Symptoms

- Deficient response to auditory stimuli
- Impaired speech development
- Loss of perception of certain frequencies (around 4,000 Hz)
- Tinnitus
- Inability to understand the spoken word

AGE ALERT

A deaf infant's behavior can appear normal and mislead the parents as well as the health care professional, especially if the infant has autosomal recessive deafness and is the first child of carrier parents.

Diagnostic Test Results

- Computed tomography scan shows vestibular and auditory pathways.
- Magnetic resonance imaging reveals acoustic tumors and brain lesions.
- Auditory brain response shows activity in auditory nerve and brain stem.
- Pure tone audiometry reveals presence and degree of hearing loss.
- Electronystagmography shows vestibular function.
- Otoscopic or microscopic examination reveals middle ear disorders and removes debris.
- Rinne and Weber's tests show whether hearing loss is conductive or sensorineural.

Treatment

Congenital Hearing Loss

- Surgery, if correctable
- Sign language, speech reading, or other effective means of developing communication
- Phototherapy and exchange transfusions for hyperbilirubinemia
- Appropriate childhood immunizations

Sudden Deafness

- Prompt identification of underlying cause, such as acoustic neuroma or noise, and appropriate treatment

Noise-Induced Hearing Loss

- Normal hearing usually restored by overnight rest after several hours' exposure to noise levels greater than 90 dB
- High-frequency hearing loss generally prevented by reducing exposure to loud noises
- Speech and hearing rehabilitation possibly required after repeated exposure to such noise, because hearing aids are seldom helpful

Presbycusis

- Amplifying sound, as with a hearing aid, helpful to some patients
- Hearing aid no help for many patients who are intolerant of loud noise

Other

- Antibiotics
- Agents to dissolve cerumen
- Decongestants
- Analgesics

CAUSES OF CONDUCTIVE HEARING LOSS

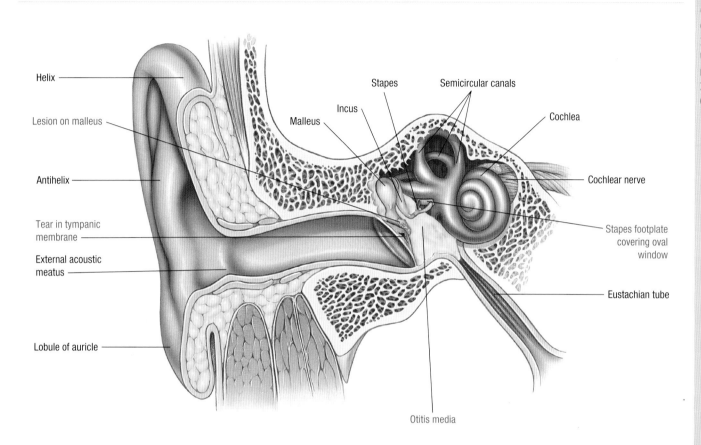

CLINICAL TIP

HOW HEARING OCCURS

- Sound vibrations strike the tympanic membrane (eardrum).
- The auditory ossicles vibrate, and the footplate of the stapes moves at the oval window.
- Movement of the oval window causes the fluid inside the scala vestibuli and scala tympani to move.
- Fluid movement against the cochlear duct sets off nerve impulses, which are carried to the brain via the cochlear nerve.

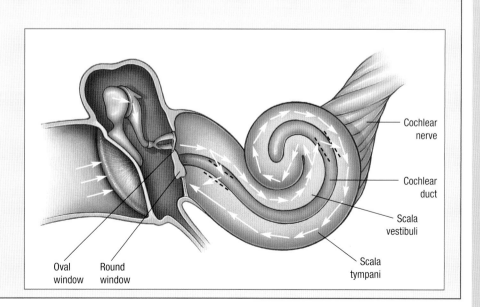

LARYNGEAL CANCER

Laryngeal cancer is cancer of the larynx or voice box in which malignant cells are found in the tissue of the larynx. The most common form of laryngeal cancer is squamous cell carcinoma (95%); rare forms include adenocarcinoma, sarcoma, and others.

Causes

Unknown

Risk Factors

- Smoking
- Alcoholism
- Chronic inhalation of noxious fumes
- Familial tendency
- History of gastroesophageal reflux disease

Pathophysiology

Laryngeal cancer may be intrinsic or extrinsic. An intrinsic tumor is on the true vocal cord and doesn't tend to spread because underlying connective tissues lack lymph nodes. An extrinsic tumor is on some other part of the larynx and tends to spread early. Laryngeal cancer is further classified according to these locations:

- *supraglottis* (false vocal cords)
- *glottis* (true vocal cords)
- *subglottis* (downward extension from vocal cords [rare]).

COMPLICATIONS
- Swallowing difficulty

Signs and Symptoms

Intrinsic Laryngeal Cancer

- Hoarseness that persists longer than 3 weeks

Extrinsic Cancer

- Lump in the throat
- Pain or burning in the throat when drinking citrus juice or hot liquid

Later Clinical Effects of Metastases

- Dysphagia
- Dyspnea
- Cough
- Enlarged cervical lymph nodes
- Pain radiating to the ear

Diagnostic Test Results

- Xeroradiography, laryngeal tomography, computed tomography scan, and laryngography confirm the presence of a mass.
- Chest X-ray identifies metastasis.
- Laryngoscopy allows definitive staging by obtaining multiple biopsy specimens to establish a primary diagnosis, to determine the extent of disease, and to identify additional premalignant lesions or second primary lesions.
- Biopsy identifies cancer cells.

Treatment

Precancerous Lesions

- Laser surgery

Early Lesions

- Surgery or radiation

Advanced Lesions

- Surgery; procedures vary with tumor size and can include cordectomy, partial or total laryngectomy, supraglottic laryngectomy, or total laryngectomy with laryngoplasty
- Laser surgery to help relieve obstruction caused by tumor growth
- Radiation and chemotherapy

Speech Rehabilitation

- If speech preservation isn't possible, may include:
  - esophageal speech
  - prosthetic devices
  - experimental surgical techniques to construct a new voice box.

Mirror view

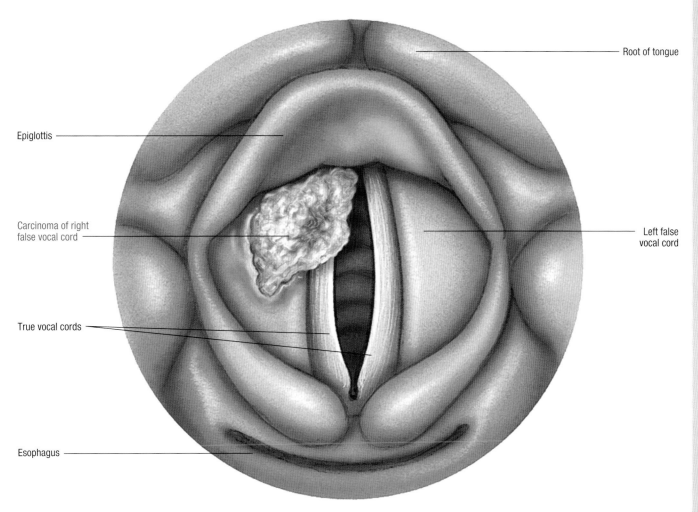

Epiglottis

Carcinoma of right false vocal cord

True vocal cords

Esophagus

Root of tongue

Left false vocal cord

MACULAR DEGENERATION

Macular degeneration — atrophy or degeneration of the macular disk — is the most common cause of legal blindness in adults. Commonly affecting both eyes, it accounts for about 12% of blindness in the United States and for about 17% of new blindness. It's one cause of severe, irreversible, and unpreventable loss of central vision in elderly patients.

AGE ALERT
Two types of age-related macular degeneration occur:

- dry, or atrophic — characterized by atrophic pigment epithelial changes; most commonly causes mild, gradual visual loss
- wet, or exudative — characterized by subretinal formation of new blood vessels (neovascularization) that cause leakage, hemorrhage, and fibrovascular scar formation; causes severe, rapid vision loss.

Causes

Primary cause unknown

Possible Contributing Factors

- Aging
- Inflammation
- Trauma
- Infection
- Poor nutrition
- Family history
- Smoking
- Cardiovascular disease

Pathophysiology

Age-related macular degeneration results from hardening and obstruction of retinal arteries, which probably reflect normal degenerative changes. The formation of new blood vessels in the macular area obscures central vision. Underlying pathologic changes occur primarily in the retinal pigment epithelium, Bruch's membrane, and choriocapillaris in the macular region.

The dry form develops as yellow extracellular deposits or drusen, which accumulate beneath the pigment epithelium of the retina; they may be prominent in the macula. Drusen are common in elderly patients. Over time, drusen grow and become more numerous. Visual loss occurs as the retinal pigment epithelium detaches and becomes atrophic.

COMPLICATIONS
- Blindness
- Macular lesions
- Nystagmus

Signs and Symptoms

- Changes in central vision due to neovascularization, such as a blank spot (scotoma) in the center of a page when reading
- Distorted appearance of straight lines caused by relocation of retinal receptors

Diagnostic Test Results

- Indirect ophthalmoscopy shows gross macular changes, opacities, hemorrhage, neovascularization, retinal pallor, drusen bodies, or retinal detachment.
- I.V. fluorescein angiography sequential photographs show leaking vessels as fluorescein dye flows into the tissues from the subretinal neovascular net.
- Amsler's grid test reveals central visual field loss.

Treatment

- Exudative form (subretinal neovascularization): laser photocoagulation
- Atrophic form: currently no cure

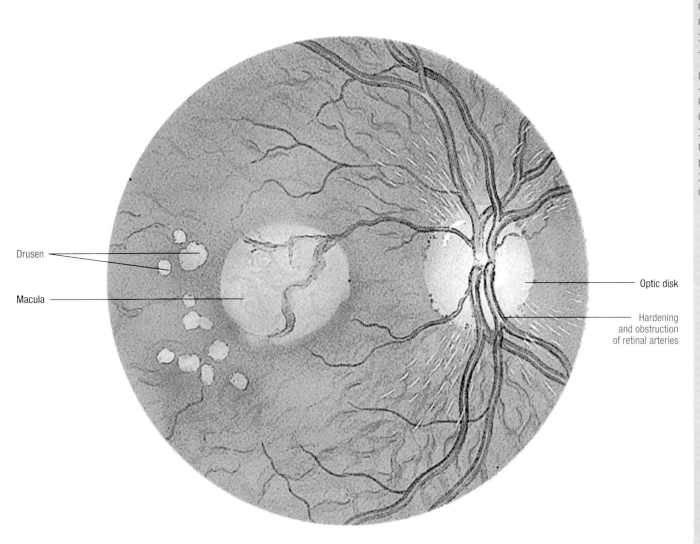

Drusen

Macula

Optic disk

Hardening
and obstruction
of retinal arteries

MÉNIÈRE'S DISEASE

Ménière's disease, a labyrinthine dysfunction also known as *endolymphatic hydrops,* causes severe vertigo, sensorineural hearing loss, and tinnitus.

AGE ALERT

Ménière's disease usually affects adults between the ages of 30 and 60 years, men slightly more often than women. It rarely occurs in children.

Usually, only one ear is involved. After multiple attacks over several years, residual tinnitus and hearing loss can be incapacitating.

Causes

Unknown but may be related to anatomic abnormalities; immune, genetic, and/or vascular etiologies

Possible Associations

- Positive family history
- Immune disorder
- Migraine headaches
- Middle ear infection
- Head trauma
- Autonomic nervous system dysfunction
- Premenstrual edema

Pathophysiology

Ménière's disease may result from overproduction or decreased absorption of endolymph — the fluid contained in the labyrinth of the ear. Accumulated endolymph dilates the saccule and cochlear duct. Dilation of the endolymphatic system occurs and the Reissner membrane often tears. The ruptured Reissner membrane causes the endolymph to escape into the perilymph, causing symptoms of Ménière's occurs.

COMPLICATIONS
- Trauma from falls
- Dehydration
- Decreased quality of life

Signs and Symptoms

- Sudden, severe spinning, whirling vertigo, lasting from 10 minutes to several hours, because of increased endolymph (attacks may occur several times a year, or remissions may last as long as several years)
- Tinnitus caused by altered firing of sensory auditory neurons; possibly, residual tinnitus between attacks
- Hearing impairment due to sensorineural loss:
  - hearing possibly normal between attacks
  - repeated attacks possible progressive cause of permanent hearing loss.
- Feeling of fullness or blockage in the ear before an attack, a result of changing sensitivity of pressure receptors
- Severe nausea, vomiting, sweating, and pallor during an acute attack because of autonomic dysfunction
- Nystagmus due to asymmetry and intensity of impulses reaching the brain stem
- Loss of balance and falling to the affected side due to vertigo

Diagnostic Test Results

- Audiometric testing shows a sensorineural hearing loss and loss of discrimination and recruitment.
- Electronystagmography reveals normal or reduced vestibular response on the affected side.
- Cold caloric testing shows impairment of oculovestibular reflex.
- Electrocochleography reveals increased ratio of summating potential to action potential.
- Brain stem–evoked response audiometry test evaluates for acoustic neuroma, brain tumor, and vascular lesions in the brain stem.
- Computed tomography scan and magnetic resonance imaging (MRI) detects acoustic neuroma as a cause of symptoms.

Treatment

During an Acute Attack

- Lying down to minimize head movement
- Avoiding sudden movements and glaring lights to reduce dizziness
- Promethazine or prochlorperazine to relieve nausea and vomiting
- Atropine to control an attack by reducing autonomic nervous system function
- Dimenhydrinate to control vertigo and nausea
- Central nervous system depressants, such as lorazepam or diazepam, to reduce excitability of vestibular nuclei
- Antihistamines, such as meclizine or diphenhydramine, to reduce dizziness and vomiting

Long-Term Management

- Diuretics, such as triamterene or acetazolamide, to reduce endolymph pressure
- Betahistine, to alleviate vertigo, hearing loss, and tinnitus
- Vasodilators, to dilate blood vessels supplying the inner ear
- Sodium restriction, to reduce endolymphatic hydrops
- Restriction of caffeine and nicotine, both shown to decrease microvascular flow in the labyrinthine system
- Antihistamines or mild sedatives, to prevent attacks
- Systemic streptomycin, to produce chemical ablation of the sensory neuroepithelium of the inner ear and thereby control vertigo in patients with bilateral disease for whom no other treatment can be considered

Disease that Persists Despite Medical Treatment or Produces Incapacitating Vertigo

- Endolymphatic drainage and shunt placement, to reduce pressure on the hair cells of the cochlea and prevent further sensorineural hearing loss
- Vestibular nerve resection in patients with intact hearing, to reduce vertigo and prevent further hearing loss
- Labyrinthectomy to relieve vertigo in patients with incapacitating symptoms and poor or no hearing (destruction of the cochlea results in a total loss of hearing in the affected ear)
- Cochlear implantation, to improve hearing in patients with profound deafness

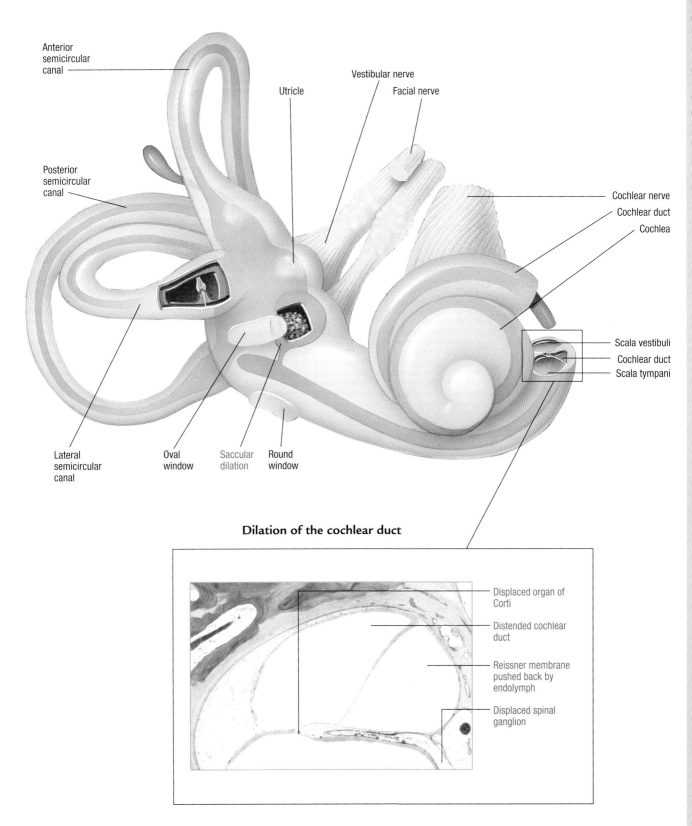

Anterior
semicircular
canal

Utricle

Vestibular nerve

Facial nerve

Cochlear nerve

Cochlear duct

Cochlea

Posterior
semicircular
canal

Scala vestibuli

Cochlear duct

Scala tympani

Lateral
semicircular
canal

Oval
window

Saccular
dilation

Round
window

Dilation of the cochlear duct

Displaced organ of
Corti

Distended cochlear
duct

Reissner membrane
pushed back by
endolymph

Displaced spinal
ganglion

OCULAR MELANOMA

Although melanoma typically develops in areas of the body that contain cells that produce melanin such as the skin, it can also occur in the pigmented area of the eye. Ocular melanoma most commonly occurs in the vascular layer of the eye called the uvea, the area between the retina and the sclera. It can occur in the iris and ciliary body (the front part of the uvea) or in the choroid layer (the back part of the uvea).

Melanoma that originates in the eye is a primary cancer, the most common primary cancer of the eye in adults. Melanoma that appears elsewhere first and then spreads to the eye is a secondary cancer. Both types of ocular melanoma are rare.

Causes

- Exact cause unknown
- Blue eye color (increased risk)
- Dysplastic nevus syndrome (possible increased risk)

Pathophysiology

Primary melanoma originates in the melanocytes of the choroid or back part of the uvea and typically begins as preexisting melanocytic nevi. Choroidal melanoma impedes circulation to the pigmented retinal epithelium. The tumors can become large before noticeable vision loss occurs, depending on the distance from the optic nerve and fovea where they originate. Seepage of fluid into the subretinal space can lead to total retinal detachment.

Choroidal melanomas ultimately result in death because of metastasis. Unfortunately, this cancer metastasizes before diagnosis. Because there are no lymphatic vessels in the eye, the cancer can only spread through the hematologic system and most often metastasizes to the liver. Other organs of metastasis include the lungs, bone, skin, and central nervous system.

COMPLICATIONS
- Metastasis
- Blindness

Signs and Symptoms

- Light flashes
- Visual blurring
- Dark spot in the visual field
- Change in the color of the iris
- Growing dark spot on the iris
- Loss of peripheral vision in the affected eye
- Visual floaters
- Red, painful eye

Diagnostic Test Results

- Ultrasound of the eye shows the tumor and helps to evaluate size and thickness to determine appropriate treatment.
- Blood tests, radiography, ultrasonography, magnetic resonance imaging, or computerized tomography scanning detects metastasis to the liver and lungs.

Treatment

- Surgery (iridectomy, iridotrabeculectomy, iridocyclectomy, choroidectomy, or enucleation)
- Radiation therapy (teletherapy or brachytherapy)
- Chemotherapy
- Interferon
- Cryotherapy or transpupillary thermotherapy (for small tumors)

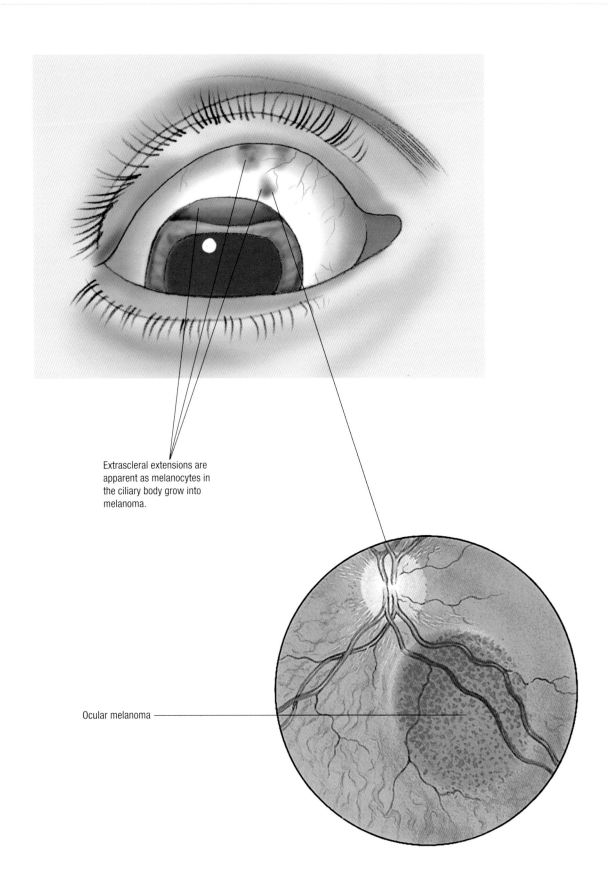

Extrascleral extensions are apparent as melanocytes in the ciliary body grow into melanoma.

Ocular melanoma

OTITIS MEDIA

Otitis media — inflammation of the middle ear — may be suppurative or secretory and acute, persistent, unresponsive, or chronic.

Acute otitis media is common in children between the ages of 6 and 36 months; its incidence rises during the winter months, paralleling the seasonal rise in nonbacterial respiratory tract infections. Prolonged accumulation of fluid within the middle ear cavity causes chronic otitis media.

Chronic suppurative otitis media may lead to scarring, adhesions, and severe structural or functional ear damage. Chronic secretory otitis media, with its persistent inflammation and pressure, may cause conductive hearing loss. It most commonly occurs in children with tympanostomy tubes or those with a perforated tympanic membrane.

Recurrent otitis media is defined as three near-acute otitis media episodes within 6 months or four episodes of acute otitis media within 1 year.

Causes

Suppurative Otitis Media (Bacterial Infection)

- Pneumococci
- *Haemophilus influenzae,* most common cause in children under 6 years of age
- *Moraxella catarrhalis*
- *Beta-hemolytic streptococci*
- Staphylococci, most common cause in children age 6 years or older
- Gram-negative bacteria

Chronic Suppurative Otitis Media

- Inadequate treatment of acute otitis episodes
- Infection by resistant strains of bacteria
- Tuberculosis (rare)

Secretory Otitis Media

- Obstruction of the eustachian tube secondary to eustachian tube dysfunction from viral infection or allergy
- Barotrauma — pressure injury caused by inability to equalize pressures between the environment and the middle ear during aircraft descent or underwater ascent

Chronic Secretory Otitis Media

- Mechanical obstruction — adenoidal tissue overgrowth or tumors
- Edema — allergic rhinitis or chronic sinus infection
- Inadequate treatment of acute suppurative otitis media

Pathophysiology

Otitis media results from disruption of eustachian tube patency. In the suppurative form, respiratory tract infection, allergic reaction, nasotracheal intubation, or positional changes allow nasopharyngeal flora to reflux through the eustachian tube and colonize the middle ear.

In the secretory form, obstruction of the eustachian tube promotes transudation of sterile serous fluid from blood vessels in the middle ear membrane.

COMPLICATIONS
- Mastoiditis
- Meningitis
- Permanent hearing loss
- Septicemia
- Abscesses
- Vertigo
- Lymphadenopathy
- Damage to middle ear structures
- Perforation of the tympanic membrane

Signs and Symptoms

Acute Suppurative Otitis Media

- Severe, deep, throbbing pain from pressure behind the tympanic membrane
- Signs of upper respiratory tract infection (sneezing, coughing)
- Mild to very high fever
- Hearing loss, usually mild and conductive
- Tinnitus, dizziness, nausea, or vomiting
- Bulging, erythematous tympanic membrane; purulent drainage in the ear canal if the tympanic membrane ruptures

Acute Secretory Otitis Media

- Severe conductive hearing loss — varies from 15 to 35 dB, depending on the thickness and amount of fluid in the middle ear cavity
- Sensation of fullness in the ear
- Popping, crackling, or clicking sounds on swallowing or with jaw movement
- Echo during speech
- Vague feeling of top-heaviness

Chronic Otitis Media

- Thickening and scarring of the tympanic membrane
- Decreased or absent tympanic membrane mobility
- Cholesteatoma (cystlike mass in middle ear)
- Painless, purulent discharge

Diagnostic Test Results

- Culture and sensitivity tests of exudate show the causative organism.
- Complete blood count reveals leukocytosis.
- Radiographic studies demonstrate mastoid involvement.
- Tympanometry detects hearing loss and evaluates the condition of the middle ear.
- Audiometry shows degree of hearing loss.
- Pneumatic otoscopy reveals decreased tympanic membrane mobility.

Treatment

- Antibiotic therapy
- Myringotomy — insertion of polyethylene tube into tympanic membrane

- Inflation of eustachian tube by performing Valsalva's maneuver several times per day
- Nasopharyngeal decongestant
- Aspiration of middle ear fluid

- Concomitant treatment of underlying cause, such as elimination of allergens, or adenoidectomy for hypertrophied adenoids
- Myringoplasty, tympanoplasty, or mastoidectomy

CLASSIFICATION AND COMMON COMPLICATIONS OF OTITIS MEDIA

Classifications

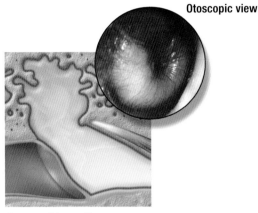

Otoscopic view

Acute otitis media
- Infected fluid in middle ear
- Rapid onset and short duration

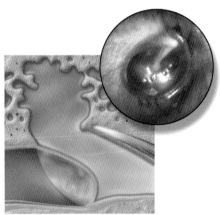

Otitis media with effusion
- Relatively asymptomatic fluid in middle ear
- May be acute, subacute, or chronic in nature

Complications

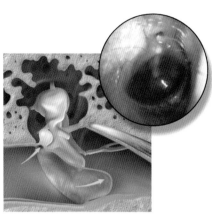

Atelectasis
- Thinning and potential collapse of tympanic membrane

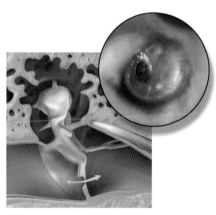

Perforation
- Hole in tympanic membrane caused by chronic negative middle ear pressure, inflammation, or trauma

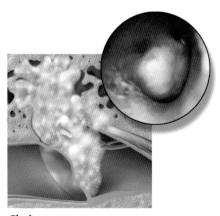

Cholesteatoma
- Mass of entrapped skin in middle ear or temporal lobe

PHARYNGITIS

Pharyngitis is an infection or irritation of the pharynx or tonsils. It is usually an infectious process of viral or bacterial origin but may also be the result of allergy, trauma, neoplasm, and toxins.

Causes

Bacterial Etiology

Bacterial throat infection caused by streptococcus pyogenes, a beta-hemolytic group A streptococci (also known as group A streptococci, GAS). Streptococcus pyogenes is the most common bacterial cause of acute bacterial pharyngitis. It is responsible for approximately 15% to 30% of pediatric cases and 5% to 10% of adult cases. It can be asymptomatic in up to 20% of school-aged children. More commonly seen during the winter and spring months.

Viral Etiology

Viral throat infection is most often caused by the rhinovirus or coronavirus but may also be caused by the Epstein-Barr virus (EBV), cytomegalovirus (CMV), herpes simplex virus (HSV), and primary HIV.

Pathophysiology

Acute pharyngitis is a sore throat caused by a bacterial or viral infection. In viral infections, it is often accompanied by cough, rhinorrhea, and coryza. With bacterial infection, cough and rhinorrhea are usually absent, and there may be whitish exudate, swollen cervical lymph nodes, and fever.

COMPLICATIONS
- Epiglottitis
- Peritonsillar abscess
- Submandibular infections
- Rheumatic heart disease
- Acute glomerulonephritis
- Toxic shock syndrome

Signs and Symptoms
- Hyperemia (redness) of the pharynx
- Whitish exudate
- Fever
- Swollen cervical lymph nodes
- Rhinorrhea
- Cough
- Coryza
- Rash

Diagnostic Test Results
- Rapid streptococcal test — positive means infection; GAS
- Throat culture to identify bacteria

Treatment
- Antibiotics if GAS
- Gargle with warm water, throat lozenges, or analgesics if viral

Suggested References

Arroyo, J. (2016). Age-related macular degeneration: Clinical presentation, etiology and diagnosis. *Uptodate.* Retrieved from https://www.uptodate.com/contents/age-related-macular-degeneration-clinical-presentation-etiology-and-diagnosis?source=see_link

Li, J. (2016). Meniere disease (idiopathic endolymphatic hydrops). *Medscape.* Retrieved from http://emedicine.medscape.com/article/1159069-overview

McCance, K. L., & Huether, S. E. (2014). *Pathophysiology: The biologic basis for disease in adults and children – study guide* (7th ed.). St. Louis, MO: The C.V. Mosby Company.

Porth, C. (2014). *Essentials of pathophysiology: Concepts of altered states* (4th ed.). Philadelphia, PA: Wolters Kluwer.

Van Meter, K., & Hubert, R. (2014). *Gould's pathophysiology for the health professions* (5th ed.). St. Louis, MO: The C.V. Mosby Company.

Waseem, M. (2016). Otitis media. *Medscape.* Retrieved from http://emedicine.medscape.com/article/994656-overview

TYPES OF CARDIAC ARRHYTHMIAS

ARRHYTHMIA AND FEATURES	CAUSES

Sinus tachycardia

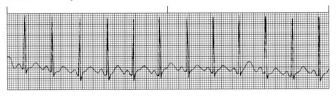

- Rhythm: atrial and ventricular regular; rate > 100 beats/minute
- Normal P wave preceding each QRS complex

- May be a normal physiologic response
- Left ventricular failure, cardiac tamponade, hyperthyroidism, anemia, hypovolemia, pulmonary embolism (PE), anterior wall myocardial infarction (MI), cardiogenic shock, pericarditis, anemia, hemorrhage
- Atropine, epinephrine, isoproterenol, quinidine, caffeine, alcohol, amphetamines, dobutamine, dopamine, or nicotine

Sinus bradycardia

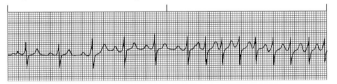

- Rhythm: atrial and ventricular regular; rate < 60 beats/minute
- Normal P waves preceding each QRS complex

- Normal in well-conditioned heart
- Increased intracranial pressure
- Increased vagal tone
- Hypothermia
- Hyperkalemia
- Hypothyroidism
- Anticholinesterase, beta-blocker, calcium channel blocker, digoxin, lithium, antiarrhythmics, or morphine

Supraventricular tachycardia (SVT)

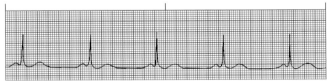

- Rhythm: atrial and ventricular regular; rate > 160 beats/minute; rarely exceeds 250 beats/minute
- P waves regular but aberrant; difficult to differentiate from preceding T wave; P waves proceed each QRS complex
- If the arrhythmia starts and stops suddenly, it's called *paroxysmal SVT*

- Intrinsic abnormality of atrioventricular (AV) conduction
- Physical or psychological stress, hypoxia, hypokalemia, cardiomyopathy, congenital heart disease, MI, valvular disease, Wolff-Parkinson-White syndrome, cor pulmonale, hyperthyroidism, or systemic hypertension
- Digoxin toxicity: use of caffeine, marijuana, or central nervous system stimulants

Atrial flutter

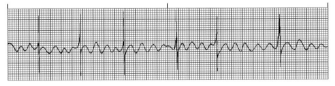

- Atrial rhythm regular; rate 250–400 beats/minute
- Ventricular rate variable, depending on degree of AV block
- No P waves; atrial activity appears as flutter waves (F waves); sawtooth P-wave configuration common in lead II
- QRS complexes uniform in shape, but often irregular in rate

- Heart failure, tricuspid or mitral valve disease, PE, cor pulmonale, inferior wall MI, sick sinus syndrome, or pericarditis
- Digoxin toxicity

(continued)

ARRHYTHMIA AND FEATURES	CAUSES

Atrial fibrillation

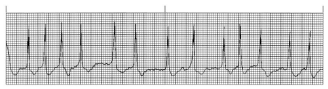

- Atrial rhythm grossly irregular; rate > 400 beats/minute
- Ventricular rate grossly irregular
- QRS complexes of uniform configuration and duration
- PR interval indiscernible
- No P waves; atrial activity appears as erratic, irregular, baseline fibrillatory waves (F waves)

- Heart failure, chronic obstructive pulmonary disease, thyrotoxicosis, constrictive pericarditis, ischemic heart disease, sepsis, PE, rheumatic heart disease, hypertension, mitral stenosis, atrial irritation, or complication of coronary bypass or valve replacement surgery
- Nifedipine and digoxin use

Junctional rhythm

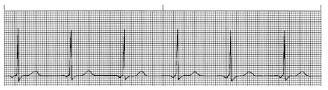

- Rhythm: regular; atrial rate 40 to 60 beats/minute; ventricular rate usually 40 to 60 beats/minute (60 to 100 beats/minute is called *accelerated junctional rhythm*)
- P waves preceding, hidden within, or after QRS complex; may be inverted if visible
- PR interval (when present) < 0.12 seconds
- QRS complex configuration and duration normal, except in aberrant conduction

- Inferior wall MI or ischemia, hypoxia, vagal stimulation, or sick sinus syndrome
- Acute rheumatic fever
- Valve surgery
- Digoxin toxicity

First-degree atrioventricular (AV) block

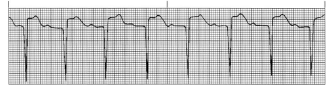

- Rhythm: atrial and ventricular regular
- PR interval > 0.20 seconds
- P wave precedes QRS complex
- QRS complex normal

- May occur in healthy persons
- Inferior wall MI or ischemia, hypothyroidism, hypokalemia, or hyperkalemia
- Digoxin toxicity: quinidine, procainamide, amiodarone, propranolol, beta-blocker, or calcium channel blocker

Second-degree AV block
Mobitz I (Wenckebach)

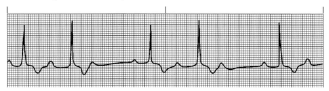

- Rhythm: atrial regular, ventricular irregular; atrial rate exceeds ventricular rate
- PR interval progressively, but only slightly, longer with each cycle until QRS complex disappears (dropped beat); PR interval shorter after dropped beat

- Inferior wall MI, cardiac surgery, acute rheumatic fever, or vagal stimulation
- Digoxin toxicity
- Propranolol, quinidine, or procainamide

ARRHYTHMIA AND FEATURES	CAUSES

Mobitz II

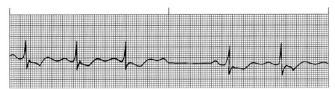

- Rhythm: atrial regular, ventricular irregular
- P-P interval constant for conducted beats
- P waves normal size and shape; some not followed by a QRS complex

- Severe coronary artery disease (CAD), anterior wall MI, or acute myocarditis
- Digoxin toxicity

Third-degree AV block
(Complete heart block)

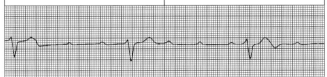

- Rhythm: atrial and ventricular regular; ventricular rate slower than atrial
- No relation between P waves and QRS complexes
- No constant PR interval
- QRS duration normal (junctional pacemaker) or wide and bizarre (ventricular pacemaker)

- Inferior or anterior wall MI, congenital abnormality, rheumatic fever, hypoxia, postoperative complication of mitral valve replacement, postprocedure complication of radiofrequency ablation in or near AV nodal tissue, Lev's disease (fibrosis and calcification that spreads from cardiac structures to the conductive tissue), or Lenègre's disease (conductive tissue fibrosis)
- Digoxin toxicity

Premature ventricular contractions (PVCs)

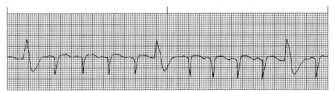

- Rhythm: atrial regular, ventricular irregular
- QRS complex premature, usually followed by a compensatory pause
- QRS complex wide and distorted, usually > 0.12 seconds
- Premature QRS complexes occurring singly, in pairs, or in threes, alternating with normal beats; focus from one or more sites
- Ominous when clustered, multifocal, or with R wave on T pattern

- Heart failure; old or acute MI, ischemia, or contusion; myocardial irritation by ventricular catheter or pacemaker; hypercapnia; hypokalemia; hypocalcemia; or hypomagnesemia
- Drug toxicity: digoxin, aminophylline, tricyclic antidepressants, beta-blockers, isoproterenol, or dopamine
- Caffeine, tobacco, or alcohol use
- Psychological stress, anxiety, pain, or exercise

Ventricular tachycardia

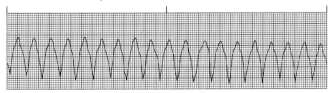

- Ventricular rate 100–220 beats/minute, rhythm usually regular
- QRS complexes wide, bizarre, and independent of P waves
- P waves not discernible
- May start and stop suddenly

- Myocardial ischemia, MI, or aneurysm; CAD; rheumatic heart disease; mitral valve prolapse; heart failure; cardiomyopathy; ventricular catheters; hypokalemia; hypercalcemia; hypomagnesemia; or PE
- Drug toxicity: digoxin, procainamide, epinephrine, or quinidine
- Anxiety

(continued)

ARRHYTHMIA AND FEATURES	CAUSES

Ventricular fibrillation

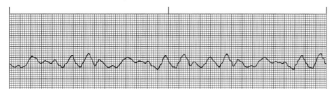

- Ventricular rhythm and rate rapid and chaotic
- QRS complexes wide and irregular; no visible P waves

- Myocardial ischemia, MI, untreated ventricular tachycardia, R-on-T phenomenon, hypokalemia, hyperkalemia, hypercalcemia, alkalosis, electric shock, or hypothermia
- Drug toxicity: digoxin, epinephrine, or quinidine

Asystole

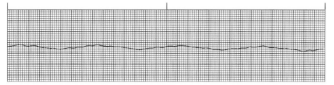

- No atrial or ventricular rate or rhythm
- No discernible P waves, QRS complexes, or T waves

- Myocardial ischemia, MI, aortic valve disease, heart failure, hypoxia, hypokalemia, severe acidosis, electric shock, ventricular arrhythmia, AV block, PE, heart rupture, cardiac tamponade, hyperkalemia, or electromechanical dissociation
- Cocaine overdose

GLOSSARY

Acanthosis nigricans Darkening of the skin on the neck or under the arms

Acidemia Abnormal acidity, or low pH, of the blood

Acidosis Condition caused by accumulation of acid or depletion of the alkaline reserve in the blood and body tissues

Acinus Any of the smallest lobules of a gland

Acromegaly Abnormal enlargement of the extremities of the skeleton caused by hypersecretion of growth hormone from the pituitary gland

Acropachy Soft tissue swelling accompanied by underlying bone changes where new bone formation occurs

Acyanotic Not characterized by or accompanied by cyanosis

Adenomyosis Invasion of the muscular wall of the uterus by glandular tissue

Afterload The force opposing ventricular contraction

Agranulocyte Leukocyte (white blood cell) not containing granules or grains; includes lymphocytes, monocytes, and plasma cells

Akinesia Absence or loss of power of voluntary movement

Alkalemia Abnormal alkalinity, or high pH, of the blood

Alkalosis Abnormal condition of body fluids resulting from accumulation of base or from loss of acid without comparable loss of base

Allele One of two or more different genes that occupy a corresponding position (locus) on matched chromosomes; allows for different forms of the same inherited characteristic

Alopecia Hair loss

Amyloidosis Disorder of unknown cause, in which insoluble protein fibers become deposited in tissues and organs, impairing their function

Anaphase Third stage of division of the nucleus in meiosis or mitosis

Anaplasia Loss of differentiation of cells; a characteristic of tumor cells

Aneurysm Sac formed by localized vasodilation of the wall of an artery or vein

Angioedema Localized edematous reaction of the dermis or subcutaneous or submucosal tissues

Angiography Radiographic examination of vessels of the body

Anion Ion carrying a negative charge

Anisocytosis Presence of erythrocytes with abnormal variations in size

Ankylosis Immobility and consolidation of a joint, often in an abnormal position; caused by disease, trauma, or surgical procedure

Anorexia Lack of or loss of appetite for food

Anovulation Absence of ovulation

Anoxia Absence of oxygen in the tissues

Antibody Immunoglobulin molecule that reacts only with the specific antigen that induced its formation in the lymph system

Antigen Foreign substance, such as a bacteria or toxin, that induces antibody formation

Anuria Complete cessation of urine formation by the kidney

Areflexia Absence of reflexes

Arnold-Chiari syndrome Congenital anomaly in which the cerebellum and medulla protrude through the foramen magnum into the spinal canal

Arousal State of being ready to respond to sensory stimulation

Arteriosclerosis Group of diseases characterized by thickening and loss of elasticity of the arterial walls

Arthralgia Pain in a joint

Arthrodesis Surgical fusion of a joint

Ascites Abnormal accumulation of serous fluid in the peritoneal cavity

Aspiration Inhalation of mucus or vomitus into the respiratory tract; suctioning of fluid or gas from a body cavity

Asterixis Motor disturbance marked by intermittent lapses of assumed posture; also known as *liver flap*

Atelectasis Collapsed or airless state of the lung; may involve all or part of the lung

Atopy Clinical hypersensitivity or allergy with a hereditary predisposition

Atrophy Decrease in size or wasting away of a cell, tissue, organ, or body part

Autoimmune disorder Disorder in which the body launches an immunologic response against itself

Autoinoculation Inoculation with microorganisms from one's own body

Autosome Any of the 22 pairs of chromosomes not concerned with determination of gender

Azotemia Excess nitrogenous waste products in the blood

Babinski's reflex Reflex action of the toes, normal during infancy, elicited by rubbing a firm substance on the sole of the foot, which results in dorsiflexion (upward bending) of the great toe and fanning of the smaller toes; after infancy, normal response is downward bending of all toes on the foot

Bacteria One-celled microorganisms that have no true nucleus and reproduce by cell division

Bactericidal Destructive to bacteria

Bacteriostatic Preventing bacteria from multiplying or growing

Bacteriuria Bacteria in the urine

Balanoposthitis Inflammation of the glans penis and prepuce

Barotrauma Injury caused by pressure

Benign Not malignant or recurrent; favorable for recovery

Biopsy Examination, usually microscopic, of tissue removed from the living body

Blepharospasm Spasm of the orbicular muscle of the eyelid that completely closes eyelids

Bone   Hard, rigid form of connective tissue constituting most of the skeleton

Bone marrow   Soft organic material filling the cavities of bones

Bradykinin   Nonpeptide kinin formed from a plasma protein; a powerful vasodilator that increases capillary permeability, constricts smooth muscle, and stimulates pain receptors

Bronchiectasis   Chronic dilation of the bronchi and bronchioles with secondary infection, usually of the lower lung lobes

Bronchiolitis   Inflammation of the bronchioles

Bruch's membrane   Support structure on the inner side of the choroid

Brudzinski's sign   In meningitis, bending the patient's neck usually produces flexion of the knee and hip

Bulla   Space filled with air or fluid

Bursa   Fluid-filled sac or cavity in connective tissue near a joint; acts as a cushion

Cachexia   State of marked ill health and malnutrition

Carcinogen   Any substance that causes cancer

Carcinoma   Malignant growth made of epithelial cells; tends to infiltrate surrounding tissues and metastasize

Cardiac output   Volume of blood ejected by the heart per minute

Carphology   Involuntary picking at the bedclothes; seen in states of great exhaustion and high fevers

Cartilage   Dense connective tissue consisting of fibers embedded in a strong, gel like substance; supports, cushions, and shapes body structures

Cation   Ion carrying a positive charge

Cell-mediated immunity   Immune response that involves effector T lymphocytes and not the production of humoral antibody

Cercaria   Final, free-swimming stage of a trematode larva

Chemonucleolysis   Injection of the enzyme chymopapain (a chemolytic agent) into a herniated intervertebral disk

Chemotaxis   Response of leukocytes to products formed in immunologic reactions, wherein leukocytes are attracted to and accumulate at the site of the reaction

Cholangioma   Tumor of the bile ducts

Cholangitis   Inflammation of a bile duct

Cholecystectomy   Excision of the gallbladder

Choledochostomy   Creation of an opening into the common bile duct for drainage

Cholestasis   Stopped or decreased bile flow

Cholesteatoma   Cystlike mass filled with desquamating debris frequently including cholesterol, which occurs most commonly in the middle ear and mastoid region

Chondrocalcinosis   Deposition of calcium salts in the cartilage of joints

Chorea   Rapid, jerky involuntary movements

Choriocapillaris   Capillary layer of the choroid

Choroid   Thin membrane that covers the eyeball and supplies blood to the retina

Chromatin   The substance of chromosomes, composed of deoxyribonucleic acid and basic proteins

Chvostek's sign   Spasm of a hyperirritable facial nerve induced by tapping the facial nerve in the region of the parotid gland

Claudication   Pain in the calves caused by reduced blood flow to the legs

Cognition   Process by which a person becomes aware of objects; includes all aspects of perception, thought, and memory

Commissurotomy   Surgical separation of adherent, thickened leaflets of the mitral valve

Complement system   Major mediator of inflammatory response; a functionally related system of 20 proteins circulating as inactive molecules

Congenital   Present at birth

Constipation   Condition in which feces in the bowel are too hard to pass easily

Cor pulmonale   Right ventricular hypertrophy with right-sided heart failure caused by pulmonary hypertension

Corrigan's pulse   Jerky pulse with full expansion and sudden collapse

Cremasteric reflex   Stimulation of the skin on the inner thigh retracts the testis on the same side

Crepitus   Crackling sound in the joints, skin, or lungs

Curettage   Scraping or collecting tissue from the wall of a body cavity

Cyanosis   Bluish discoloration of the skin and mucous membranes caused by reduced hemoglobin in the blood

Cystitis   Inflammation of the urinary bladder

Cytokines   Nonantibody proteins, secreted by inflammatory leukocytes and some nonleukocytic cells, that act as intercellular mediators

Cytology   The study of cells, their origin, structure, function, and pathology

Cytotoxic   Destructive to cells

Debridement   Removal of all foreign material and diseased and devitalized tissue from or adjacent to a traumatic or infected lesion until surrounding healthy tissue is exposed

Decortication   Surgical removal of the thick coating over an organ, such as the lung or kidney

Demyelination   Destruction of a nerve's myelin sheath; prevents normal conduction

Diabetic ketoacidosis   Complication of diabetes mellitus that results from by-products of fat metabolism (ketones) when glucose isn't available as a fuel source in the body

Diaphoresis   Perspiration, especially profuse perspiration

Diarrhea   Frequent evacuation of watery stools caused by rapid movement of intestinal contents; results in poor absorption of water, nutritive elements, and electrolytes

Differentiation   Process of cells maturing into specific types

Diffusion   Spontaneous movement of molecules or other particles in a solution

Diplegia   Paralysis of like parts on either side of the body

Diploid   Cell with a full set of genetic material; a human diploid cell has 46 chromosomes

Diplopia   Double vision

Disjunction   Separation of chromosomes during cell division

Divarication   Separation into two parts or branches; bifurcation

Diverticula   Pockets of tissue that push out from the colon walls

Dominant gene   Gene that produces an effect in an organism regardless of the state of the corresponding allele

Dressler's syndrome   Pericarditis that develops weeks to several months after myocardial infarction or open heart surgery

Dysarthria   Imperfect articulation of speech caused by disturbances of muscular control

Dyscrasia   Condition related to a disease, usually referring to an imbalance of component elements

Dysphagia   Difficulty swallowing

Dysplasia   Alteration in size, shape, and organization of adult cells

Dyspnea   Labored or difficult breathing

Dysthymia   Depression

Dysuria   Painful or difficult urination

Eclampsia   Potentially life-threatening disorder of pregnancy characterized by seizures, hypertension, generalized edema, and proteinuria

Ejection fraction   Measure of ventricular contractility

Embolism   Sudden obstruction of a blood vessel by a foreign substance or a blood clot

Empyema   Accumulation of pus in a body cavity

Endocrine   Pertaining to internal hormone secretion by glands

Endogenous   Occurring inside the body

Endolymph   Fluid within the membranous labyrinth of the ear

Endotoxin   Toxin associated with the outer membranes of certain gram-negative bacteria

Epistaxis   Hemorrhage from the nose, usually caused by rupture of small vessels

Erythema marginatum   Nonpruritic, macular, transient rash on the trunk or inner aspects of the upper arms or thighs, that gives rise to red lesions with blanched centers

Erythrocyte   Red blood cell; carries oxygen to the tissues and removes carbon dioxide from them

Erythropoiesis   Production of red blood cells or erythrocytes

Estrogen   Female sex hormone

Exacerbation   Increase in the severity of a disease or any of its symptoms

Exanthem   Rash or skin eruption

Exocrine   External or outward secretion of a gland

Exogenous   Occurring outside the body

Exotoxin   Potent toxin formed and excreted by a bacterial cell and found in the surrounding medium

Extracellular fluid   Fluid in the spaces outside the cells

Fetor hepaticus   Musty, sweetish breath characteristic of hepatic disease

Fulguration   Destruction of tissue by high-frequency electricity

Fungate   Funguslike growth; growing rapidly like a fungus

Fungus   Nonphotosynthetic microorganism that reproduces asexually by cell division

Furunculosis   Occurrence of furuncles serially over weeks or months

Gait ataxia   Unsteady, uncoordinated walk, with a wide base and the feet turned out, coming down first on the heel and then on the toes with a double tap

Gap junctions   Channels through which ions and other small molecules pass

Gastrectomy   Excision of the stomach or a portion of it

Gastrostomy   Creation of an opening into the stomach for the purpose of administering food or fluids

Genome   Total of all genetic information included in a set of unreplicated chromosomes

Gibson murmur   Continuous murmur heard throughout systole and diastole in older children and adults caused by shunting of blood from the aorta to the pulmonary artery

Gland   Organ composed of specialized cells that produce a secretion used in some other body part

Glomerulopathy   Any disease of the renal glomeruli

Glomerulosclerosis   Glomerular disease characterized by hardening of focal and segmental areas of the glomerulus

Glomerulus   Network of twisted capillaries in the nephron, the basic unit of the kidney; brings blood and waste products carried by blood to the nephron

Glucagon   Hormone released during the fasting state that increases blood glucose concentration

Gluconeogenesis   Formation of glucose from molecules that aren't carbohydrates, such as amino acids and glycerol

Glycogenolysis   Splitting of glycogen in the liver, yielding glucose

Glycosuria   Presence of glucose in the urine

Goblet cells   Mucus-secreting cells of the epithelial lining of the small intestine and respiratory passages

Granulocyte   Any cell containing granules, especially a granular leukocyte (white blood cell)

Granuloma   Any small nodular aggregation of mononuclear inflammatory cells or a similar collection of modified macrophages resembling endothelial cells, usually surrounded by lymphocytes, often with multinucleated giant cells

Gubernaculum   Fibromuscular band that connects the testes to the scrotal floor

Hamartoma   Benign tumorlike nodule composed of an overgrowth of mature cells and tissues normally present in the affected part

Haploid   Having half the normal number of chromosomes

Heberden's nodules   Small, hard nodules on the distal interphalangeal joints of the fingers in osteoarthritis

Hematemesis   Vomiting of blood

Hematoma   Localized collection of blood, usually clotted, in an organ, space, or tissue

Hematopoiesis   Production of red blood cells in the bone marrow

Hematuria   Blood in the urine

Hemochromatosis   Disorder of iron metabolism with excess deposition of iron in the tissues, bronze skin pigmentation, cirrhosis, and diabetes mellitus

Hemoglobin   Protein in erythrocytes that transports oxygen

Hemolysis   Red blood cell destruction

Hemostasis   Complex process whereby platelets, plasma, and coagulation factors interact to control bleeding

Hepatojugular reflux   Distention of the jugular vein induced by manual pressure over the liver

Hepatoma   Any tumor of the liver

Heterozygous   Genes having different alleles at the same site (locus)

Hirsutism   Abnormal hairiness

Histamine   An amine found in all body tissues that induces capillary dilation, which increases capillary permeability, lowers blood pressure, and causes contraction of most smooth muscle tissue, increased gastric acid secretion, and increased heart rate; also a mediator of immediate hypersensitivity

Homeostasis   Dynamic, steady state of internal balance in the body

Homologous genes   Gene pairs sharing a corresponding structure and position

Homozygous   Genes that have identical alleles for a given trait

Hormone   Chemical substance produced in the body that has a specific regulatory effect on the activity of specific cells or organs

Humoral immunity   Form of immunity in which B lymphocytes and plasma cells produce antibodies to foreign agents (antigens) and stimulate T lymphocytes to attack them (cellular immunity)

Hyperplasia   Excessive growth of normal cells that causes an increase in the volume of a tissue or organ

Hyperpnea   Increase in depth of breathing, which may be accompanied by an increased respiratory rate

Hyperreflexia   Exaggeration of reflexes

Hypertonic   Having an osmotic pressure greater than that of the solution with which it's compared

Hypertrichosis   Excessive hair growth

Hypertrophy   Increase in volume of tissue or organ caused by enlargement of existing cells

Hypervolemia   Abnormal increase in the volume of circulating fluid in the body

Hypoplasia   Incomplete development or underdevelopment of an organ or tissue

Hypotonia   Abnormally low tonicity or strength

Hypotonic   Having an osmotic pressure lower than that of the solution with which it's compared

Hypovolemia   Abnormally low volume of circulating fluid in the body

Hypoxia   Reduction of oxygen in body tissues to below normal levels

Idiopathic   Occurring without known cause

Ileal conduit   Use of a segment of the ileum for the diversion of urinary flow from the ureters

Ileus   Failure of appropriate forward movement of bowel contents

Immunodeficiency   Disorder caused by inadequate immune response; caused by hypoactivity or decreased numbers of lymphoid cells

Immunoglobulin   Serum protein synthesized by lymphocytes and plasma cells that has known antibody activity

Intention tremor   Tremor occurring when one attempts voluntary movement

Interphase   Interval between two successive cell divisions

Interstitial fluid   Fluid between cells in tissues

Intertrigo   Erythematous skin eruption in such areas as the creases of the neck, folds of the groin and axillae, and beneath pendulous breasts

Intracellular fluid   Fluid inside each cell

Intrapleural   Within the pleura

Ion   Atom or group of atoms having a positive or negative electric charge

Ischemia   Decreased blood supply to a body organ or tissue

Isotonic   Solution having the same tonicity as another solution with which it's compared

Jaundice   Yellow discoloration of skin, sclera, mucous membranes, and excretions caused by hyperbilirubinemia and deposition of bile pigments

Joint   Intersection of two or more bones; most provide motion and flexibility

Karyotype   Chromosomal arrangement of the cell nucleus

Kernig's sign   Sign of meningitis in which a patient in supine position can easily and completely extend the leg; patient in sitting position or lying with the thigh flexed upon the abdomen can't completely extend leg

Ketones   By-products of fat metabolism when glucose isn't available

Ketonuria   Excess of ketones in the urine

Koilonychia   Abnormally thin nails that are concave from side to side, with the edges turned up

Korotkoff sound   Sound heard during auscultation of blood pressure

Kupffer's cells   Large, phagocytic cells lining the walls of the hepatic sinusoids

Kussmaul's respirations   Dyspnea characterized by increased rate and depth of respirations, panting, and labored respiration; seen in metabolic acidosis

Kussmaul's sign   Increased jugular vein distention on inspiration; caused by restricted right-sided filling

Kyphoscoliosis   Forward and lateral curvature of the spine

Lasègue's sign   In sciatica, pain in the back and leg elicited by passive raising of the heel from the bed with the knee straight

Leukapheresis   Selective removal of leukocytes from withdrawn blood, which is then retransfused into the donor

Leukocyte   White blood cell that protects the body against microorganisms causing disease

Leukocytosis   Increase in the number of leukocytes in the blood; generally caused by infection

Leukopenia   Reduction in the number of leukocytes in the blood

Leukotrienes   Group of compounds derived from unsaturated fatty acids; extremely potent mediators of immediate hypersensitivity reactions and inflammation

Lichenification   Thickening and hardening of the skin

Ligament   Band of fibrous tissue that connects bones or cartilage, provides stability, strengthens joints, and limits or facilitates movement

Locus   Location on a chromosome

Lymph node   Structure that filters the lymphatic fluid that drains from body tissue and is later returned to the plasma

Lymphadenitis   Inflammation of one or more lymph nodes

Lymphedema   Chronic swelling of a body part from accumulation of interstitial fluid secondary to obstruction or surgical removal of lymphatic vessels or lymph nodes

Lymphocytes   Leukocytes produced by lymphoid tissue that participate in immunity

Lysozyme   Enzyme that can kill microorganisms or microbes

Macroglossia   Excessive size of the tongue

Macrophages   Highly phagocytic cells that are stimulated by inflammation

Malignant   Condition that becomes progressively worse and results in death

Megakaryocyte   Platelet precursor; the giant cell of bone marrow

Megaloureter   Congenital ureteral dilation without demonstrable cause

Meiosis   Process of cell division by which reproductive cells are formed

Menorrhagia   Heavy or prolonged menses

Merozoite   Stage in the life cycle of the malaria parasite

Mesorchium   Fold in the tissue between the testis and epididymis

Metabolic acidosis   Acidosis resulting from accumulation of keto acids in the blood at the expense of bicarbonate

Metabolic alkalosis   Disturbance in which the acid-base status shifts toward the alkaline because of uncompensated loss of acids, ingestion or retention of excess base, or potassium depletion

Metaphase Stage of cell division in which the chromosomes, each consisting of two chromatids, are arranged in the equatorial plane of the spindle

Metaplasia Change in adult cells to a form abnormal for that tissue

Metastasis Transfer of disease via pathogenic microorganisms or cells from one organ or body part to another not directly associated with it

Metrorrhagia Episodes of vaginal bleeding between menses

Microembolus Embolus of microscopic size

Micturition Urination

Mitosis Ordinary process of cell division in which each chromosome with all its genes reproduces itself exactly

Monocyte Mononuclear, phagocytic leukocyte

Monoplegia Paralysis of a single part

Monosomy Presence of one chromosome less than the normal number

Morbidity Condition of having a disease

Morphea Condition in which connective tissue replaces skin and sometimes subcutaneous tissues

Mortality Ratio of the total number of deaths to the total population

Mucolytic Agent that acts by destroying mucus

Muscle Bundle of long slender cells, or fibers, that has the power to contract and produce movement

Mutation Permanent change in genetic material

Myalgia Muscle pain

Myectomy Excision of a muscle

Myelomatous cells Increased number of immature plasma cells

Myolysis Degeneration of muscle tissue

Myomectomy Removal of tumors in the uterine muscle

Myotomy Cutting or dissection of a muscle

Myxedema Condition resulting from advanced hypothyroidism or deficiency of thyroxine

Nausea Unpleasant sensation with the tendency to vomit

Necrosis Cell or tissue death

Neoplasm Abnormal growth in which cell multiplication is uncontrolled and progressive

Nephrolithiasis Condition marked by the presence of renal calculi

Nephron Structural and functional unit of the kidney that forms urine

Neuritis Inflammation of a nerve

Neurolysis Freeing of nerve fibers by cutting the nerve sheath longitudinally

Neuron Highly specialized conductor cell that receives and transmits electrochemical nerve impulses

Neutropenia Neutrophil deficiency in the blood

Neutrophil Granular leukocyte

Nevus Circumscribed, stable malformation of the skin and oral mucosa

Nondisjunction Failure of chromosomes to separate properly during cell division; causes an unequal distribution of chromosomes between the two resulting cells

Nystagmus Involuntary, rapid, rhythmic movement of the eyeball

Obstipation Intractable constipation

Oculogyric crises Eyelids are fixed upward with involuntary tonic movements

Oligomenorrhea Abnormally infrequent menses

Oliguria Diminished urine secretion

Omentum Fold of the peritoneum between the stomach and adjacent abdominal organs

Onychia Inflammation of the nail bed

Onycholysis Distal nail separated from the bed

Oophoritis Inflammation of the ovary

Opisthotonos Spasm in which the head and heels arch backward and the body bows forward

Opportunistic infection Infection striking people with altered, weakened immune systems; caused by microorganism that doesn't ordinarily cause disease but becomes pathogenic under certain conditions

Ophthalmoplegia Ocular paralysis

Optic neuritis Inflammation of the optic nerve

Orchiectomy Excision of a testis

Orchiopexy Surgical fixation of an undescended testis in the scrotum

Organelle Structure in the cytoplasm that performs a specific function

Orthopnea Ability to breathe easily only in the upright position

Orthostatic hypotension Fall in blood pressure that occurs upon standing or when standing motionless in a fixed position

Osmolality Concentration of a solution expressed in terms of osmoles of solute per kilogram of solvent

Osmolarity Concentration of a solution expressed in terms of osmoles of solute per liter of solution

Osseous Of the nature or quality of bone

Osteoblasts Bone-forming cells

Osteoclasts Giant, multinuclear cells that reabsorb material from previously formed bones, tear down old or excess bone structure, and allow osteoblasts to rebuild new bone

Osteotomy Surgical division and realignment of bone

Ostium primum Opening in the lower portion of the membrane dividing the embryonic heart into right and left sides

Pancarditis Concurrent myocarditis, pericarditis, and endocarditis

Pancytopenia Abnormal depression of all the cellular elements of blood

Panmyelosis Proliferation of all the elements of the bone marrow

Papilledema Inflammation and edema of the optic nerve; associated with increased intracranial pressure

Paracentesis Surgical puncture of a cavity for the aspiration of fluid

Parametritis Inflammation of the parametrium

Paresthesia Abnormal burning or prickling sensation

Paronychia Inflammation of the folds of tissue around the fingernail

Paroxysmal nocturnal dyspnea Respiratory distress related to posture (reclining at night) usually associated with heart failure and pulmonary edema

Pericardiectomy Surgical creation of an opening to remove accumulated fluid from the pericardial sac

Pericardiocentesis Needle aspiration of the pericardial cavity

Perilymph Fluid in the space separating the membranous and osseous labyrinths of the ear

Periosteum Specialized connective tissue covering all bones and possessing bone-forming potential

Perseveration Abnormally persistent replies to questions

Petechiae Minute, round purplish red spots caused by intradermal or submucosal hemorrhage

Phagocyte   Cell that ingests microorganisms, other cells, and foreign materials

Phagocytosis   Engulfing of microorganisms, other cells, and foreign material by a phagocyte

Phlebectomy   Removing a varicose vein through small incisions in the skin

Phlebography   Radiographic examination of a vein

Photoplethysmography   Plethysmographic determination in which the intensity of light reflected from the skin surface and the red cells below is measured to determine the blood volume of the respective area

Pilosebaceous   Pertaining to the hair follicles and sebaceous glands

Plasmapheresis   Removal of plasma from withdrawn blood and retransfusion of the formed elements into the donor

Plethora   Edema and blood vessel distention

Polycythemia   Increase in the total red cell mass of the blood

Polydipsia   Excessive thirst

Polygenic traits   Determined by several different genes

Polymenorrhea   Menstrual cycle of less than 18 days

Polyphagia   Excessive ingestion of food

Polyuria   Excessive excretion of urine

Preload   Volume of blood in the ventricle at the end of diastole

Presbycusis   Progressive, symmetrical, bilateral sensorineural hearing loss, usually of high-frequency tones, caused by loss of hair cells in the organ of Corti

Pretibial edema   Nonpitting edema of the anterior surface of the legs, dermopathy

Prognathism   Projection of the jaw

Prophase   First stage of cell replication in meiosis or mitosis

Prostaglandins   Group of fatty acids that stimulate contractility of the uterine and other smooth muscle and have the ability to lower blood pressure, regulate acid secretion in the stomach, regulate body temperature and platelet aggregation, and control inflammation and vascular permeability

Protease inhibitor   Drug that binds to and blocks the action of the human immunodeficiency virus protease enzyme

Proteinuria   Excess of serum proteins in the urine

Pruritus   Itching

Ptosis   Paralytic drooping of the upper eyelid

Pulsus bisferiens   Peripheral pulse with a characteristic double impulse

Pulsus paradoxus   Drop in systemic blood pressure that's greater than 15 mm Hg and coincides with inspiration

Pyloroplasty   Plastic surgery of the pylorus to create larger communication between the stomach and duodenum

Pyrosis   Heartburn

Pyuria   Pus in urine

Quadriplegia   Paralysis of all four limbs

Quincke's sign   Alternate blanching and flushing of the skin

Recessive gene   Gene that doesn't express itself in the presence of its dominant allele

Red blood cell   Erythrocyte

Remission   Abatement of a disease's symptoms

Remyelination   Healing of demyelinated nerves

Renin   Enzyme produced by the kidneys in response to an actual decline in extracellular fluid volume

Resistance   Opposition to airflow in the lung tissue, chest wall, or airways; opposition to blood flow in the circulatory system

Respiratory acidosis   Acidosis resulting from impaired ventilation and retention of carbon dioxide

Respiratory alkalosis   Alkalosis caused by excessive excretion of carbon dioxide through the lungs

Romberg's sign   Tendency of a patient to sway while standing still with feet close together and eyes closed

Rubella syndrome   Exposure of a nonimmune mother to rubella during the first trimester of pregnancy

Salpingitis   Inflammation of the fallopian tubes

Sclerodactyly   Scleroderma of the fingers and toes

Sebum   Oily secretion of the sebaceous glands

Sepsis   Pathologic state resulting from microorganisms or their poisonous products in the bloodstream

Serositis   Inflammation of a serous membrane

Serotonin   Hormone and neurotransmitter that inhibits gastric acid secretion, stimulates smooth muscle, and produces vasoconstriction

Shunt   Passage or anastomosis between two natural channels

Specific gravity   Weight of a substance compared with the weight of an equal amount of water

Status asthmaticus   Particularly severe episode of asthma

Steatorrhea   Excess fat in the feces caused by a malabsorption syndrome

Stenosis   Constriction or narrowing of a passage or orifice

Stratum corneum epidermidis   Dead top layer of the skin

Stroke volume   Amount of blood pumped out of the heart in a single contraction

Subcutaneous emphysema   Crackling beneath the skin on palpation

Subluxation   Incomplete or partial dislocation

Surfactant   Mixture of phospholipids that reduces the surface tension of pulmonary fluids and contributes to the elastic properties of pulmonary tissue

Sympathectomy   Excision or interruption of some portion of the sympathetic nervous pathway

Synovectomy   Removal of destructive, proliferating synovium, usually, in the wrists, knees, and fingers

Synovial fluid   Viscous, lubricating substance secreted by the synovial membrane, which lines the cavity between the bones of free-moving joints

Telophase   Last of the four stages of mitosis or of the two divisions of meiosis

Tendon   Fibrous cord of connective tissue that attaches the muscle to bone or cartilage and enables bones to move when skeletal muscles contract

Tenotomy   Surgical cutting of the tendon

Teratogens   Agents or factors that can harm the developing fetus by causing congenital structural or functional defects

Thoracentesis   Surgical puncture and drainage of the thoracic cavity

Thrombocytopenia   Decreased number of platelets in circulating blood

Thrombocytosis   Excessive number of platelets in circulating blood

Thrombus   Blood clot

Thymoma   Tumor on the thymus gland

Tinea cruris   Fungal infection of the groin

Tinel's sign   Tingling over the median nerve on light percussion

Tophi   Accumulations of urate salts; occur throughout the body in gout

Torticollis   Abnormal contraction of the cervical muscles, producing torsion of the neck

Transcription   Synthesis of ribonucleic acid using a deoxyribonucleic acid template

Transient ischemic attack   Brief episode of neurologic deficit resulting from cerebral ischemia

Translocation   Alteration of a chromosome by attachment of a fragment to another chromosome or a different portion of the same chromosome

Trisomy   Presence of an extra chromosome

Trousseau's sign   Carpal spasm

Truss   Elastic, canvas, or metallic device for retaining a reduced hernia within the abdominal cavity

Vagotomy   Surgical interruption of the impulses carried by the vagus nerve or nerves

Vasculitis   Inflammation of a vessel

Ventriculoatrial shunt   Drains fluid from the brain's lateral ventricle into the right atrium of the heart, where the fluid enters the venous circulation

Ventriculoperitoneal shunt   Transports excess fluid from the lateral ventricle into the peritoneal cavity

Virus   Microscopic, infectious parasite that contains genetic material and needs a host to replicate

Vitiligo   Absence of pigmentation

Wilms' tumor   Rapidly developing malignant mixed tumor of the kidneys, made up of embryonal elements; occurs mainly in children before age 5

X-linked   Inheritance pattern in which single gene disorders are passed through sex chromosomes

Xanthoma   A papule, nodule, or plaque in the skin caused by lipid deposits

INDEX

Note: Page numbers followed by "t" denote tables.

Cleft lip/palate, 36t, 432–433
Closed pneumothorax, 114
Cluster headache, 152
Coagulative necrosis, 6
Coarctation of the aorta, 56
Cochlear duct, in Ménière's disease, 449
Codons, 28
Cold, common, 128
Colitis
    granulomatous, 186–187
    spastic, 212–213
    ulcerative, 228–229
Colles' fracture, 243
Colonic polyps, 182–183
Colorectal cancer, 184–185
Comedones, of acne, 405
Common cold, 128
    complications of, 129
Compensation, in acid-base imbalance, 41
Compensatory hyperplasia, 5
Compensatory stage, of shock, 82
Complex-partial seizures, 150
Compression test
    for carpal tunnel syndrome, 250
    manual, for varicose veins, 86
Computed tomography (CT) scan, in cancer
        diagnosis, 14
Conduction, as cell function, 4
Conductive hearing loss, 443
Condyloma acuminatum, 428
Condylomata acuminata, 364
Congenital anomalies, 29
Congenital defects, of heart, 56–59
Congenital hearing loss, 442
Congenital hydrocele, 346–347
Congenital megacolon, 204–205
Conjunctivitis, 20t, 434–435
    manifestations of, 435
Connective tissue cells, 4
Consumption coagulopathy, 272–273
Contact dermatitis, 412–413
Convalescence
    as disease stage, 7
Corneal ulcer, 436–437
Coronary arteries, 61
    atherosclerosis and, 60–61
Coronary artery disease, 60–61
Coronavirus, 124
Corpus luteum cysts, ovarian, 352
Cortisol
    deficiency, in adrenal hypofunction,
        302–303
    excess, in Cushing's syndrome, 304–305
Coryza, acute, 128
Coup/contrecoup injury, 132
Crescentic glomerulonephritis, 386–387
Cretinism, infantile, 318
Crohn's disease, 186–187
    bowel changes in, 187
Cryptorchidism, 334–335
Cushing's disease, 304
Cushing's syndrome, 304–305
    manifestations of, 304
Cystic fibrosis, 33t, 102–103
    systemic changes in, 103
Cystic fibrosis transmembrane regulator
        (CFTR), 102
Cystitis, 384–385

Cysts
    breast, 331
    ovarian, 352–353
Cytomegalovirus, 23t
Cytoplasm, 3
    in cancer, 11
Cytoskeleton, 3
    in cancer, 11

D

Deafness, 442–443
Deep vein thrombosis, 62–63, 118
Deep veins
    of knee, 63
Deep veins, of leg, 63
Defense mechanisms, weakened, as infection
        risk factor, 17
Defibrination syndrome, 272–273
Deficit injury, cell, 6
Dementia, Alzheimer's, 134–135
Demyelination
    in multiple sclerosis, 160–161
    peripheral nerve, 150–151
Deoxyribonucleic acid (DNA), 3, 25
Depression, 146–147
    brain changes in, 147
    pediatric symptoms, 146
Dermatitis
    atopic, 406–407
    contact, 412–413
Dermoid cysts, ovarian, 353
Descending aortic aneurysm, 48
Developmental dysplasia of hip, 232–233
    signs of, 233
Developmental factors, in infection, 17
Diabetes insipidus, 306–307
    laboratory values for, 307t
    mechanism of deficiency
Diabetes mellitus, 308–309
    type 1, 308–309
    type 2, 308–309
Diagonal artery, 61
Diaphoresis, 18
Diaphragm, in hiatal hernia, 202–203
Diastolic dysfunction, in heart failure, 66
Dietary factors, as cancer risk factor, 9
Differentiation, cancer cells and, 11
Digitate wart, 428
Dilated cardiomyopathy, 54–55
Diploid cells, 27
Disease
    defined, 6
    illness vs., 6
    stages of, 6
Dissecting aortic aneurysm, 48–49
Disseminated intravascular coagulation,
        272–273
Diverticular disease, 188–189
Diverticulitis, 188
Diverticulosis, 188
DNA sequences, 25
Dominant gene, 29
Dopamine levels, in Parkinson's disease,
        164–165
Down syndrome, 37t
Dry gangrene, 6
Dry macular degeneration, 446
Duchenne's muscular dystrophy, 234–235

Ductal carcinoma
    infiltrating, 329
    in situ, 329
Dysfunctional uterine bleeding, 370–371
Dysplasia, 5
    in cancer, 12

E

Ectopic pregnancy, 336–337
Ectropion, 438–439
Eczema, atopic, 406–407
Edema
    fluid balance and, 39–40
    pulmonary, 116–117
Edematous pancreatitis, 222
Edward's syndrome, 37t
Effector, homeostasis and, 6
Elbow
    fracture of, 243
    tendinopathy, 257
Electrical burn, 408
Electrolyte balance, 40–41
    disorders of, 42–43t
    pathophysiologic concepts, 39–43
Electrolytes, 38
    characteristics of major, 39t
    normal values for, 39t
Embolism
    pulmonary, 118–119
    in stroke, 170–171
Emphysema, 100–101
    lung changes in, 101
Emphysematous pyelonephritis, 394
Empyema, 110
Encephalopathy, hepatic, 216
Endemic goiter, 322
Endocarditis, 64–65
Endolymphatic hydrops, 448–449
Endometrial cancer, 338–339
    progress of, 339
Endoplasmic reticulum, 3
Endoscopy, in cancer diagnosis, 14
Enteritis, regional, 186
Entropion, 438–439
Environmental carcinogens, 29
Environmental factors, in infection, 17
Environmental teratogens, 29
Ependymal cells, 4
Epigenetics, 29
Epilepsy, 148–149
    types of seizures, 149
Epileptogenic focus, 148
Epispadias, 348–349
Epithelial cells, 4
Erectile dysfunction, 342–343
Erythema migrans, 418–419
Erythrocyte sedimentation rate, in infection
        diagnosis, 19
Erythrodermic psoriasis, 422
Esophageal stricture, 196
Esophagitis, 196
Esophagus
    in achalasia, 174–175
    cancer of, 190–191
    in gastroesophageal reflux disease, 196–197
Estrogen, in dysfunctional uterine bleeding,
        370
Ewing's sarcoma, 238